VOLUME NINETY FOUR

VITAMINS AND HORMONES

Endocrine Disrupters

VOLUME NINETY FOUR

VITAMINS AND HORMONES

Endocrine Disrupters

Series Editor

GERALD LITWACK, PhD

Toluca Lake, North Hollywood, California

ELSEVIER

AMSTERDAM • BOSTON • HEIDELBERG • LONDON
NEW YORK • OXFORD • PARIS • SAN DIEGO
SAN FRANCISCO • SINGAPORE • SYDNEY • TOKYO
Academic Press is an imprint of Elsevier

Cover photo credit:
Delfosse V., Grimaldi M., le Maire A., Bourguet W. and Balaguer P.
Nuclear Receptor Profiling of Bisphenol-A and its Halogenated Analogues
Vitamins and Hormones (2014) **94**, pp. 229-252

Academic Press is an imprint of Elsevier
32 Jamestown Road, London, NW1 7BY, UK
The Boulevard, Langford Lane, Kidlington, Oxford, OX5 1GB, UK
Linacre House, Jordan Hill, Oxford OX2 8DP, UK
225 Wyman Street, Waltham, MA 02451, USA
525 B Street, Suite 1800, San Diego, CA 92101-4495, USA

First edition 2014

ISBN: 978-0-12-800095-3
ISSN: 0083-6729

For information on all Academic Press publications
visit our website at store.elsevier.com

Printed and bound by CPI Group (UK) Ltd, Croydon, CR0 4YY

14 15 16 17 11 10 9 8 7 6 5 4 3 2 1

CONTENTS

Contributors *xiii*
Preface *xvii*

1. Endocrine-Disrupting Chemicals and Human Growth and Maturation: A Focus on Early Critical Windows of Exposure **1**

Julie Fudvoye, Jean-Pierre Bourguignon, and Anne-Simone Parent

1. Introduction 2
2. Challenges in Evidencing Endocrine Disruption 2
3. Endocrine-Disrupting Chemicals and Fetal Growth 4
4. EDCs and Sexual Differentiation 5
5. EDCs and Puberty 8
6. EDCs and Brain Development 9
7. EDC and Energy Balance 14
8. Epigenetic Perspective on the Developmental Effects of EDCs 16
9. Conclusion 17

References 18

2. Agricultural Pesticides and Precocious Puberty **27**

Samim Ozen, Damla Goksen, and Sukran Darcan

1. Introduction 27
2. Puberty 28
3. Precocious Puberty 29
4. The Effects of EDs on Puberty 30
5. Organochlorine Pesticides and Puberty 33
6. DDT and DDE 34
7. Methoxychlor 35
8. Endosulfans 36
9. Vinclozolin 37
10. Acetochlor 37
11. Conclusion 37

References 38

3. Endocrine-Disrupting Chemicals: Elucidating Our Understanding of Their Role in Sex and Gender-Relevant End Points **41**

Cheryl A. Frye

1. Introduction 43

2. Endocrine Disruption May Underlie Negative Effects of Contaminants 45
3. Adverse Health Consequences of Lifelong EDC Exposure 45
4. Signficance of Investigating EDC Effects on Neurodevelopmental Processes 47
5. Hormones' Effects to Organize Neural Systems and Behavioral Processes 48
6. Developmental EDC Exposure Alters Reproductive Development and Behavior 48
7. Exposure to EDCs in Adulthood Also Effects Reproductive Parameters 50
8. EDCs in Adulthood Influence Sexually Dimorphic Brain Morphology 51
9. Do EDCs Influence Sex Differences in Nonreproductive Behaviors? 52
10. Effects of EDCs on Sexually Dimorphic, Nonreproductive Behaviors 54
11. Potential Mechanisms by which EDCs May Produce Their Effects 57
12. Several Factors May Bear upon Estrogenicity of Compounds 59
13. Effects of EDCs on Uterotropic Activity 60
14. Importance of Examining EDC Effects on Whole-Animal Estrogenic Measures 61
15. Effects of EDCs on E_2 Metabolism 62
16. Androgenic/Antiandrogenic Effects of EDCs 64
17. Effects of EDCs via Traditional Intracellular Steroid Receptors 65
18. Other Substrates to Consider for Actions of EDCs 66
19. Preliminary Studies 68
20. Organized Reproductive Parameters: Immature Rats 68
21. Organized and Activated Reproductive Parameters: Peripubertal and Maturation Measures 69
22. Organized and Activated Reproductive Parameters: Effects in Adults 72
23. Strategy: EDC Effects on Reproductive Parameters: A Biomarker of Effects 75
24. Organized and/or Activated Nonreproductive Sexually Dimorphic Behaviors 75
25. Suggested Experiments Moving Forward 79
26. Approach: The Importance of Integration of Reproductive and Nonreproductive Measures 79
27. Approach: Examining Effects of EDC Exposure Throughout Development 79
28. Suggestions for Future Work Examining Mechanisms of EDCs Effects 80
29. Logistical Factors for Experimental Control and Power 81
30. Summary 82
31. Conclusions 84
Acknowledgment 85
References 85

4. Ovarian Toxicity from Reactive Oxygen Species **99**

Ulrike Luderer

1. Ovarian Follicular Development and Its Hormonal Regulation 100

2. Reactive Oxygen Species and Oxidative Stress 103
3. Hormonal Regulation of and Effects of Depleting or Enhancing Ovarian Antioxidants 104
4. Oxidative Stress Occurs in the Ovarian Follicles When the Normal Hormonal Support for Follicular Survival is Removed 108
5. Effects of Exogenous H_2O_2 on Ovarian Follicles and Granulosa Cells 109
6. Involvement of ROS in Ovarian Toxicity Caused by Chemical Toxicants 109
7. Involvement of ROS in Ovarian Toxicity Caused by Ionizing Radiation 118
8. Summary and Conclusions 120
References 120

5. Low-Dose Effects of Hormones and Endocrine Disruptors 129

Laura N. Vandenberg

1. Introduction 130
2. What is Meant by "Low Dose?" 131
3. Hormones Act at Low Doses 133
4. The "Rules" of Hormones are Obeyed by EDCs: Implications for Low-Dose Chemical Exposures 136
5. NTP Panel's Findings on Low-Dose Effects: 2000–2002 138
6. The NTP Panel's Assessment: Low-Dose Effects of Specific Chemicals 140
7. Updates to the NTP Panel Report on Low-Dose Effects 142
8. BPA and the Prostate: A Low-Dose Case Study 143
9. Additional Low-Dose Findings: Evidence from Laboratory Animals and Human Populations 145
10. Traditional Toxicology Studies are Not Designed to Detect Low-Dose Effects 146
11. Low-Dose Effects: Biological Changes are Not Necessarily Adverse 148
12. Real World EDC Exposures: Mixture Effects 150
13. Nonmonotonic Dose Responses 151
14. Conclusions 152
References 153

6. Contamination from Endocrine Disrupters of the General Population at Low and High Concentrations 167

Miquel Porta, José Pumarega, Magda Gasull, and Tomàs Lopez

1. Introduction 168
2. How to Implement the Indicator? An Example 172
3. Results of the Implementation of the Indicator 175
4. Discussion 183
References 189

7. Reproductive Toxicities of Methoxychlor Based on Estrogenic Properties of the Compound and Its Estrogenic Metabolite, Hydroxyphenyltrichloroethane **193**

Hiroaki Aoyama and Robert E. Chapin

1. Introduction 194
2. Estrogenicity of Methoxychlor and Its Active Metabolite, HPTE 195
3. Reproductive and Developmental Toxicities of Methoxychlor 199
4. Conclusion 206

Acknowledgment 207
References 207

8. Epigenetic Effects of Methoxychlor and Vinclozolin on Male Gametes **211**

Ariane Paoloni-Giacobino

1. Introduction 212
2. Epigenetics 213
3. Imprinting 213
4. Environmental Changes Affect Imprinting 215
5. Imprinting Defects and Male Infertility 215
6. Endocrine Disruptors and Male Infertility 216
7. Conclusion and Perspectives 223

References 224

9. Nuclear Receptor Profiling of Bisphenol-A and Its Halogenated Analogues **229**

Vanessa Delfosse, Marina Grimaldi, Albane le Maire, William Bourguet, and Patrick Balaguer

1. Introduction 230
2. Estrogen Receptors 232
3. Estrogen-Related Receptor γ 236
4. Androgen Receptor 239
5. Peroxysome Proliferator-Activated Receptor γ 240
6. Thyroid Receptors 243
7. Pregnane X Receptor 243
8. Conclusions 245

Acknowledgments 245
References 246

10. Long-Lasting Effects of Neonatal Bisphenol A Exposure on the Implantation Process **253**

Jorgelina Varayoud, Jorge G. Ramos, Mónica Muñoz-de-Toro, and Enrique H. Luque

1. Introduction 254
2. Uterine Implantation of the Embryo 255
3. Endocrine Disruptors and the Developmental Programming Hypothesis 259
4. Endocrine Disruption and Female Fertility 269
5. Conclusions 270

Acknowledgments 270
References 270

11. The Obesogen Tributyltin **277**

Felix Grün

1. The Obesogen Hypothesis 277
2. Organotins Environmental Exposure 281
3. Mechanisms of Cellular Organotin Toxicity 285
4. Nuclear Hormone Receptors as Organotin Targets 291
5. TBT and Disrupted Adipose Biology 297
6. Epigenetic Perturbations in Adipogenesis and Metabolic Set Points 303
7. Conclusion and Perspective 308

Acknowledgments 311
References 312

12. Human Testicular Insulin-Like Factor 3 and Endocrine Disrupters **327**

Katrine Bay and Ravinder Anand-Ivell

1. Introduction 328
2. INSL3: Expression and Regulation 328
3. Functions of INSL3 331
4. INSL3 and Endocrine Disrupters 336
5. Conclusions and Future Directions 341

References 341

13. Environmental Pollutants and Hydroxysteroid Dehydrogenases **349**

Leping Ye, Jingjing Guo, and Ren-Shan Ge

1. Introduction 350
2. 3β-Hydroxysteroid Dehydrogenase/Isomerase 352

3. 11β-Hydroxysteroid Dehydrogenase 358
4. 17β-Hydroxysteroid Dehydrogenase 370
5. 20α-Hydroxysteroid Dehydrogenase 375
6. Summary and Conclusion 377
Acknowledgments 377
References 378

14. Cadmium Effects on the Thyroid Gland **391**

Snezana A. Jancic and Bojan Z. Stosic

1. Introduction 392
2. Cadmium 393
3. Structural and Functional Organization of the Thyroid Gland 397
4. Cadmium and the Thyroid Gland 401
5. Molecular Mechanism of Cadmium Influence 409
6. Conclusions and Future Directions 417
References 417

15. A Recombinant PPRE-Driven Luciferase Bioassay for Identification of Potential PPAR Agonists **427**

Feng-Yuan Tsai, Yi-Ting Cheng, and Tsui-Chun Tsou

1. Introduction 428
2. Materials 428
3. Methods 431
4. Notes 433
Acknowledgment 434
References 434

Index *437*

CONTRIBUTORS

Ravinder Anand-Ivell
Division of Animal Science, School of Biosciences, University of Nottingham, UK

Hiroaki Aoyama
Toxicology Division, Institute of Environmental Toxicology, Joso, Ibaraki, Japan

Patrick Balaguer
Institut de Recherche en Cancérologie de Montpellier; Institut National de la Santé et de la Recherche Médicale U896; Institut régional du Cancer de Montpellier, and Universités Montpellier 1, Montpellier, France

Katrine Bay
University Department of Growth and Reproduction, Rigshospitalet, Copenhagen, Denmark

William Bourguet
Centre de Biochimie Structurale, Institut National de la Santé et de la Recherche Médicale U1054; Centre National de la Recherche Scientifique, Unité Mixte de Recherche 5048, and Universités Montpellier 1 and 2, Montpellier, France

Jean-Pierre Bourguignon
Developmental Neuroendocrinology Unit, GIGA Neurosciences, University of Liège, CHU, Liège, Belgium

Robert E. Chapin
Developmental and Reproductive Toxicology, Drug Safety R&D, Pfizer, Inc., Groton, Connecticut, USA

Yi-Ting Cheng
Laboratory of Molecular Toxicology, Division of Environmental Health and Occupational Medicine, National Health Research Institutes, Zhunan, Miaoli, Taiwan

Sukran Darcan
Department of Pediatric Endocrinology, Ege University School of Medicine, Izmir, Turkey

Vanessa Delfosse
Centre de Biochimie Structurale, Institut National de la Santé et de la Recherche Médicale U1054; Centre National de la Recherche Scientifique, Unité Mixte de Recherche 5048, and Universités Montpellier 1 and 2, Montpellier, France

Cheryl A. Frye
Department of Psychology; Department of Biological Sciences; The Center for Neuroscience Research, and The Center for Life Sciences Research, The University at Albany-SUNY, Albany, New York, and Department of Chemistry; IDeA Network of Biomedical Excellence (INBRE), and Institute of Arctic Biology, University of Alaska Fairbanks, Fairbanks, Alaska, USA

Julie Fudvoye
Developmental Neuroendocrinology Unit, GIGA Neurosciences, University of Liège, CHU, Liège, Belgium

Magda Gasull
Unit of Clinical and Molecular Epidemiology of Cancer, Hospital del Mar Institute of Medical Research—IMIM, Barcelona, Catalonia, and CIBER en Epidemiología y Salud Pública (CIBERESP), Spain

Ren-Shan Ge
The 2nd Affiliated Hospital and Research Academy of Reproductive Biomedicine of Wenzhou Medical University, Wenzhou, Zhejiang, PR China

Damla Goksen
Department of Pediatric Endocrinology, Ege University School of Medicine, Izmir, Turkey

Marina Grimaldi
Institut de Recherche en Cancérologie de Montpellier; Institut National de la Santé et de la Recherche Médicale U896; Institut régional du Cancer de Montpellier, and Universités Montpellier 1, Montpellier, France

Felix Grün
The Center for Complex Biological Systems, University of California Irvine, Irvine, California, USA

Jingjing Guo
The 2nd Affiliated Hospital and Research Academy of Reproductive Biomedicine of Wenzhou Medical University, Wenzhou, Zhejiang, PR China

Snezana A. Jancic
Department of Pathology, Institute for Pathology, Faculty of Medical Sciences, University of Kragujevac, Kragujevac, Serbia

Albane le Maire
Centre de Biochimie Structurale, Institut National de la Santé et de la Recherche Médicale U1054; Centre National de la Recherche Scientifique, Unité Mixte de Recherche 5048, and Universités Montpellier 1 and 2, Montpellier, France

Tomàs Lopez
Unit of Clinical and Molecular Epidemiology of Cancer, Hospital del Mar Institute of Medical Research—IMIM, Barcelona, Catalonia; School of Medicine, Universitat Autònoma de Barcelona, Barcelona, and CIBER en Epidemiología y Salud Pública (CIBERESP), Spain

Ulrike Luderer
Medicine, Developmental and Cell Biology, and Public Health, University of California Irvine, Irvine, California, USA

Enrique H. Luque
Laboratorio de Endocrinología y Tumores Hormonodependientes, School of Biochemistry and Biological Sciences, Universidad Nacional del Litoral, Santa Fe, Argentina

Mónica Muñoz-de-Toro
Laboratorio de Endocrinología y Tumores Hormonodependientes, School of Biochemistry and Biological Sciences, Universidad Nacional del Litoral, Santa Fe, Argentina

Samim Ozen
Department of Pediatric Endocrinology, Ege University School of Medicine, Izmir, Turkey

Ariane Paoloni-Giacobino
Department of Genetic Medicine and Development, and Swiss Center for Applied Human Toxicology, University of Geneva Medical School, Geneva, Switzerland

Anne-Simone Parent
Developmental Neuroendocrinology Unit, GIGA Neurosciences, University of Liège, CHU, Liège, Belgium

Miquel Porta
Unit of Clinical and Molecular Epidemiology of Cancer, Hospital del Mar Institute of Medical Research—IMIM, Barcelona, Catalonia; School of Medicine, Universitat Autònoma de Barcelona, Barcelona, and CIBER en Epidemiología y Salud Pública (CIBERESP), Spain, and Gillings School of Global Public Health, University of North Carolina at Chapel Hill, Chapel Hill, North Carolina, USA

José Pumarega
Unit of Clinical and Molecular Epidemiology of Cancer, Hospital del Mar Institute of Medical Research—IMIM, Barcelona, Catalonia, and CIBER en Epidemiología y Salud Pública (CIBERESP), Spain

Jorge G. Ramos
Laboratorio de Endocrinología y Tumores Hormonodependientes, School of Biochemistry and Biological Sciences, Universidad Nacional del Litoral, Santa Fe, Argentina

Bojan Z. Stosic
PhD student (Serbian Armed Forces), Faculty of Medical Sciences, University of Kragujevac, Kragujevac, Serbia

Feng-Yuan Tsai
Laboratory of Molecular Toxicology, Division of Environmental Health and Occupational Medicine, National Health Research Institutes, Zhunan, Miaoli, Taiwan

Tsui-Chun Tsou
Laboratory of Molecular Toxicology, Division of Environmental Health and Occupational Medicine, National Health Research Institutes, Zhunan, Miaoli, Taiwan

Laura N. Vandenberg
Department of Public Health, Division of Environmental Health Sciences, University of Massachusetts - Amherst, Amherst, Massachusetts, USA

Jorgelina Varayoud
Laboratorio de Endocrinología y Tumores Hormonodependientes, School of Biochemistry and Biological Sciences, Universidad Nacional del Litoral, Santa Fe, Argentina

Leping Ye
The 2nd Affiliated Hospital and Research Academy of Reproductive Biomedicine of Wenzhou Medical University, Wenzhou, Zhejiang, PR China

PREFACE

Advances in technology have been accompanied by the development of chemicals (pesticides) to control insects that normally infect crops as well as herbicides. Contamination of the food chain and in the air we breath has resulted wide scale in the inhalation and consumption of chemicals, many of which can affect the human endocrine system. The results of research in this area have led to the withdrawal of some of these pesticides from use in the field so as to minimize these effects on crop workers; however, there are currently toxic compounds in the atmosphere, in the food we consume, and in the water we drink. In this volume, many of the endocrine-disrupting chemicals are reviewed. Effects on sexual development and function represent an important group of disrupting effects. Human growth and development are targeted. These chemicals affect receptors and enzymes, and many of these aspects are reviewed in the contributions that follow.

The first group of contributions represents general aspects of endocrine disrupters. In the second group, the effects of these chemicals concern specific endpoints. To begin, J. Fudvoye, J.-P. Bourguignon, and A.-S. Parent relate "Endocrine-disrupting chemicals and human growth and maturation: a focus on early critical windows of exposure." Then, S. Ozen, D. Goksen, and S. Darcan detail the "Agricultural pesticides and precocious puberty." "Endocrine-disrupting chemicals: Elucidating our understanding of their role in sex and gender-relevant endpoints" is the topic of C.A. Frye. U. Luderer discusses "Ovarian toxicity from reactive oxygen species." L.N. Vandenberg reports on "Low-dose effects of hormones and endocrine disrupters," and M. Porta, J. Pumarega, M. Gasull, and T. Lopez follow with "Contamination from endocrine disrupters of the general population at low and high concentrations."

In the second group of papers, H. Aoyama and R.E. Chapin review "Reproductive toxicities of methoxychlor based on estrogenic properties of the compound and its estrogenic metabolite, hydroxyphenyltrichloroethane." A. Paoloni-Giacobino discusses "Epigenetic effects of methoxychlor and vinclozolin on male gametes." "Nuclear receptor profiling of bisphenol-A and its halogenated analogues" is the subject of the work contributed by V. Delfosse, M. Grimaldi, A. le Maire, W. Bourguet, and P. Balaguer. The "Long-lasting effects of neonatal bisphenol A exposure on the implantation process" is the review by J. Varayoud,

J.G. Ramos, M. Munoz-de-Toro, and E.H. Luque. F. Grün reports on "The obesogen tributyltin." K. Bay and R. Anand-Ivell have as their topic "Human testicular insulin-like factor 3 and endocrine disrupters." "Environmental pollutants and hydroxysteroid dehydrogenases" is the subject of L. Ye, J. Guo, and R.-S. Ge. S. Jancic and B. Stosic address "Cadmium effects on the thyroid gland." In the final chapter, F.-Y. Tsai, Y.-T. Cheng, and T.-C. Tsou describe "A recombinant PPRE-driven luciferase bioassay for identification of potential PPAR agonists."

Helene Kabes and Mary Ann Zimmerman of Elsevier (in the United Kingdom) were instrumental in the processing of the assembled chapters.

The figure on the cover of the book was supplied by Dr. William Bourguet, one of the authors of the chapter by V. Delfosse, M. Grimaldi, A. le Maire, W. Bourguet, and P. Balaguer entitled "Nuclear receptor profiling of bisphenol-A and its halogenated analogues." The figure depicts the crystal structure of the estrogen receptor (gray molecular surface and yellow helices) bound to bisphenol-A (orange).

Gerald Litwack
Toluca Lake, North Hollywood
July 26, 2013

CHAPTER ONE

Endocrine-Disrupting Chemicals and Human Growth and Maturation: A Focus on Early Critical Windows of Exposure

Julie Fudvoye, Jean-Pierre Bourguignon, Anne-Simone Parent[1]
Developmental Neuroendocrinology Unit, GIGA Neurosciences, University of Liège, CHU, Liège, Belgium
[1]Corresponding author: e-mail address: asparent@ulg.ac.be

Contents

1. Introduction 2
2. Challenges in Evidencing Endocrine Disruption 2
3. Endocrine-Disrupting Chemicals and Fetal Growth 4
4. EDCs and Sexual Differentiation 5
5. EDCs and Puberty 8
6. EDCs and Brain Development 9
   6.1 Disruption of thyroid function and brain development 11
   6.2 Disruption of sex steroid action and brain development 12
7. EDC and Energy Balance 14
8. Epigenetic Perspective on the Developmental Effects of EDCs 16
9. Conclusion 17
References 18

Abstract

Endocrine-disrupting chemicals (EDCs) are exogenous substances that interfere with hormone synthesis, metabolism, or action. In addition, some of them could cause epigenetic alterations of DNA that can be transmitted to the following generations. Because the developing organism is highly dependent on sex steroids and thyroid hormones for its maturation, the fetus and the child are very sensitive to any alteration of their hormonal environment. An additional concern about that early period of life comes from the shaping of the homeostatic mechanisms that takes place also at that time with involvement of epigenetic mechanisms along with the concept of fetal origin of health and disease. In this chapter, we will review the studies reporting effects of EDCs on human development. Using a translational approach, we will review animal studies that can shed light on some mechanisms of action of EDCs on the developing organism. We will focus on the major hormone-dependent stages of development: fetal growth, sexual differentiation, puberty, brain development, and energy balance. We will also discuss the possible epigenetic effects of EDCs on human development.

Vitamins and Hormones, Volume 94
ISSN 0083-6729
http://dx.doi.org/10.1016/B978-0-12-800095-3.00001-8

1. INTRODUCTION

Endocrine-disrupting chemicals (EDCs) are exogenous substances that interfere with hormone synthesis, metabolism, or action. Moreover, it appears that some of them could cause epigenetic alterations of the DNA that can be transmitted to the following generations. Animal and human studies have brought evidence that EDCs affect male and female reproduction, thyroid function, and control of energy balance. They could increase the risk of breast or prostate cancer as well as the risk of metabolic syndrome (Diamanti-Kandarakis et al., 2009). Because the developing organism is highly dependent on sex steroids and thyroid hormones for its maturation, the fetus and the child are very sensitive to any alteration of their hormonal environment. An additional concern about that early period of life comes from the shaping of the homeostatic mechanisms that takes place also at that time with involvement of epigenetic mechanisms along with the concept of fetal origin of health and disease (Gluckman, Hanson, & Low, 2011). Most studies have identified the perinatal period as a specific window of sensitivity. However, most of the reported effects were observed later in life. A review of the existing literature underlines the need for identification of early markers of exposure to EDCs. In this chapter, we will review the studies reporting effects of EDCs on human development. Using a translational approach, we will review animal studies that can shed light on some mechanisms of action of EDCs on the developing organism. We will focus on the major hormone-dependent stages of development: fetal growth, sexual differentiation, puberty, brain development, and energy balance. We will also discuss the possible epigenetic effects of EDCs on human development.

2. CHALLENGES IN EVIDENCING ENDOCRINE DISRUPTION

Before we discuss the different aspects of growth and maturation that are possibly altered by endocrine disruption, it is important to be aware of some challenges (Table 1.1) that we face in this area and that are relevant to all the specific aspects we will discuss later. Because the persistence of EDCs in the body and the environment is highly variable between few days such as for bisphenol A (BPA) (Rudel et al., 2011) and several decades such as for

Table 1.1 Challenges in the demonstration of endocrine disruption

1. Variable persistence in the body and the environment
2. Variable effects depending on the critical periods and duration of exposure
3. Simultaneous action at different interrelated levels of endocrine systems
4. Low-dose mixtures consistent with human exposure not conforming to simple additive models
5. Nonmonotonic dose–response relationship
6. Variable latency between exposure and effects including multigenerational impact

1,1-dichloro-2,2-bis (p-chlorophenyl) ethane (DDE) (Kirman, Aylward, Hays, Krishnan, & Nong, 2011), linking any disorder with previous EDC exposure is most difficult especially when latency is long between exposure and manifestation of health consequences. Also, the effects of EDCs can vary depending on the critical periods and duration of exposure. As will be discussed in the next sections, prenatal and early postnatal life is a period characterized by organization of the mechanisms that will drive homeostatic processes such as control of reproduction and energy balance. Obviously, EDC interference during those organizing periods could have much more severe consequences than later in life. Among the features of endocrine systems, they involve a cascade of activation or inhibition at different levels where EDCs play disturbing roles. We will see illustrations with puberty and reproduction that can be altered by effects at the hypothalamic–pituitary level as well as in target tissues (e.g., breasts). This also applies to energy balance through involvement of hypothalamic centers as well as fat tissue. Moreover, the physiological feedback systems through factors such as sex steroids and leptin, respectively, will also be disturbed by EDCs. Further challenges come from observations that are inconsistent with classical toxicology: Low-dose mixtures that are consistent with human exposure can have effects not conforming to simple additive models (Christiansen et al., 2012; Kortenkamp, 2008); the dose–response relationship can be nonmonotonic such as seen for BPA with U-shaped dose–response curves (Vandenberg et al., 2012). For both reasons, setting a threshold dose for EDC effects has become meaningless. A final issue is the highly variable latency between exposure and effects including multigenerational impact.

3. ENDOCRINE-DISRUPTING CHEMICALS AND FETAL GROWTH

Data concerning EDCs effects on fetal growth are scarce. However, one can hypothesize that fetal growth could be altered by endocrine disruption. Indeed, several EDCs cross the placental barrier and accumulate in the embryo or amniotic fluid (Diamanti-Kandarakis et al., 2009). The fetus is particularly sensitive to the effects of EDCs because of its dependency on hormones for development (Diamanti-Kandarakis et al., 2009). Moreover, animal studies have shown that most biotransformation enzymes are not produced until after birth (Pottenger et al., 2000), which means that fetuses might be exposed longer to higher concentration of EDCs. Clearance of BPA from fetal circulation, for instance, is slower than from maternal circulation (Takahashi & Oishi, 2000). It remains very complex to evaluate the effects of prenatal exposure to EDCs on fetal growth in human. Most studies focus on correlations between birth weight and serum or urinary levels of EDCs during pregnancy or at birth. Because of some limitations discussed later, few studies have identified a link between prenatal exposure to EDCs and fetal growth. We will review here some of the most significant human data as well as supporting animal studies.

For BPA, for instance, few studies have been published and lead to various results. Miao et al. have shown that maternal exposure to BPA in the workplace was associated with decreased birth weight (Miao et al., 2011b) after adjusting for confounding factors. BPA exposure during pregnancy was evaluated through personal air-sampling measurements and exposure history. Chou et al. (2011) reported an increased risk of low birth weight in male newborn exposed prenatally to higher levels of BPA, while Padmanabhan did not report any effect of BPA neither on birth weight nor on length (Padmanabhan et al., 2008). In both studies, prenatal exposure to BPA was evaluated through a single measurement of BPA in maternal or cord blood. Philippat et al. have shown an association between urinary BPA concentration (in one urinary sample between 24 and 30 weeks of gestation) and birth weight following an inverse U shape (Philippat et al., 2012). However, serial urinary measurements before and during pregnancy have been shown to be highly variable and this variability was even increased during pregnancy (Braun et al., 2011a). Given this variability, it appears that more than one sample may be necessary to adequately classify gestational exposure to BPA especially because the half-life is short and the clearance rate is rather rapid as opposed to other EDCs. Rudel et al. (2011) showed that urinary excretion of BPA fell significantly 2–3 days after changing habits regarding food, drinks, and containers. In addition, for feasibility reasons, most studies focus on one or a few compounds and might miss exposure to other EDCs. Another limitation of current epidemiological studies is the studied parameters: most studies focus on birth weight, while they might oversee more subtle effects of EDCs on body composition.

Some epidemiological studies have identified a negative correlation between exposure to polybrominated diphenyl ethers (PBDEs) and birth weight. PBDEs are flame-retardant chemicals used in the manufacture of infant products, furniture, and electronics. Ninety-seven percent of the American population appears to be contaminated by those persistent EDCs (Sjödin et al., 2008). Animal studies have shown that PBDEs disrupt thyroid function and alter behavior and memory (Herbstman et al., 2010). A prospective study in a population of 286 pregnant women with low income living in California showed that higher concentrations of PBDEs in maternal serum during pregnancy were associated with lower birth weight. Each 10-fold increase in concentrations of BDE-47, BDE-99, and BDE-100 was associated with a 115 g decrease in birth weight (Harley et al., 2011). Other smaller studies had similarly shown that higher concentrations of PBDEs were associated with a higher risk of delivering lower birth weight infants (Chao, Wang, Lee, Wang, & Päpke, 2007; Wu et al., 2010). Some human studies, however, did not identify any effects of PBDE exposure on birth weight (Mazdai, Dodder, Abernathy, Hites, & Bigsby, 2003; Tan, Loganath, Chong, & Obbard, 2009). Animal models have not reported an effect of PBDEs on birth weight but identified a decreased weight gain of offspring during the postnatal period, which is comparable to the third trimester of pregnancy in human (Kodavanti et al., 2010). The tested doses were however elevated and difficult to translate into relevant environmental exposure.

4. EDCs AND SEXUAL DIFFERENTIATION

Sexual differentiation depends on prenatal hormonal environment. Therefore, exposure to EDCs may be associated with disorders of development of the reproductive system by altering this hormonal environment. Cryptorchidism and hypospadias in the male newborn and low sperm counts and increased risk of testicular germ cell cancer in young adult males belong to a lifelong spectrum of disorders caused by early impairment of testicular function. This association of disorders has been proposed as the testicular dysgenesis syndrome (TDS) (Skakkebaek, Rajpert-De Meyts, & Main, 2001). TDS appears to involve deficient testosterone (androgen) production by the fetal testis (Sharpe & Shakkebaek, 2008). Indeed, it has been shown that normal development of the male reproductive system depends on the crucial role of androgen within an early fetal time window, called the masculinization programming window (Welsh et al., 2008), which influences the reproductive capacity throughout life. Thus, EDCs, which interfere with the synthesis or action of androgens, can have deleterious consequences for the developing male genital tract and appear to be risk factors for TDS (Bay, Asklund, Skakkebaek, & Andersson, 2006).

Several animal experimental studies have confirmed this hypothesis, especially using the phthalates, a group of anti-androgenic compound present in personal care products, coating of pharmaceutical products, and soft plastics. Male offspring of pregnant rats exposed to 250 mg/kg or more of monobenzyl phthalate, a major metabolite of butyl benzyl phthalate, on days 15–17 of pregnancy had an increased incidence of undescended testes and a decreased anogenital distance, a marker of androgenic impregnation (Ema, Miyawaki, Hirose, & Kamata, 2003). Likewise, Fisher et al. reported a TDS-like condition after fetal rat exposure to phthalate esters (Fisher, Macpherson, Marchetti, & Sharpe, 2003). The effects of phthalates on male sexual development in rats result from alterations of Leydig cell function leading to androgen insufficiency, which can be responsible of hypospadias or cryptorchidism. Swan et al., in 2005, have demonstrated a similarly reduced androgenization after phthalate exposure in humans since boys whose mother had elevated prenatal phthalate exposure, measured through phthalate urinary concentration, had shorter anogenital distance and impaired testicular descent (Swan et al., 2005). Main et al. (2006) reported that free testosterone levels at age 1–3 months were negatively correlated with monoethyl phthalate (MEP) levels in breast milk collected during that period. A reduced Leydig cell response to LH was suggested by the increasing LH/free testosterone ratio in relation to milk MEP levels (Main et al., 2006). Though these findings suggest similar mechanisms in both rodents and humans, recent studies indicate possible differences in testicular sensitivity to phthalate effects among humans and rodents. Given the difficulty to evaluate the production of testosterone by the human fetal testis, Mitchell et al. (2012) and Heger et al. (2012) used a xenograft model to evaluate the effects of phthalates on steroidogenesis of human fetal testis. They used second-trimester human fetal testes xenografts, which were exposed to phthalates for 1–4 days or 21 days. There was no difference in serum testosterone levels or in the seminal vesicles weight between xenograft model exposed to DBP or MBP and controls (Mitchell et al., 2012). Heger et al. (2012) reported that steroidogenesis was suppressed in rodent xenograft but not in human xenografts in such conditions. Germ cell alterations however were observed in human xenografts.

Data concerning BPA are controversial. In animal studies, perinatal BPA exposure has been shown to lead to decreased levels of testicular testosterone (Richter et al., 2007) or impaired fertility (Salian, Doshi, & Vanage, 2009). These data are consistent with two human epidemiological studies highlighting the negative effect of BPA on the male reproductive function, by modifying sex hormone concentrations (Galloway et al., 2010; Meeker, Calafat, & Hauser, 2010). However, other animal and human studies have reported conflicting results when studying effect of BPA on male reproductive tract. Indeed, in human, an association between maternal exposure to BPA during pregnancy and a shorter anogenital distance in male offspring has been shown (LaRocca, Boyajian, Brown, Smith, & Hixon, 2011), while cord blood BPA levels are not different between normal and cryptorchid boys (Ema et al., 2001). In rodents, several studies have reported that BPA exposure *in utero* had no effect on the adult male reproductive system (Fénichel et al., 2012; Kobayashi, Ohtani, Kubota, & Miyagawa, 2010; Meeker et al., 2010; Miao et al., 2011a).

Interestingly, one recent study has evaluated the effects of perinatal exposure to BPA and diethylhexyl phthalate on gonadal development of male mice. Using a mixture of EDCs (DEHP and BPA) better illustrates the synergistic effects of a combination of EDCs as encountered in the environment (Xi et al., 2012). Significant reduction in testicular weight and/or epididymal sperm count was identified in immature and mature animals on postnatal days 15 and 42. Serum testosterone levels were also decreased. These authors however used doses of EDCs that were higher than those relevant for human exposure and mixture effects.

We discussed earlier the peripheral effects of EDCs on sexual differentiation. However, brain sexual differentiation should not been ignored because of its sensitivity to hormonal environment and its significance for reproduction. It is well established that testosterone secreted by the fetal and neonatal testis is involved in brain sexual differentiation, most likely after it has been converted to estradiol by aromatase in specific brain regions during critical periods of development (Rubin et al., 2006). Thus, perinatal exposure to BPA could alter sex steroid action in the rodent brain and disrupt the development of sexually dimorphic pathways. This concept is confirmed by data available in animals. Kubo et al. demonstrated that BPA exposure during prenatal and postnatal period abolished the sex differences in open-field behavior in mice. Likewise, it increases the size of the locus coeruleus (LC) in males and decreases LC volume in females (Kubo et al., 2003). Rubin et al. also identified an effect of BPA on brain sexual differentiation since exposure to low doses of BPA decreased the sexually dimorphic population of tyrosine hydroxylase (TH) neurons in the rostral periventricular preoptic area, an important brain region for estrous cyclicity and estrogen-positive feedback (Rubin et al., 2006). Similarly, a decreased sexual dimorphism in the number of corticotropin-releasing hormone neurons in the bed nucleus of the stria terminalis has been shown after BPA exposure, whereas there was no effect in the preoptic area (Funabashi, Kawaguchi, Furuta, Fukushima, & Kimura, 2004). Moreover, Tando et al. have shown that BPA exposure can affect brain development in a sex-specific manner. Indeed, a significant reduction in the total volume and density of dopaminergic neurons in the substantia nigra (SN) is observed only in adult female offspring after maternal BPA treatment during pregnancy and lactation (Tando et al., 2007). The cited studies underline the need to focus on both sexes when studying EDCs in order to identify sexual dimorphism in sensitivity to endocrine disruption.

5. EDCs AND PUBERTY

The effects of EDCs on puberty have been investigated mainly through variations in pubertal timing with emphasis on the onset of sexual maturation. Therefore, our current knowledge may miss some additional effects such as changes in age at occurrence of regular (ovulatory) cycles. As stated earlier, the appraisal of EDC effects on puberty is complex due to involvement of possible effects on peripheral target organs such as uterus and breast in females and penis in males as well as effects on neuroendocrine control of maturation through hypothalamic–pituitary maturation. Second, pubertal timing can be influenced by exposure close to the time of puberty or during the process of puberty as well as much earlier in life since pubertal timing is one among the parameters programmed during fetal/neonatal life. The published human observations after exposure that was estimated to have occurred pre- or neonatally are summarized in Table 1.2 and those after postnatal exposure in Table 1.3. The data are scarce and it appears that

Table 1.2 Effect of prenatal or early postnatal exposure to EDCs on timing of breast development and menarche

Pubertal timing	**Early**		**Normal**		**Delayed**	
Event	**Breast**	**Menarche**	**Breast**	**Menarche**	**Breast**	**Menarche**
DDE (+DDT)	Krstevska-Konstantinova et al. (2001)	Vasiliu, Muttineni, and Karmaus (2004)				
PCBs				Vasiliu et al. (2004), Yang et al. (2005)		
Dioxins				Leijs et al. (2008), Warner et al. (2004)	Leijs et al. (2008)	
Mixture of pesticides	Wohlfahrt-Veje et al. (2012)					

no firm conclusion can be drawn. It is of note that, except in conditions of accidental massive exposure to a single class of EDCs, mixtures are likely involved in most conditions. Therefore, measurement of particular compounds and study of a compound in relation to pubertal timing may involve some biases.

6. EDCs AND BRAIN DEVELOPMENT

Several studies have reported that prenatal or early postnatal exposure to some EDCs is associated with alterations of cognitive or motor functions in children. Knowing the fundamental role played by thyroid hormones and sex steroids in cortex development, one can hypothesize that disruption of those hormones could cause alteration of the development of the cerebral cortex and of its functions later in life. We will review here the human data suggesting a causal effect for endocrine disrupters on impairment of cortical functions and approach some EDC mechanisms of action using animal models.

Table 1.3 Effect of postnatal exposure to EDCs on timing of breast development and menarche

Pubertal timing	Early		Normal		Delayed	
Event	**Breast**	**Menarche**	**Breast**	**Menarche**	**Breast**	**Menarche**
DDE(+DDT)		Ouyang et al. (2005)	Wolff et al. (2008)	Denham et al. (2005)		
PCBs	Denham et al. (2005)	Denham et al. (2005)	Den Hond et al. (2002), Wolff et al. (2008)	Den Hond et al. (2002)		
Dioxins				Den Hond et al. (2002)	Den Hond et al. (2002)	
Phthalates	Colon et al. (2000), Wolff et al. (2010)		Lomenick et al. (2010), Frederiksen et al. (2012)		Pubarche: Frederiksen et al. (2012)	
Soy phytoestrogens			Strom et al. (2001)	Strom et al. (2001)	Wolff et al. (2008, 2010)	

6.1. Disruption of thyroid function and brain development

Thyroid hormones are known to be essential for brain development. They regulate progenitor proliferation and differentiation, neuron migration, and dendrite outgrowth (Parent, Naveau, Gerard, Bourguignon, & Westbrook, 2011). Even mild thyroid hormone insufficiency in humans can produce measurable deficits in cognitive functions (Zoeller & Rovet, 2004). Thyroid hormone action is mediated by two classes of nuclear receptors (Forrest & Vennström, 2000) that exhibit differential spatial and temporal expressions in the brain, suggesting that thyroid hormones have variable functions during brain development (Horn & Heuer, 2010). This differential expression of thyroid hormone receptors explains the critical period of thyroid hormone action on brain development as suggested by models of maternal hypothyroidism or congenital hypothyroidism (Zoeller & Rovet, 2004). Depending on the timing of onset of hypothyroidism, the offspring will display problems of visual attention, gross or fine motor skills, or language and memory skills. Similarly, one can hypothesize that disruption of thyroid function by EDCs will have different effects based on the timing of exposure. However, few studies focused on that aspect.

Polychlorinated biphenyls (PCBs) form a group of widespread environmental contaminants composed of 209 different congeners used in a wide variety of applications. Their production was banned in the 1970s but PCBs are still present in the environment due to their high stability. PCBs were among the first EDCs identified as responsible for alterations of cognitive functions. Indeed, impaired memory and altered learning abilities have been associated with prenatal exposure to EDCs in humans and rodents (Schantz, Widholm, & Rice, 2003). In animal models, perinatal exposure to PCBs has been consistently associated with a decrease of thyroid hormone concentration in maternal serum as well as pup serum (Brouwer et al., 1998). Some but not all epidemiological studies in human have found an association between PCB body burden and thyroid hormone levels (Langer, 2008). This disruption of thyroid function could explain some of the effects of PCBs on the developing brain. Indeed, animal models have shown that the ototoxic effects of PCBs could be partially ameliorated by thyroxin replacement and PCBs seem to alter some of the developmental processes in the cortex and the cerebellum that are dependent on thyroid hormones (Diamanti-Kandarakis et al., 2009). However, recent publications raise important issues. First, PCBs produce paradoxical effects on the thyroid system; PCBs reduce serum T_4 but increase the expression of some genes regulated by TH (Zoeller, Dowling, & Vas, 2000). Second, while some report agonistic actions of PCBs on the TH receptor (Gauger et al., 2007), others report antagonistic actions (Koibuchi & Iwasaki, 2006). Although this appears paradoxical, it is consistent with *in vivo* studies showing that PCBs can exert different actions on TH response genes in the developing brain (Bansal & Zoeller, 2008). In addition, as suggested by *in vitro* models, some congeners can have direct toxic effects on neurons through alterations of neurotransmission or intracellular signaling, independent of disruption of thyroid hormones.

PBDEs are semivolatile and migrate into house dust, placing the young children at risk of higher exposure (Stapleton et al., 2008). Animal studies suggest that pre- and postnatal exposure to different PBDE congeners causes long-lasting behavioral alterations, in particular alterations of motor activity and cognitive behavior (reviewed in Costa & Giordano, 2007). As it is the case for other EDCs, some windows of susceptibility have been identified during pre- and postnatal brain development (Eriksson, Viberg, Jakobsson, Orn, & Fredriksson, 2002; Kuriyama & Chahoud, 2004). Recent studies have shown that exposure to PBDEs causes alteration of thyroid hormone levels in pregnant women (Chevrier et al., 2010) and infants (Herbstman et al., 2008) as it is the case in rodents. Only very few studies, however, have focused on the molecular or cellular effects of perinatal exposure to PBDEs *in vivo*. Viberg et al. have reported a decrease of cholinergic nicotinic receptors in the hippocampus after exposure to BDE-99 and BDE-153 (Viberg, Fredriksson, & Eriksson, 2003). However, the link between such a decrease and the behavioral effects of PBDEs is still unclear. Other teams have reported that exposure to PBDEs reduced hippocampal long-term potentiation and decreased brain-derived neurotrophic factor expression in the brain (Viberg, Mundy, & Eriksson, 2008). While several studies have reported negative effect of PBDEs on brain development and cognitive function in animals, there is relatively little information about adverse health effects of PBDEs in humans. Some very recent studies have identified a correlation between prenatal exposure to PBDEs and alteration of cognitive functions. Eskenazi et al. have reported that both prenatal and early postnatal PBDE exposures were associated with poorer attention and fine motor coordination and cognition in a cohort of 300 school-age children at 5 and 7 years of age (Eskenazi et al., 2012).

6.2. Disruption of sex steroid action and brain development

Sex steroids also play a major role during brain development. Androgens and estrogens sculpt the gender-specific differences of brain regions involved in behavior, learning, memory, mood, and socialization. Both androgens and estrogens stimulate progenitor proliferation in the cortex and hippocampus. However, it has been shown in the hippocampus that androgens preferably support neurogenesis, whereas estrogens promote gliogenesis (Zhang, Konkle, Zup, & McCarthy, 2008). Estrogens and aromatizable androgens also regulate dendritic outgrowth, synaptic function, and neuronal connectivity. Because several EDCs affect estrogen and androgen receptors directly or indirectly through an effect on sex steroid biosynthesis, it is important to examine the effects of those EDCs on development of the cerebral cortex, the hippocampus, and the hypothalamus. As an illustration, we will summarize here some of the effects of BPA on behavior and cognitive functions in animals and humans. As developed earlier in this chapter, BPA has been shown to alter sexually dimorphic behaviors such as aggression, anxiety, and exploration in rodents (Palanza, Gioiosa, vom Saal, & Parmigiani, 2008; vom Saal et al., 2007). Sexually dimorphic disorders such as autism, attention deficit, or hyperactivity could be correlates of these animal behaviors and might be related to early exposure to EDCs. Braun et al. (2011a) studied a prospective cohort of 244 mothers and their 3-year-old children. BPA exposure was evaluated by measuring BPA levels in maternal urine at 16 and 26 weeks of gestation as well as BPA urinary levels in the children at 1, 2, and 3 years of age. Each 10-fold increase in gestational BPA exposure was associated with more anxious and depressed behavior and poorer emotional control in the 3-year-old children (Braun et al., 2011b). Effects appeared to be sexually different since girls, for example, exhibited increased hyperactivity, while boys exhibited decreased hyperactivity after gestational exposure to BPA. It is not known however if those effects will persist later in life. Those results illustrate the importance of the window of exposure since behavior appeared to be affected by prenatal exposure to BPA but not by postnatal exposure.

One can hypothesize that perinatal exposure to EDCs could lead to alterations of the development of brain circuits and an increased risk of neurodevelopmental deficits. Indeed, the developing brain is remarkably malleable. Such plasticity is advantageous in that it allows the refinement of the basic organization in response to the surrounding environment. However, this plasticity also can be maladaptive in that these critical developmental periods are extremely vulnerable to disruption as illustrated by neurodevelopmental disorders such as autism or fetal alcohol syndrome. Such diseases often are characterized by a disruption of functional brain circuits in the setting of grossly normal brain morphology. Animal models could be used to identify cellular or molecular markers of EDCs effects. Indeed, the synapse is the fundamental unit responsible for formation of brain circuitry and thus should serve as a sensitive indicator of disruption by EDCs. Leranth et al. have shown that adult exposure to BPA prevents the synaptogenic response to estradiol in hippocampus and prefrontal cortex in ovariectomized nonhuman primates (Leranth et al., 2008a) and antagonizes spine formation induced by estrogens and testosterone in limbic areas in gonadectomized female and male rats (Leranth et al., 2008b; MacLusky et al., 2005). Those data were obtained after BPA exposure during adult life. A more recent study, however, showed that gestational exposure to BPA reduced the number of dopamine neurons in the midbrain and the number of spine synapses in the hippocampus, while no effects were observed when the animals were exposed during the juvenile period (Elsworth et al., 2013).

7. EDC AND ENERGY BALANCE

The concept of developmental or fetal origin of adult disease was developed by Barker at the end of the 1980s. He showed that nutritional status during early life is linked to an increased risk of cardiovascular disease in early-adult life and premature death as a consequence (Barker & Osmond, 1986; Barker, 2004). Several studies initially focused on the correlation between fetal growth (often assessed by the birth weight) and the predisposition to adult disease, in particular metabolic disorders. Thereby, it has been shown that low birth weight is correlated with a major risk to develop insulin resistance (Hales et al., 1991), metabolic syndrome (Barker et al., 1993), and obesity (Ravelli, Van Der Meulen, Osmond, Barker, & Bleker, 1999) during adulthood.

The possible implication of EDCs during pregnancy in the development of diseases in adulthood was first evocated in the early 1970s, after millions of pregnant women were prescribed DES (diethylstilbestrol). Indeed, daughters of woman treated by DES, a pharmaceutical estrogen given to prevent miscarriages, had an increased incidence of vaginal adenocarcinoma and benign reproductive lesions (Herbst, Ulfelder, & Poskanzer, 1971).

All these data highlight intrauterine and early postnatal life as critical periods for future health. According to this idea, one can hypothesize that the significant increase of obesity and metabolic syndrome incidence might be linked to perinatal disrupting factors acting as predisposition factors. Exposure to EDCs perinatally, by altering hormonal environment, could be associated with disorders of energy balance throughout subsequent life.

This hypothesis has been evocated in several animal studies. Significant data have been obtained for DES and BPA. Howdeshell et al. showed that pregnant mice fed with BPA (2.4 μg/kg/day on 11–17 days of gestation) had heavier pups than control mice (Howdeshell, Hotchkiss, Thayer, Vandenbergh, & vom Saal, 1999). This finding was confirmed in 2001, by Rubin, who exposed pregnant rat to BPA (0.1 mg BPA/kg/day or 1.2 mg BPA/kg/day) and observed an increase in body weight of the male and female offspring, an increase that was more persistent in females than males (Rubin et al., 2001). BPA has also been shown to reduce glucose tolerance and increase insulin resistance in male offspring at 6 months of age (Alonso-Magdalena et al., 2010). Interestingly, some studies suggest that these changes in glucose regulation are persistent in adult offspring and are worsened if the offspring is fed with a high-fat diet (Wei et al., 2011). The data of Ryan et al., however, are not consistent with this findings since they have shown that BPA exposure during pregnancy (0.25 μg/kg/day) results in accelerated growth early in life but does not result in impaired glucose regulation in adulthood, even when the mice are maintained on a high-fat diet (Ryan et al., 2010).

In addition to altering glucose tolerance, BPA appears to affect adipogenesis very early in life. Female pups born from dams exposed to 1 mg/L of BPA in drinking water during gestation and lactation showed adipocyte hypertrophy and overexpression of lipogenic genes such PPAR-γ, SREBP-1C, SCD-1, and C/EBP-ALPHA (Somm et al., 2009). Masuno et al., using 3T3-L1 cells, a preadipocyte cell line that differentiates into mature adipocytes, have shown that BPA leads to an accelerated differentiation into adipocytes, causing high accumulation of triglycerides and lipoprotein lipase (Masuno, Iwanami, Kidani, Sakayama, & Honda, 2005; Wang, Sun, Hou, Pan, & Li, 2012). More recently, the effect of BPA on adipogenesis has been confirmed by Sargis et al., who assessed the ability of BPA (100 nM) to activate the glucocorticoid receptor and thereby increase lipid accumulation and expression of adipocytic proteins in mature adipocytes (Sargis, Johnson, Choudhuryl, & Bradyl, 2010).

In addition, exposure to BPA, at 10 nM, 1 μM, and 80 μM, increased the mRNA expression and enzymatic activity of 11β-HSD1, an enzyme that converts the inactive hormone cortisone to the active hormone cortisol in adipose tissues and promotes adipogenesis (Masuno et al., 2002). Interestingly, BPA at low doses (1 and 10 nM) also decreases adiponectin production from human adipose tissue (Hugo et al., 2008). Adiponectin is an adipocyte-specific hormone that increases insulin sensitivity and reduces tissue inflammation (Whitehead, Richards, Hickman, Macdonald, & Prins, 2006). Similarly, it has been shown that release of IL-6 and TNF alpha, two inflammatory cytokines involved to obesity, is stimulated by BPA exposure (Ben-Jonathan, Hugo, & Brandebourg, 2009).

Effects of BPA on energy balance are also suggested by studies in humans. A large cross-sectional study in human, by Lang et al., has shown that higher urinary BPA concentrations in adults were associated with diagnosis of cardiovascular disease and diabetes and abnormal concentrations of three liver enzymes (gamma-glutamyltransferase (GGT), alkaline phosphatase, and lactate dehydrogenase) (Lang et al., 2008; Vom Saal & Myers, 2008). However, measurements of BPA were made in adults and do not bring any information about the critical perinatal period identified in animals. A recent study in children showed that incidence of obesity was increased among children who had higher urinary BPA concentrations (Trasande, Attina, & Blustein, 2012). However, it is difficult to correlate BPA exposure and BPA urinary excretion. Moreover, the causal link remains difficult to establish. Indeed, obese children could, for instance, consume more BPA-contaminated food such as canned sodas, which would explain their higher urinary BPA levels. Further longitudinal studies are thus necessary in humans in order to determine if gestational and postnatal exposure to BPA could lead to an increased risk of metabolic syndrome later in life.

8. EPIGENETIC PERSPECTIVE ON THE DEVELOPMENTAL EFFECTS OF EDCs

Epigenetics refers to heritable alterations that are not due to changes in DNA sequence. Rather, epigenetic modifications, such as DNA methylation and histone modification, alter DNA accessibility and chromatin structure, thereby regulating patterns of gene expression. This mechanism appears as an adaptive response to insults during the developmental period, such as variations in maternal diet or sex steroids (Fowden & Forhead, 2009; Lillycrop et al., 2007). For example, it has been recently proposed that maternal undernutrition could cause epigenetic changes in the proopiomelanocortin (POMC) and glucocorticoid receptor genes in the fetal hypothalamus (Stevens, Begum, & White, 2011). POMC-derived peptides synthesized in neurons of the hypothalamus play a central role in the control of energy homeostasis (Coll, Sadaf, Challis, Yeo, & O'Rahylly, 2004).

EDCs, by interfering with the nutritional and/or hormonal environment during fetal life, may interfere with epigenetic programming, which can be passed from one cell generation to another and persist in adulthood (MClachlan, 2001; Anway, Cupp, Uzumcu, & Skinner, 2005). Moreover, epigenetic modifications, when they occur in the gonads, can be transmitted to the next generations as illustrated by Anway et al. (2005).

Some studies have reported the effects of prenatal BPA exposure on epigenetic mechanisms. Dolinoy et al., using the Agouti viable yellow mouse model, have shown that BPA exposure during pregnancy led to DNA hypomethylation of the offspring epigenome. Interestingly, this effect can be counteracted by maternal dietary supplementation (diet enriched with methyl group donors) (Dolinoy, Huang, & Jirtle, 2007). It will be necessary to examine the correlation between BPA-induced epigenetic alterations, modification in gene expression, and phenotype expression. But the absence of hypomethylation when supplementing maternal dietary during pregnancy suggests possible means for reducing risk of disease. Other studies supported epigenetic effects of BPA. Bromer et al. have shown that *in utero* exposure to high doses of BPA increased the expression of the homeobox gene Hoxa 10 in the uterus of female offspring at 2 weeks of age. This was correlated with significant demethylation of specific CpG sites in the Hoxa 10 gene, a gene necessary for uterus development. It is interesting to note that Hoxa 10 DNA methylation was not altered in adult mice treated with these doses of BPA. It highlights the great vulnerability of the fetus and the existence of a critical developmental window for the epigenetic effects of EDCs (Bromer, Zhou, Taylor, Doherty, & Taylor, 2010). Other studies have shown an association between *in utero* exposure to BPA and hypomethylation of specific sites in genes involved in cancer development (Ho, Tang, Belmonte de Frausto, & Prins, 2006).

9. CONCLUSION

The fetus and child are particularly exposed to EDCs. Indeed, several of those EDCs cross the placental barrier or accumulate in maternal milk. Moreover, childhood behavior such as crawling or placing objects in their mouth increases exposure. Because of its high dependence on sex steroids and thyroid hormones for its maturation, the developing organism is very sensitive to any alteration of its hormonal environment. Epidemiological studies have reported effects of EDCs on major hormone-dependent stages of development: fetal growth, sexual differentiation, puberty, brain development, and energy balance. However, the epidemiological data concerning the EDCs effects on the developing fetus and child are relatively scarce. Besides the challenges listed in Table 1.1, epidemiological studies present several other difficulties. Accurate quantification of exposure throughout pregnancy and childhood is difficult as described for BPA. In addition, for practical reasons, most epidemiological studies have to focus on one group of compounds and ignore other EDCs or risk factors. Genetic susceptibility to endocrine disruption or the effect of associated stresses of other nature is still to be studied.

An analysis of the literature underlines the need for identifying early and fine markers of EDC effects. Animal models can help to unravel the mechanisms of action of EDCs and discover new markers that could underlie alterations of function.

REFERENCES

Alonso-Magdalena, P., Vieira, E., Soriano, S., Menes, L., Burks, D., Quesada, I., et al. (2010). Bisphenol A exposure during pregnancy disrupts glucose homeostasis in mothers and adult male offspring. *Environmental Health Perspectives*, *118*, 1243–1250.

Anway, M. D., Cupp, A. S., Uzumcu, M., & Skinner, M. K. (2005). Epigenetic transgenerational actions of endocrine disruptors and male fertility. *Science*, *308*, 1466–1469.

Bansal, R., & Zoeller, R. T. (2008). Polychlorinated Biphenyls (Aroclor 1254) do not uniformly produce agonist actions on thyroid hormone responses in the developing rat brain. *Endocrinology*, *149*, 4001–4008.

Barker, D. J. (2004). The developmental origins of adult disease. *Journal of the American College of Nutrition*, *23*, 588–595.

Barker, D. J. P., Hales, C. N., Fall, C. H. D., Osmond, C., Phipps, K., & Clark, P. M. S. (1993). Type 2 (non-insulin-dependent) diabetes mellitus, hypertension and hyperlipidaemia (syndrome X): Relation to reduced fetal growth. *Diabetologia*, *36*, 62–67.

Barker, D. J. P., & Osmond, C. (1986). Infant mortality, childhood nutrition, and ischaemic heart disease in England and Wales. *The Lancet*, *1*, 1077–1081.

Bay, K., Asklund, C., Skakkebaek, N. E., & Andersson, A. M. (2006). Testicular dysgenesis syndrome: Possible role of endocrine disrupters. *Best Practice & Research. Clinical Endocrinology & Metabolism*, *20*, 77–90.

Ben-Jonathan, N., Hugo, E. R., & Brandebourg, T. D. (2009). Effects of bisphenol A on adipokine release from human adipose tissue: Implications for the metabolic syndrome. *Molecular and Cellular Endocrinology*, *304*, 49–54.

Braun, J., Kalkbrenner, E., Calafat, A., Bernert, J., Ye, X., Silva, M., et al. (2011a). Variability and predictors of urinary Bisphenol A concentrations during pregnancy. *Environmental Health Perspectives*, *119*, 131–137.

Braun, J. M., Kalkbrenner, A. E., Calafat, A. M., Yolton, K., Ye, X., Dietrich, K. N., et al. (2011b). Impact of early-life bisphenol A exposure on behaviour and executive function in children. *Pediatrics*, *128*, 873–882.

Bromer, J. G., Zhou, Y., Taylor, M. B., Doherty, L., & Taylor, H. S. (2010). Bisphenol-A exposure in utero leads to epigenetic alterations in the developmental programming of uterine estrogen response. *FASEB Journal*, *24*, 2273–2280.

Brouwer, A., Morse, D. C., Lans, M. C., Schuur, A. G., Murk, A. J., Klasson-Wheler, E., et al. (1998). Interactions of persistent environmental organohalogens with the thyroid hormones system: Mechanisms and possible consequences for animal and human health. *Toxicology and Industrial Health*, *14*, 59–84.

Chao, H. R., Wang, S. L., Lee, W. J., Wang, Y. F., & Päpke, O. (2007). Levels of polybrominated diphenyl ethers (PBDEs) in breast milk from central Taiwan and their relation to infant birth outcome and maternal menstruation effects. *Environment International*, *33*, 239–245.

Chevrier, J., Harley, K. G., Bradman, A., Gharbi, M., Sjödin, A., & Eskenazi, B. (2010). Polybrominated diphenyl ether (PBDE) flame retardants and thyroid hormone during pregnancy. *Environmental Health Perspectives*, *118*, 1444–1449.

Chou, W. C., Chen, J. L., Lin, C. F., Chen, Y. C., Shih, F. C., & Chuang, C. Y. (2011). Biomonitoring of bisphenol A concentrations in maternal and umbilical cord blood in regard to birth outcomes and adipokine expression: A birth cohort study in Taiwan. *Environmental Health*, *3*, 10–94.

Christiansen, S., Kortenkamp, A., Axelstad, M., Boberg, J., Scholze, M., Jacobsen, P. R., et al. (2012). Mixtures of endocrine disrupting contaminants modelled on human high end exposures: An exploratory study in rats. *International Journal of Andrology*, *35*, 303–316.

Coll, A. P., Farooqi, I. S., Challis, B. G., Yeo, G. S., & O'Rahylly, S. (2004). Proopiomelanocortin and energy balance: Insights from human and murine genetics. *Journal of Clinical Endocrinology and Metabolism*, *89*, 2557–2562.

Colon, I., Caro, D., Bourdony, C. J., & Rosario, O. (2000). Identification of phthalate esters in the serum of young Puerto Rican girls with premature breast development. *Environmental Health Perspectives*, *108*, 895–900.

Costa, L. G., & Giordano, G. (2007). Developmental neurotoxicity of polybrominated diphenyl ether (PBDE) flame retardants. *Neurotoxicology*, *28*, 1047–1067.

Denham, M., Schell, L. M., Deane, G., Gallo, M. V., Ravenscroft, J., & DeCaprio, A. P. (2005). Relationship of lead, mercury, mirex, dichlorodiphenyldichloroethylene, hexachlorobenzene, and polychlorinated biphenyls to timing of menarche among Akwesasne Mohawk girls. *Pediatrics*, *115*, 127–134.

Den Hond, E., Roels, H. A., Hoppenbrouwers, K., Nawrot, T., Thijs, L., Vandermeulen, C., et al. (2002). Sexual maturation in relation to polychlorinated aromatic hydrocarbons: Sharpe and Skakkebaek's hypothesis revisited. *Environmental Health Perspectives*, *110*, 771–776.

Diamanti-Kandarakis, E., Bourguignon, J. P., Giudice, L., Hauser, R., Prins, G., Soto, A., et al. (2009). Endocrine-disrupting chemicals: An endocrine society scientific statement. *Endocrine Reviews*, *30*, 293–342.

Dolinoy, D. C., Huang, D., & Jirtle, R. L. (2007). Maternal nutrient supplementation counteracts bisphenol A-induced DNA hypomethylation in early development. *Proceedings of the National Academy of Sciences of the United States of America*, *104*, 13056–13061.

Elsworth, J. D., Jentsch, J. D., Vandevoort, C. A., Roth, R. H., Jr, D. E., & Leranth, C. (2013). Prenatal exposure to bisphenol A impacts midbrain dopamine neurons and hippocampal spine synapses in non-human primates. *Neurotoxicology*, *35*, 113–120.

Ema, M., Fujii, S., Furukawa, M., Kiguchi, M., Ikka, T., & Harazono, A. (2001). Rat two-generation reproductive toxicity study of bisphenol A. *Reproductive Toxicology*, *15*, 505–523.

Ema, M., Miyawaki, E., Hirose, A., & Kamata, E. (2003). Decreased anogenital distance and increased incidence of undescended testes in fetuses of rats given monobenzyl phthalate, a major metabolite of butyl benzyl phthalate. *Reproductive Toxicology, 17*, 407–412.

Eriksson, P., Viberg, H., Jakobsson, E., Orn, U., & Fredriksson, A. (2002). A brominated flame retardant, 2,2′,4,4′,5-pentabromodiphenyl ether: Uptake, retention, and induction of neurobehavioral alterations in mice during a critical phase of neonatal brain development. *Toxicological Sciences, 67*, 98–103.

Eskenazi, B., Chevrier, J., Rauch, S. A., Kogut, K., Harley, K. G., Johnson, C., et al. (2012). In utero and childhood polybrominated diphenyl ether (PBDE) exposures and neurodevelopment in the CHAMACOS study. *Environmental Health Perspectives, 121*, 257–262.

Fénichel, P., Déchaux, H., Harthe, C., Gal, J., Ferrari, P., Pacini, P., et al. (2012). Unconjugated bisphenol A cord blood levels in boys with descended or undescended testes. *Human Reproduction, 27*, 983–990.

Fisher, J. S., Macpherson, S., Marchetti, N., & Sharpe, R. M. (2003). Human 'testicular dysgenesis syndrome': A possible model using in-utero exposure of the rat to dibutyl phthalate. *Human Reproduction, 18*, 1383–1394.

Forrest, D., & Vennström, B. (2000). Functions of thyroid hormone receptors in mice. *Thyroid, 10*, 41–52.

Fowden, A. L., & Forhead, A. J. (2009). Hormones as epigenetic signals in developmental programming. *Experimental Physiology, 94*, 607–625.

Frederiksen, H., Sørensen, K., Mouritsen, A., Aksglaede, L., Hagen, C. P., Petersen, J. H., et al. (2012). High urinary phthalate concentration associated with delayed pubarche in girls. *International Journal of Andrology, 35*, 216–226.

Funabashi, T., Kawaguchi, M., Furuta, M., Fukushima, A., & Kimura, F. (2004). Exposure to bisphenol A during gestation and lactation causes loss of sex difference in corticotropin-releasing hormone-immunoreactive neurons in the bed nucleus of the stria terminalis of rats. *Psychoneuroendocrinology, 29*, 475–485.

Galloway, T., Cipelli, R., Guralnik, J., Ferrucci, L., Bandinelli, S., Corsi, A. M., et al. (2010). Daily bisphenol A excretion and associations with sex hormone concentrations: Results from the InCHIANTI adult population study. *Environmental Health Perspectives, 118*, 1603–1608.

Gauger, K. J., Giera, S., Sharlin, D. S., Bansal, R., Iannacone, E., & Zoeller, R. T. (2007). Polychlorinated biphenyls 105 and 118 form thyroid hormone receptor agonists after cytochrome P4501A1 activation in rat pituitary GH3 cells. *Environmental Health Perspectives, 115*, 1623–1630.

Gluckman, P. D., Hanson, M. A., & Low, F. M. (2011). The role of developmental plasticity and epigenetics in human health. *Birth Defects Research. Part C, Embryo Today, 93*, 12–18.

Hales, C. N., Barker, D. J., Clark, P. M., Cox, L. J., Fall, C., Osmond, C., et al. (1991). Fetal and infant growth and impaired glucose tolerance at age 64. *BMJ, 303*, 1019–1022.

Harley, K. G., Chevrier, J., Aguilar, Schall R., Sjödin, A., Bradman, A., & Eskenazi, B. (2011). Association of prenatal exposure to polybrominated diphenyl ethers and infant birth weight. *American Journal of Epidemiology, 174*, 1166–1174.

Heger, N. E., Hall, S. J., Sandrof, M. A., McDonnell, E. V., Hensley, J. B., McDowell, E. N., et al. (2012). Human fetal testis xenografts are resistant to phthalate-induced endocrine disruption. *Environmental Health Perspectives, 120*, 1137–1143.

Herbst, A. L., Ulfelder, H., & Poskanzer, D. C. (1971). Adenocarcinoma of vagina. Association of maternal stilbestrol therapy with tumor appearance in young women. *The New England Journal of Medicine, 284*, 878–881.

Herbstman, J. B., Sjodin, A., Apelberg, B. J., Witter, F. R., Halden, R. U., Patterson, D. G., et al. (2008). Birth delivery mode modifies the associations between prenatal polychlorinated biphenyl (PCB) and polybrominated diphenyl ether (PBDE) and neonatal thyroid hormone levels. *Environmental Health Perspectives, 116*, 1376–1382.

Herbstman, J. B., Sjödin, A., Kurzon, M., Lederman, S. A., Jones, R. S., & Rauh, V. (2010). Prenatal exposure to PBDEs and neurodevelopment. *Environmental Health Perspectives, 118*, 712–719.

Ho, S. M., Tang, W. Y., Belmonte de Frausto, J., & Prins, G. S. (2006). Developmental exposure to estradiol and bisphenol A increases susceptibility to prostate carcinogenesis and epigenetically regulates phosphodiesterase type 4 variant 4. *Cancer Research, 66*, 5624–5632.

Horn, S., & Heuer, H. (2010). Thyroid hormone action during brain development: More questions than answers. *Molecular and Cellular Endocrinology, 315*, 19–26.

Howdeshell, K. L., Hotchkiss, A. K., Thayer, K. A., Vandenbergh, J. G., & vom Saal, F. S. (1999). Exposure to bisphenol A advances puberty. *Nature, 401*, 763–764.

Hugo, E. R., Brandebourg, T. D., Woo, J. G., Loftus, J., Wesley, Alexander J., & Ben-Jonathan, N. (2008). Bisphenol A at environmentally relevant doses inhibits adiponectin release from human adipose tissue explants and adipocytes. *Environmental Health Perspectives, 116*, 1642–1647.

Kirman, C. R., Aylward, L. L., Hays, S. M., Krishnan, K., & Nong, A. (2011). Biomonitoring equivalents for DDT/DDE. *Regulatory Toxicology and Pharmacology, 60*, 172–180.

Kobayashi, K., Ohtani, K., Kubota, H., & Miyagawa, M. (2010). Dietary exposure to low doses of bisphenol A: Effects on reproduction and development in two generations of C57BL/6J mice. *Congenital Anomalies (Kyoto), 50*, 159–170.

Kodavanti, P. R., Coburn, C. G., Moser, V. C., MacPhail, R. C., Fenton, S. E., Stoker, T. E., et al. (2010). Developmental exposure to a commercial PBDE mixture, DE-71: Neurobehavioral, hormonal, and reproductive effects. *Toxicological Sciences, 116*, 297–312.

Koibuchi, N., & Iwasaki, T. (2006). Regulation of brain development by thyroid hormone and its modulation by environmental chemicals. *Endocrine Journal, 53*, 295–303.

Kortenkamp, A. (2008). Low dose mixture effects of endocrine disrupters: Implications for risk assessment and epidemiology. *International Journal of Andrology, 31*, 233–240.

Krstevska-Konstantinova, M., Charlier, C., Craen, M., Du Caju, M., Heinrichs, C., de Beaufort, C., et al. (2001). Sexual precocity after immigration from developing countries to Belgium: Evidence of previous exposure to organochlorine pesticides. *Human Reproduction, 16*, 1020–1026.

Kubo, K., Arai, O., Omura, M., Watanabe, R., Ogata, R., & Aou, S. (2003). Low dose effects of bisphenol A on sexual differentiation of the brain and behavior in rats. *Neuroscience Research, 45*, 345–356.

Kuriyama, S. N., & Chahoud, I. (2004). In utero exposure to low-dose 2,3′,4,4′,5-pentachlorobiphenyl (PCB 118) impairs male fertility and alters neurobehavior in rat offspring. *Toxicology, 202*, 185–197.

Lang, I. A., Galloway, T. S., Scarlett, A., Henley, W. E., Depledge, M., Wallace, R. B., et al. (2008). Association of urinary bisphenol A concentration with medical disorders and laboratory abnormalities in adults. *JAMA, 300*, 1303–1310.

Langer, P. (2008). Persistent organochlorinated pollutants (PCB, DDE, HCB, dioxins, furans) and the thyroid. *Endocrine Regulations, 42*, 79–104.

LaRocca, J., Boyajian, A., Brown, C., Smith, S. D., & Hixon, M. (2011). Effects of in utero exposure to bisphenol A or diethylstilbestrol on the adult male reproductive system. *Birth Defects Research. Part B, Developmental and Reproductive Toxicology, 92*, 526–533.

Leijs, M. M., Koppe, J. G., Olie, K., van Aalderen, W. M. C., de Voogt, P., Vulsma, T., et al. (2008). Delayed initiation of breast development in girls with higher prenatal dioxin exposure; a longitudinal cohort study. *Chemosphere, 73*, 999–1004.

Leranth, C., Hajszan, T., Szigeti-Buck, K., Bober, J., & MacLusky, N. J. (2008a). Bisphenol A prevents the synaptogenic response to estradiol in hippocampus and prefrontal cortex

of ovariectomized nonhuman primates. *Proceedings of the National Academy of Science of the United States of America, 105*, 14187–14191.
Leranth, C., Szigeti-Buck, K., MacLusky, N. J., & Hajszan, T. (2008b). Bisphenol A prevents the synaptogenic response to testosterone in the brain of adult male rats. *Endocrinology, 149*, 988–994.
Lillycrop, K. A., Slater-Jefferies, J. L., Hanson, M. A., Godfrey, K. M., Jackson, A. A., & Burdge, G. C. (2007). Induction of altered epigenetic regulation of the hepatic glucocorticoid receptor in the offspring of rats fed a protein-restricted diet during pregnancy suggests that reduced DNA methyltransferase-1 expression is involved in impaired DNA methylation and changes in histone modifications. *British Journal of Nutrition, 97*, 1064–1073.
Lomenick, J. P., Calafat, A. M., Melguizo Castro, M. S., Mier, R., Stenger, P., Foster, M. B., et al. (2010). Phthalate exposure and precocious puberty in females. *The Journal of Pediatrics, 156*, 221–225.
MacLusky, N. J., Hajszan, T., & Leranth, C. (2005). The environmental estrogen bisphenol A inhibits estradiol-induced hippocampal synaptogenesis. *Environmental Health Perspectives, 113*, 675–679.
Main, K. M., Mortensen, G. K., Kaleva, M. M., Boisen, K. A., Damgaard, I. N., Chellakooty, M., et al. (2006). Human breast milk contamination with phthalates and alterations of endogenous reproductive hormones in infants three months of age. *Environmental Health Perspectives, 114*, 270–276.
Masuno, H., Iwanami, J., Kidani, T., Sakayama, K., & Honda, K. (2005). Bisphenol A accelerates terminal differentiation of 3T3-L1 cells into adipocytes through the phosphatidylinositol 3-kinase pathway. *Toxicological Sciences, 84*, 319–327.
Masuno, H., Kidani, T., Sehiya, K., Sakayama, K., Shiosaka, T., Yamamoto, H., et al. (2002). Bisphenol A in combination with insulin can accelerate the conversion of 3T3-L1 fibroblasts to adipocytes. *Journal of Lipid Research, 43*, 676–684.
Mazdai, A., Dodder, N. G., Abernathy, M. P., Hites, R. A., & Bigsby, R. M. (2003). Polybrominated diphenyl ethers in maternal and fetal blood samples. *Environmental Health Perspectives, 111*, 1249–1252.
Mclachlan, J. A. (2001). Environmental signaling: What embryos and evolution teach us about endocrine disrupting chemicals. *Endocrine Reviews, 22*, 319–341.
Meeker, J. D., Calafat, A. M., & Hauser, R. (2010). Urinary bisphenol A concentrations in relation to serum thyroid and reproductive hormone levels in men from an infertility clinic. *Environmental Science and Technology, 44*, 1458–1463.
Miao, M., Yuan, W., He, Y., Zhou, Z., Wang, J., Gao, E., et al. (2011a). In utero exposure to bisphenol-A and anogenital distance of male offspring. *Birth Defects Research. Part A, Clinical and Molecular Teratology, 91*, 867–872.
Miao, M., Yuan, W., Zhu, G., He, X., & Li, D. K. (2011b). In utero exposure to bisphenol-A and its effect on birth weight of offspring. *Reproductive Toxicology, 32*, 64–68.
Mitchell, R. T., Childs, A. J., Anderson, R. A., van den Driesche, S., Saunders, P. T., McKinnell, C., et al. (2012). Do phthalates affect steroidogenesis by the human fetal testis? Exposure of human fetal testis xenografts to di-*n*-butyl phthalate. *Journal of Clinical Endocrinology and Metabolism, 97*, 341–348.
Ouyang, F., Perry, M. J., Venners, S. A., Chen, C., Wang, B., Yang, F., et al. (2005). Serum DDT, age at menarche, and abnormal menstrual cycle length. *Occupational and Environmental Medicine, 62*, 878–884.
Padmanabhan, V., Siefert, K., Ransom, S., Johnson, T., Pinkerton, J., Anderson, L., et al. (2008). Maternal bisphenol-A levels at delivery: A looming problem? *Journal of Perinatology, 28*, 258–263.
Palanza, P., Gioiosa, L., vom Saal, F. S., & Parmigiani, S. (2008). Effects of developmental exposure to bisphenol A on brain and behavior in mice. *Environmental Sciences, 108*, 150–157.

Parent, A. S., Naveau, E., Gerard, A., Bourguignon, J. P., & Westbrook, G. L. (2011). Early developmental actions of endocrine disruptors on the hypothalamus, hippocampus, and cerebral cortex. *Journal of Toxicology and Environmental Health, 14*, 328–345.

Philippat, C., Mortamais, M., Chevrier, C., Petit, C., Calafat, A. M., Ye, X., et al. (2012). Exposure to phthalates and phenols during pregnancy and offspring size at birth. *Environmental Health Perspectives, 120*, 464–470.

Pottenger, L. H., Domoradski, J. Y., Markham, D. A., Hansen, S. C., Cagen, S. Z., & Waechter, J. M., Jr. (2000). The relative bioavailability and metabolism of bisphenol A in rats is dependent upon the route of administration. *Toxicological Sciences, 54*, 3–18.

Ravelli, A. C., Van Der Meulen, J. H., Osmond, C., Barker, D. J., & Bleker, O. P. (1999). Obesity at the age of 50 y in men and women exposed to famine prenatally. *American Journal of Clinical Nutrition, 70*, 811–816.

Richter, C., Birnbaum, L., Farabollini, F., Newbold, R. R., Rubin, B., Talsness, C. E., et al. (2007). In vivo effects of Bisphenol A in laboratory rodent studies. *Reproductive Toxicology, 24*, 199–224.

Rubin, B. S., Lenkowski, J. R., Schaeberle, C. M., Vandenberg, L. N., Ronsheim, P. M., & Soto, A. M. (2006). Evidence of altered brain sexual differentiation in mice exposed perinatally to low, environmentally relevant levels of bisphenol A. *Neuroendocrinology, 147*, 3681–3691.

Rubin, B. S., Murray, M. K., Damassa, D. A., King, J. C., & Soto, A. M. (2001). Perinatal exposure to low doses of bisphenol A affects body weight, patterns of estrous cyclicity and plasma LH levels. *Environmental Health Perspectives, 109*, 675–680.

Rudel, R. A., Gray, J. M., Engel, C. L., Rawsthorne, T. W., Dodson, R. E., Ackerman, J. M., et al. (2011). Food packaging and bisphenol A and bis(2-ethyhexyl) phthalate exposure: Findings from a dietary intervention. *Environmental Health Perspectives, 119*, 914–920.

Ryan, K. R., Haller, A. M., Sorrel, J. E., Woods, S. C., Jandacek, R. J., & Seeley, R. J. (2010). Perinatal exposure to Bisphenol-A and the development of metabolic syndrome in CD-1 Mice. *Endocrinology, 151*, 2603–2612.

Salian, S., Doshi, T., & Vanage, G. (2009). Neonatal exposure of male rats to bisphenol A impairs fertility and expression of sertoli cell junctional proteins in the testis. *Toxicology, 265*, 56–67.

Sargis, R. M., Johnson, D. N., Choudhuryl, R. A., & Bradyl, M. J. (2010). Endocrine disruptors promote adipogenesis in the 3T3-L1 cell line through glucocorticoid receptor activation. *Obesity, 18*, 1283–1288.

Schantz, S. L., Widholm, J. J., & Rice, D. C. (2003). Effects of PCB exposure on neuropsychological function in children. *Environmental Health Perspectives, 111*, 357–376.

Shakkebaek, N. E., Rajpert-De, Meyts E., & Main, K. M. (2001). Testicular dysgenesis syndrome: An increasingly common developmental disorder with environmental aspects. *Human Reproduction, 16*, 972–978.

Sharpe, R. M., & Skakkebaek, N. E. (2008). Testicular dysgenesis syndrome: Mechanistic insights and potential new downstream effects. *Fertility and Sterility, 89*, 33–38.

Sjödin, A., Wong, L. T., Jones, R. S., Park, A., Zhang, Y., Hodge, C., et al. (2008). Serum concentrations of polybrominated diphenyl ethers (PBDEs) and polybrominated biphenyl (PBB) in the United States population: 2003–2004. *Environmental Science and Technology, 42*, 1377–1384. http://dx.doi.org/10.1021/es702451p.

Somm, E., Schwitzgebel, V. M., Toulotte, A., Cederroth, C. R., Combescure, C., Nef, S., et al. (2009). Perinatal exposure to bisphenol A alters early adipogenesis in the rat. *Environmental Health Perspectives, 117*, 1549–1555.

Stapleton, H. M., Sjodin, A., Jones, R. S., Niehoser, S., Zhang, Y., & Patterson, D. G. (2008). Serum levels of polybrominated diphenyl ethers (PBDEs) in foam recyclers and carpet installers working in the United States. *Environmental Science and Technology*, *42*, 3453–3458.

Stevens, A., Begum, G., & White, A. (2011). Epigenetic changes in the hypothalamic proopiomelanocortin gene: A mechanism linking maternal undernutrition to obesity in the offspring? *European Journal of Pharmacology*, *660*, 194–201.

Strom, B. L., Schinnar, R., Ziegler, E. E., Barnhart, K. T., Sammel, M. D., Macones, G. A., et al. (2001). Exposure to soy-based formula in infancy and endocrinological and reproductive outcomes in young adulthood. *JAMA*, *286*, 807–814.

Swan, S. H., Main, K. M., Liu, F., Stewart, S. L., Kruse, R. L., Calafat, A. M., et al. (2005). Decrease in anogenital distance among male infants with prenatal phthalate exposure. *Environmental Health Perspectives*, *113*, 1056–1061.

Takahashi, O., & Oishi, S. (2000). Disposition of orally administered 2,2-bis(4-hydroxyphenyl)propane (bisphenol A) in pregnant rats and the placental transfer to fetuses. *Environmental Health Perspectives*, *108*, 931–935.

Tan, J., Loganath, A., Chong, Y. S., & Obbard, J. P. (2009). Exposure to persistent organic pollutants in utero and related maternal characteristics on birth outcomes: A multivariate data analysis approach. *Chemosphere*, *74*, 428–433.

Tando, S., Itoh, K., Yaoi, T., Ikeda, J., Fujiwara, Y., & Fushiki, S. (2007). Effects of pre- and neonatal exposure to bisphenol A on murine brain development. *Brain and Development*, *29*, 352–356.

Trasande, L., Attina, T. M., & Blustein, J. (2012). Association between urinary bisphenol A concentration and obesity prevalence in children and adolescents. *JAMA*, *308*, 1113–1121.

Vandenberg, L. N., Colborn, T., Hayes, T. B., Heindel, J. J., Jacobs, D. R., Jr., Lee, D. H., et al. (2012). Hormones and endocrine-disrupting chemicals: Low-dose effects and nonmonotonic dose responses. *Endocrine Reviews*, *33*, 378–455.

Vasiliu, O., Muttineni, J., & Karmaus, W. (2004). In utero exposure to organochlorines and age at menarche. *Human Reproduction*, *19*, 1506–1512.

Viberg, H., Fredriksson, A., & Eriksson, P. (2003). Neonatal exposure to polybrominated diphenyl ether (PBDE 153) disrupts spontaneous behaviour, impairs learning and memory, and decreases hippocampal cholinergic receptors in adult mice. *Toxicology and Applied Pharmacology*, *192*, 95–106.

Viberg, H., Mundy, W., & Eriksson, P. (2008). Neonatal exposure to decabrominated diphenyl ether (PBDE 209) results in changes in BDNF, CaMKII and GAP-43, biochemical substrates of neuronal survival, growth, and synaptogenesis. *Neurotoxicology*, *29*, 152–159.

vom Saal, F. S., Akingbemi, B. T., Belcher, S. M., Birnbaum, L. S., Crain, D. A., Eriksen, M., et al. (2007). Chapel Hill bisphenol A expert panel consensus statement: Integration of mechanisms, effects in animals and potential to impact human health at current levels of exposure. *Reproductive Toxicology*, *24*, 131–138.

Vom Saal, F. S., & Myers, J. (2008). Bisphenol A and risk of metabolic disorders. *JAMA*, *300*, 1353–1355.

Wang, J., Sun, B., Hou, M., Pan, X., & Li, X. (2012). The environmental obesogen bisphenol A promotes adipogenesis by increasing the amount of 11β-hydroxysteroid dehydrogenase type 1 in the adipose tissue of children. *International Journal of Obesity*, *37*(7), 999–1005.

Warner, M., Samuels, S., Mocarelli, P., Gerthou, P. M., Needham, L., Patterson, D. G., et al. (2004). Serum dioxin concentrations and age at menarche. *Environmental Health Perspectives*, *112*, 1289–1292.

Wei, J., Lin, Y., Li, Y., Ying, C., Chen, J., Song, L., et al. (2011). Perinatal exposure to bisphenol A at reference dose predisposes offspring to metabolic syndrome in adult rats on a high-fat diet. *Endocrinology*, *152*, 3049–3061.

Welsh, M., Saunders, P., Fisken, M., Scott, M., Hutchison, G., Smith, L., et al. (2008). Identification in rats of a programming window for reproductive tract masculinization, disruption of which leads to hypospadias and cryptorchidism. *Journal of Clinical Investigation, 118*, 1479–1490.

Whitehead, J. P., Richards, A. A., Hickman, I. J., Macdonald, G. A., & Prins, J. B. (2006). Adiponectin—A key adipokine in the metabolic syndrome. *Diabetes, Obesity & Metabolism, 8*, 264–280.

Wohlfahrt-Veje, C., Andersen, H. R., Jensen, T. K., Grandjean, P., Skakkebæk, N. E., & Main, K. M. (2012). Smaller genitals at school age in boys whose mothers were exposed to non-persistent pesticides in early pregnancy. *International Journal of Andrology, 35*, 273–282.

Wolff, M. S., Britton, J. A., Boguski, L., Hochman, S., Maloney, N., Serra, N., et al. (2008). Environmental exposures and puberty in inner-city girls. *Environmental Research, 107*, 393–400.

Wolff, M. S., Teitelbaum, S. L., Pinney, S. M., Windham, G., Liao, L., Biro, F., et al. (2010). Investigation of relationships between urinary biomarkers of phytoestrogens, phthalates, and phenols and pubertal stages in girls. *Environmental Health Perspectives, 118*, 1039–1046.

Wu, K., Xu, X., Liu, J., Guo, Y., Li, Y., & Huo, X. (2010). Polybrominated diphenyl ethers in umbilical cord blood and relevant factors in neonates from Guiyu, China. *Environmental Science and Technology, 44*, 813–819.

Xi, W., Wan, H. T., Zhao, Y. G., Wong, M. H., Giesy, J. P., & Wong, C. K. (2012). Effects of perinatal exposure to bisphenol A and di(2-ethylhexyl)-phthalate on gonadal development of male mice. *Environmental Science and Pollution Research International, 19*, 2515–2527.

Yang, C. Y., Yu, M. L., Wuo, H. R., Lai, T. J., HSu CC, C. C., Lambert, G., et al. (2005). The endocrine and reproductive function of the female Yucheng adolescents prenatally exposed to PCBs/PCDFs. *Chemosphere, 61*, 355–360.

Zhang, J. M., Konkle, A. T., Zup, S. L., & McCarthy, M. M. (2008). Impact of sex and hormones on new cells in the developing rat hippocampus: A novel source of sex dimorphism? *European Journal of Neuroscience, 27*, 791–800.

Zoeller, R. T., Dowling, A. L. S., & Vas, A. (2000). Developmental exposure to polychlorinated biphenyls exerts thyroid hormone-like effects on the expression of RC3/ Neurogranin and myelin basic protein messenger ribonucleic acids in the developing rat brain. *Endocrinology, 141*, 181–189.

Zoeller, R. T., & Rovet, J. (2004). Timing of thyroid hormone action in the developing brain: Clinical observations and experimental findings. *Journal of Neuroendocrinology, 16*, 809–818.

CHAPTER TWO

Agricultural Pesticides and Precocious Puberty

Samim Ozen[1], Damla Goksen, Sukran Darcan
Department of Pediatric Endocrinology, Ege University School of Medicine, Izmir, Turkey
[1]Corresponding author: e-mail address: samimozen@gmail.com

Contents

1. Introduction 27
2. Puberty 28
3. Precocious Puberty 29
4. The Effects of EDs on Puberty 30
5. Organochlorine Pesticides and Puberty 33
6. DDT and DDE 34
7. Methoxychlor 35
8. Endosulfans 36
9. Vinclozolin 37
10. Acetochlor 37
11. Conclusion 37
References 38

Abstract

The onset and course of puberty is under the control of the neuroendocrine system. Factors affecting the regulation of timing and order of this system's functions may alter the onset and course of puberty. Several environmental endocrine disruptors (EDs) with significant influences on the normal course of puberty have been identified. Despite the numerous animal and human studies on EDs that may extensively affect human health, there are still several issues that need to be clarified. This chapter discusses the effects of pesticides, which constitute a significant portion of disruptors and have been increasingly used in agriculture, on precocious puberty.

1. INTRODUCTION

Recent studies have shown that there is a trend toward earlier onset of puberty in children. Although reasons for this trend remain unclear, the prevailing view involves a complex interaction between genetic, endocrine,

Vitamins and Hormones, Volume 94
ISSN 0083-6729
http://dx.doi.org/10.1016/B978-0-12-800095-3.00002-X

and environmental factors. The ever-increasing industrialization has caused a rapid and significant increase in environmental pollutants. A proportion of these environmental pollutants are natural and synthetic chemicals that have certain effects on the endocrine system. These chemicals that have negative effects on the endocrine system are called endocrine disruptors (EDs). EDs exert their effects by binding to relevant hormone receptors, disturbing cell signaling pathways, directly affecting the central neuroendocrine system, inhibiting hormone synthesis, or causing toxic effects to relevant organs. Certain EDs that affect pubertal development in humans have been identified, such as phytoestrogens, topical and natural estrogens, pesticides, industrial chemicals, and phthalates. It has first been noticed in 1990 that EDs can cause precocious puberty (PP) in humans (Buck Louis et al., 2008; Den Hond & Schoeters, 2006; Jacobson-Dickman & Lee, 2009; McLachlan, Simpson, & Martin, 2006; Nebesio & Pescovitz, 2007; Schoeters, Den Hond, Dhooge, Van Larebeke, & Leijs, 2008). Subsequently, numerous studies with animals and humans were conducted on the effects of EDs on the onset and course of puberty, which lead to the banning of certain chemicals. This chapter will discuss the effects of agricultural pesticides, which constitute a significant portion of EDs and have been increasingly used in recent years in parallel to the industrialization in agriculture, on PP development.

2. PUBERTY

Puberty is a complex developmental process characterized by rapid physiological alterations that lead to maturation of sexual characteristics, acceleration of growth, and attainment of reproductive capacity. This sensitive developmental interval constitutes the transition from a nonreproductive to a reproductive state. Puberty is initiated during late childhood with maturation of the hypothalamic–pituitary–gonadal axis and requires extensive interplay among a variety of hormones. There are a number of dramatic changes in reproductive hormones during this period, particularly estrogen in females and androgens in males. Considering that most EDs act as estrogen or may exhibit antagonistic effects to estrogen or androgen receptors, such exposure has been implicated as provoking pubertal abnormalities in humans by interrupting normal hormonal activity (Nebesio & Pescovitz, 2007; Schoeters et al., 2008).

3. PRECOCIOUS PUBERTY

PP is characterized by the early development of secondary sexual characteristics at the age of 8 in girls and 9 in boys. It is also defined as the onset of puberty symptoms at an earlier age, that is, 2.5 standard deviations below the expected mean age, exhibiting persistent and progressive characteristics. PP includes the development of secondary sexual characteristics at an earlier age than expected, rapid bone growth, decrease in predicted final height, changes in body fat distribution, and psychosocial changes (Berberoglu, 2009; Carel & Leger, 2008). A number of studies have shown that the onset of puberty could be as early as 7.7 years in girls and 7.6 years in boys. Although there is still no consensus on this matter, the age range of 7–8 years can be defined as the gray area. The onset of puberty in girls within this age range is described with terms such as "early normal puberty," "rapid progressive thelarche variant," and "premature puberty" (Berberoglu, 2009; Carel & Leger, 2008; Herman-Giddens, 2007; Parent et al., 2003).

Observed more frequently in girls, PP can cause significant problems, such as psychosocial issues, short stature, and increased risk of breast cancer in adulthood. Therefore, early diagnosis and treatment is necessary. PP is diagnosed by determining early secondary sexual characteristics, accelerated body growth, and advanced bone age, as well as increased levels of gonadotropins and/or sex steroids. Cases in which breast development alone is observed without advanced bone age or accelerated body growth are referred to as isolated early thelarche. Even though these cases are regarded as variants of norms, they might still develop PP later on (Berberoglu, 2009; Carel & Leger, 2008; Herman-Giddens, 2007; Parent et al., 2003). In a population study conducted in Denmark, PP was determined at a rate of 0.2% in girls and 0.01–0.02% in boys. Only half of these were determined to be actual early puberty cases. When evaluated according to the definition of early puberty, considering that puberty symptoms by PP are observed with 2.5 standard deviations below the mean age, the expected frequency should have been 0.6%. This difference may be due to insufficient determination of patients (Teilman, Pedersen, Jensen, Skakkebaek, & Jull, 2005).

PP can be categorized as either gonadotropin-dependent (central/true) or gonadotropin-independent (peripheral/pseudopuberty). In gonadotropin-dependent PP, the hypothalamic–pituitary–gonadal (HPG) axis is activated, as also observed in physiological puberty. On the other hand, in gonadotropin-independent puberty, the HPG axis is suppressed, and PP is not dependent on gonadotropin secretion. This group of PP is dependent on endogenous and/or exogenous sex steroids (Berberoglu, 2009; Carel & Leger, 2008).

4. THE EFFECTS OF EDs ON PUBERTY

Recent studies have shown that while the menarcheal age in girls remains unchanged, onset of puberty shifted 1–2 years earlier compared to the past years. The triggering mechanism of the early onset of puberty remains unclear. However, it is believed that this early onset is due to a complex interaction between genetic, hormonal, and environmental factors. EDs, one of the environmental factors, are blamed more intensely in the recent years (Buck Louis et al., 2008; Den Hond & Schoeters, 2006; Jacobson-Dickman & Lee, 2009; McLachlan et al., 2006; Nebesio & Pescovitz, 2007; Schoeters et al., 2008). Theoretically, hormones or substances with hormone-disrupting capability may interfere with pubertal development by actions at different levels, including the neuroendocrine hypothalamic–pituitary axis, the gonads, and peripheral target organs such as breasts, hair follicles, and genitals. In the brain, EDs may act by the stimulation of estrogen-sensitive nuclei, including hypothalamic neurons, thereby releasing kisspeptin and promoting the maturation of the hypothalamus causing earlier onset of puberty, or even PP. However, other compounds could act by gonadotropin inhibition through negative feedback. It is also possible that EDs have direct effects on both the body weight and the endocrine system of the HPG axis (Stahlhut, Van Wijngaarden, Dye, Cook, & Swan, 2007). Steroids from the adrenal glands also play a role for normal progression of puberty, including pubic hair development. Potentially, a dysfunction of the adrenal gland caused by EDs may influence the estrogenic hormonal milieu and thereby also influence pubertal development (Ulleras, Ohlsson, & Oskarsson, 2008). A potential mechanism of ED action at the HPG axis has been described in rats (Rasier, Parent, Gerard, Lebrethon, & Bourguignon, 2007). Animals were exposed to DDT or beta-estradiol, and GnRH pulsatile secretion was increased. Furthermore, an *in vitro* study showed amplification of the glutamate-evoked secretion of GnRH after exposure to DDT and E2 (Rasier et al., 2008).

A significant portion of environmental EDs consist of pesticides used in agriculture. Pesticides have a long history of global use and have a broad spectrum of applications in agricultural and commercial pest control. Insecticides are one of the most widely used classes of pesticides. Other classes of pesticides include herbicides and fungicides, which target unwanted plants and fungi, respectively. While these agents have been useful for eradicating undesirable pests and disease vectors, pesticides also have unintended actions on nontargeted species, including humans, and recent studies have shown that even extremely low levels of exposure can cause damage to the developing reproductive axis (McLachlan et al., 2006; Nebesio & Pescovitz, 2007; Schoeters et al., 2008).

Table 2.1 shows the major pesticides that can affect the endocrine system. Certain pesticides can accumulate in the environment over time and can enter the human body through water, air, food sources, and objects used in work and home settings. In addition, studies have also shown that pesticides can pass from the mother to the fetus through the placenta and to the baby through the mother's milk (Buck Louis et al., 2008; Jacobson-Dickman & Lee, 2009; McLachlan et al., 2006; Nebesio & Pescovitz, 2007; Schoeters et al., 2008).

The effects of pesticides on the endocrine system are agonistic or antagonistic due to their hormone-like characteristics. Their effects on puberty are estrogenic, antiestrogenic, androgenic, and antiandrogenic and directly on the GnRH system (Buck Louis et al., 2008; McLachlan et al., 2006; Nebesio & Pescovitz, 2007; Schoeters et al., 2008).

These chemicals exert their estrogenic effects by directly binding to estrogen receptors, increasing aromatase activity and sensitivity to estrogen or increasing endogenous estrogen production through the GnRH system, which can eventually cause PP. The antiestrogenic and androgenic effects of these chemicals are often expressed through the inhibition of aromatase enzyme activity and the steroidogenic enzyme production system. Lastly, they exert their antiandrogenic effects by suppressing testicular steroidogenesis and blocking androgen receptors. Ultimately, depending on the types of effects they exert, pesticides can cause PP, delayed puberty, and disorders of sexual differentiation (Abaci, Demir, Bober, & Buyukgebiz, 2009; Buck Louis et al., 2008; Kandarakis et al., 2009; Massart, Parrino, Seppia,

Table 2.1 Major pesticides that affect the endocrine system

Pesticides	Dichlorodiphenyltrichloroethane (DDT), methoxychlor, endosulfan, 2,4-dichlorophenoxyacetic acid, alachlor, aldicarb, amitrole, atrazine, benomyl, dibromochloropropane, carbaryl, chlordane, ethyl parathion, heptachlor, kepone, ketoconazole, lindane, methomyl, permethrin, malathion, trifluralin, vinclozolin

Federico, & Saggese, 2006; Roy, Chakraborty, & Chakraborty, 2009). The classification of some pesticides in terms of their effects on puberty is presented in Table 2.2.

Most of these substances cannot be broken down and rendered ineffective by the body and are generally accumulated in fat tissue, which causes them to remain in the body for long periods of time exerting harmful effects. The period of time that the body is exposed to EDs during lifetime is crucial in terms of their harmful effects. Furthermore, the dosage and exposure duration are also important with regard to the consequences of these negative effects. As exposure duration and dosage increase, the negative effects can be more severe (Buck Louis et al., 2008; Den Hond & Schoeters, 2006;

Table 2.2 Classification of some pesticides according to their effects on the reproductive system

Type of effect	Pesticide	References
Estrogenic	Dichlorodiphenyltrichloroethane (DDT) and its metabolites	Nebesio and Pescovitz (2007)
	Methoxychlor	Gray, Ostby, Cooper, and Kelce (1999)
	Methoprene	Roy et al. (2009) and Kandarakis et al. (2009)
	Endosulfan	Jørgensen et al. (2000)
Antiestrogenic	Prochloraz	Vinggaard, Nellemann, Dalgaard, Jørgensen, and Andersen (2002)
Androgenic	Unknown	
Antiandrogenic	Dichlorodiphenyldichloroethylene (DDE)	Kelce et al. (1995) and Wolf et al. (1999)
	Vinclozolin	Gray et al. (2001) and Eustache et al. (2009)
	Endosulfan	Eroschenko and Cooke (1990) and Wade, Desaulniers, Leingartner, and Foster (1997)
Inhibition of aromatase	Prochloraz	Vinggaard et al. (2002)

Jacobson-Dickman & Lee, 2009; McLachlan et al., 2006; Nebesio & Pescovitz, 2007; Schoeters et al., 2008).

There are still a very limited number of studies with animals and humans on the role of pesticides in PP. These chemicals cause PP symptoms by exerting estrogenic effects, which might be accomplished through increasing estrogenic effects, antiandrogenic effects, and GnRH production (Buck Louis et al., 2008; Den Hond & Schoeters, 2006; Jacobson-Dickman & Lee, 2009; McLachlan et al., 2006; Nebesio & Pescovitz, 2007; Schoeters et al., 2008).

In a study by Wohlfahrt-Veje et al. (2012) conducted in Denmark, it was shown that breast development was earlier in individuals exposed to nonpersistent pesticides prenatally compared to the control group. In the same study, it was also revealed that endogenous gonadotropin levels were normal and androgen levels were increased in early breast development cases. The authors suggested that pesticides accelerated the formation of estrogens from androgens by increasing aromatase activity, which in turn caused early breast development. Ozen et al. (2012) evaluated the effects of pesticides on premature breast development. Forty-five girls with premature breast development, living in a rural area where greenhouse cultivation is the main income; 16 girls with early puberty, living in the city center; and 33 girls who had no signs of puberty were included in the study. Endosulfan 1, endosulfan 2, endosulfan sulfate, methoxychlor, vinclozolin, 4,4-dichlorodiphenyldichloroethylene (DDE), 4,4-dichlorodiphenyltrichloroethane (DDT), and 2,4-DDT were evaluated in the serum and adipose tissues of the groups using gas chromatography–mass spectrometry. With the exception of 4,4′-DDE, the pesticides studied were undetectable in the serum and adipose tissue samples. The levels of basal luteinizing hormone (LH), stimulated LH, and follicle-stimulating hormone and the long axis of the uterus and both ovaries were significantly different in the girls who had premature thelarche and detectable 4,4′-DDE levels compared to the girls who had premature thelarche and undetectable 4,4′-DDE levels in the serum and adipose tissues. The presence and levels of pesticides in serum and adipose tissues were not related to PP. The mechanisms that lead to PP may also result in obesity, and obesity may be the underlying cause for PP in this group (Ozen et al., 2012).

5. ORGANOCHLORINE PESTICIDES AND PUBERTY

Organochlorine pesticides are lipophilic, accumulating in fatty tissues and remaining in the body for years. Organochlorine pesticides include certain agents, such as DDT, methoxychlor, dicofol, heptachlor, chlordane, endosulfan, aldrin, dieldrin, endrin, and mirex. Humans are predominantly exposed to organochlorine pesticides as residues on produce or through pest control. Individuals working directly with insecticides come into direct contact through inhalation and skin (Dickerson, Cunningham, & Gore, 2012).

6. DDT AND DDE

DDT and similar chemicals have been long known to have estrogenic effects. In a study by Gellert, Heinrichs, and Swerdloff (1972), DDT homologues were shown to cause early puberty through their estrogenic effects in female mice. In the 1980s, after a vast quantity of DDT and dicofol was accidentally spilled into Lake Apopka in Florida, the male crocodiles were observed to have smaller phalli, lower serum testosterone levels, abnormal gonad structures, and higher concurrent serum DDT levels (Semenza, Tolbert, Rubin, Guillette, & Jackson, 1997).

Numerous studies have been conducted on the effects of DDT, of which the estrogenic effects have already been proven, and its metabolite DDE on the pubertal development in children. The use of DDT, a pesticide, and its metabolites, which have been used extensively in agriculture, has been banned in many countries after determining their negative effects. In their study, Vasiliu et al. (2004) had determined that menarche occurred 1 year earlier in girls who had been exposed to high levels of DDT/DDE during the intrauterine period. In another study, Krstevska-Konstantinova et al. (2001) determined that the PP rate was 80 times higher in girls who immigrated to Belgium compared to the natives and that these girls had significantly high serum DDE levels. Ouyang et al. (2005) studied newly married female textile workers in China by measuring serum DDT/DDE concentrations. A 10 ng/g increase in exposure was associated with 0.2 years earlier onset of menarche. Because exposure occurred after pubertal development was complete, the causal order of exposure–puberty cannot be established since pubertal development may have affected the metabolism/distribution of DDT or other behaviors that influenced DDT exposure. Denham et al. (2005) conducted a cross-sectional study among girls who were aged 10–17 years and resided in the Mohawk Nation along the United States/Canadian border to assess serum concentrations and self-reported menarcheal status. No association was observed between DDT exposure and menarche despite the authors' assumption that current serum concentrations were indicative of *in utero* and lactational exposures, given the long-standing concern regarding consumption of contaminated fish among this population. Gladen, Ragan, and Rogan (2000) conducted a prospective cohort study of boys and girls who resided in North Carolina in relation to DDE concentrations that were previously measured in their mothers' serum, the cord serum, and the placenta (averaged for *in utero* exposure). Concentrations in breast milk were also determined (lactational exposure). Puberty-timing measures, Tanner stages (boys and girls), and menarche were assessed by annual questionnaires. For boys, no association was observed for either *in utero* or lactational DDE exposure. Among girls, there was no association with age at menarche; however, there was a suggestion of an association of higher *in utero* or lactational exposure and earlier breast and pubic hair development that was not statistically significant. Gaspari, Paris, Jeandel, and Sultan (2011) reported breast development and menstruation alongside enlargement of the uterus in a 4-month-old girl. Along with the patient, gas chromatography results revealed p.p′DDD, p.p′DDT, lindane, and endosulfan in the plasma of the parents, who had a dramatic decrease in libido, and early sexual maturation in this case, whose parents were farmers, was associated with estrogenic pesticides.

It was hypothesized that early and temporary exposure to weakly estrogenic DDT in developing countries, where the exposure is still high, could stimulate hypothalamic maturation, while the pituitary gonadotropins are inhibited via negative feedback that prevents manifestation of central maturation. Migration causes withdrawal from the EDC, and the consequent pituitary inhibition disappears, allowing the hypothalamic maturation to turn on the pituitary–ovarian cascade of pubertal events, that is, central puberty (Rasier, Toppari, Parent, & Bourguignon, 2006).

7. METHOXYCHLOR

Methoxychlor, a chemical that belongs to the organochlorine group, is still being extensively used in agriculture as a pesticide. It has been shown to exert estrogenic effects in a number of animal studies (Ashby & Lefevre, 2000; Eroschenko & Cooke, 1990; Gray et al., 1999; Masutomi et al., 2003). Early vaginal dilatation was observed in female mice administered with methoxychlor following the termination of receiving breast milk. PP was also observed in female mice that received methoxychlor, an antiandrogenic and estrogenic agent (Ashby & Lefevre, 2000). It has been proven to disrupt reproductive behavior and functions due to its estrogenic effects in male mice (Gray et al., 1999). In their study, conducted in a region where greenhouse cultivation and methoxychlor use were extensive, Ozen et al. (2012) did not detect this pesticide in the fatty tissue and serum samples of girls with early breast development. The authors suggested that this may be due to the fact that methoxychlor is a water-soluble chemical that does not accumulate in the body.

8. ENDOSULFANS

It has been known that endosulfan and its derivatives, which are widely used in agriculture, have antiandrogenic and estrogenic effects (Buck Louis et al., 2008; Den Hond & Schoeters, 2006; Jacobson-Dickman & Lee, 2009; McLachlan et al., 2006; Nebesio & Pescovitz, 2007; Schoeters et al., 2008). Studies with animals have revealed that endosulfan exerted estrogenic effects and inhibited FSH, LG, and testosterone levels (Singh & Pandley, 1990; Wade et al., 1997). Studies on the relationship between endosulfan-group pesticides, which have been banned in many developed countries due to their toxic effects, and puberty in humans are still insufficient. In the first human study on this matter, conducted by Ozen et al. (2012), levels of the endosulfan-group pesticides endosulfan 1 (endosulfan-alpha), endosulfan 2 (endosulfan-beta), and endosulfan sulfate were measured in the serum and fatty tissue samples of girls with early breast development. While the rate of early breast development was determined to be 10% in this region, there was no evidence of the aforementioned endosulfan-group pesticides in the serum and/or fatty tissue samples. The authors suggested that the absence of these pesticides in the samples may be due to the fact that they were not being used extensively in this region at the time of the study and that these pesticides do not have significant accumulation properties as DDT and its metabolites have. There is a need for further studies on this matter. In a different study conducted in India with a total of 117 boys aged between 10 and 19 years, significant retardation of pubertal development and five times higher rate of testicular abnormalities (undescended testes, congenital hydrocele, and congenital inguinal hernia) were observed in boys, who were exposed to high levels of endosulfan, compared to the control group. The authors suggested that endosulfans exerted these effects by disrupting sex hormone synthesis (Saiyed et al., 2003). This pesticide is highly likely to cause PP in girls while exerting antiandrogenic effects in boys. There is a need for wide-population study on this matter.

9. VINCLOZOLIN

The antiandrogenic effects of vinclozolin have mostly been observed in male animals (Blystone et al., 2009). Although the estrogenic effects of this chemical used extensively in agriculture remain unclear, it has been reported that it can exert estrogen-like effects through antiandrogenic effects and estrogen receptor-alpha (Khurana, Ranmal, & Ben-Jonathan, 2000). Ozen et al. (2012) found no relationship between vinclozolin and PP in their study. However, pubertal disorders may develop through changes in sex hormone synthesis and effects due to frequent and intensive exposure to this nonpersistent pesticide.

10. ACETOCHLOR

In a study with female Wistar rats and the herbicide called acetochlor, it has been shown that acetochlor can cause earlier vaginal dilatation through estrogen receptors. Researchers noted that this persistent pollutant might be an ED with estrogenic effects (Rollerova, Wsolova, & Urbancikova, 2011). In a similar study by Rollerova, Gasparova, Wsolova, and Urbancikova (2000), an increased estrogen receptor binding activity was observed in the uterus of rats that were given with acetochlor. There are no human studies with this herbicide.

11. CONCLUSION

Animal and human studies on the relationship between PP and pesticides that have been increasingly used in recent years are still insufficient. It is still unclear through which mechanisms these chemicals cause PP. However, these chemicals can indirectly affect and change the normal physiological functions of the HPG axis by directly disrupting gonadotropin secretion or feedback mechanisms. It should be kept in mind that the time of exposure is as important as exposed dose, duration of exposure, and age for pesticides to be able to disrupt endocrine functions. Many other pesticides that have not been discussed in this chapter can potentially have harmful effects on pubertal development. There is a need for advanced population studies on this topic.

Conflict of Interest: The authors declare there is no conflict of interest in this chapter.

REFERENCES

Abaci, A., Demir, K., Bober, E., & Buyukgebiz, A. (2009). Endocrine disruptors—With special emphasis on sexual development. *Pediatric Endocrinology Reviews, 6*, 464–475.

Ashby, J., & Lefevre, P. A. (2000). The peripubertal male rat assay as an alternative to the Hershberger castrated male rat assay for the detection of anti-androgens, oestrogens and metabolic modulators. *Journal of Applied Toxicology, 20*, 35–47.

Berberoglu, M. (2009). Precocious puberty and normal variant puberty: Definition, etiology, diagnosis and current management. *Journal of Clinical Research in Pediatric Endocrinology, 1*, 164–174.

Blystone, C. R., Lambright, C. S., Cardon, M. C., Furr, J., Rider, C. V., Hartig, P. C., et al. (2009). Cumulative and antagonistic effects of a mixture of the antiandrogens vinclozolin and iprodione in the pubertal male rat. *Toxicological Sciences, 111*, 179–188.

Buck Louis, G. M., Gray, L. E., Jr., Marcus, M., Ojeda, S. R., Pescovitz, O. H., Witchel, S. F., et al. (2008). Environmental factors and puberty timing: Expert panel research needs. *Pediatrics, 121*, 192–207.

Carel, J. C., & Leger, J. (2008). Precocious puberty. *The New England Journal of Medicine, 358*, 2366–2377.

Denham, M., Schell, L. M., Deane, G., Gallo, M. V., Ravenscroft, J., & DeCaprio, A. P. (2005). Akwesasne task force on the environment: Relationship of lead, mercury, mirex, dichlorodiphenyldichloroethylene, hexachlorobenzene, and polychlorinated biphenyls to timing of menarche among Akwesasne Mohawk girls. *Pediatrics, 115*(2), 127–134.

DenHond, E., & Schoeters, G. (2006). Endocrine disrupters and human puberty. *International Journal of Andrology, 29*, 264–271.

Dickerson, S. M., Cunningham, S. L., & Gore, A. C. (2012). Reproductive neuroendocrine targets of developmental exposure to endocrine disruptors. In E. D. Kandarakis & A. C. Gore (Eds.), *Endocrine disruptors and puberty* (pp. 49–117). New York, NY: Humana Press.

Eroschenko, V. P., & Cooke, P. S. (1990). Morphological and biochemical alterations in reproductive tracts of neonatal female mice treated with the pesticide methoxychlor. *Biology of Reproduction, 42*(3), 573–583.

Eustache, F., Mondon, F., Canivenc-Lavier, M. C., Lesaffre, C., Fulla, Y., Berges, R., et al. (2009). Chronic dietary exposure to a low-dose mixture of genistein and vinclozolin modifies the reproductive axis, testis transcriptome, and fertility. *Environmental Health Perspectives, 117*(8), 1272–1279.

Gaspari, L., Paris, F., Jeandel, C., & Sultan, C. (2011). Peripheral precocious puberty in a 4-month-old girl: Role of pesticides. *Gynecological Endocrinology, 27*(9), 721–724.

Gellert, R. J., Heinrichs, W. L., & Swerdloff, R. S. (1972). DDT homologues: Estrogen-like effects on the vagina, uterus and pituitary of the rat. *Endocrinology, 91*(4), 1095–1100.

Gladen, B. C., Ragan, N. B., & Rogan, W. J. (2000). Pubertal growth and development and prenatal and lactational exposure to polychlorinated biphenyls and dichlorodiphenyl dichloroethene. *Journal of Pediatrics, 136*(4), 490–496.

Gray, L. E., Jr., Ostby, J., Cooper, R. L., & Kelce, W. R. (1999). The estrogenic and antiandrogenic pesticide methoxychlor alters the reproductive tract and behavior without affecting pituitary size or LH and prolactin secretion in male rats. *Toxicology and Industrial Health, 15*, 37–47.

Gray, L. E., Ostby, J., Furr, J., Wolf, C. J., Lambright, C., Parks, L., et al. (2001). Effects of environmental antiandrogens on reproductive development in experimental animals. *Human Reproduction Update*, 7(3), 248–264.

Herman-Giddens, M. E. (2007). Puberty is starting earlier in the 21st century. In O. H. Pescovitz & E. C. Walvoord (Eds.), *When puberty is precocious: Scientific and clinical aspects* (pp. 105–136). Totowa, NJ: Humana press.

Jacobson-Dickman, E., & Lee, M. M. (2009). The influence of endocrine disruptors on pubertal timing. *Current Opinion in Endocrinology, Diabetes, and Obesity, 16*, 25–30.

Jørgensen, M., Vendelbo, B., Skakkebaek, N. E., & Leffers, H. (2000). Assaying estrogenicity by quantitating the expression levels of endogenous estrogen-regulated genes. *Environmental Health Perspectives, 108*(5), 403–412.

Kandarakis, E. D., Bourguignon, J. P., Giudice, L. C., Hauser, R., Prins, G. S., Soto, A. M., et al. (2009). Endocrine-disrupting chemicals: An Endocrine Society scientific statement. *Endocrine Reviews, 30*, 293–342.

Kelce, W. R., Stone, C. R., Laws, S. C., Gray, L. E., Kemppainen, J. A., & Wilson, E. M. (1995). Persistent DDT metabolite p,p'-DDE is a potent androgen receptor antagonist. *Nature, 375*(6532), 581–585.

Khurana, S., Ranmal, S., & Ben-Jonathan, N. (2000). Exposure of newborn male and female rats to environmental estrogens: Delayed and sustained hyperprolactinemia and alterations in estrogen receptor expression. *Endocrinology, 141*, 4512–4517.

Krstevska-Konstantinova, M., Charlier, C., Craen, M., Du Caju, M., Heinrichs, C., de Beaufort, C., et al. (2001). Sexual precocity after immigration from developing countries to Belgium: Evidence of previous exposure to organochlorine pesticides. *Human Reproduction, 16*, 1020–1026.

Massart, F., Parrino, R., Seppia, P., Federico, G., & Saggese, G. (2006). How do environmental estrogen disruptors induce precocious puberty? *Minerva Pediatrica, 58*, 247–254.

Masutomi, N., Shibutani, M., Takagi, H., Uneyama, C., Takahashi, N., & Hirose, M. (2003). Impact of dietary exposure to methoxychlor, genistein, or diisononyl phthalate during the perinatal period on the development of the rat endocrine/reproductive systems in later life. *Toxicology, 192*(2–3), 149–170.

McLachlan, J. A., Simpson, E., & Martin, M. (2006). Endocrine disrupters and female reproductive health. *Best Practice & Research Clinical Endocrinology & Metabolism, 20*, 63–75.

Nebesio, T. D., & Pescovitz, O. H. (2007). The role of endocrine disruptors in pubertal development. In O. H. Pescovitz & E. C. Walvoord (Eds.), *When puberty is precocious: Scientific and clinical aspects* (p. 468). Totowa, NJ: Humana press.

Ouyang, F., Perry, M. J., Venners, S. A., Chen, C., Wang, B., Yang, F., et al. (2005). Serum DDT, age at menarche, and abnormal menstrual cycle length. *Occupational and Environmental Medicine, 62*, 878–884.

Ozen, S., Darcan, S., Bayindir, P., Karasulu, E., Simsek, D. G., & Gurler, T. (2012). Effects of pesticides used in agriculture on the development of precocious puberty. *Environmental Monitoring and Assessment, 184*(7), 4223–4232.

Parent, A. S., Teilmann, G., Juul, A., Skakkebaek, N. E., Toppari, J., & Bourguignon, J. P. (2003). The timing of normal puberty and the age limits of sexual precocity: Variations around the world, secular trends, and changes after migration. *Endocrine Reviews, 24*, 668–693.

Rasier, G., Parent, A. S., Gerard, A., Denooz, R., Lebrethon, M. C., Charlier, C., et al. (2008). Mechanisms of interaction of endocrine-disrupting chemicals with glutamate-evoked secretion of gonadotropin-releasing hormone. *Toxicological Sciences, 102*, 33–41.

Rasier, G., Parent, A. S., Gerard, A., Lebrethon, M. C., & Bourguignon, J. P. (2007). Early maturation of gonadotropin-releasing hormone secretion and sexual precocity after exposure of infant female rats to estradiol or dichlorodiphenyltrichloroethane. *Biology of Reproduction, 77*, 734–742.

Rasier, G., Toppari, J., Parent, A. S., & Bourguignon, J. P. (2006). Female sexual maturation and reproduction after prepubertal exposure to estrogens and endocrine disrupting chemicals: A review of rodent and human data. *Molecular and Cellular Endocrinology, 254–255*, 187–201.

Rollerova, E., Gasparova, Z., Wsolova, L., & Urbancikova, M. (2000). Interaction of acetochlor with estrogen receptor in the rat uterus. Acetochlor—Possible endocrine modulator? *General Physiology and Biophysics, 19*(1), 73–84.

Rollerova, E., Wsolova, L., & Urbancikova, M. (2011). Neonatal exposure to herbicide acetochlor alters pubertal development in female wistar rats. *Toxicology Mechanisms and Methods, 21*(5), 406–417.

Roy, J. R., Chakraborty, S., & Chakraborty, T. R. (2009). Estrogen-like endocrine disrupting chemicals affecting puberty in humans—A review. *Medical Science Monitor, 15*, 137–145.

Saiyed, H., Dewan, A., Bhatnagar, V., Shenoy, U., Shenoy, R., Rajmohan, H., et al. (2003). Effect of endosulfan on male reproductive development. *Environmental Health Perspectives, 111*(16), 1958–1962.

Schoeters, G., Den Hond, E., Dhooge, W., Van Larebeke, N., & Leijs, M. (2008). Endocrine disruptors and abnormalities of pubertal development. *Basic & Clinical Pharmacology & Toxicology, 102*, 168–175.

Semenza, J. C., Tolbert, P. E., Rubin, C. H., Guillette, L. J., Jr., & Jackson, R. J. (1997). Reproductive toxins and alligator abnormalities at Lake Apopka, Florida. *Environmental Health Perspectives, 105*, 1030–1032.

Singh, S. K., & Pandley, R. S. (1990). Effect of sub-chronic endosulfan exposures on plasma gonadotrophins, testosterone, testicular testosterone and enzymes of androgen biosynthesis in rat. *Indian Journal of Experimental Biology, 28*, 953–956.

Stahlhut, R. W., Van Wijngaarden, E., Dye, T. D., Cook, S., & Swan, S. H. (2007). Concentrations of urinary phthalate metabolites are associated with increased waist circumference and insulin resistance in adult U.S. males. *Environmental Health Perspectives, 115*, 876–882.

Teilman, G., Pedersen, C. B., Jensen, T. K., Skakkebaek, N. E., & Jull, A. (2005). Prevalence and incidence of precocious pubertal development in Denmark: An epidemiologic study based on national registries. *Pediatrics, 116*, 1323–1328.

Ulleras, E., Ohlsson, A., & Oskarsson, A. (2008). Secretion of cortisol and aldosterone as a vulnerable target for adrenal endocrine disruption—Screening of 30 selected chemicals in the human H295R cell model. *Journal of Applied Toxicology, 28*, 1045–1053.

Vasiliu, O., Muttineni, J., & Karmaus, W. (2004). *In utero* exposure to organochlorines and age at menarche. *Human Reproduction, 19*, 1506–1512.

Vinggaard, A. M., Nellemann, C., Dalgaard, M., Jørgensen, E. B., & Andersen, H. R. (2002). Antiandrogenic effects *in vitro* and *in vivo* of the fungicide prochloraz. *Toxicological Sciences, 69*(2), 344–353.

Wade, M. G., Desaulniers, D., Leingartner, K., & Foster, W. G. (1997). Interaction between endosulphan and dieldrin on estrogen-mediated processes *in vitro* and *in vivo*. *Reproductive Toxicology, 11*, 791–798.

Wohlfahrt-Veje, C., Andersen, H. R., Schmidt, I. M., Aksglaede, L., Sørensen, K., Juul, A., et al. (2012). Early breast development in girls after prenatal exposure to non-persistent pesticides. *International Journal of Andrology, 35*(3), 273–282.

Wolf, C., Jr., Lambright, C., Mann, P., Price, M., Cooper, R. L., Ostby, J., et al. (1999). Administration of potentially antiandrogenic pesticides (procymidone, linuron, iprodione, chlozolinate, p,p'-DDE, and ketoconazole) and toxic substances (dibutyl- and diethylhexyl phthalate, PCB 169, and ethane dimethane sulphonate) during sexual differentiation produces diverse profiles of reproductive malformations in the male rat. *Toxicology and Industrial Health, 15*(1-2), 94–118.

CHAPTER THREE

Endocrine-Disrupting Chemicals: Elucidating Our Understanding of Their Role in Sex and Gender-Relevant End Points

Cheryl A. Frye[1]
Department of Psychology, The University at Albany-SUNY, Albany, New York, USA
Department of Biological Sciences, The University at Albany-SUNY, Albany, New York, USA
The Center for Neuroscience Research, The University at Albany-SUNY, Albany, New York, USA
The Center for Life Sciences Research, The University at Albany-SUNY, Albany, New York, USA
Department of Chemistry, University of Alaska Fairbanks, Fairbanks, Alaska, USA
IDeA Network of Biomedical Excellence (INBRE), University of Alaska Fairbanks, Fairbanks, Alaska, USA
Institute of Arctic Biology, University of Alaska Fairbanks, Fairbanks, Alaska, USA
[1]Corresponding author: e-mail address: cheryl.a.frye@albany.edu

Contents

1. Introduction 43
   1.1 Sources of environmental contaminants 44
2. Endocrine Disruption May Underlie Negative Effects of Contaminants 45
3. Adverse Health Consequences of Lifelong EDC Exposure 45
   3.1 Cancer 46
   3.2 Heart disease 46
   3.3 Neurodegenerative diseases 47
   3.4 Other considerations 47
4. Signficance of Investigating EDC Effects on Neurodevelopmental Processes 47
5. Hormones' Effects to Organize Neural Systems and Behavioral Processes 48
6. Developmental EDC Exposure Alters Reproductive Development and Behavior 48
   6.1 Diethylstilbestrol 48
   6.2 Reproductive dysfunction 49
7. Exposure to EDCs in Adulthood Also Effects Reproductive Parameters 50
8. EDCs in Adulthood Influence Sexually Dimorphic Brain Morphology 51
9. Do EDCs Influence Sex Differences in Nonreproductive Behaviors? 52
   9.1 Cognitive dysfunction 52
10. Effects of EDCs on Sexually Dimorphic, Nonreproductive Behaviors 54
   10.1 Spatial memory 54
   10.2 Rough-and-tumble play 55
   10.3 Emotional reactivity 55
   10.4 Stress 56
11. Potential Mechanisms by which EDCs May Produce Their Effects 57
   11.1 Progress limitations 58

Vitamins and Hormones, Volume 94
ISSN 0083-6729
http://dx.doi.org/10.1016/B978-0-12-800095-3.00003-1

12. Several Factors May Bear upon Estrogenicity of Compounds 59
12.1 Mixtures 59
12.2 Additivity 60
12.3 Concentrations 60
13. Effects of EDCs on Uterotropic Activity 60
14. Importance of Examining EDC Effects on Whole-Animal Estrogenic Measures 61
15. Effects of EDCs on E_2 Metabolism 62
16. Androgenic/Antiandrogenic Effects of EDCs 64
17. Effects of EDCs via Traditional Intracellular Steroid Receptors 65
18. Other Substrates to Consider for Actions of EDCs 66
18.1 ERα and ERβ 66
18.2 Other intracellular and membrane steroid receptors 66
18.3 Relevant brain areas 67
19. Preliminary Studies 68
20. Organized Reproductive Parameters: Immature Rats 68
20.1 Perinatal androgen surge 69
20.2 Anogenital distance 69
21. Organized and Activated Reproductive Parameters: Peripubertal and Maturation Measures 69
21.1 Accessory structures 70
21.2 Puberty 70
21.3 Estrous cycle/sperm motility 70
21.4 E_2 and androgen levels 70
21.5 E_2 receptors 72
22. Organized and Activated Reproductive Parameters: Effects in Adults 72
22.1 Manifestation of sexual responsiveness 73
22.2 Fertility and fecundity 73
23. Strategy: EDC Effects on Reproductive Parameters: A Biomarker of Effects 75
24. Organized and/or Activated Nonreproductive Sexually Dimorphic Behaviors 75
24.1 Spatial performance 76
24.2 Rough-and-tumble play 77
24.3 Emotional reactivity 78
25. Suggested Experiments Moving Forward 79
26. Approach: The Importance of Integration of Reproductive and Nonreproductive Measures 79
27. Approach: Examining Effects of EDC Exposure Throughout Development 79
28. Suggestions for Future Work Examining Mechanisms of EDCs Effects 80
28.1 Activational effects in adults 80
28.2 Rationale for use of females in second-generation studies 80
28.3 Organizational effects in offspring 81
28.4 Organizational and activational effects in offspring 81
29. Logistical Factors for Experimental Control and Power 81
29.1 Controlling for cohort and maternal behavior effects 81
29.2 Random assignment to sets of dependent measures 82
30. Summary 82
30.1 Other considerations 84

31. Conclusions 84
Acknowledgment 85
References 85

Abstract

Endocrine-disrupting chemicals (EDCs) are diverse and pervasive and may have significant consequence for health, including reproductive development and expression of sex-/gender-sensitive parameters. This review chapter discusses what is known about common EDCs and their effects on reproductively relevant end points. It is proposed that one way that EDCs may exert such effects is by altering steroid levels (androgens or 17-estradiol, E_2) and/or intracellular E_2 receptors (ERs) in the hypothalamus and/or hippocampus. Basic research findings that demonstrate developmentally sensitive end points to androgens and E_2 are provided. Furthermore, an approach is suggested to examine differences in EDCs that diverge in their actions at ERs to elucidate their role in sex-/gender-sensitive parameters.

1. INTRODUCTION

Reproductive dysfunction among adults and emotional, attentional, and behavioral disorders among children are on the rise. Sperm counts and fertility have declined in the last 50 years (Carlesen, Giwercman, Keiding, & Skakkebaek, 1992). Incidence of attention-deficit hyperactivity disorder (ADHD) and autism has increased in the last 30 years (Schettler, 2001). These increases in reproductive dysfunction and developmental disorders may be due to increased exposure to environmental contaminants, although there is controversy about the relationship between exposure and these effects.

Many contaminants in the environment, including polychlorinated biphenyls (PCBs), dioxins, and metals, accumulate in exposed individuals and may have adverse consequences due to effects as endocrine-disrupting chemicals (EDCs). EDCs may have effects by altering steroid levels (androgens or 17β-estradiol, E_2) and/or intracellular E_2 receptors (ERs) in the hypothalamus and/or hippocampus.

Steroid hormones, during critical periods of development, organize sexual dimorphisms in brain and behavior and give rise to sex differences in later responses to steroid hormones. EDCs can profoundly disrupt reproductive responses following adult exposure and result in pervasive effects that extend throughout the life of their offspring. This demonstrates endocrine disruption, bioaccumulation, and cross-generational neurodevelopmental effects of EDCs. Many nonreproductive behaviors, such as spatial performance, activity, and arousal, are also sexually dimorphic and organized and activated by steroid hormones. Thus, EDCs may affect reproductive and the aforementioned nonreproductive parameters by altering E_2 levels and/or ER binding in the hypothalamus and/or hippocampus. The following paper describes our preliminary work on basic effects of reproductive parameters, effects of EDCs, and some of the future directions and work that could be done to address the defining questions of how EDS may change phenotypes and health outcomes.

Results from the literature and preliminary data will be presented that demonstrate our use of a whole-animal model to begin to investigate effects of exposure (in adulthood and/or development) to EDCs on steroid levels (androgens and E_2), actions at ERs (in hypothalamus and hippocampus), and reproductive-sensitive measures (anogenital distance, accessory structure weight, onset of puberty and sexual maturity, and reproductive behavior) and nonreproductive behaviors (spatial performance, play behavior, and arousal) throughout development. That being said, a challenge with EDCs is their nature and mixture. Examination of all EDCs is beyond the scope of our investigation at this time. However, some EDCs that are commonly considered and required further investigation are indicated later.

1.1. Sources of environmental contaminants

Contaminants, which are manufactured or are unintentional by-products of human activity, have pervasive effects on exposed individuals. Many are persistent exogenous substances that are highly lipophyllic. These environmental contaminants include PCBs, dioxins, mixtures of polycyclic aromatic hydrocarbons, crude, and refined petroleum products. These manufactured contaminants exist as mixtures of several congeners in the environment: they are ubiquitous and persistent and bioaccumulate in the body. Other sources of contaminants are used, combustion and/or incineration of products, which can result in contamination with lead and mercury and other heavy metals. These contaminants bioaccumulate in exposed individuals.

There are varied sources of environmental contaminants. Typical human exposure occurs with environmental contamination of the food chain, especially freshwater fish and meat, and occupational exposure. Fish, in particular, often contain significant amounts of methylmercury (Clarkson, 1983), which can damage the nervous system, especially in developing fetus. Pregnant women have been encouraged to limit their fish consumption (Schober et al., 2003). A family of industrial PCB compounds often sold as mixtures (Aroclor) are still found in significant quantities in the environment, although their manufacture in the United States was banned in 1977. In certain uses, PCBs can partially oxidize and themselves become contaminated by extremely toxic compounds, such as polychlorinated dibenzofurans (PCDFs). In some areas, PCB levels in drinking water ranged from 100 to 450 ng/l; in food products, levels were over 200 mg/kg fresh weight (WHO, 1989). PCB levels in occupationally exposed workers ranged from 2.2 to 290 ppm in adipose tissue (WHO, 1989), and blood concentrations in capacitor manufacturing workers were up to 3.5 μg/ml (Wolff, 1985).

There are other sources of contaminants. Pesticides and herbicides, such as dichlorodiphenyltrichloroethane (DDT) and methoxychlor, also get into the environment and have adverse consequences. Contaminants, such as bisphenol A (BPA), are present in plastics, including beverage and food storage containers. Many textiles contain contaminants, such as flame retardants, including tetrabromobisphenol A and polybrominated diphenyl ethers. Some individuals have also been exposed to contaminants with adverse effects due to medical (diethylstilbestrol, DES), dental (diglycidyl methacrylate), or dietary (phytoestrogens) interventions. Although effects of some of these specific EDS are considered, the approach discussed later is common sequelae on phenotype.

2. ENDOCRINE DISRUPTION MAY UNDERLIE NEGATIVE EFFECTS OF CONTAMINANTS

A common feature of many environmental contaminants is their estrogenic effects. Some contaminants can alter production of E_2 and/or androgens or act as agonists or antagonists for intracellular or membrane ERs (DiLorenzo et al., 2002). Thus, the term "endocrine-disrupting chemicals" (EDCs) in this chapter is used to refer to contaminants with these effects. *An important question considered here is the extent to which EDCs' actions to alter E_2 levels and/or ER binding in the hypothalamus or hippocampus mitigates effects on reproductive or nonreproductive processes.*

3. ADVERSE HEALTH CONSEQUENCES OF LIFELONG EDC EXPOSURE

Exposure to EDCs is associated with increased risk of cancer, cardiovascular disease, and/or neurodegenerative disease (Carpenter et al., 1998; see Fig. 3.1).

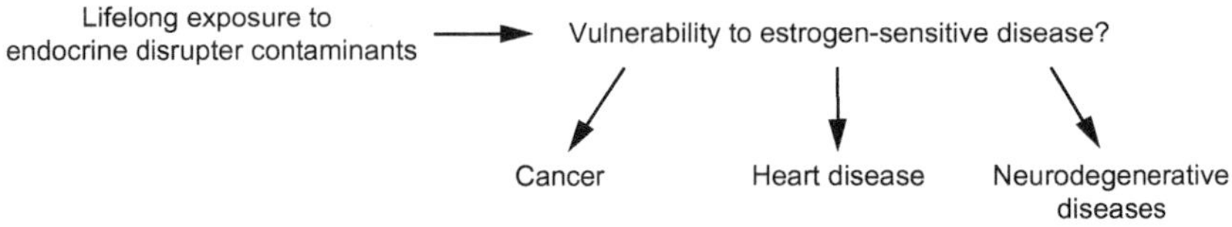

Figure 3.1 There are potential pervasive, negative effects of endocrine disrupters on steroid sensitive tissues, which may confer risk to disease states, such as cancer, heart disease, and neurodegenerative disorders.

3.1. Cancer

Contaminants, such as metals and estrogenic compounds, may be carcinogenic. Arsenic, cadmium, chromium, and thorium are known carcinogens. Beryllium, lead, nickel, and selenium are probable carcinogens. Lifetime exposure to estrogens is also a significant risk factor for breast cancer (Bernstein & Ross, 1993; Toniolo, 1997). Serum E_2 levels and rates of E_2 excretion are increased in breast cancer patients compared with controls (Bernstein & Ross, 1993; Goldin et al., 1986; Key, Chen, Wang, Pike, & Boreham, 1990; Shimizu, Ross, Bernstein, Pike, & Henderson, 1990; Ursin et al., 2001). Although some studies have found elevated levels of EDCs, such as PCBs and DDT, in tissues from women with breast cancer (Dewailly, Ayotte, Brisson, & Dodin, 1994; Dewailly, Ryan, et al., 1994; Guttes et al., 1998; Wolff, Toniolo, Lee, Rivera, & Dubin, 1993), others have not (Hunter et al., 1997; Kreiger et al., 1994; Lopez-Carrillo et al., 1997; Unger, Kiaer, Blichert-Toft, Olsen, & Clausen, 1984; van't Veer et al., 1997). These divergent reports may be due to higher levels of exposure increasing genetic susceptibility to breast cancer (Fielden et al., 2001). Women with a high PCB body burden, and a variant allele associated with E_2 metabolism and related to breast cancer incidence, had a higher incidence of breast cancer. However, there was no significant association between PCB concentration and breast cancer among women who did not have the variant allele (Moysich et al., 1999). Thus, exposure to EDCs may amplify negative health consequences in vulnerable individual or populations.

3.2. Heart disease

Serum lipids are elevated in PCB- (Baker et al., 1980; Calvert, Willie, Sweeney, Fingerhut, & Halperin, 1996; Kreiss, 1985; Smith et al., 1982; Stehr-Green, Welty, Steele, & Steinberg, 1986) or dioxin-exposed (Calvert et al., 1996) populations. Animals exposed to 2,3,7,8-tetrachlorodibenzo-*p*-dioxin

(TCDD) have increased serum triglycerides (Schiller et al., 1985). The increased lipid levels reflect altered liver function, which may increase risk of heart disease. Morbidity from ischemic heart disease increased dose-dependently with exposure to polychlorinated dioxin and furan exposure (Flesch-Janys et al., 1995).

3.3. Neurodegenerative diseases

Although metals are not the sole or primary risk factor, aluminum, iron, and lead have long been implicated in amyotrophic lateral sclerosis (ALS), Parkinson's disease, and Alzheimer's disease (AD). Occupational exposure to metals increases the risk of ALS five- to eightfold (Strickland, Smith, Dolliff, Goldman, & Roelofs, 1996). AD is more common in urban than rural areas and in developed than developing countries (Prince, 2000), where there may be differential lead exposure. Lead increases neuronal damage (Savolainen, Loikkanen, Eerikainen, & Naarala, 1998) through generation of reactive oxygen species (ROS).

These data suggest that EDCs can have profound health consequences that typically afflict individuals later in life and may represent effects of cumulative, lifelong exposure.

3.4. Other considerations

Also of interest are effects of contaminants that may alter the behavior, biochemistry, and/or physiology of the organism without profound effects to cause overt disease or mortality. EDCs may contribute to reduced IQ, decreased fertility, and altered sex hormone balance/metabolism (ATSDR, 1993). The development period on which exposure to EDCs occurs may be critical for the expression of effects. The following discusses differences in developmental exposure timing to EDCs.

4. SIGNFICANCE OF INVESTIGATING EDC EFFECTS ON NEURODEVELOPMENTAL PROCESSES

EDCs may have particularly significant effects on neurodevelopmental processes. EDCs accumulate in fatty tissues of exposed individuals, are readily transferred across the placenta prenatally, and are expressed in breast milk. This perinatal exposure may have particularly deleterious effects on development. Indeed, there is growing recognition of the increased incidence of behavioral, cognitive, and/or emotional disturbances in children in the past 30 years, which has been proposed to be related to increased exposure to

EDCs (Safer, Zito, & Fine, 1996). The following discussion provides evidence that exposure to EDCs during development may result in permanent, lifelong differences in sexual function and reproductive ability, as well as cognitive function and/or emotional reactivity/arousal.

5. HORMONES' EFFECTS TO ORGANIZE NEURAL SYSTEMS AND BEHAVIORAL PROCESSES

Gonad development, sex determination, and reproductive success of offspring are highly dependent on sex hormone systems. The developing organism is exquisitely sensitive to alterations in hormone function. In the early embryonic state, the gonads of human males and females are morphologically identical. Sexual differentiation begins under hormonal influence during the fifth and sixth weeks of fetal development, and thus, alterations in hormones during this highly sensitive period can have profound consequences. The balance of estrogens and androgens is critical for normal development, growth, and functioning of the reproductive system. Although especially important during development, this balance is important throughout life for the preservation of normal feminine or masculine traits, as well as the expression of some sexually dimorphic behaviors (sex, spatial performance, and arousal).

EDCs affect the production of sex steroid hormones, such as estrogens and androgens (Golden et al., 1998; Vincent, Bradshaw, Booth, Seegmiller, & Allen, 1992; Vreugdenhil, Hack, Draguhn, & Jefferys, 2002). Normal sexual development and behavior depends upon neural systems that are "organized" perinatally by these hormones during critical or sensitive periods of development and would also be vulnerable to the effects of EDCs (Fitch & Denenberg, 1998; Hutchison, 1997).

6. DEVELOPMENTAL EDC EXPOSURE ALTERS REPRODUCTIVE DEVELOPMENT AND BEHAVIOR

Evidence suggests that people or animals exposed perinatally to EDCs have altered reproductive development and behavior (see Fig. 3.2).

6.1. Diethylstilbestrol

Disruption of the sex steroid system during fetal stages of life results in profound adverse developmental reproductive effects, as is well known from the effects of DES (Brouwer et al., 1999; Golden et al., 1998; Newbold, 1995).

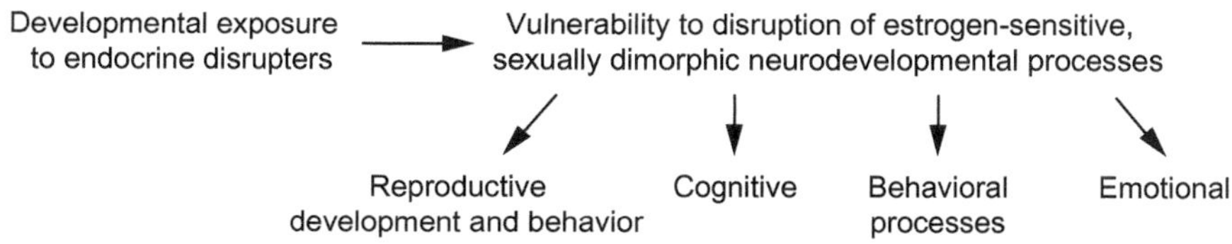

Figure 3.2 Proposed negative effects of exposure to endocrine disrupters during development in people and in animals. The focus here is on vulnerability to sexually dimorphic processes that are estrogen-sensitive, such as reproductive, cognitive, and emotional development and associated behavioral processes.

DES, a synthetic estrogen that was used in the 1950s and 1960s to prevent miscarriage, is an EDC. This synthetic estrogen caused a series of developmental abnormalities of both male and female genital systems, as well as a rare form of vaginal cancer. *In utero* exposure to DES resulted in hypospadia, microphallus, infertility, and testicular and prostate tumors of male offspring. Females exposed *in utero* to DES had ovarian cysts, malformations of the cervical canal, infertility, ovarian tumors, and/or vaginal adenocarcinoma.

6.2. Reproductive dysfunction

Episodes of intoxication with PCBs in Japan and Taiwan produced reproductive anomalies in exposed offspring. In 1979, over 2000 persons in Taiwan were intoxicated by heat-degraded PCBs that had contaminated their cooking oil (Hsu et al., 1985). Exposed victims developed skin disorders, peripheral neuropathy, and other neurological problems (called Yu-Cheng "oil disease") caused by and by their heat-degraded products, PCDFs (Kashimoto et al., 1985). Males born to exposed mothers have decreased penis length (Guo, Hse, & Lambert, 1996) and girls reach puberty at a younger age than unexposed girls (Carpenter, Shen, Nguyen, Le, & Lininger, 2001; Pauwels, Covaci, Delbeke, Punjabi, & Schepens, 1999). Similar patterns have been seen in Tanner stage development among girls environmentally exposed to EDCs (Schell, Burnitz, & Gallo, 2012).

Animal models have demonstrated adverse effects of other EDCs, due to perinatal exposure. TCDD exposure to rat pups during development caused changes in both male and female gonad development, reduction in sperm counts, abnormal sperm, and changes in sexual behavior, such as demasculinization and feminization of male offspring (Brouwer et al., 1999; Gray, Kelce, Monosson, Ostby, & Birnbaum, 1995; Peterson, Theobald, & Kimmel, 1993). Lactational exposure of rats to Aroclor 1254 (8, 32, or 64 mg/kg to dams) decreased mating behavior, reproductive success, and ventral prostate and testicular weights of male pups in adulthood (Brouwer et al., 1999; Sager, 1983). Females that were exposed had delayed puberty, decreased uterine weight, impaired fertility, and irregular estrous cycles (Brouwer et al., 1999; Sager & Girard, 1994). Also, acute exposure to Aroclor 1254 (from neonatal days 1 to 7) significantly reduced lordosis quotients of adult female rats in both paced and nonpaced testing paradigm (Chung, Nunez, & Clemens, 2001).

Quails are also particularly sensitive to effects of exogenous E_2 administration during development. The administration of methoxychlor in doses that would be analogous to less than 10 ppm (which is considered safe in the environment) to eggs of hatching Japanese quail, or to parents, impaired sexual behavior of adult male offspring, as well as altered hypothalamic catecholamines and plasma steroid hormones (Ottinger et al., 2003). Also, bobwhite quail exposed to methoxychlor during the perinatal period requires longer to achieve sexual maturity (Ottinger et al., 2003). DDT administered to quail eggs resulted in impaired sexual behavior, reduced cloacal gland area, and lowered plasma T concentration in males (Halldin, Axelsson, & Brunstrom, 2003).

These data clearly indicate that developmental exposure to EDCs can adversely affect sexual development of people and animals; however, there are different effects depending upon the EDCs and when in development exposure occurs. Therefore, we consider the next effects of EDCs exposure at different point in development and the consequences for reproductive development and behavior, as well as E_2 levels and hypothalamic ER binding.

7. EXPOSURE TO EDCs IN ADULTHOOD ALSO EFFECTS REPRODUCTIVE PARAMETERS

In adulthood, "activational" effects of sex hormones include facilitating, modulating, or inhibiting the function of neural circuits organized during development. To date, there has been much less investigation of the activational effects of EDCs compared to their organizational effects. Typically, EDCs are accumulated in biological tissue in an ongoing manner, and circumscribed exposure is not common. However, there have been two incidents of profound and acute exposure via cooking oil contamination (Hsu et al., 1985). Also, even limited consumption of game fish (7–15 meals) during a single fishing season has been demonstrated to result in profound accumulation in biological tissues (Schwartz, Jacobson, Fein,

Jacobson, & Price, 1983). Therefore, the extent to which exposure during adulthood may influence previously established sexually dimorphic behaviors is of interest and will be discussed.

EDCs influence rodent sex behavior. The administration of Aroclor 1221 or 1254 during adulthood affected the timing of female sexual behavior of rats (Chung & Clemens, 1999). Exposure of rats to lead acetate in drinking water results in decreased sperm count (McGivern, Sokol, & Berman, 1991; Ronis, Gandy, & Badger, 1998; Sokol, Madding, & Swerdloff, 1985), decreased gonadotropin-stimulated testosterone (T) production (Thoreux-Manlay, Le Goascogne, Segretain, Jegou, & Pinon-Lataillade, 1995; Thoreux-Manlay, Pinon-Lataillade, Coffigny, Soufir, & Masse, 1995), and decreased serum T production (Hsu, Hsu, Liu, Chen, & Guo, 1998). Not surprisingly, EDC exposure may also influence fertility.

EDCs can alter reproductive responses of adults. Men with infertility had significantly higher tetra- and pentachlorinated biphenyls, DDE, DDT, and lindane than controls (Pines, Cucos, Ever-Handani, & Ron, 1987); however, another study found no relationship between PCB levels and sperm profile (Emmett, Maroni, Schmith, Levin, & Jefferys, 1988). Lead exposure reduces sperm count, semen volume, and sperm motility and increases infertility (Apostoli, Kiss, Porru, Bonde, & Vanhoorne, 1998; Lancranjan, Popescu, GAvanescu, Klepsch, & Serbanescu, 1975; Telisman et al., 2000). EDC effects on women's fertility have not been well investigated. In collaboration with Drs. Lawrence Schell and Mia Gallo, we are currently investigating how menstrual cyclicity may be influenced by EDCs' body burden. The following discusses some of what is known about effects of EDC exposure on reproductive parameters, sexual behaviors, and fertility of adult female and male rats. Also, effects on offspring of EDC exposed and nonexposed female rats will be examined in adulthood.

8. EDCs IN ADULTHOOD INFLUENCE SEXUALLY DIMORPHIC BRAIN MORPHOLOGY

There is a robust sex difference in the volume of the sexually dimorphic nucleus of the preoptic area, an important brain region for sexual behavior, with male rats typically having larger volumes than females. Exposure to phytoestrogens in adulthood may in part maintain this sexual dimorphism in brain morphology. When male and female rats are switched from a phytoestrogen-rich diet to a phytoestrogen-free diet in adulthood, this sex difference is abrogated (Lephart et al., 2002).

Together, these data demonstrate that perinatal and adult exposure to EDCs can negatively affect sexual development, reproductive function, and sexual dimorphisms in the brain. Because there has been little systematic investigation of the organizational and/or activational effects of EDCs on these parameters in animal models, it is necessary to further and determine the extent to which E_2 and/or ER actions in the hypothalamus mediate these effects.

9. DO EDCs INFLUENCE SEX DIFFERENCES IN NONREPRODUCTIVE BEHAVIORS?

Steroid hormones also play a critical role in neurodevelopment that influences not only reproductive but also nonreproductive behaviors that show sex differences (Fitch & Denenberg, 1998; Matsumoto, 1991). Specific behavioral differences in nonreproductive behaviors between males and females include differences in spatial learning, play, exploration, activity levels, novelty-seeking behavior, and emotional reactivity (Goy & McEwen, 1980). These sex dimorphisms are thought to reflect adaptive differences for behavioral strategies in coping as a result of sexual selection. Moreover, these sexually dimorphic behaviors may be relevant for concerns regarding increased developmental, cognitive, or emotional disabilities over the past 30 years (Schettler, 2001). Also, behaviors are particularly sensitive measures of effects of EDCs. To date, there has been little investigation of the effects of PCBs on sexually dimorphic nonreproductive behaviors (Weiss, 2002). It is necessary to consider effects of EDCs on these sex differences and on E_2 levels and hippocampal ER binding.

9.1. Cognitive dysfunction

EDCs can alter cognitive development. Some, but not all, studies have shown a predictive relationship between prenatal PCB exposure and cognitive development in infancy through preschool years (Darvill, Lonky, Reihman, Stewart, & Pagano, 2000; Jacobson, Fein, Jacobson, Schwartz, & Dowler, 1985, Jacobson, Jacobson, & Humphrey, 1990; Patandin et al., 1999). Animals exposed pre- or postnatally to PCBs have deficits in executive functions (Levin, Schantz, & Bowman, 1992), reversal learning (Schantz, Levin, Bowman, Heironimus, & Laughlin, 1989), working memory (Roegge, Seo, Crofton, & Schantz, 2000), fixed-interval responding, and response inhibition (Rice, 1997, 1999).

Chronic exposure to lead affects behavioral development in children and other vertebrates, even at blood levels below the "community action level" of 10 gm/dl (Garavan, Morgan, Levitsky, Hermer-Vazquez, & Strupp, 2000; Walkowiak et al., 1998). Among the effects reported in children are changes in activity levels (Mendelsohn et al., 1998; 10–25 M/dl), sensory function (Altmann et al., 1998; 1.4–17.4 gm/dl), attention (Walkowiak et al., 1998; 95% of subjects below 9 gm/dl), and cognitive function (Lanphear, Dietrich, Auinger, & Cox, 2000; 98% below 10 gm/dl); for reviews, see Banks, Ferretti, and Shucard (1997) and Nevin (2000). Indeed, exposure of young children to lead or PCBs results in a decrement in IQ of 5–7 points that is not reversible (Wang et al., 1992; Needleman et al., 1979; Rogan et al., 2001). Effects of other EDCs on sensory, attention, and cognitive function have not been as extensively investigated. However, adults who eat a significant amount of contaminated fish suffer from some cognitive deficits, attributed in different regions to methylmercury (Lebel et al., 1998) and to PCBs (Schantz et al., 2001). Pesticide exposure also has adverse effects on neurobehavioral functioning. Children exposed to pesticides had significantly less ability to draw a human form, and they demonstrated a variety of motor deficits for simple tasks (Guillette, Meza, Aquilar, Soto, & Enedina, 1998).

EDCs have direct effects on nervous system function. Long-term potentiation (LTP), a form of synaptic plasticity used as a model system for study of cognitive potential, is altered by PCBs and lead (Altmann et al., 1993; Carpenter, Arcaro, & Spink, 2002; Carpenter, Hussain, Berger, Lombardo, & Park, 2002; Hori, Busselberg, Matthews, Parsons, & Carpenter, 1993; Nguyen, Abel, Kandel, & Bourtchouladze, 2000; Niemi, Audi, Bush, & Carpenter, 1998). Developmental exposure to commercial PCB mixtures, such as Aroclor, produces a persistent impairment in LTP and neurobehavioral deficits (Gilbert & Crofton, 1999; Hany, Lilienthal, Roth-Harer, et al., 1999; Hany, Lilienthal, Sarasin, et al., 1999). The protein kinase C (PKC)-signaling pathway is involved in the modulation of learning, memory, and motor behavior and may be a target of E_2's actions. PCBs also alter PKC signaling (Chen, Ma, Paul, Spencer, & Ho, 1997; Narita, Aoki, Ozaki, Yajima, & Suzuki, 2001; Van der Zee, Kroon, Nieweg, van de Merwe, & Kampinga, 1997). Although the findings indicated earlier provide evidence that EDCs can alter cognitive performance, these measures of cognition are neither sexually dimorphic nor E_2- or ER-dependent (see Frye, Paris, Walf, & Rusconi, 2011 for comprehensive review). Therefore, data are lacking on mechanisms of EDCs on these measures of cognitive performance. As such, evidence that EDCs alter spatial performance is discussed in the succeeding text.

10. EFFECTS OF EDCs ON SEXUALLY DIMORPHIC, NONREPRODUCTIVE BEHAVIORS

10.1. Spatial memory

There are sex-specific effects of perinatal PCB and dioxin exposure on spatial learning. Yu-Cheng boys that were prenatally exposed to high levels of PCBs and PCDFs when their mothers were accidentally exposed to these contaminants in rice oil show more disrupted cognitive development, mainly spatial function, than did exposed girls (Guo, Lai, Chen, & Hsu, 1995; Vreugdenhil et al., 2002). In animal studies, spatial learning that favors males is mediated by perinatal exposure to androgens (Williams & Meck, 1991). The sparse existing literature suggests that developmental exposure to EDCs can affect spatial performance. Gestational and lactational exposure to ortho-substituted PCBs produces spatial deficits at adolescence in male mice or adulthood in male rats (Palanza, 2003; Schantz, Moshtaghian, & Ness, 1995). Japanese quail exposed to Aroclor 1254 (200 ppm) from 7 to 15 days of age had deficits in avoidance responding as adults (Kreitzer & Heinz, 1974). Similarly, rats exposed to Fenclor 42 during lactation had acquisition deficits in an active avoidance task (Pantaleoni et al., 1988). These data suggest that developmental exposure to EDCs disrupts spatial memory.

Exposure during adulthood to EDCs can also have activational effects on spatial memory. Females exposed to a phytoestrogen-rich diet exhibit "masculinized" spatial performance in a radial arm maze, while males fed with a phytoestrogen-free diet show "feminized" performance (Lund & Lephart, 2001). These data suggest that adult exposure to EDCs also disrupts spatial memory.

An important question is what are the mechanisms by which developmental and/or adult exposure to EDCs alters spatial performance. There is evidence for sex differences in spatial performance and activational effects of E_2 in adulthood to alter spatial performance of rats. Systemic or intrahippocampal administration of E_2 improves spatial performance of female rats (Frye & Rhodes, 2002). Further, E_2's actions at intracellular ERs in the hippocampus of adults do not seem to be required to mediate these effects on spatial performance; however, the extent to which ERs mediate sex differences in spatial performance has not been investigated.

Thus, we next examine the effects and mechanisms (E_2 and/or hippocampal ER dependency) of developmental and/or adult exposure to various EDCs for their effects on spatial memory.

10.2. Rough-and-tumble play

In addition to spatial cognition, rough-and-tumble play is another sexually dimorphic nonreproductive behavior that may be influenced by EDCs. Young boys and male rodents show a significantly greater incidence of rough-and-tumble play than do their female counterparts (Collaer & Hines, 1995; Ward & Stehm, 1991). Girls that are masculinized due to DES exposure or congenital adrenal hyperplasia show more rough-and-tumble tomboyish behavior than do their nonmasculinized sisters (Berenbaum et al., 2000; Reinisch & Sanders, 1984). Consistent with this, girls exposed to PCBs perinatally showed more masculinized play behavior and boys exposed to PCBs show more feminized play behavior (Linn & Petersen, 1985; Voyer, Voyer, & Bryden, 1995; Vreugdenhil et al., 2002). The developmental effects of EDCs in animal models have also been reported. Female offspring exposed to BPA had a masculinization of rough-and-tumble play (Dessi-Fulgheri, Porrini, & Farabollini, 2002). Notably, the sex difference in rough-and-tumble play is not dependent on activational effects of gonadal hormones. Castration or other postnatal endocrine manipulation does not affect this behavior (Goy & Phoenix, 1972), which may be ER-dependent. *Therefore, we will examine the effects of EDCs on rough-and-tumble play behavior and concomitant hypothalamic ER binding in our proposed research.*

10.3. Emotional reactivity

Children exposed to PCBs, lead, or mercury showed inattention, hyperactivity, and disordered and/or mildly antisocial behavior (Needleman et al., 1979; Schettler, 2001; Yu et al., 1994). In animal models, developmental exposure to EDCs produces similar effects. Mice exposed to BPA or methoxychlor perinatally (from gestation day 11 to postpartum day 8) showed a reversal of sex differences at periadolescence in exploratory activity in a novel open field, elevated plus maze, and social interactions with a conspecific (Palanza, 2003). This was due to females being more sensitive to effects of exposure to the EDCs (Palanza, 2003).

Adult exposure to EDCs can also have activational effects on motor behavior, exploration, and anxiety. Exposure to a phytoestrogen-rich diet feminizes male rats' exploratory behavior in the plus maze (Lund & Lephart, 2001). Although there has not been a great deal of investigation of the effects of EDCs on these measures, these data suggest that activity, exploration, and effect are altered by EDCs.

An important question is what are the mechanisms by which developmental and/or adult exposure to EDCs alters motor behavior, exploration, and anxiety. There are sex differences in motor behavior, exploration, and anxiety that are mediated in part by E_2 in adulthood. Females that have high endogenous levels of E_2, or are administered with E_2, demonstrate more activity, exploratory behavior in open field, and less anxiety in the plus maze and in social interaction tasks than do males or females with low levels of E_2 (Frye, Petralia, & Rhodes, 2000). These data suggest that E_2 can have activational effects on motor behavior, exploration, and anxiety. The ER dependency of these effects has not been systematically investigated.

10.4. Stress

To our knowledge, there are few published reports of the effects of EDCs on stress reactivity. However, there is evidence (discussed in the succeeding text) that E_2 may mitigate stress responsiveness.

Female rats with high hormone levels are more responsive when subjected to stress than are their female counterparts with low hormone levels or male rats. First, there are sex differences in the response of rodents to stressful stimuli. Female rats have increased stress responses compared to males. Female rats have increased corticosterone levels in response to less robust stress stimuli than do male rats (Figueiredo, Dolgas, & Herman, 2002). Also, female rats have impairments in conditioning, decreased punished drinking, and increased defensive behaviors and analgesia compared to male rats (Aloisi, Ceccarelli, & Lupo, 1998; Pericic & Pivac, 1996; Shepherd, Blanchard, Weiss, Rodgers, & Blanchard, 1992; Wood & Shors, 1998). Second, the behavioral response of females to stressful stimuli varies across the estrous cycle. During proestrus when E_2 levels peak, females have increased responsiveness to stressors, as indicated by greater corticosteroid levels; impairments in conditioned responses; increased ulcer severity; and increased estrous cycle disruption compared to females in other estrous cycle stages (Matysek, 1989; Pare & Redei, 1993; Shors, Lewczyk, Pacynski, Mathew, & Pickett, 1998; Viau & Meaney, 1991). Third, the removal of circulating E_2 via ovariectomy attenuates stress-induced sex differences in corticosterone responses, learning impairments, and analgesia (Bodnar, Romero, & Kramer, 1988; Romero, Mounho, Lauer, Born, & Burchiel, 1997; Ryan & Maier, 1988; Viau & Meaney, 1991; Wood & Shors, 1998). Fourth, E_2 replacement reinstates increased response to stress in ovx rats (Ryan & Maier, 1988; Sternberg et al., 1995; Viau & Meaney, 1991).

It has been proposed that these sex/hormone differences in stress responsiveness may be due to E_2's effects on the hypothalamic–pituitary–adrenal (HPA) axis (Figueiredo et al., 2002). The ER dependency of E_2's effects on stress is not known.

There are reported increases in behavioral and/or emotional disorders in the last 30 years (Safer et al., 1996), which may be related to greater developmental exposure to EDCs (Pimentel et al., 1995). Notably, there are significant increases in the incidence of ADHD and autism (Goldman, Genel, Bezman, & Slanetz, 1998; Schettler, 2001). Males are more vulnerable to these disorders, which have salient motor and arousal components. Thus, the increase in the incidence of these disorders may reflect effects of EDCs on male-typical levels of arousal and/or stress responsiveness. This idea has not been systematically investigated; however, we consider the developmental and activational effects of EDCs on various measures of arousal, as well as stress responsiveness, will be considered as changes in corticosteroid levels.

11. POTENTIAL MECHANISMS BY WHICH EDCs MAY PRODUCE THEIR EFFECTS

The results discussed earlier suggest that EDCs can influence sexual development, reproductive behavior, and other sexually dimorphic behaviors, such as spatial memory, rough-and-tumble play, and emotional reactivity. Further investigation is needed to establish and characterize these effects. The putative mechanisms by which EDCs may have these effects also need to be explored. A review of potential actions of EDCs follows. This discussion focuses on EDC effects to alter E_2 levels and/or actions at ERs; however, it is important to notice that the site specificity of these effects has not been systematically addressed or has been related to the functional effects of EDCs. Therefore, we will relate effects of EDCs on reproductive processes, spatial performance, motor behavior, exploration, and anxiety to effects on E_2 levels and ER binding. Reproductive responses are expected to be mediated by changes in E_2 and/or ERs in the hypothalamus. The hippocampus is essential for spatial performance, motor behavior, exploration, and anxiety.

An important question is whether EDCs interact with endogenous estradiol. This is relevant not only for women of reproductive age, who have high and fluctuating E_2 levels, but also especially for children, postmenopausal women, and men, whose E_2 levels are low.

Although PCBs have long been known to be estrogenic (Bitman, Cecil, & Harris, 1972; Ecobichon & MacKenzie, 1974; Gellert, 1978; Nelson, 1974), EDCs vary in their estrogenic effects. Attempts to establish a relationship between PCBs and their estrogenic/antiestrogenic actions have not reached a consensus (Hansen, 1998). The lower chlorinated mixtures tend to have more estrogenic potential than do the more highly chlorinated mixtures (Bitman, Cecil, & Harris, 1972; Ecobichon & MacKenzie, 1974; Gellert, 1978; Kramer, Helferich, Bergman, Klasson-Wehler, & Giesy, 1997; Nelson, 1974). Aroclor 1242 is weakly estrogenic (Bitman, Cecil, & Harris; Dewailly, Ayotte, et al., 1994; Dewailly, Ryan, et al., 1994; Ecobichon & MacKenzie, 1974; Jansen, Cooke, Porcelli, Liu, & Hansen, 1993; Li, Zhao, & Hansen, 1994; Nesaretnam, Corcoran, Dils, & Darbre, 1996; Soontornchat, Li, Cooke, & Hansen, 1994). Many infrequently reported lightly chlorinated congeners are active (or share characteristics with active but environmentally irrelevant congeners) in estrogenicity assays. Some persistent higher chlorinated and/or coplanar PCBs are antiestrogenic (Jansen et al., 1993; Moore et al., 1997; Safe et al., 1991).

11.1. Progress limitations

Rate-limiting factors elucidating the role of EDS in etiopathophysiology and the expression of phenotypes and health outcomes have been due to a variety of EDSs and exposure. Indeed, challenge to ascertain effects of EDS via estrogen signaling or other factors is the ubiquity and heterogeneity of commonly considered EDS and diverse effects on estrogen signaling. Some of the common EDCs and their different effects on estrogenic parameters are indicated later.

1. *Aroclor 1242* is a PCB mixture that may increase E_2 levels and/or ER binding (Jansen et al., 1993). If adult and/or developmental exposure to Aroclor 1242 increases E_2 levels, hypothalamic/hippocampal ER binding, *and* reproductive or nonreproductive processes, respectively, then these behaviors may be E_2- and/or ER-dependent and these mechanisms may underlie Aroclor 1242's effects.

2. *Aroclor 1260* is a PCB mixture that may decrease androgen/E_2 levels *and* ER binding (Andric et al., 2000). If adult and/or developmental exposure to Aroclor 1260 decreases E_2 levels, blocks ER activity in the hypothalamus and hippocampus, *and* disrupts reproductive and nonreproductive processes, then this would suggest that Aroclor 1260 may have these effects through its actions as an ER antagonist.
3. *PCB 52* is a PCB congener that may have ER agonist effects (Hansen, 1998). If PCB 52 increases ER binding in the hypothalamus and enhances reproductive processes, without substantive alterations in E_2 levels, then this would suggest that these effects of PCB 52 are due to actions at ERs rather than E_2 levels. Nonreproductive behaviors are somewhat ER-independent; therefore, PCB 52 would not be expected to substantially alter hippocampal ERs, spatial performance, activity, and/or arousal.
4. *PCB 77* is a congener that may increase E_2 levels *but* have ER antagonist actions (Hansen, 1998). If PCB 77 increases E_2 but decreases hypothalamic ER binding, then only E_2- and not ER-dependent reproductive processes would be altered. If hippocampal ERs are blocked, ER-independent spatial performance and arousal would still be expected to be increased.
5. *Lead* is a heavy metal that may decrease androgen/E_2 levels without altering ERs (Pillai, Laxmipriya, Rawal, & Gupta, 2002). If lead decreases E_2 and disrupts E_2-dependent reproductive and nonreproductive processes, without substantive alterations in hypothalamic or hippocampal ERs, then this would provide further support that lead and/or other EDCs' actions cannot be completely accounted for by ER activity.

Traditional methods of behavioral neuroendocrinology are of great value to ascertain effects and mechanisms of different EDCs. EDC effects on reproductive parameters and nonreproductive behaviors should be characterized. The extent to which these effects are due to altering E_2 levels and/or ERs in the hypothalamus and/or hippocampus can then be elucidated.

12. SEVERAL FACTORS MAY BEAR UPON ESTROGENICITY OF COMPOUNDS

12.1. Mixtures

A factor that may contribute to the lack of established structure/function relationships for EDCs and estrogenic effects is that many PCBs are mixtures of compounds that have different estrogenic activities. For example, two Chinese PCB mixtures, PCB3 and PCB5 (which are similar in congener composition to US Aroclors 1242 and 1254, respectively), were estrogenic at nanomolar levels. All previous reports have suggested that individual PCB congeners and mixtures are only estrogenic in the micromolar range and show no effects at nanomolar and picomolar levels.

12.2. Additivity

The total activities of mixtures of individually weakly estrogenic organochlorines are additive. Weakly estrogenic compounds may produce additive effects with low levels of steroidal estrogens. In support, a yeast reporter gene assay for BPA and DDT was used to investigate the combined action of weakly estrogenic chemicals with estradiol. Mixtures of weakly estrogenic compounds contributed to an estrogenic effect when the endogenous estradiol levels were very low and the EDC concentrations were high, which is most likely to occur in children (Rajapakse, Shimizu, Payne, & Busija, 2001).

12.3. Concentrations

Whether a mixture of weakly estrogenic chemicals results in estrogenic activity also depends on the concentration of individual compounds. A mixture of PCBs prepared to reflect the PCB congeners and concentrations routinely detected in human breast milk was estrogenic (Hany, Lilienthal, Roth-Harer, et al., 1999; Hany, Lilienthal, Sarasin, et al., 1999). Female rats whose mothers received the PCB mixture had increased uterine weights at 21 days old. Other PCB mixtures tested at similar concentrations were not estrogenic.

13. EFFECTS OF EDCs ON UTEROTROPIC ACTIVITY

In addition, differences between E_2-sensitive measures may also be problematic. *In vitro* ER-binding studies may not accurately predict gene expression, ER-dependent responses in other tissues (Feldman, 1997), or *in vivo* estrogenic actions (Ashby et al., 1997; Feldman, 1997; Li, 1997; Moore et al., 1997). *Therefore, in the succeeding text, we consider the effects of different EDCs in a relatively circumspect assay of uterine growth.*

E_2 has profound proliferative effects that mediate growth and development. Uterotropic activity in immature female or ovariectomized (ovx) adult female rodents has been an accepted standard of estrogenic activity. Male, as well as female, reproductive tissues are sensitive to endogenous estradiol and EDCs (Allen et al., 1997; Cooke, Young, Hess, & Cunha, 1991; Feldman, 1997; Jansen et al., 1993; Li, 1997; Seegal, Brosch, & Okoniewski, 1997; Steinmetz, Brown, Allen, Bigsby, & Ben-Jonathan, 1997; Sundaresan, Weiss, Bauer-Dantoin, & Jameson, 1997; Vom Saal et al., 1997). However, although the uterotropic response increases with estradiol levels (Kramer et al., 1997), some PCBs demonstrate nonmonotonic uterotropic responses (Li, 1996; Li et al., 1994; Nesaretnam et al., 1996; Sajid, 1996; Vom Saal et al., 1997).

Some would argue that uterotropic responses are a relatively insensitive assay. Effects of EDCs on uterine growth may not be predictive of other reproductive tract changes or ER-dependent responses in other tissues (Ashby et al., 1997; Feldman, 1997; Kupfer, 1988). For example, effects of EDCs on uterotropic activity may not predict estrogenic or ER-mediated effects of EDCs in the brain. Actions of EDCs in the brain likely mediate some of the more relevant effects of EDCs for people. *Therefore, we will consider effects of EDCs on E_2 levels and ER binding in brain areas, such as the hypothalamus and hippocampus, which are most relevant for functions under investigation (reproductive processes, spatial performance, and arousal, respectively).*

Despite the arguable insensitivity of this end point, a significant effect at modest dosages confirms at least the potential for weak estrogenic activity of EDCs.

14. IMPORTANCE OF EXAMINING EDC EFFECTS ON WHOLE-ANIMAL ESTROGENIC MEASURES

The reported estrogenic/antiestrogenic activity of PCBs is highly variable and may be response-specific because of the nature of the assays employed. Other measures of estrogenic activity may be more sensitive than *in vitro* ER-binding studies or *in vivo* uterotropic responses. Perinatal exposure to low doses of BPA in drinking water affected several E_2-sensitive measures including body weight, estrous cycle patterns, and plasma luteinizing hormone levels in adult rats (Rubin, Murray, Damassa, King, & Soto, 2001). The concentrations used were below those that produced a uterotropic response in ovx females. This suggests that whole-animal, physiological, E_2-responsive measures may be more sensitive than are tissue-specific responses. *Therefore, effects of EDCs on whole-animal physiology and behavior will be considered with effects of EDCs on tissue-specific responses (e.g., E_2 levels and ER* *binding) in brain areas thought to be important for reproductive (hypothalamus) and nonreproductive (hippocampus) behaviors.*

15. EFFECTS OF EDCs ON E_2 METABOLISM

EDCs may have effects on E_2 metabolism in a number of ways. First, as discussed earlier, some EDCs can alter serum lipid concentrations. Cholesterol is the precursor for the production of E_2 and other steroid hormones (see Fig. 3.3). Second, there is also evidence that some EDCs can alter metabolism enzymes that are necessary for converting cholesterol to steroid hormones. Numerous compounds can activate one of the P450

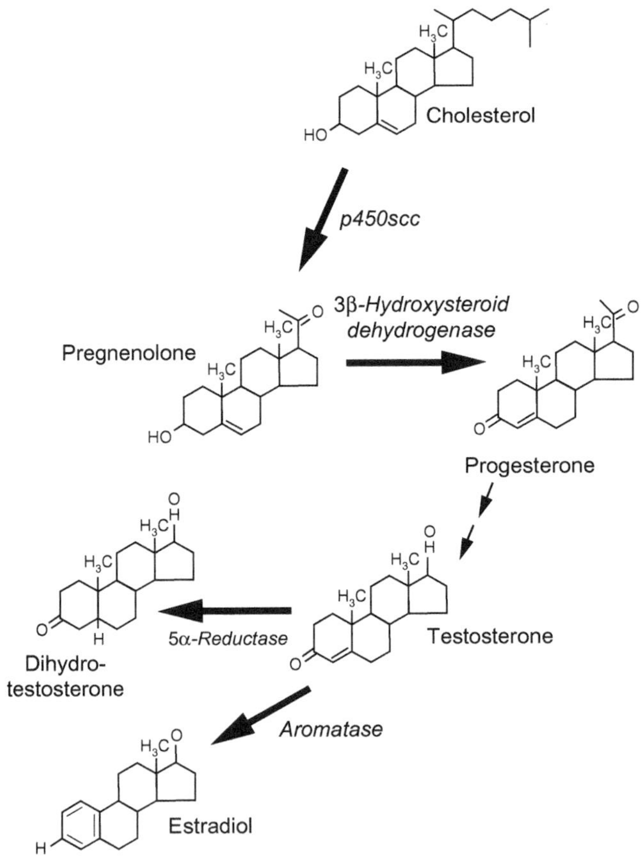

Figure 3.3 Metabolism pathway of steroid hormones. All steroids have cholesterol as a precursor that is metabolized to other precursors, such as progesterone, to eventually form testosterone and then estradiol.

cytochromes (P450 or CYP): these enzymes are involved in the metabolism of most steroid hormones and EDCs. Steroid hormones and EDCs also induce P450s. Environmental contaminants may contain chemicals that induce P450s, are metabolized by P450s, or both. Induction of CYP occurs when EDCs, such as TCDD, bind the aromatic hydrocarbon receptor (AhR). There is a firm link between PCBs, enzyme induction, and AhR effects (Namkung, Porubek, Neslon, & Juchau, 1995). The binding of EDCs with AhR can result in antiestrogenic activity through increased metabolism and depletion of endogenous E_2 (Spink, Lincoln, Dickerman, & Gierthy, 1990). Elevated levels of CYP enzymes, primarily expressed not only in the liver but also in the brain and other tissues, result in increased E_2 metabolism and excretion. Alternatively, compounds that are metabolized by P450s may result in a net estrogenic effect if they inhibit endogenous estrogens from being metabolized.

Altered rates of estradiol metabolism are observed in animals exposed to PCBs. Coplanar PCBs like TCDD activate AhR, causing the induction of CYP, which catalyzes the metabolism of many PCB congeners and other endogenous hormones, including estradiol (Hayes et al., 1996; Spink et al., 1994). Estradiol can be oxidized at several positions, and the products are reactive, rapidly metabolized further, and excreted. Measurement of the 2- and 4-hydroxylated metabolites indicates the relative activity of the two forms of P450. When metabolism of estradiol is increased, functional levels fall and an altered estrogenic function ensues. A number of the ortho-substituted PCBs, but not the coplanars, produce enzyme induction (Parkinson et al., 1983).

The profound effects of PCBs on enzymes and the enhanced activities of some primary metabolites may readily influence the outcome of *in vivo* tests (Korach, Sarver, Chae, McLachlan, & McKinney, 1988; Li & Hansen, 1996; Li et al., 1997; Safe, 1994). Some individual pesticides, PCBs, and their metabolites are estrogenic *in vitro* and *in vivo* but only at high, micromolar concentrations (Arcaro, Vakharia, Yang, & Gierthy, 1998; Fielden et al., 1997; Jansen et al., 1993; Korach et al., 1988; Li & Hansen, 1995; Soto et al., 1995). These effects on enzyme changes may account for some of the nonlinearity in dose–response relationships of EDCs (Li & Hansen, 1997; Li et al., 1994; Nagel et al., 1994; Soontornchat et al., 1994; Vom Saal et al., 1997).

Whole-animal preparations may be particularly sensitive to the effects of EDCs because EDCs may produce some of their estrogenic responses by altering endogenous E_2 metabolism and some *in vitro* models may lack these essential metabolism enzymes. In support, many EDCs have no measurable estrogenic/antiestrogenic activity in simple *in vitro* systems yet produce significant activity *in vivo*.

The effects of EDCs on enzyme induction and endogenous E_2 levels neither are completely established nor have brain area-specific responses been examined. For this reason, it is still important to monitor effects of EDCs on E_2 levels in individual experiments (Dragnev et al., 1994; Li & Hansen, 1997; Van der Oost et al., 1994). Therefore, a whole-animal model approach should be considered so that endogenous plasma and central E_2 levels are accounted for.

16. ANDROGENIC/ANTIANDROGENIC EFFECTS OF EDCs

Antiandrogenic activity has been noted for a number of EDCs. Perinatal exposure to antiandrogens can be detected in laboratory animals as a decrease in anogenital distance, nipple retention, hypospadias, delay in preputial separation, decrease in sex accessory gland weights, and inhibition of endogenous gene expression. The antiandrogenic effects of estrogens are detectable *in vivo* in male laboratory animals as alterations in mating behavior, serum levels of luteinizing hormone, and spermatogenesis.

Estrogens can produce antiandrogenic effects by the inhibition of testicular androgen secretion via blocking secretion of luteinizing hormone or by direct suppression of T synthesis by Leydig cells. High levels of PCB-inducible androstenedione formation have also been found (Machala et al., 1998). PCB exposure reduced testicular microsomal P450s and affected androstenedione formation and 16β-hydroxylation of T. Mitochondrial CYP, the rate-limiting enzyme of steroidogenesis, was inhibited by 50% in testes of animals exposed to EDCs (Haake-McMillan & Safe, 1991). Adult male rats given single doses of TCDD exhibited decreases in plasma T and dihydrotestosterone concentrations by 90% and 75%, respectively, and decreased seminal vesicle and ventral prostate weights (Moore, Potter, Theobald, Robinson, & Peterson, 1985). In addition, PCB126 can suppress 5α-reduction of T or progesterone in liver microsomes (Yoshihara et al., 1982). Notably, our lab has demonstrated that 5α-reduced metabolites have profound effects to mediate sexually dimorphic behaviors (Frye, 2001a, 2001b). Moreover, 5α-reduced metabolites seem to mitigate many of the behavioral effects of their parent compounds (precursors). *Therefore, levels of T and its 5α-reduced metabolites associated with EDC exposure should be considered.*

17. EFFECTS OF EDCs VIA TRADITIONAL INTRACELLULAR STEROID RECEPTORS

Steroid hormones are lipid molecules with limited solubility in plasma and are accordingly carried through the plasma compartment to target cells by specific plasma transporter proteins. Each transporter protein has a specific ligand-binding domain for its associated hormone. It is generally accepted that the "free" form of the steroid hormone, and not the conjugate of the hormone with its plasma transport protein, enters target cells and binds with the appropriate receptor. Receptors for the steroid hormones are proteins located primarily in the cell nucleus or partitioned between the cytoplasm and the nucleus. The unoccupied steroid receptors may reside in the cell as heterodimeric complexes with the 90 kDa heat-shock protein, which prevents the receptor from binding with the DNA until the receptor has first bound with its steroid hormone. Once the hormone binds to the receptor, the hormone receptor complexes with the heterodimeric heat-shock protein and undergoes a conformational change and is activated. The activated receptor binds with DNA at a specific site, initiating gene transcription and eventually resulting in a specific biological response (e.g., protein proliferation and tissue restructuring; see Fig. 3.4). This traditional view of steroid hormone

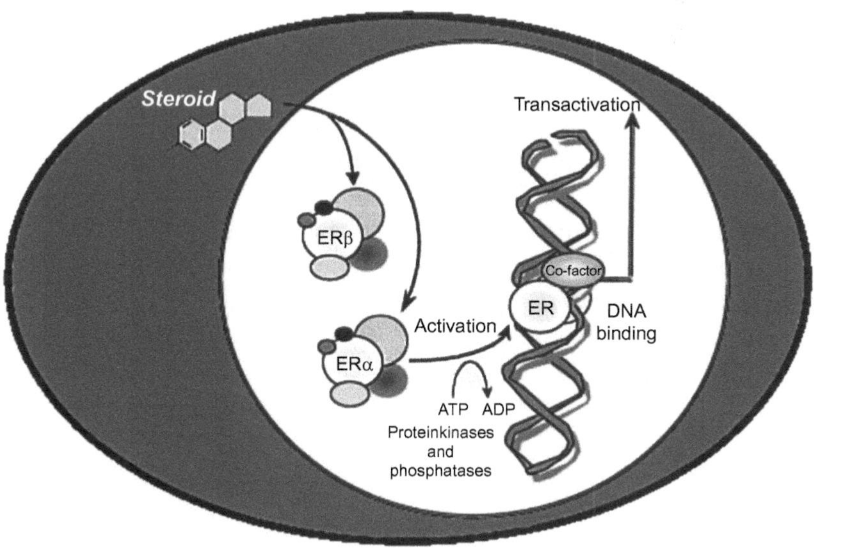

Figure 3.4 Example of traditional effects of steroid hormones at their cognate steroid receptors, which act as transcription factors. In this example, effects of steroid hormones, such as estradiol, to bind estrogen receptor (ER) subtypes, referred to as ERα and ERβ, are shown.

action occurs through a series of feedback mechanisms involving both hormone production and receptor levels in target tissues.

EDCs could interfere at any of the steps described earlier to alter physiology and/or behavior. However, most recent investigations have focused on binding of EDCs to the ER. A chemical mixture may contain a number of estrogenic compounds that agonistically bind the ER, enhancing the response of endogenous estrogens, or it may contain a number of antiestrogens that antagonistically bind the ER, inhibiting the normal action of endogenous estrogens. Some estrogenic compounds in chemical mixtures may exert an overall estrogenic response not by binding to the ER but rather by binding to E_2 plasma transport proteins, resulting in "free" endogenous E_2. A mixture containing both estrogenic and antiestrogens may have no net biological response in the organism. Further, there may be tissue-specific responses between the brain and other substrates and among different CNS sites.

18. OTHER SUBSTRATES TO CONSIDER FOR ACTIONS OF EDCs

The multiplicity of estrogenic mechanisms may result in reported inconsistencies of EDC effects. Attempts to establish estrogenic actions of PCBs may have failed to reach a consensus because data generated to date are not reliable due to the many and variable actions of PCBs interacting with the many and variable responses of E_2-sensitive targets.

18.1. ERα and ERβ

There are at least two distinct ERs isoforms, ERα and ERβ, with significant differences in the ligand-binding domain, which may result in different affinities for EDCs (Kuiper et al., 1997). There may be different cell-specific responses at even the same ER to different ligands due to different receptor-associated proteins required for transcriptional activity by the entire complex. (Feldman, 1997; Jensen, Jacobson, Walf, & Frye, 2010; Katzenellenbogen, 1996; Katzenellenbogen, Iwamoto, Heiman, Lan, & Katzenellenbogen, 1978; McDonnell, Clemm, Hermann, Goldman, & Pike, 1995; McDonnell & Norris, 1997).

18.2. Other intracellular and membrane steroid receptors

In addition to actions via ERs, EDCs may also have their actions via other cognate, intracellular steroid receptors. PCBs can mediate responses of two orphan receptors of the nuclear receptor family, the constitutive androstane

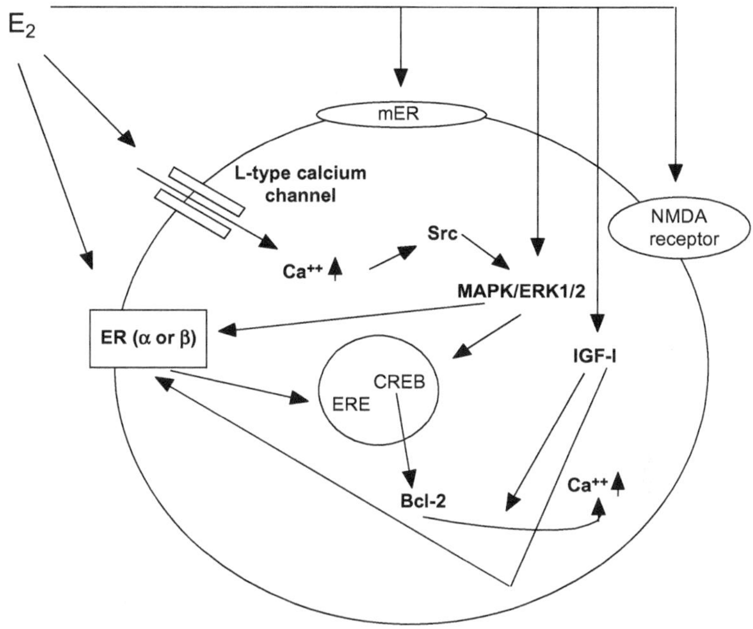

Figure 3.5 Beyond traditional actions solely through intracellular cognate estrogen receptors (ERs; ERα and ERβ), steroids, such as estradiol, and estradiol-mimetics (endocrine disrupters) may have novel actions involving membrane bound ERs, other neurotransmitter systems (e.g., NMDA receptor), and signal transduction cascades (e.g., growth factors, MAPK).

receptor and the pregnane X receptor (Wei, Zhang, Dowhan, Han, & Moore, 2002). Further, there is accumulating evidence for steroid receptors on neuronal membranes that specifically bind estrogens and/or progestins (Toran-Allerand et al., 2002). We have recently reported that bending to membrane progestin receptors mediates sexually dysmorphic responses of rats (Frye et al., 2012).

Like E_2, EDCs may have steroid receptor-independent actions through numerous other substrates, such as signal transduction pathways, calcium influx, and/or neurotransmitter receptors, such as NMDA receptors (see Fig. 3.5). Our lab has been investigating the extent to which E_2's actions via ER and non-ER mechanisms mediate E_2-dependent behaviors.

18.3. Relevant brain areas

It should be noted that the endocrine parameters and reproductive behaviors to be investigated are all mediated by the hypothalamus. However, the non-reproductive behaviors to be examined are mediated, at least in part, by the hippocampus. To date, there has been little investigation in a whole-animal model of the effects of EDCs on E_2 levels and/or activity at intracellular ERs in the brain. Thus, changes in E_2 levels and ER activity in the hypothalamus and hippocampus, concomitant with alterations in endocrine parameters and reproductive behavior and nonreproductive behavior, respectively, are needed to elucidate tissue specificity of EDCs' functions and mechanisms.

19. PRELIMINARY STUDIES

Animal models have been used extensively to characterize processes underlying the development of sexual dimorphic phenotypes. In people, the critical period for androgen sensitivity occurs *in utero*, whereas, in rodents, the critical period for androgen exposure is shortly after parturition. Many studies have been conducted that demonstrate the postnatal androgen surge in male rodents has an essential masculinizing effect. Male rodents are readily feminized by perinatal removal of the testes, the primary endogenous source of masculinizing androgens. Also, female rodents can be readily masculinized by perinatal administration of exogenous androgens or estrogens. These manipulations have revealed the many reproductive and nonreproductive phenotypes that differential androgen exposure during this perinatal critical period can give rise to. In the succeeding text is a review of some of the sex differences in these measures reported in the literature *and* observed in our laboratory. Evidence that these measures are sensitive to perinatal and/or adult exposure to E_2-like compounds is also discussed. Measures are presented in the developmental order in which they are typically manifest. These are the types of measures that EDC effects and mechanisms can and should be examined in.

20. ORGANIZED REPRODUCTIVE PARAMETERS: IMMATURE RATS

There are many measures of reproductive development, which are organized and sexually dimorphic (see Fig. 3.6).

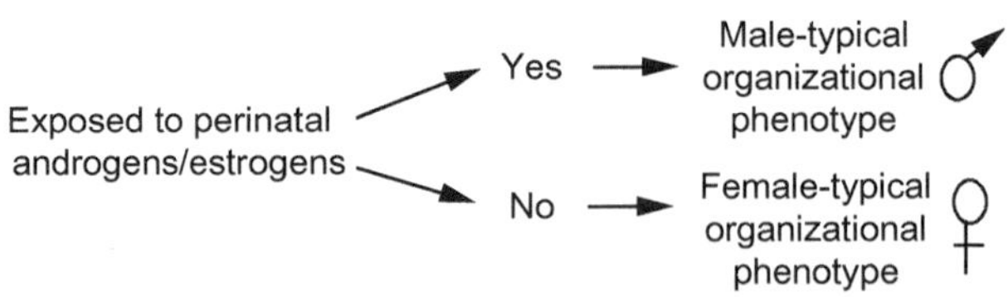

Figure 3.6 Model of organizational effects of androgens/estrogens.

20.1. Perinatal androgen surge

As discussed earlier, male rodents are androgenized by a perinatal T surge and females are feminized by the lack of perinatal T. The effects of exposure to EDCs on the perinatal androgen surge have not been reported. However, the extensive evidence that this perinatal androgen surge is critical for organizing male and female sexual dimorphisms of rodents, in conjunction with data showing EDCs alter sexually dimorphic parameters, suggests further investigation is warranted.

20.2. Anogenital distance

Males have a markedly longer anogenital distance than do females (see Table 3.1; Beatty, 1979). Perinatal castration of males reduces anogenital distance and administering female rats T perinatally increases their anogenital distance (Hotchkiss, Ostby, Vandenburgh, & Gray, 2002). Perinatal exposure to EDCs has a masculizing effect to increase the anogenital distance of female offspring (Wang, Fang, Nunez, & Clemens, 2002) and a feminizing effect in male rats to reduce anogenital distance of male offspring (Ema & Miyawaki, 2002; Hellwig, van Ravenzwaay, Mayer, & Gembardt, 2000).

21. ORGANIZED AND ACTIVATED REPRODUCTIVE PARAMETERS: PERIPUBERTAL AND MATURATION MEASURES

In addition to organizing physiology and behavior, the perinatal androgen surge also establishes male- and female-typical patterns of responsiveness to gonadotropins at puberty, which result in primary secretion and responsiveness by females to E_2 and by males to androgens.

Table 3.1 Typical developmental time periods for androgen surges (present in males, but not female) rodents and greater associated anogenital distance in males compared to females prepuberty (Beatty, 1979)

	Developmental age	Females	Males
Perinatal androgen surge	0–2 days of age	Absent	Present
Anogenital distance	0–21 days of age	7.3 ± 0.3 mm at 21 days	10.3 ± 0.3 mm at 21 days

21.1. Accessory structures

The weight of sexually dimorphic accessory structures is typically less in immature rats than in rats after puberty. With reproductive maturity, and exposure to gonadal hormones, the accessory structures will increase in weight. In immature rats, the administration of E_2 to females or androgens to males can produce the same proliferative effects that are observed at puberty. Prenatal exposure to EDCs has a disruptive effect to reduce the increase in uterine and seminal vesicle weights that are observed at puberty in rats compared to rats administered vehicle (Sager & Girard, 1994, Kuriyama & Chahoud, 2004). These data suggest that developmental exposure to EDCs may interfere with some of the proliferative effects of steroids.

21.2. Puberty

Age of vaginal opening in females and descent of the testes in males are used as indices of onset of puberty (see Table 3.2). In general, female rats undergo puberty prior to males. These measures of onset of puberty are sensitive to perinatal androgens and gestational exposure to EDCs. Advanced age of vaginal opening has been reported following *in utero* exposure to BPA (Tinwell et al., 2002) and postnatal exposure to ethinyl estradiol, DES, and methoxychlor (Kim et al., 2002). Thus, EDCs can alter onset of puberty.

21.3. Estrous cycle/sperm motility

Estrous cycle duration in females and sperm motility in males can be used as a marker of sexual maturity/gonadotropin responsiveness (see Table 3.2). Female rats typically cycle every 4–5 days (Asdell, 1964). Both estrous cycle length and sperm motility are altered by exposure to EDCs. Estrous cycle duration of adult females is lengthened (Sager & Girard, 1994) and sperm motility of adult males is decreased (Hsu, Holsen, & Hopke, 2003) with exposure to PCBs. Thus, EDCs can alter sex differences in sexual maturation.

21.4. E_2 and androgen levels

There are sex differences in circulating levels of gonadal hormones. Typically, females have higher estradiol levels and males have higher T levels (see Table 3.2). At puberty, both males and females display pulsatile release of gonadotropin-releasing hormone (GnRH) from the hypothalamus. In response to hypothalamic GnRH, both male and female rats release LH in a pulsatile fashion from the anterior pituitary. In females, the pulse

Table 3.2 Typical developmental time periods and effects of steroids in female and male rodents for accessory structure weight, onset of puberty, sexual maturity–gonad function, sexual maturity–estrogen levels, sexual maturity–testosterone (T) levels, sexual maturity–hypothalamic estrogen receptor (ER) binding

		Observed effect			
		Females		**Males**	
Accessory structure weight	30 days of age	Ovaries and fallopian tubes with vehicle—34 ± 6 mg	Ovaries and fallopian tubes with estrogen administered—56 ± 8 mg	Testes, vas deferens, prostrate, glands with vehicle—66 ± 5 mg	Testes, vas deferens, prostrate, glands with vehicle—93 + 12 mg
Onset of puberty	30–37 days of age	Vaginal opening at 31 days of age		Testes descend—~36 days of age	
Sexual maturity–gonad function	37+ days	Estrous cycle duration = 4 days		Increased sperm motility	
Sexual maturity–estrogen levels	37+ days	Diestrus—8.2 pg/ml	Proestrus—33.7 pg/ml	Less than 2 ng/ml	
Sexual maturity–T levels	37+ days	Diestrus—serum $T = 0.1$ ng/ml	Proestrus—serum $T = 0.6$ ng/ml	Serum $T = 4.8 + 1.7$ ng/ml	
Sexual maturity–hypothalamic ER binding	37+ days	Diestrus—~20 occupancy	Proestrus—~50% occupancy	~21% occupancy	

frequency and amplitude increases around ovulation, as negative feedback mechanisms are temporarily overwhelmed by increasing E_2 concentrations and positive feedback mechanisms are engaged to result in cyclic variations in E_2 and progestins. In males, the potential for cycling of hormones that is seen in females is destroyed when the blood T concentrations of male rat pups approach that of adult concentrations about 6 h after birth. (This may occur by early exposure to androgens destroying the neural connections between surge and pulse generators.) This results in a clear sexual dimorphism that males have a more tonic release of T in response to LH and FSH and females have a more cyclic E_2 and progestin response to LH and FSH. Exposure to EDCs can alter endogenous levels of gonadal hormones. As previously discussed, estradiol and T are reduced in PCB-exposed female and male rats (Hsu et al., 2003; Kaya et al., 2002), which may reduce sexual dimorphism in levels and responses to these steroid hormones.

21.5. E_2 receptors

There are sex differences in ERs in the hypothalamus and hippocampus, which may underlie sexual dimorphisms in E_2 and androgen responsiveness. As discussed earlier, EDCs can alter ER binding, which may thereby disrupt some sexual dimorphisms in E_2 and androgen responsiveness. Notably, most effects of EDCs on ERs have been examined in the uterus not in the brain.

22. ORGANIZED AND ACTIVATED REPRODUCTIVE PARAMETERS: EFFECTS IN ADULTS

As the material reviewed earlier indicates, perinatal androgen exposure causes lifelong masculinization of physiology, including the pattern of hormone secretion and response in adulthood (see Fig. 3.7). These permanent organizational effects of hormones during developmental give rise to, and can be contrasted with, the reversible behavioral influences of steroid hormones in adulthood, which are termed activational effects of hormones.

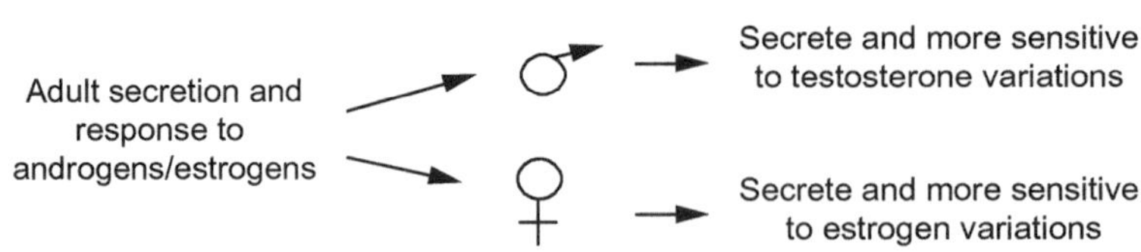

Figure 3.7 Model of activational effects of androgens/estrogens.

The activational effects of hormones on adult behavior are temporary and may wane soon after the hormone is metabolized.

22.1. Manifestation of sexual responsiveness

Lordosis behavior of female rats and mounting behavior of male rats are classic sexually dimorphic, reproductive behaviors of adult rodents (see Table 3.3; Frye & Erskine, 1990). Prenatal androgen exposure results in male-typical mounting behavior in the presence of adequate androgens and sexually receptive females in adulthood. In the absence of perinatal androgens, there is a response to E_2 in adulthood with lordosis to male-typical sexual stimuli. Like other sexually dimorphic behaviors that are organized and activated by steroid hormones, this sex-specific pattern can be reversed by castrating males perinatally or administering females androgens perinatally (Phoenix, Goy, & Resko, 1959).

Developmental or adult exposure to EDCs alters sexually dimorphic, sexual behaviors. Perinatal administration of Aroclor 1254 decreases mounting of male rats and lordosis incidence and intensity of female rats in adulthood (Brouwer et al., 1999; Chung et al., 2001; Sager, 1983). Administration of Aroclor 1221 or 1254 during adulthood disrupted the typical pattern of the female sexual behavior of rats (Chung & Clemens, 1999) and decreased male sexual responses (Hsu et al., 1998; McGivern et al., 1991; Thoreux-Manlay, Le Goascogne, et al., 1995; Thoreux-Manlay, Pinon-Lataillade, et al., 1995). How EDCs have such effects has not been examined.

22.2. Fertility and fecundity

Fertility and fecundity are also important measures of reproductive function. We, and others, have demonstrated that adult female rats that are able to control or "pace" their sexual contacts have greater lordosis intensity, exhibit greater luteal activation in response to mating, are more likely to become pregnant, and have larger litters, than do females that are not able to control their sexual contacts (Erskine, 1985, 1989; Frye & Erskine, 1990). Perinatal or adult stress manipulations to females can interfere with this typical adult pattern of fertility and fecundity (Frye & Orecki, 2002a, 2002b). Also, there is evidence that prenatal exposure to EDCs reduces reproductive success (Sager & Girard, 1994). Virgin females mated with males exposed through lactation to PCBs had a significantly lower proportion of ovulated eggs that implanted, a significantly lower number of live fetuses, and a

Table 3.3 Sex differences in activational effects of steroids between for reproductive behavior (measured by lordosis quotients and ratings—LQs, and LRs—in female rats and number of mounts in male rats), fertility (rates of impregnation), and fecundity (litter size)

	Developmental age	Observed effect			
		Females in behavioral estrus		**Males**	
Reproductive behavior	60–90 days of age	10 paced	10 nonpaced	10 paced	10 nonpaced
		$LQ = 99.9 \pm 0.1\%$ $LR = 1.94 \pm 0.08$	$LQ = 98.8 + 1.2$ $LR = 1.68 \pm 0.19$	29.0 ± 6.3	8.5 ± 3.2
Fertility measure	60–90 days of age	10 paced	10 nonpaced	10 paced	10 nonpaced
		40% of females have >8 days of diestrous smears; 43% pregnant	8% of females have >8 days of diestrous smears; 11% pregnant	42.8% impregnated	0% impregnated
Fecundity measure	60–90 days of age	10 paced	10 nonpaced	10 paced	10 nonpaced
		14 pups/litter	11 pups/litter	14 pups/ litter	11 pups litter

Greater responses for all of these reproductive measures are noted in a seminatural paced mating situation versus when females are not permitted to pace (control the timing of sexual contacts with males) significantly higher rate of resorption than females mated with controls (Sager, 1983). The effects of females' exposure to EDCs have not been extensively investigated. Therefore, we will examine effects of developmental and/or adult exposure to EDCs by males and females on these various parameters of reproductive success.

23. STRATEGY: EDC EFFECTS ON REPRODUCTIVE PARAMETERS: A BIOMARKER OF EFFECTS

Because organizational and activational effects of steroid hormones have established effects on the reproductive parameters discussed earlier, the effects of EDCs on these various parameters may be particularly informative. The effects of the investigated compounds on the various, classic reproductive parameters may enable to characterize the effects and thereby use them as indices or benchmarks to reveal the extent of endocrine disruption. Also, by examining these reproductive parameters throughout development, we will be able to begin to discern lifelong effects of perinatal exposure and differentiate those from acute activational exposure in already organized individuals. Indeed, the most salient effects of EDCs are often observed when administered during development; however, the critical periods of exposure for their effects need to be established. Thus, the strategy of using multiple, established reproductive parameters as biomarkers will enable the investigation of EDC effects on neurodevelopmental, sexually dimorphic nonreproductive behaviors in the most meaningful way.

24. ORGANIZED AND/OR ACTIVATED NONREPRODUCTIVE SEXUALLY DIMORPHIC BEHAVIORS

It has been proposed that the increased incidence in cognitive, behavioral, and/or emotional disruptions in children over the past 30 years may be related to developmental exposure to EDC contaminants (Schettler, 2001). It is necessary to directly test the exposure to EDCs (during development and/or adulthood) to alter cognitive, behavioral, and emotional parameters. As will be reviewed later, the aforementioned indices are sexually dimorphic and sensitive to endocrine manipulations. Although there has not been extensive investigation of EDC effects in these models, the data available are mentioned where appropriate.

24.1. Spatial performance

The most robust sex difference reported in cognitive performance is spatial performance. The sex differences in spatial performance that favor males are organized by perinatal androgens. Castrating males attenuates the sex differences and perinatal androgen administration to females results in a male-typical pattern of spatial performance (Williams & Meck, 1991). The sex difference is observed prepubertally. In the object recognition task, 30-day-old male rats have a better memory for a familiar object and thus spend more time investigating a novel object than do females (see Table 3.4).

In general, adult male rodents also exhibit better performance in the inhibitory avoidance task compared to adult females. Males require fewer trials to criterion than do females in the step-down inhibitory avoidance task (Podhorna et al., 2002; also see Table 3.4). Additionally, male rodents typically outperform females in the water maze task (Kanit et al., 2000; Kavaliers, Ossenkopp, Galea, & Kolb, 1998). Males learn the location of the hidden platform faster (see Table 3.4) and spend more time in the previously correct quadrant of the water maze than do females (Kavaliers et al., 1998). Notably, in adulthood, sex differences in spatial performance are more pronounced when the activational effects of hormones are also considered. For example, castration of adult males reduces the sex difference favoring males, as does examining the performance of female rats in high androgen phases of the cycle (Kritzer, McLaughlin, Smirlis, & Robinson, 2001).

Performance of male and female rats on spatial tasks is altered with exposure to EDCs. Male and female rats perinatally exposed to Aroclor 1254 made significantly more total errors in a spatial reversal task than did vehicle-administered controls (Widholm et al., 2001). Additionally, prenatal

Table 3.4 Sex differences in cognitive performance of rats across development (prepuberty, 30 days of age; young adulthood/peripuberty, 60 days of age; and later adulthood, 90 days of age)

	Developmental age	Observed effect	
		Females	**Males**
Object recognition	30 days of age	2.8 ± 1.1 s investigating novel object	22.0 ± 1.8 s investigating novel object
Inhibitory avoidance	60 days of age	91.6 ± 70.2 s crossover latency	207.8 ± 31.1 s crossover latency
Water maze	90 days of age	112.3 ± 4.0 s to find hidden platform	63.8 ± 7.0 s to find hidden platform

exposure to individual PCB congeners (#28, 118, and 153) resulted in slower acquisition of the T-maze delayed spatial alternation task by female rats (Schantz et al., 1995). These data suggest that spatial performance is sexually dimorphic and can be altered by developmental exposure to EDCs. Effects of adult exposure on spatial performance have not been extensively reported. *Therefore, spatial performance of rats exposed to EDCs either developmentally, in adulthood, or both, in the object recognition, inhibitory avoidance, and water maze tasks should be examined systematically. This will enable developmental effects in spatial performance to be observed. Also, if EDCs have effects by altering E_2 and/or ERs in the hippocampus will be investigated.*

24.2. Rough-and-tumble play

One sexually dimorphic behavior that is only organized and not activated by hormones is play behavior. Male juvenile rats typically engage in more rough-and-tumble play than do females (Meaney, 1989; Pellis, Field, Smith, & Pellis, 1997; see Table 3.5). Males initiate more playful contacts than do females (Pellis & Pellis, 1990; Thor & Holloway, 1983) and male pairs have a greater frequency of play fights than do female pairs (Pellis & Pellis, 1990). This difference in play behavior depends on the actions of sex hormones perinatally. Castration of males at birth reduces the later frequency of play fighting to female-typical levels and perinatal androgenization of females raises the levels of play fighting to near male-typical frequencies (Meaney, Aitken, Jensen, McGinnis, & McEwen, 1985; Thor & Holloway, 1986). Effects of EDCs on rough-and-tumble play have also been observed. Female offspring exposed to BPA perinatally had a masculinization of rough-and-tumble play behavior (Dessi-Fulgheri et al., 2002). These data suggest that rough-and-tumble play is sexually dimorphic and this effect can be reversed by exposure to EDCs. Because play behavior of juvenile rats is robustly and sexually dimorphic and is only organized by steroid hormones, it can be used as a sensitive measure to determine how EDCs may perturb normal developmental, behavioral patterns independent of activational effects.

Table 3.5 Sex differences are notes in rats (prepuberty, 30 days of age) for rough and tumble play behavior

	Developmental age	Observed effect	
		Females	**Males**
Rough-and-tumble play	30 days of age	32.5 ± 2.3 s total play	67.0 ± 24.1 s total play

24.3. Emotional reactivity

There are robust sex differences in indices of arousal/emotional reactivity in rodents that are both organized and activated by steroid hormones. Prepubertally, females are more active than males (see Table 3.6) and perinatal androgenization of females reverses this effect (Beatty, 1979). These sex differences are amplified by activational effects of steroid hormones. There are marked sex differences in behavioral arousal, such that adult females, with high E_2 levels, typically have increased locomotor activity and E_2-dependent anxiolytic behavior compared to females with low E_2 levels and/or intact males (see Table 3.4; Frye et al., 2000). Females also show greater stress hormone responses than do males: these effects are thought to be mitigated by actions of E_2 on the HPA.

Although there has not been extensive investigation, there is evidence that EDCs may alter the typical sexually dimorphic pattern of effects on anxiety behavior. Male rats exposed to phytoestrogens in their diet exhibit elevated plus-maze behavior that is more similar to that of females (Lund & Lephart, 2001). These data suggest that emotional reactivity/arousal is different for males and females and that exposure to EDCs may influence this behavior. Experiments should further explore the effects of EDCs on various indices of emotional reactivity/arousal throughout development. This will enable us to discern if effects of EDCs in these measures are likely organizational, activational, or both.

Table 3.6 Sex differences in emotional reactivity, measured by activity levels and corticosterone in circulation, of female and male rats across development (prepuberty, 30 days of age; young adulthood/peripuberty, 60 days of age; and later adulthood, 90 days of age)

	Developmental age	Observed effect	
		Females	**Males**
Horizontal crossings	30 days of age	267 ± 82 beam breaks	125 ± 26 beam breaks
Open field	60 days of age	162 ± 9 total squares entered	115 ± 16 total squares entered
Elevated plus maze	90 days of age	104 ± 9 s on open arms	38 ± 9 s on open arms
Corticosterone	90 days of age	300 ng/ml	175 ng/ml

25. SUGGESTED EXPERIMENTS MOVING FORWARD

To investigate the estrogenic/antiestrogenic effects of EDCs, it is necessary to consider known indices of reproductive development and behavior, in conjunction with several nonreproductive sexually dimorphic behaviors, discussed earlier. As the pilot data show, there are sex differences in these various reproductive and nonreproductive parameters at different points in development. The following section describes experimental approaches that can be used and provides rationale, justification, and details for such an approach.

26. APPROACH: THE IMPORTANCE OF INTEGRATION OF REPRODUCTIVE AND NONREPRODUCTIVE MEASURES

An important aspect of the effective research on EDCs will be the unique examination of effects of different EDCs on reproductive *and* nonreproductive parameters at analogous points throughout development. Previous research has demonstrated (1) that EDCs can alter reproductive phenotypes and (2) that there are sex differences and hormone effects on nonreproductive behavior. However, there has been very little investigation of EDC effects on hormone-sensitive nonreproductive measures—cognitive performance, behavioral effects, and emotional arousal (which have relevance for neurodevelopmental disorders). Effects of EDCs on reproductive phenotypes will be used as biomarkers to reveal the extent to which their effects on nonreproductive behaviors may be due to disruptions of endocrine systems throughout development. As indicated earlier, our preliminary data indicate that there are sex differences in each of the measures to be utilized. Thus, if such differences are diminished, reversed, or increased with exposure to EDCs, this would suggest that EDC exposure interfered with the modulatory effects of sex hormones on neurodevelopment.

27. APPROACH: EXAMINING EFFECTS OF EDC EXPOSURE THROUGHOUT DEVELOPMENT

The model system described earlier could answer questions about whether exposure to the different EDCs to be investigated alters reproductive and nonreproductive end points throughout development; however, the effects of exposure at different points in the life span should be considered.

28. SUGGESTIONS FOR FUTURE WORK EXAMINING MECHANISMS OF EDCs EFFECTS

The investigation of the functional effects of EDCs throughout development should be extended to E_2 levels and ER binding in the hypothalamus and hippocampus. This whole-animal model can be used to determine EDCs mechanisms in the hypothalamus and hippocampus to mediate reproductive and nonreproductive functions, respectively.

28.1. Activational effects in adults

Adult male or female intact rats should be administered different EDCs (exposed) or vehicles (not exposed). Following 2 weeks of daily exposure (and cycling), nontested rats could be used primarily for tissue collection. In these rats, physiological parameters, such as brain and/or plasma levels of contaminants, E_2, and androgens; hypothalamic and hippocampal ER binding; weight of reproductive tissues; cyclicity; and sperm levels, could be determined. Other groups of exposed and nonexposed male and female rats could be mated with nonexposed stimulus rats. The effects of the EDCs on reproductive behavior (mounting latency in males; lordosis quotients and ratings and pacing in females) and consequences (percent impregnated; number of pups produced with 10 paced and 10 nonpaced intromissions) could be determined. Other groups of exposed and nonexposed male and female rats could be tested for spatial performance (object recognition, inhibitory avoidance, and/or water maze tasks) and emotional reactivity (horizontal crossing, open field, elevated plus-maze tasks, and corticosterone levels). It would not be advantageous to examine rough-and-tumble play because it is a behavior that is not activated by steroid hormones and is only manifest peripubertally.

28.2. Rationale for use of females in second-generation studies

Generational studies could be utilized so that only dams exposed to contaminants because their body burdens may have a salient effect on offspring, due to placental and/or lactational exposure. Further, exposure of adult males to some EDCs decreases sperm production and T levels (Andric et al., 2000); thus, exposed males as parents would not be used to avoid any potential confound and to focus on examination on differential exposure of pups via dams. Further, more experiments looking at second-generation effects in female offspring are needed. Few studies have been conducted perhaps due to the complexity of accounting for estrous cycle variations.

28.3. Organizational effects in offspring

After behavioral testing, all adult, female rats that were exposed or not to EDCs could be mated with stimulus male rats (not been exposed to EDCs). These females can serve as dams for our neurodevelopmental, second-generation studies, in which the relative contributions of adult exposure of dams, gestational, lactational, and/or postweaning exposure on neurodevelopmental effects in offspring, are examined. The effects of exposure to EDCs during these various critical periods on reproductive parameters, spatial performance, play behavior, and/or emotional reactivity of male and female offspring throughout development will be compared.

28.4. Organizational and activational effects in offspring

Comparisons of maternal exposure will inform about organizational effects of maternal body burden, placental, and/or lactational exposure of EDCs on neurodevelopmental processes in male and female offspring. Another important question is whether additional, activational exposure to EDCs as adults has further detrimental effects. To address this, rats can be randomly assigned to receive no further exposure to EDCs. The other half of these groups will receive exposure to the same contaminant as adults. Comparing effects in offspring exposed only during development, versus in development and as adults, will reveal the routes of exposure, critical periods, and/or consequences of EDC exposure. Further, comparisons across generations, between adult behavior of parents (just exposed during adulthood), with their offspring exposed during development and/or adulthood, will elucidate the additive potential for detrimental effects of EDC exposure on neurodevelopment. Thus, the experimental design to be utilized will be very powerful. It will enable multiple comparisons within and across generations to reveal exposures to EDCs that have the most salient effects on neurodevelopmental processes.

29. LOGISTICAL FACTORS FOR EXPERIMENTAL CONTROL AND POWER

29.1. Controlling for cohort and maternal behavior effects

Based upon our extensive experience examining gestational manipulations' effects on steroid action, several important logistical factors are needed to produce the clearest, most interpretable results (Frye & Orecki, 2002a, 2002b). These include controlling for cohort and potential maternal behavior effects between litters. All litters should be culled to 12 pups (6 females and 6 males). This will ensure that no differences in litter size or composition contribute to variability in maternal behavior (Moore & Power, 1992). To control for cohort effects, one male and one female offspring from each litter will be randomly assigned to one of six measurement conditions. Thus, each litter will be randomly represented by a male and female in each measurement condition so that we ensure there are no possible litter confounds.

29.2. Random assignment to sets of dependent measures

There can be six sets of dependent measures. Three sets of measures will involve tissues collected from rats at 0, 30, or 60–90 days of age. Rats' tissues can be collected at 30 days of age and they can be assessed for rough-and-tumble play prior to this tissue collection. These tissues can be utilized to determine brain and/or plasma levels of contaminants, E_2, and androgens; hypothalamic ER binding; weight of reproductive tissues; cyclicity; and sperm levels throughout development. The other three dependent measure conditions can be for reproductive behavior, spatial performance, and emotional reactivity. In the animals used for reproductive measures, onset of puberty and maturity can be determined. In adulthood, sexual responses (lordosis in females and mounting in males) in paced and nonpaced mating paradigms can be examined, as will percentage of rats impregnated and number of offspring. The animals can be tested for spatial performance to have object recognition, inhibitory avoidance, and water maze performance examined at 30, 60, and 90 days of age, respectively. Those rats in which emotional arousal can be examined may be tested for horizontal crossing activity, open field behavior, and plus-maze performance at 30, 60, and 90 days of age, respectively. This can be followed by tissue collection for the determination of plasma corticosterone levels, estrogen levels, and estrogen-binding parameters.

30. SUMMARY

People are exposed to multiple chemicals, which may have diverse effects. The number of chemicals that people are exposed to has increased threefold between the 1940s and the 1990s (Pimentel et al., 1995). Some 80,000 chemicals are in use today and nearly 10% are recognized toxicants.

Although individuals are exposed to multiple chemicals, even single chemical compounds can have multiple effects due to actions of the chemical itself, as well as actions of its metabolic products, which may or may not be similar to the parent compound.

PCBs are examples of chemicals that may have multiple effects for several reasons. First, exposure to chemicals often occurs to mixtures of these chemicals that may exhibit complex synergistic or antagonistic interactions. PCBs were made as commercial mixtures with varying degrees of chlorination. Aroclors are complex PCB mixtures that vary in their estrogenic activity in part due to their chlorine content. In general, compounds with lower chlorination (<48%) are estrogenic and bind competitively to ERs and increase uterine weights (Bitman & Cecil, 1970; Ecobichon & MacKenzie, 1974; Gellert, 1978; Jansen et al., 1993; Korach et al., 1988; Nelson, 1974). We will examine effects of PCB mixtures Aroclors 1242 and 1260, which are expected to have estrogenic and antiestrogenic effects, respectively, based upon their chlorination. Second, individual PCB congeners are subject to metabolism within the body, which can alter the number and positions of chlorine (Carpenter et al., 1998; Phillips et al., 1989) and thereby their estrogenicity. Effects of individual congeners, PCBs 52 and 77, will be examined, for their estrogenic and antiestrogenic activity, respectively. PCBs have been studied extensively for their effects on reproductive parameters. A significant contribution of our investigation of these compounds will be to determine their effects on other sexually dimorphic behaviors, such as spatial cognition, behavior, and emotional arousal.

Conversely, many studies have focused on the cognitive effects of lead exposure. There is evidence for lead to alter reproductive parameters; however, this has received much less attention. For example, lead can alter E_2 metabolism and can cause delayed pubertal development in rats of both sexes (Der, Fahim, Hilderbrand, & Fahim, 1974; Kimmell, Grant, Sloan, & Gladen, 1980; McGivern et al., 1991; Ronis et al., 1998). Thus, a significant contribution of our investigation of lead will be to determine its effects on reproductive parameters, in addition to effects on spatial cognition and emotional arousal and other behavioral processes.

Thus, we can investigate specificity of these compounds by comparing the effects of PCB mixtures and individual congeners with varying estrogenic capacity, that have known effects on reproduction, but not cognition or affect. Also, lead has known effects on cognition, but not reproduction or affect. *Thus, comparing different EDC effects on various behavioral processes,*

E_2 levels, and ER binding will advance the field and elucidate the mechanisms in different brain areas by which EDCs may have their functional effects.

30.1. Other considerations

Depending on the results of each compound investigated, and the time and resources available, there are other investigations that could be pursued. First, it is necessary to further characterize the effects of the proposed contaminants by examining other dose regimens on the parameters and behaviors indicated. Second, it is necessary to investigate other possible non-ER mechanisms by which these contaminants may have their actions. Finally, it would be fruitful to examine effects of adult or developmental exposure to EDCs on behavior into senescence.

31. CONCLUSIONS

Known effects and mechanisms of EDS have been previewed. Further, proposed investigation of EDCs in systematic cross-generational studies has been suggested to advance the field. The mechanisms for these EDCs' functional effects on reproductive processes, spatial performance, and arousal could be revealed.

The experiments that will address several shortcomings that have been previously identified as needing to be filled in the EDC field are suggested (Brouwer et al., 1995; Brouwer et al., 1999). First, there is a need to examine effects of EDC mixtures, as well as congeners, in sexually mature animals, prior to, during, and after pregnancy. The experimental paradigm suggested will examine effects of exposures in adulthood, through pregnancy and lactation, and throughout the offspring's development. The experiments would also enable comparisons to be made between effects of some mixtures versus individual congeners and compare their effects with the non-PCB EDC lead. Second, there is a need to examine the effects of EDCs that have the most direct relevance for people. Studies suggested utilize developmental test batteries as indices of reproductive, cognitive, and emotional processes that are directly relevant for people. Also, compounds will be investigated that people are directly exposed to. Third, animal studies using functional/developmental assessments are needed that include long-term follow-up with equal emphasis on behavior and reproductive end points. The suggested research utilizes end points of reproductive indices, as well as reproductive and nonreproductive behaviors. The investigation of EDC effects in whole-animal models and with behavioral end points is particularly appropriate because behaviors are very sensitive to hormones and will reveal with effects of EDCs that are most relevant for people. Throughout the second generation, long-term effects may extend to adulthood and into aging and senescence (as possible). Further, most of the prior research has focused on reproductive parameters that are primarily mediated by the hypothalamus. Nonreproductive behaviors can be examined to reveal effects mediated by the hippocampus. Fourth, measurement of levels of contaminants and their modes of action should be performed in target tissues throughout development to identify critical periods, effects, and processes. This should be accomplished in future studies. Tissues can be collected in adults administered with contaminants and their offspring exposed at different points in development. Tissues can be collected around birth, prepubertally, and in adulthood so that levels of contaminants and their effects on steroid hormone levels and steroid receptors can be determined. This will enable the identification of coincident effects on these measures concomitant with changes in functional end points throughout development.

The suggested research will fill a void in the EDC literature and will expand the current knowledge about basic sex differences and their biological underpinnings. The compounds suggested to investigate have varying effects on androgen/E_2 levels and ER activity. Thus, comparing effects of these various compounds on developmental processes and behaviors that are known to be sexually dimorphic will reveal the importance of altered androgen/E_2 levels, and ER activity, for the mediation of these established sex differences.

ACKNOWLEDGMENT

Assistance provided by Drs. Alicia Walf and Madeline Rhodes is greatly appreciated.

REFERENCES

Allen, D. L., Mitchner, N. A., Uveges, T. E., Nephew, K. P., Khan, S., & Ben-Jonathan, N. (1997). Cell-specific induction of c-fos expression in the pituitary gland by estrogen. *Endocrinology, 138*(5), 2128–2135.

Aloisi, A. M., Ceccarelli, I., & Lupo, C. (1998). Behavioural and hormonal effects of restraint stress and formalin test in male and female rats. *Brain Research Bulletin, 47*(1), 57–62.

Altmann, L., Sveinsson, K., Kramer, U., Weishoff-Houben, M., Turfeld, M., Winneke, G., et al. (1998). Visual functions in 6-year-old children in relation to lead and mercury levels. *Neurotoxicology and Teratology, 20*(1), 9–17.

Altmann, L., Weinsberg, F., Sveinsson, K., Lilienthal, H., Wiegand, H., & Winneke, G. (1993). Impairment of long-term potentiation and learning following chronic lead exposure. *Toxicology Letters, 66*(1), 105–112.

Andric, S. A., Kostic, T. S., Dragisic, S. M., Andric, N. L., Stojilkovic, S. S., & Kovacevic, R. Z. (2000). Acute effects of polychlorinated biphenyl-containing and -free transformer fluids on rat testicular steroidogenesis. *Environmental Health Perspectives*, *108*(10), 955–959.

Apostoli, P., Kiss, P., Porru, S., Bonde, J. P., & Vanhoorne, M. (1998). Male reproductive toxicity of lead in animals and humans ASCLEPIOS Study Group. *Occupational and Environmental Medicine*, *55*(6), 364–374.

Arcaro, K. F., Vakharia, D. D., Yang, Y., & Gierthy, J. F. (1998). Lack of synergy of weakly estrogenic hydroxylated polychlorinated biphenyls and pesticides. *Environmental Health Perspectives*, *106*(S4), 1041–1046.

Asdell, S. A. (1964). *Patterns of mammalian reproduction*. Ithaca, NY: Cornell University Press.

Ashby, J., Lefevre, P. A., Odum, J., Tinwell, H., Kennedy, S. J., Beresford, N., et al. (1997). Failure to confirm estrogenic activity for benzoic acid and clofibrate: Implications for lists of endocrine-disrupting agents. *Regulatory Toxicology and Pharmacology*, *26*(1 Pt 1), 96–101.

ATSDR, (1993). Priority health conditions. An integrated strategy to evaluate the relationship between illness and exposure to hazardous substances. In J. A. Lybarger, R. F. Spengler, & C. T. DeRosa (Eds.), Atlanta, GA: Agency for Toxic Substances and Disease Registry.

Baker, E. L., Jr., Landrigan, P. J., Glueck, C. J., Zack, M. M., Jr., Liddle, J. A., Burse, V. W., et al. (1980). Metabolic consequences of exposure to polychlorinated biphenyls (PCB) in sewage sludge. *American Journal of Epidemiology*, *112*(4), 553–563.

Banks, E. C., Ferretti, L. E., & Shucard, D. W. (1997). Effects of low level lead exposure on cognitive function in children: A review of behavioral, neuropsychological and biological evidence. *Neurotoxicology*, *18*(1), 237–281.

Beatty, W. W. (1979). Gonadal hormones and sex differences in nonreproductive behaviors in rodents: Organizational and activational influences. *Hormones and Behavior*, *12*(2), 112–163.

Berenbaum, F., Le Gars, L., Toussirot, E., Sanon, A., Bories, C., Kaplan, G., et al. (2000). Marked elevation of serum N-acetyl-beta-D-hexosaminidase activity in rheumatoid rheumatoid arthritis. *Clinical and Experimental Rheumatology*, *18*(1), 63–66.

Bernstein, L., & Ross, R. K. (1993). Endogenous hormones and breast cancer risk. *Epidemiologic Reviews*, *15*(1), 48–65.

Bitman, J., & Cecil, H. C. (1970). Estrogenic activity of DDT analogs and polychlorinated biphenyls. *Journal of Agricultural and Food Chemistry*, *18*(6), 1108–1112.

Bitman, J., Cecil, H. C., & Harris, S. J. (. 1972). Biological effects of polychlorinated biphenyls in rats and quail. *Environ Health Perspect.*, *1*, 145–149Apr.

Bodnar, R. J., Romero, M. T., & Kramer, E. (1988). Organismic variables and pain inhibition: Roles of gender and aging. *Brain Research Bulletin*, *21*(6), 947–953.

Brouwer, A., Ahlborg, U. G., Van den Berg, M., Birnbaum, L. S., Boersma, E. R., Bosveld, B., et al. (1995). Functional aspects of developmental toxicity of polyhalogenated aromatic hydrocarbons in experimental animals and human infants. *European journal of pharmacology*, *293*(1), 1–40.

Brouwer, A., Longnecker, M. P., Birnbaum, L. S., Cogliano, J., Kostyniak, P., Moore, J., et al. (1999). Characterization of potential endocrine-related health effects at low-dose levels of exposure to PCBs. *Environmental Health Perspectives*, *107*(Suppl. 4), 639–649.

Calvert, G. M., Willie, K. K., Sweeney, M. H., Fingerhut, M. A., & Halperin, W. E. (1996). Evaluation of serum lipid concentrations among U.S. workers exposed to 2,3,7,8-tetrachlorodibenzo-p-dioxin. *Archives of Environmental Health*, *51*(2), 100–107.

Carlesen, E., Giwercman, A., Keiding, N., & Skakkebaek, N. E. (1992). Evidence for decreasing quality of semen during the past 50 years. *British Medical Journal*, *305*, 609–613.

Carpenter, D. O., Arcaro, K., Bushu, B., Niemi, W. D., Pang, S., & Vakharia, D. D. (1998). Human health and chemical mixtures: An overview. *Environmental Health Perspectives, 106*(6), 1263–1270.

Carpenter, D. O., Arcaro, K., & Spink, D. (2002). Understanding the human health effects of chemical mixtures. *Environmental Health Perspectives, 110*, 25–42.

Carpenter, D. O., Hussain, R. J., Berger, D. F., Lombardo, J. P., & Park, H. Y. (2002). Electrophysiologic and behavioral effects of perinatal and acute exposure of rats to lead and polychlorinated biphenyls. *Environmental Health Perspectives, 110*(Suppl. 3), 377–386.

Carpenter, D. O., Shen, Y., Nguyen, T., Le, L., & Lininger, L. L. (2001). Incidence of endocrine disease among residents of New York areas of concern. *Environmental Health Perspectives, 109*(Suppl. 6), 845–851.

Chen, H. H., Ma, T., Paul, I. A., Spencer, J. L., & Ho, I. K. (1997). Developmental lead exposure and two-way active avoidance training alter the distribution of protein kinase C activity in the rat hippocampus. *Neurochemical Research, 22*(9), 1119–1125.

Chung, Y. W., & Clemens, L. G. (1999). Effects of perinatal exposure to polychlorinated biphenyls on development of female sexual behavior. *Bulletin of Environmental Contamination and Toxicology, 62*(6), 664–670.

Chung, Y. W., Nunez, A. A., & Clemens, L. G. (2001). Effects of neonatal polychlorinated biphenyl exposure on female sexual behavior. *Physiology and Behavior, 74*(3), 363–370.

Clarkson, T. W. (1983). Methylmercury toxicity to the mature and developing nervous system: Possible mechanism. In B. Sarker (Ed.), *Biological aspects of metals and metal-related diseases* (pp. 183–197). New York: Raven Press.

Collaer, M. L., & Hines, M. (1995). Human behavioral sex differences: A role for gonadal hormones during early development? *Psychological Bulletin, 118*(1), 55–107.

Cooke, P. S., Young, P., Hess, R. A., & Cunha, G. R. (1991). Estrogen receptor expression in developing epididymis, efferent ductules, and other male reproductive organs. *Endocrinology, 128*(6), 2874–2879.

Darvill, T., Lonky, E., Reihman, J., Stewart, P., & Pagano, J. (2000). Prenatal exposure to PCBs and infant performance on the fagan test of infant intelligence. *Neurotoxicology, 21*(6), 1029–1038.

Der, R., Fahim, Z., Hilderbrand, D., & Fahim, M. (1974). Combined effects of lead and low protein diet on growth, sexual development and metabolism in female rats. *Research Communication in Chemical Pathology and Pharmacology, 9*, 723–738.

Dessi-Fulgheri, F., Porrini, S., & Farabollini, F. (2002). Effects of perinatal exposure to bisphenol A on play behavior of female and male juvenile rats. *Environmental Health Perspectives, 110*(Suppl. 3), 403–407.

Dewailly, E., Ayotte, P., Brisson, J., & Dodin, S. (1994). Breast cancer and organochlorines. *Lancet, 344*(8938), 1707–1708.

Dewailly, E., Ryan, J. J., Laliberte, C., Bruneau, S., Weber, J. P., Gingras, S., et al. (1994). Exposure of remote maritime populations to coplanar PCBs. *Environmental Health Perspectives, 102*(Suppl. 1), 205–209.

Di Lorenzo, D., Villa, R., Biasiotto, G., Belloli, S., Ruggeri, G., Albertini, A., et al. (2002). Isomer-specific activity of dichlorodyphenyltrichloroethane with estrogen receptor in adult and suckling estrogen reporter mice. *Endocrinology, 143*(12), 4544–4551.

Dragnev, K. H., Beebe, L. E., Jones, C. R., Fox, S. D., Thomas, P. E., Nims, R. W., et al. (1994). Subchronic dietary exposure to Aroclor 1254 in rats: Accumulation of PCBs in liver, blood, and adipose tissue and its relationship to induction of various hepatic drug-metabolizing enzymes. *Toxicology and Applied Pharmacology, 125*, 111–122.

Ecobichon, D. J., & MacKenzie, D. O. (1974). The uterotropic activity of commercial and isomerically-pure chlorobiphenyls in the rat. *Research Communications in Chemical Pathology and Pharmacology, 9*(1), 85–95.

Ema, M., & Miyawaki, E. (2002). Effects on development of the reproductive system in male offspring of rats given butyl benzyl phthalate during late pregnancy. *Reproductive Toxicology, 16*(1), 71–76.

Emmett, E. A., Maroni, M., Schmith, J. M., Levin, B. K., & Jefferys, J. (1988). Studies of transformer repair workers exposed to PCBs: I. Study design, PCB concentrations, questionnaire, and clinical examination results. *American Journal of Industrial Medicine, 13*(4), 415–427.

Erskine, M. S. (1985). Effects of paced coital stimulation on estrus duration in intact cycling rats and ovariectomized and ovariectomized-adrenalectomized hormone-primed rats. *Behavioral Neuroscience, 99*(1), 151–161.

Erskine, M. S. (1989). Solicitation behavior in the estrous female rat: A review. *Hormones and Behavior, 23*(4), 473–502.

Feldman, D. (1997). Estrogens from plastic—Are we being exposed? *Endocrinology, 138*(5), 1777–1779.

Fielden, M. R., Chen, I., Chittim, B., Safe, S. H., & Zacharewski, T. R. (1997). Examination of the estrogenicity of 2,4,6,2',6'-pentachlorobiphenyl (PCB 104), its hydroxylated metabolite 2,4,6,2',6'-pentachloro-4-biphenylol (HO-PCB 104), and a further chlorinated derivative, 2,4,6,2',4',6'-hexachlorobiphenyl (PCB 155). *Environmental health perspectives, 105*(11), 1238–1248.

Fielden, M. R., Halgren, R. G., Tashiro, C. H., Yeo, B. R., Chittim, B., Chou, K., et al. (2001). Effects of gestational and lactational exposure to Aroclor 1242 on sperm quality and in vitro fertility in early adult and middle-aged mice. *Reproductive Toxicology, 15*(3), 281–292.

Figueiredo, H. F., Dolgas, C. M., & Herman, J. P. (2002). Stress activation of cortex and hippocampus is modulated by sex and stage of estrus. *Endocrinology, 143*(7), 2534–2540.

Fitch, R. H., & Denenberg, V. H. (1998). A role for ovarian hormones in sexual differentiation of the brain. *Behavioral and Brain Sciences, 21*(3), 311–327.

Flesch-Janys, D., Berger, J., Gurn, P., Manz, A., Nagel, S., Waltsgott, H., et al. (1995). Exposure to polychlorinated dioxins and furans (PCDD/F) and mortality in a cohort of workers from a herbicide-producing plant in Hamburg, Federal Republic of Germany. *American Journal of Epidemiology, 142*(11), 1165–1175.

Frye, C. A. (2001a). The role of neurosteroids and non-genomic effects of progestins and androgens in mediating sexual receptivity of rodents. *Brain Research. Brain Research Reviews, 37*(1–3), 201–222.

Frye, C. A. (2001b). The role of neurosteroids and nongenomic effects of progestins in the ventral tegmental area in mediating sexual receptivity of rodents. *Hormones and Behavior, 40*(2), 226–233.

Frye, C. A., Bo, E., Calamandrei, G., Calzà, L., Dessì-Fulgheri, F., Fernández, M., et al. (2012). Endocrine disrupters: A review of some sources, effects, and mechanisms of actions on behaviour and neuroendocrine systems. *Journal of Neuroendocrinology, 24*(1), 144–159.

Frye, C. A., & Erskine, M. S. (1990). Influence of time of mating and paced copulation on induction of pseudopregnancy in cyclic female rats. *Journal of Reproduction and Fertility, 90*(2), 375–385.

Frye, C. A., & Orecki, Z. A. (2002a). Prenatal stress alters reproductive responses of rats in behavioral estrus and paced mating of hormone-primed rats. *Hormones and Behavior, 42*(4), 472–483.

Frye, C. A., & Orecki, Z. A. (2002b). Prenatal stress produces deficits in socio-sexual behavior of cycling, but not hormone-primed, Long-Evans rats. *Pharmacology, Biochemistry, and Behavior, 73*(1), 53–60.

Frye, C. A., Paris, J. J., Walf, A. A., & Rusconi, J. C. (2011). Effects and mechanisms of 3α,5α,-THP on emotion, motivation, and reward functions involving Pregnane Xenobiotic Receptor. *Frontiers in Neuroscience, 5*, 136.

Frye, C. A., Petralia, S. M., & Rhodes, M. E. (2000). Estrous cycle and sex differences in performance on anxiety tasks coincide with increases in hippocampal progesterone and 3alpha,5alpha-THP. *Pharmacology, Biochemistry, and Behavior, 67*(3), 587–596.

Frye, C. A., & Rhodes, M. E. (2002). Enhancing effects of estrogen on inhibitory avoidance performance may be in part independent of intracellular estrogen receptors in the hippocampus. *Brain Research, 956*(2), 285–293.

Garavan, H., Morgan, R. E., Levitsky, D. A., Hermer-Vazquez, L., & Strupp, B. J. (2000). Enduring effects of early lead exposure: Evidence for a specific deficit in associative ability. *Neurotoxicology and Teratology, 22*(2), 151–164.

Gellert, R. J. (1978). Uterotrophic activity of polychlorinated biphenyls (PCB) and induction of precocious reproductive aging in neonatally treated female rats. *Environmental Research, 16*(1–3), 123–130.

Gilbert, M. E., & Crofton, K. M. (1999). Developmental exposure to a commercial PCB mixture (Aroclor 1254) produces a persistent impairment in long-term potentiation in the rat dentate gyrus in vivo. *Brain Research, 850*(1–2), 87–95.

Golden, R. J., Noller, K. L., Titus-Ernstoff, L., Kaufman, R. H., Mittendorf, R., Stillman, R., et al. (1998). Environmental endocrine modulators and human health: An assessment of the biological evidence. *Critical Reviews in Toxicology, 28*(2), 109–227.

Goldin, B. R., Adlercreutz, H., Gorbach, S. L., Woods, M. N., Dwyer, J. T., Conlon, T., et al. (1986). The relationship between estrogen levels and diets of Caucasian American and Oriental immigrant women. *American Journal of Clinical Nutrition, 44*(6), 945–953.

Goldman, L. S., Genel, M., Bezman, R. J., & Slanetz, P. J. (1998). Diagnosis and treatment of attention-deficit/hyperactivity disorder in children and adolescents. Council on Scientific Affairs, American Medical Association. *JAMA, 279*(14), 1100–1107.

Goy, R. W., & McEwen, B. S. (1980). *Sexual differentiation of the brain*. Cambridge: MIT Press.

Goy, R. W., & Phoenix, C. H. (1972). The effects of testosterone propionate administered before birth on the development of behavior in genetic female rhesus monkeys. *UCLA Forum in Medical Sciences, 15*, 193–201.

Gray, L. E., Jr., Kelce, W. R., Monosson, E., Ostby, J. S., & Birnbaum, L. S. (1995). Exposure to TCDD during development permanently alters reproductive function in male Long Evans rats and hamsters: Reduced ejaculated and epididymal sperm numbers and sex accessory gland weights in offspring with normal androgenic status. *Toxicology and Applied Pharmacology, 131*(1), 108–118.

Guillette, E. A., Meza, M. M., Aquilar, M. G., Soto, A. D., & Enedina, I. (1998). An anthropological approach to the evaluation of preschool children exposed to pesticides in Mexico. *Environmental Health Perspectives, 106*, 347–353.

Guo, Y. L., Hse, C. C., & Lambert, G. H. (1996). Effects of environmental chemicals (EC) on sexual maturation. *Pediatric Research, 39*, 74.

Guo, Y. L., Lai, T. J., Chen, S. J., & Hsu, C. C. (1995). Gender-related decrease in Raven's progressive matrices scores in children prenatally exposed to polychlorinated bophenyis and related contaminants. *Environmental Contamination and Toxicology, 55*, 8–13.

Guttes, S., Failing, K., Neumann, K., Kleinstein, J., Georgii, S., & Brunn, H. (1998). Chlororganic pesticides and polychlorinated biphenyls in breast tissue of women with benign and malignant breast disease. *Archives of Environmental Contamination and Toxicology, 35*(1), 140–147.

Haake-McMillan, J. M., & Safe, S. H. (1991). Neonatal exposure to Aroclor 1254: Effects on adult hepatic testosterone hydroxylase activities. *Xenobiotica, 21*(4), 481–489.

Halldin, K., Axelsson, J., & Brunstrom, B. (2003). Effects of endocrine modulators on sexual differentiation and reproductive function Japanese quail. In *2nd International meeting steroids and nervous system, Torino, Italy* (p. 13).
Hansen, L. G. (1998). Stepping backward to improve assessment of PCB congener toxicities. *Environmental Health Perspectives, 106*(Suppl. 1), 171–189.
Hany, J., Lilienthal, H., Roth-Harer, A., Ostendorp, G., Heinzow, B., & Winneke, G. (1999). Behavioral effects following single and combined maternal exposure to PCB 77 (3,4,3',4'-tetrachlorobiphenyl) and PCB 47 (2,4,2',4'-tetrachlorobiphenyl) in rats. *Neurotoxicology and Teratology, 21*(2), 147–156.
Hany, J., Lilienthal, H., Sarasin, A., Roth-Harer, A., Fastabend, A., Dunemann, L., et al. (1999). Developmental exposure of rats to a reconstituted PCB mixture or aroclor 1254: Effects on organ weights, aromatase activity, sex hormone levels, and sweet preference behavior. *Toxicology and Applied Pharmacology, 158*(3), 231–243.
Hayes, C. L., Spink, D. C., Spink, B. C., Cao, J. Q., Walker, N. J., & Sutter, T. R. (1996). 17 Beta-estradiol hydroxylation catalyzed by human cytochrome P450 1B1. *Proceedings of the National Academy of Sciences of the United States of America, 93*(18), 9776–9781.
Hellwig, J., van Ravenzwaay, B., Mayer, M., & Gembardt, C. (2000). Pre- and postnatal oral toxicity of vinclozolin in Wistar and Long-Evans rats. *Regulatory Toxicology and Pharmacology, 32*(1), 42–50.
Hori, N., Busselberg, D., Matthews, M. R., Parsons, P. J., & Carpenter, D. O. (1993). Lead blocks LTP by an action not at NMDA receptors. *Experimental Neurology, 119*(2), 192–197.
Hotchkiss, A. K., Ostby, J. S., Vandenburgh, J. G., & Gray, L. E., Jr. (2002). Androgens and environmental antiandrogens affect reproductive development and play behavior in the Sprague-Dawley rat. *Environmental Health Perspectives, 110*(Suppl. 3), 435–439.
Hsu, Y. K., Holsen, T. M., & Hopke, P. K. (2003). Locating and quantifying PCB sources in Chicago: Receptor modeling and field sampling. *Environmental Science and Technology, 37*(4), 681–690.
Hsu, P. C., Hsu, C. C., Liu, M. Y., Chen, L. Y., & Guo, Y. L. (1998). Lead-induced changes in spermatozoa function and metabolism. *Journal of Toxicology and Environmental Health. Part A, 55*(1), 45–64.
Hsu, S. T., Ma, C. I., Hsu, S. K., Wu, S. S., Hsu, N. H., Yeh, C. C., et al. (1985). Discovery and epidemiology of PCB poisoning in Taiwan: A four-year followup. *Environmental Health Perspectives, 59*, 5–10.
Hunter, D. J., Hankinson, S. E., Laden, F., Colditz, G. A., Manson, J. E., Willett, W. C., et al. (1997). Plasma organochlorine levels and the risk of breast cancer. *The New England Journal of Medicine, 337*(18), 1253–1258.
Hutchison, J. B. (1997). Gender-specific steroid metabolism in neural differentiation. *Cellular and Molecular Neurobiology, 17*(6), 603–626.
Jacobson, S. W., Fein, G. G., Jacobson, J. L., Schwartz, P. M., & Dowler, J. K. (1985). The effect of intrauterine PCB exposure on visual recognition memory. *Child Development, 56*(4), 853–860.
Jacobson, J. L., Jacobson, S. W., & Humphrey, H. E. (1990). Effects of in utero exposure to polychlorinated biphenyls and related contaminants on cognitive functioning in young children. *Journal of Pediatrics, 116*(1), 38–45.
Jansen, H. T., Cooke, P. S., Porcelli, J., Liu, T. C., & Hansen, L. G. (1993). Estrogenic and antiestrogenic actions of PCBs in the female rat: In vitro and in vivo studies. *Reproductive Toxicology, 7*(3), 237–248.
Jensen, E. V., Jacobson, H. I., Walf, A. A., & Frye, C. A. (2010). Estrogen action: A historic perspective on the implications of considering alternative approaches. *Physiology and Behavior, 99*(2), 151–162.

Kanit, L., Taskiran, D., Yilmaz, O. A., Balkan, B., Demirgoren, S., Furedy, J. J., et al. (2000). Sexually dimorphic cognitive style in rats emerges after puberty. *Brain Research Bulletin*, *52*(4), 243–248.

Kashimoto, T., Miyata, H., Fukushima, S., Kunita, N., Ohi, G., & Tung, T. C. (1985). PCBs, PCQs and PCDFs in blood of yusho and yu-cheng patients. *Environmental Health Perspectives*, *59*, 73–78.

Katzenellenbogen, B. S. (1996). Estrogen receptors: Bioactivities and interactions with cell signaling pathways. *Biology of Reproduction*, *54*(2), 287–293.

Katzenellenbogen, B. S., Iwamoto, H. S., Heiman, D. F., Lan, N. C., & Katzenellenbogen, J. A. (1978). Stilbestrols and stilbestrol derivatives: Estrogenic potency and temporal relationships between estrogen receptor binding and uterine growth. *Molecular and Cellular Endocrinology*, *10*(1), 103–113.

Kavaliers, M., Ossenkopp, K. P., Galea, L. A., & Kolb, B. (1998). Sex differences in spatial learning and prefrontal and parietal cortical dendritic morphology in the meadow Microtus pennsylvanicus. *Brain Research*, *810*(1–2), 41–47.

Kaya, H., Hany, J., Fastabend, A., Roth-Harer, A., Winneke, G., & Lilienthal, H. (2002). Effects of maternal exposure to a reconstituted mixture of polychlorinated biphenyls on sex-dependent behaviors and steroid hormone concentrations in rats: Dose-response relationship. *Toxicology and Applied Pharmacology*, *178*(2), 71–81.

Key, T. J., Chen, J., Wang, D. Y., Pike, M. C., & Boreham, J. (1990). Sex hormones in women in rural China and in Britain. *British Journal of Cancer*, *62*(4), 631–636.

Kim, H. S., Shin, J. H., Moon, H. J., Kim, T. S., Kang, I. H., Seok, J. H., et al. (2002). Evaluation of the 20-day pubertal female assay in Sprague-Dawley rats treated with DES, tamoxifen, testosterone, and flutamide. *Toxicological Sciences*, *67*(1), 52–62.

Kimmell, C. A., Grant, L. D., Sloan, C. S., & Gladen, B. C. (1980). Chronic low-level lead toxicity in the rat. *Toxicology and Applied Pharmacology*, *56*, 28–41.

Korach, K. S., Sarver, P., Chae, K., McLachlan, J. A., & McKinney, J. D. (1988). Estrogen receptor-binding activity of polychlorinated hydroxybiphenyls: Conformationally restricted structural probes. *Molecular Pharmacology*, *33*(1), 120–126.

Kramer, V. J., Helferich, W. G., Bergman, A., Klasson-Wehler, E., & Giesy, J. P. (1997). Hydroxylated polychlorinated biphenyl metabolites are anti-estrogenic in a stably transfected human breast adenocarcinoma (MCF7) cell line. *Toxicology and Applied Pharmacology*, *144*(2), 363–376.

Kreiger, N., Wolff, M. S., Hiatt, R. A., Rivera, M., Vogelman, J., & Orentreich, N. (1994). Breast cancer and serum organochlorines: A prospective study among white, black and Asian women. *Journal of the National Cancer Institute*, *86*, 589–599.

Kreiss, K. (1985). Studies on populations exposed to polychlorinated biphenyls. *Environmental Health Perspectives*, *60*, 193–199.

Kreitzer, J. F., & Heinz, G. H. (1974). The effect of sublethal dosages of five pesticides and a polychlorinated biphenyl on the avoidance response on Coturnix quail chicks. *Environmental Pollution*, *6*, 21–29.

Kritzer, M. F., McLaughlin, P. J., Smirlis, T., & Robinson, J. K. (2001). Gonadectomy impairs T-maze acquisition in adult male rats. *Hormones and Behavior*, *39*(2), 167–174.

Kuiper, G. G., Carlsson, B., Grandien, K., Enmark, E., Haggblad, J., Nilsson, S., et al. (1997). Comparison of the ligand binding specificity and transcript tissue distribution of estrogen receptors alpha and beta. *Endocrinology*, *138*(3), 863–870.

Kupfer, D. (1988). Critical evaluation of methods for detection and assessment of estrogenic compounds in mammals: Strengths and limitations for applications to risk assessment. *Reproductive Toxcology*, *1*, 147–153.

Kuriyama, S. N., & Chahoud, I. (2004). In utero exposure to low-dose 2,3',4,4',5-pentachlorobiphenyl (PCB 118) impairs male fertility and alters neurobehavior in rat offspring. *Toxicology*, *202*(3), 185–197.

Lancranjan, I., Popescu, H. I., GAvanescu, O., Klepsch, I., & Serbanescu, M. (1975). Reproductive ability of workmen occupationally exposed to lead. *Archives of Environmental Health, 30*(8), 396–401.

Lanphear, B. P., Dietrich, K., Auinger, P., & Cox, C. (2000). Cognitive deficits associated with blood lead concentrations <10 microg/dL in US children and adolescents. *Public Health Reports, 115*(6), 521–529.

Lebel, J., Mergler, D., Branches, F., Lucotte, M., Amorim, M., Larribe, F., et al. (1998). Neurotoxic effects of low-level methylmercury contamination in the Amazonian Basin. *Environmental Research, 79*(1), 20–32.

Lephart, E. D., West, T. W., Weber, K. S., Rhees, R. W., Setchell, K. D., Adlercreutz, H., et al. (2002). Neurobehavioral effects of dietary soy phytoestrogens. *Neurotoxicology and Teratology, 24*(1), 5–16.

Levin, E. D., Schantz, S. L., & Bowman, R. E. (1992). Use of the lesion model for examining toxicant effects on cognitive behavior. *Neurotoxicology and Teratology, 14*(2), 131–141.

Li, M. H., & Hansen, L. G. (1995). Uterotropic and enzyme induction effects of 2,2',5-trichlorobiphenyl. *Bulletin of Environmental Contamination and Toxicology, 54*(4), 494–500.

Li, M. H., & Hansen, L. G. (1996). Enzyme induction and acute endocrine effects in prepubertal female rats receiving environmental PCB/PCDF/PCDD mixtures. *Environmental Health Perspectives, 104*(7), 712–722.

Li, S., Washburn, K. A., Moore, R., Uno, T., Teng, C., Newbold, R. R., et al. (1997). Developmental exposure to diethylstilbestrol elicits demethylation of estrogen-responsive lactoferrin gene in mouse uterus. *Cancer Research, 57*(19), 4356–4359.

Li, M. H., Zhao, Y. D., & Hansen, L. G. (1994). Multiple dose toxicokinetic influence on the estrogenicity of 2,2',4,4',5,5'-hexachlorobiphenyl. *Bulletin of Environmental Contamination and Toxicology, 53*(4), 583–590.

Linn, M. C., & Petersen, A. C. (1985). Emergence and characterization of sex differences in spatial ability: A meta-analysis. *Child Development, 56*(6), 1479–1498.

Lopez-Carrillo, L., Blair, A., Lopez-Cervantes, M., Cebrian, M., Rueda, C., Reyes, R., et al. (1997). Dichlorodiphenyltrichloroethane serum levels and breast cancer risk: A case-control study from Mexico. *Cancer Research, 57*(17), 3728–3732.

Lund, T. D., & Lephart, E. D. (2001). Manipulation of prenatal hormones and dietary phytoestrogens during adulthood alter the sexually dimorphic expression of visual spatial memory. *BMC Neuroscience, 2*(1), 21.

Machala, M., Neca, J., Drabek, P., Ulrich, R., Sabatova, V., Nezveda, K., et al. (1998). Effects of chronic exposure to PCBs on cytochrome P450 systems and steroidogenesis in liver and testis of bulls (Bos taurus). *Comparative Biochemistry and Physiology. Part A, Molecular & Integrative Physiology, 120*(1), 65–70.

Matsumoto, T. (1991). Endocrinological approach to symptoms and diagnosis of disorders of calcium metabolism. *Nihon Naika Gakkai Zasshi, 80*(3), 337–341.

Matysek, M. (1989). Studies on the effect of stress on the estrus cycle in rats. *Annales Universitatis Mariae Curie Sklodowska [Med], 44*, 143–149.

McDonnell, D. P., Clemm, D. L., Hermann, T., Goldman, M. E., & Pike, J. W. (1995). Analysis of estrogen receptor function in vitro reveals three distinct classes of antiestrogens. *Molecular Endocrinology, 9*(6), 659–669.

McDonnell, D. P., & Norris, J. D. (1997). Analysis of the molecular pharmacology of estrogen receptor agonists and antagonists provides insights into mechanism of action of estrogen in bone. *Osteoporosis International*, 7(Suppl. 1), S29–S34.

McGivern, R. F., Sokol, R. Z., & Berman, N. G. (1991). Prenatal lead exposure in the rat during the third week of gestation: Long-term behavioral, physiological, and anatomical effects associated with reproduction. *Toxicology and Applied Pharmacology, 110*(2), 206–215.

Meaney, M. J. (1989). The sexual differentiation of social play. *Psychiatric Developments*, 7(3), 247–261.

Meaney, M. J., Aitken, D. H., Jensen, L. K., McGinnis, M. Y., & McEwen, B. S. (1985). Nuclear and cytosolic androgen receptor levels in the limbic brain of neonatal male and female rats. *Brain Research*, *355*(2), 179–185.

Mendelsohn, A. L., Dreyer, B. P., Fierman, A. H., Rosen, C. M., Legano, L. A., Kruger, H. A., et al. (1998). Low-level lead exposure and behavior in early childhood. *Pediatrics*, *101*(3), E10.

Moore, M., Mustain, M., Daniel, K., Chen, I., Safe, S., Zacharewski, T., et al. (1997). Antiestrogenic activity of hydroxylated polychlorinated biphenyl congeners identified in human serum. *Toxicology and Applied Pharmacology*, *142*(1), 160–168.

Moore, R. W., Potter, C. L., Theobald, H. M., Robinson, J. A., & Peterson, R. E. (1985). Androgenic deficiency in male rats treated with 2,3,7,8-tetrachlorodibenzo-p-dioxin. *Toxicology and Applied Pharmacology*, *79*(1), 99–111.

Moore, C. L., & Power, K. L. (1992). Variation in maternal care and individual differences in play, exploration, and grooming of juvenile Norway rat offspring. *Developmental Psychobiology*, *25*(3), 165–182.

Moysich, K. B., Shields, P. G., Freudenheim, J. L., Schisterman, E. F., Vena, J. E., Kostyniak, P., et al. (1999). Polychlorinated biphenyls, cytochrome P4501A1 polymorphism, and postmenopausal breast cancer risk. *Cancer Epidemiology, Biomarkers and Prevention*, *8*(1), 41–44.

Nagel, S. C., vom Saal, F. S., Thayer, K. A., Dhar, M. G., Boechler, M., & Welshons, V. (1994). Relative binding affinity-serum modified access (RBA-SMA) assay predicts the relative in vivo bioactivity of the xenoestrogens bisphenol A and octylphenol. *Environmental Health Perspectives*, *105*, 70–76.

Namkung, M. J., Porubek, D. J., Neslon, S. D., & Juchau, M. R. (1995). Regulation of aromatic oxidation of estradiol-17b in maternal hepatic, fetal hepatic and placental tissues: Comparative effects of a series of inducing agents. *Journal of Steroid Biochemistry*, *22*, 563–567.

Narita, M., Aoki, T., Ozaki, S., Yajima, Y., & Suzuki, T. (2001). Involvement of protein kinase Cgamma isoform in morphine-induced reinforcing effects. *Neuroscience*, *103*(2), 309–314.

Needleman, H. L., Gunnoe, C., Leviton, A., Reed, R., Peresie, H., Maher, C., et al. (1979). Deficits in psychologic and classroom performance of children with elevated dentine lead levels. *The New England Journal of Medicine*, *300*(13), 689–695.

Nelson, J. A. (1974). Effects of dichlorodiphenyltrichloroethane (DDT) analogs and polychlorinated biphenyl (PCB) mixtures on 17beta-(3H)estradiol binding to rat uterine receptor. *Biochemical Pharmacology*, *23*(2), 447–451.

Nesaretnam, K., Corcoran, D., Dils, R. R., & Darbre, P. (1996). 3,4,3',4'-Tetrachlorobiphenyl acts as an estrogen in vitro and in vivo. *Molecular Endocrinology*, *10*(8), 923–936.

Nevin, R. (2000). How lead exposure relates to temporal changes in IQ, violent crime, and unwed pregnancy. *Environmental Research*, *83*(1), 1–22.

Newbold, R. (1995). Cellular and molecular effects of developmental exposure to diethylstilbestrol: Implications for other environmental estrogens. *Environmental Health Perspectives*, *103*(Suppl. 7), 83–87.

Nguyen, P. V., Abel, T., Kandel, E. R., & Bourtchouladze, R. (2000). Strain-dependent differences in LTP and hippocampus-dependent memory in inbred mice. *Learning and Memory*, 7(3), 170–179.

Niemi, W. D., Audi, J., Bush, B., & Carpenter, D. O. (1998). PCBs reduce long-term potentiation in the CA1 region of rat hippocampus. *Experimental Neurology*, *151*(1), 26–34.

Ottinger, M. A., Hazelton, J., Wu, J., Ruscio, M., Thompson, N., Quinn, M., et al. (2003). Assessing the consequences of dietary methoxychlor: Neuroendocrine and behavioral measures. In *2nd International meeting steroids and nervous system, Torino, Italy* (p. 10).

Palanza, P. (2003). Impact of environmental Estrogen on sexually dimorphic behavioral systems in mice. In *2nd International meeting steroids and nervous system, Torino, Italy* (p. 15).
Pantaleoni, G. C., Fanini, D., Sponta, A. M., Palumbo, G., Giorgi, R., & Adams, P. M. (1988). Effects of maternal exposure to polychlorobiphenyls (PCBs) on F1 generation behavior in the rat. *Fundamental and Applied Toxicology, 11*(3), 440–449.
Pare, W. P., & Redei, E. (1993). Sex differences and stress response of WKY rats. *Physiology and Behavior, 54*(6), 1179–1185.
Parkinson, A., Thomas, P. E., Ryan, D. E., Reik, L. M., Safe, S. H., Robertson, L. W., et al. (1983). Differential time course of induction of rat liver microsomal cytochrome P-450 isozymes and epoxide hydrolase by Aroclor 1254. *Archives of Biochemistry and Biophysics, 225*(1), 203–215.
Patandin, S., Lanting, C. I., Mulder, P. G., Boersma, E. R., Sauer, P. J., & Weisglas-Kuperus, N. (1999). Effects of environmental exposure to polychlorinated biphenyls and dioxins on cognitive abilities in Dutch children at 42 months of age. *Journal of Pediatrics, 134*(1), 33–41.
Pauwels, A., Covaci, A., Delbeke, L., Punjabi, U., & Schepens, P. J. (1999). The relation between levels of selected PCB congeners in human serum and follicular fluid. *Chemosphere, 39*(14), 2433–2441.
Pellis, S. M., Field, E. F., Smith, L. K., & Pellis, V. C. (1997). Multiple differences in the play fighting of male and female rats. Implications for the causes and functions play. *Neuroscience and Biobehavioral Reviews, 21*(1), 105–120.
Pellis, S. M., & Pellis, V. C. (1990). Differential rates of attack, defense, and counterattack during the developmental decrease in play fighting by male and female rats. *Developmental Psychobiology, 23*(3), 215–231.
Pericic, D., & Pivac, N. (1996). Effects of diazepam on conflict behaviour and on plasma corticosterone levels in male and female rats. *Naunyn-Schmiedeberg's Archives of Pharmacology, 353*(4), 369–376.
Peterson, R. E., Theobald, H. M., & Kimmel, G. L. (1993). Developmental and reproductive toxicity of dioxins and related compounds: Cross-species comparisons. *Critical Reviews in Toxicology, 23*(3), 283–335.
Phillips, D. L., Smith, A. B., Burse, V. W., Steele, G. K., Needham, L. L., & Hannon, W. H. (1989). Half-life of polychlorinated biphenyls in occupationally exposed workers. *Archives of Environmental Health, 44*, 351–354.
Phoenix, C. H., Goy, R. W., & Resko, J. A. (1959). Psychosocial differentiation as a function of androgenic stimulation. In M. Diamond (Ed.), *Perspectives in reproduction and sexual behavior.* Bloomington, IN: Indiana University Press.
Pillai, A., Laxmipriya, Rawal, A., & Gupta, S. (2002). Effect of low level exposure of lead and cadmium on hepatic estradiol metabolism in female rats. *Indian Journal of Experimental Biology, 40*(7), 807–811.
Pimentel, D., Tort, M., D'Anna, L., Krawic, A., Gerger, J., Rossman, J., et al. (1995). Ecology of increasing disease: Population growth and environmental degradation. *Biosciences, 48*, 817–826.
Pines, A., Cucos, S., Ever-Handani, P., & Ron, M. (1987). Some organochlorine insecticide and polychlorinated biphenyl blood residues in infertile males in the general Israeli population of the middle 1980's. *Archives of Environmental Contamination and Toxicology, 16*(5), 587–597.
Podhorna, J., McCabe, S., & Brown, R. E. (2002). Male and female C57BL/6 mice respond differently to diazepam challenge inlearning tasks. *Pharmacology, biochemistry, and behavior, 72*(1–2), 13–21.
Prince, M. (2000). Dementia in developing countries. A consensus statement from the 10/66 Dementia Research Group. *International Journal of Geriatric Psychiatry, 15*(1), 14–20.

Rajapakse, N., Shimizu, K., Payne, M., & Busija, D. (2001). Isolation and characterization of intact mitochondria from neonatal rat brain. *Brain Research. Brain Research Protocols*, *8*(3), 176–183.

Reinisch, J. M., & Sanders, S. A. (1984). Prenatal gonadal steroidal influences on gender-related behavior. *Progress in Brain Research*, *61*, 407–416.

Rice, D. C. (1997). Effect of postnatal exposure to a PCB mixture in monkeys on multiple fixed interval-fixed ratio performance. *Neurotoxicology and Teratology*, *19*, 915–928.

Rice, D. C. (1999). Behavioral impairment produced by low-level postnatal PCB exposure in monkeys. *Environmental Research*, *80*, S113–S121.

Roegge, C. S., Seo, B. W., Crofton, K. M., & Schantz, S. L. (2000). Gestational-lactational exposure to Aroclor 1254 impairs radial-arm maze performance in male rats. *Toxicological Sciences*, *57*(1), 121–130.

Rogan, W. J., Dietrich, K. N., Ware, J. H., Dockery, D. W., Salganik, M., Radcliffe, J., et al. (2001). The effect of chelation therapy with succimer on neuropsychological development in children exposed to lead. *The New England Journal of Medicine*, *344*(19), 1421–1426.

Romero, D. L., Mounho, B. J., Lauer, F. T., Born, J. L., & Burchiel, S. W. (1997). Depletion of glutathione by benzo(a)pyrene metabolites, ionomycin, thapsigargin, and phorbol myristate in human peripheral blood mononuclear cells. *Toxicology and Applied Pharmacology*, *144*, 62–69.

Ronis, M. J., Gandy, J., & Badger, T. (1998). Endocrine mechanisms underlying reproductive toxicity in the developing rat chronically exposed to dietary lead. *Journal of Toxicology and Environmental Health. Part A*, *54*(2), 77–99.

Rubin, B. S., Murray, M. K., Damassa, D. A., King, J. C., & Soto, A. M. (2001). Perinatal exposure to low doses of bisphenol A affects body weight, patterns of estrous cyclicity, and plasma LH levels. *Environmental Health Perspectives*, *109*(7), 675–680.

Ryan, S. M., & Maier, S. F. (1988). The estrous cycle and estrogen modulate stress-induced analgesia. *Behavioral Neuroscience*, *102*(3), 371–380.

Safe, S. H. (1994). Polychlorinated biphenyls (PCBs): Environmental impact, biochemical and toxic responses, and implications for risk assessment. *Critical Reviews in Toxicology*, *24*(2), 87–149, Review.

Safe, S., Astroff, B., Harris, M., Zacharewski, T., Dickerson, R., Romkes, M., et al. (1991). 2,3,7,8-Tetrachlorodibenzo-p-dioxin (TCDD) and related compounds as antioestrogens: Characterization and mechanism of action. *Pharmacology and Toxicology*, *69*(6), 400–409.

Safer, D. J., Zito, J. M., & Fine, E. M. (1996). Increased methylphenidate usage for attention deficit disorder in the 1990s. *Pediatrics*, *98*(6 Pt 1), 1084–1088.

Sager, D. B. (1983). Effect of postnatal exposure to polychlorinated biphenyls on adult male reproductive function. *Environmental Research*, *31*(1), 76–94.

Sager, D. B., & Girard, D. M. (1994). Long-term effects on reproductive parameters in female rats after translactational exposure to PCBs. *Environmental Research*, *66*(1), 52–76.

Sajid, T. M. (1996). *Enzyme induction and acute endocrine effects of PCB 95 and PCB 99 in immature female rats.* Maters Thesis, Urbana, IL: University of Illinois at Urbana-Champaign.

Savolainen, K. M., Loikkanen, J., Eerikainen, S., & Naarala, J. (1998). Interactions of excitatory neurotransmitters and xenobiotics in excitotoxicity and oxidative stress: Glutamate and lead. *Toxicology Letters*, *102–103*, 363–367.

Schantz, S. L., Gasior, D. M., Polverejan, E., McCaffrey, R. J., Sweeney, A. M., Humphrey, H. E., et al. (2001). Impairments of memory and learning in older adults exposed to polychlorinated biphenyls via consumption of Great Lakes fish. *Environmental Health Perspectives*, *109*(6), 605–611.

Schantz, S. L., Levin, E. D., Bowman, R. E., Heironimus, M. P., & Laughlin, N. K. (1989). Effects of perinatal PCB exposure on discrimination-reversal learning in monkeys. *Neurotoxicology and Teratology*, *11*(3), 243–250.

Schantz, S. L., Moshtaghian, J., & Ness, D. K. (1995). Spatial learning deficits in adult rats exposed to ortho-substituted PCB congeners during gestation and lactation. *Fundamental and Applied Toxicology*, *26*(1), 117–126.

Schell, L. M., Burnitz, K. K., & Gallo, M. V. (2012). Growth as a mirror: Is endocrine disruption challenging Tanner's concept? *Annals of Human Biology*, *39*(5), 361–371.

Schettler, T. (2001). Toxic threats to neurologic development of children. *Environmental Health Perspectives*, *109*(6), 813–816.

Schiller, C. M., Adcock, C. M., Moore, R. A., & Walden, R. (1985). Effect of 2,3,7,8-tetrachlorodibenzo-p-dioxin (TCDD) and fasting on body weight and lipid parameters in rats. *Toxicology and Applied Pharmacology*, *81*(2), 356–361.

Schober, S. E., Sinks, T. H., Jones, R. L., Bolger, P. M., McDowell, M., Osterloh, J., et al. (2003). Blood mercury levels in US children and women of childbearing age, 1999-2000. *JAMA*, *289*(13), 1667–1674.

Schwartz, P. M., Jacobson, S. W., Fein, G., Jacobson, J. L., & Price, H. A. (1983). Lake Michigan fish consumption as a source of polychlorinated biphenyls in human cord serum, maternal serum, and milk. *American Journal of Public Health*, *73*(3), 293–296.

Seegal, R. F., Brosch, K. O., & Okoniewski, R. J. (1997). Effects of in utero and lactational exposure of the laboratory rat to 2,4,2',4'- and 3,4,3',4'-tetrachlorobiphenyl on dopamine function. *Toxicology and Applied Pharmacology*, *146*(1), 95–103.

Shepherd, J. K., Blanchard, D. C., Weiss, S. M., Rodgers, R. J., & Blanchard, R. J. (1992). Morphine attenuates antipredator ultrasonic vocalizations in mixed-sex rat colonies. *Pharmacology, Biochemistry, and Behavior*, *41*(3), 551–558.

Shimizu, H., Ross, R. K., Bernstein, L., Pike, M. C., & Henderson, B. E. (1990). Serum oestrogen levels in postmenopausal women: Comparison of American whites and Japanese in Japan. *British Journal of Cancer*, *62*(3), 451–453.

Shors, T. J., Lewczyk, C., Pacynski, M., Mathew, P. R., & Pickett, J. (1998). Stages of estrous mediate the stress-induced impairment of associative learning in the female rat. *Neuroreport*, *9*(3), 419–423.

Smith, A. B., Schloemer, J., Lowry, L. K., Smallwood, A. W., Ligo, R. N., Tanaka, S., et al. (1982). Metabolic and health consequences of occupational exposure to polychlorinated biphenyls. *British Journal of Industrial Medicine*, *39*(4), 361–369.

Sokol, R. Z., Madding, C. E., & Swerdloff, R. S. (1985). Lead toxicity and the hypothalamic-pituitary-testicular axis. *Biology of Reproduction*, *33*(3), 722–728.

Soontornchat, S., Li, M. H., Cooke, P. S., & Hansen, L. G. (1994). Toxicokinetic and toxicodynamic influences on endocrine disruption by polychlorinated biphenyls. *Environmental Health Perspectives*, *102*(6–7), 568–571.

Soto, A. M., Sonnenschein, C., Chung, K. L., Fernandez, M. F., Olea, N., & Serrano, F. O. (1995). The E-SCREEN assay as a tool to identify estrogens: An update on estrogenic environmental pollutants. *Environmental Health Perspectives*, *103*(Suppl. 7), 113–122.

Spink, D. C., Hayes, C. L., Young, N. R., Christou, M., Sutter, T. R., Jefcoate, C. R., et al. (1994). The effects of 2,3,7,8-tetrachlorodibenzo-p-dioxin on estrogen metabolism in MCF-7 breast cancer cells: Evidence for induction of a novel 17 beta-estradiol 4-hydroxylase. *The Journal of Steroid Biochemistry and Molecular Biology*, *51*(5–6), 251–258.

Spink, D. C., Lincoln, D. W., 2nd., Dickerman, H. W., & Gierthy, J. F. (1990). 2,3,7,8-Tetrachlorodibenzo-p-dioxin causes an extensive alteration of 17 beta-estradiol metabolism in MCF breast tumor cells. *Proceedings of the National Academy of Sciences of the United States of America*, *87*(17), 6917–6921.

Stehr-Green, P. A., Welty, E., Steele, G., & Steinberg, K. (1986). Evaluation of potential health effects associated with serum polychlorinated biphenyl levels. *Environmental Health Perspectives*, *70*, 255–259.

Steinmetz, R., Brown, N. G., Allen, D. L., Bigsby, R. M., & Ben-Jonathan, N. (1997). The environmental estrogen bisphenol A stimulates prolactin release in vitro and in vivo. *Endocrinology*, *138*(5), 1780–1786.

Sternberg, W. F., Mogil, J. S., Kest, B., Page, G. G., Leong, Y., Yam, V., et al. (1995). Neonatal testosterone exposure influences neurochemistry of non-opioid swim stress-induced analgesia in adult mice. *Pain, 63*(3), 321–326.
Strickland, D., Smith, S. A., Dolliff, G., Goldman, L., & Roelofs, R. I. (1996). Amyotrophic lateral sclerosis and occupational history. A pilot case-control study. *Archives of Neurology, 53*(8), 730–733.
Sundaresan, S., Weiss, J., Bauer-Dantoin, A. C., & Jameson, J. L. (1997). Expression of ryanodine receptors in the pituitary gland: Evidence for a role in gonadotropin-releasing hormone signaling. *Endocrinology, 138*(5), 2056–2065.
Telisman, S., Cvitkovic, P., Jurasovic, J., Pizent, A., Gavella, M., & Rocic, B. (2000). Semen quality and reproductive endocrine function in relation to biomarkers of lead, cadmium, zinc, and copper in men. *Environmental Health Perspectives, 108*(1), 45–53.
Thor, D. H., & Holloway, W. R., Jr. (1983). Scopolamine blocks play fighting behavior in juvenile rats. *Physiology and Behavior, 30*(4), 545–549.
Thor, D. H., & Holloway, W. R., Jr. (1986). Social play soliciting by male and female juvenile rats: Effects of neonatal androgenization and sex of cagemates. *Behavioral Neuroscience, 100*(2), 275–279.
Thoreux-Manlay, A., Le Goascogne, C., Segretain, D., Jegou, B., & Pinon-Lataillade, G. (1995). Lead affects steroidogenesis in rat Leydig cells in vivo and in vitro. *Toxicology, 103*(1), 53–62.
Thoreux-Manlay, A., Pinon-Lataillade, G., Coffigny, H., Soufir, J. C., & Masse, R. (1995). Prenatal or lactational exposure of male rats to lead acetate. Effect on reproductive function. *Bulletin of Environmental Contamination and Toxicology, 54*(2), 266–272.
Tinwell, H., Lefevre, P. A., Moffat, G. J., Burns, A., Odum, J., Spurway, T. D., et al. (2002). Confirmation of uterotrophic activity of 3-(4 methylbenzylidine)camphor in the immature rat. *Environmental Health Perspectives, 110*(5), 533–536.
Toniolo, P. G. (1997). Endogenous estrogens and breast cancer risk: The case for prospective cohort studies. *Environmental Health Perspectives, 105*(Suppl. 3), 587–592.
Toran-Allerand, C. D., Guan, X., MacLusky, N. J., Horvath, T. L., Diano, S., Singh, M., et al. (2002). ER-X: A novel, plasma membrane-associated, putative estrogen receptor that is regulated during development and after ischemic brain injury. *The Journal of Neuroscience, 22*(19), 8391–8401.
Unger, M., Kiaer, H., Blichert-Toft, M., Olsen, J., & Clausen, J. (1984). Organochlorine compounds in human breast fat from deceased with and without breast cancer and in a biopsy material from newly diagnosed patients undergoing breast surgery. *Environmental Research, 34*(1), 24–28.
Ursin, G., Wilson, M., Henderson, B. E., Kolonel, L. N., Monroe, K., Lee, H. P., et al. (2001). Do urinary estrogen metabolites reflect the differences in breast cancer risk between Singapore Chinese and United States African-American and white women? *Cancer Research, 61*(8), 3326–3329.
Van der Oost, R., van Gastel, L., Worst, D., Hanraads, M., Stumalay, K., van Scooten, F. J., et al. (1994). Biochemical markers in feral roach (Rutilus rutilus) in relation to the bioaccumulation of organic trace pollutants. *Chemosphere, 29*, 801–817.
Van der Zee, J., Kroon, B. B., Nieweg, O. E., van de Merwe, S. A., & Kampinga, H. H. (1997). Rationale for different approaches to combined melphalan and hyperthermia in regional isolated perfusion. *European Journal of Cancer, 33*(10), 1546–1550.
van't Veer, P., Lobbezoo, I. E., Martin-Moreno, J. M., Guallar, E., Gomez-Aracena, J., Kardinaal, A. F., et al. (1997). DDt (dicophane) and postmenopausal breast cancer in Europe case-control study. *British Medical Journal, 315*, 81–85.
Viau, V., & Meaney, M. J. (1991). Variations in the hypothalamic-pituitary-adrenal response to stress during the estrous cycle in the rat. *Endocrinology, 129*(5), 2503–2511.
Vincent, D. R., Bradshaw, W. S., Booth, G. M., Seegmiller, R. E., & Allen, S. D. (1992). Effect of PCB and DES on rat monoamine oxidase, acetylcholinesterase, testosterone, and estradiol ontogeny. *Bulletin of Environmental Contamination and Toxicology, 48*(6), 884–893.

Vom Saal, F. S., Timmbes, B. G., Montano, M. M., Palanza, P., Thayer, K. A., Nagel, S. C., et al. (1997). Prostate enlargement in mice due to fetal exposure to low doses of estradiol or diethylstilbestrol and opposite effects at high doses. *Proceedings of the National Academy of Sciences of the United States of America, 94*(5), 2056–2061.
Voyer, D., Voyer, S., & Bryden, M. P. (1995). Magnitude of sex differences in spatial abilities: A meta-analysis and consideration of critical variables. *Psychological Bulletin, 117*(2), 250–270.
Vreugdenhil, M., Hack, S. P., Draguhn, A., & Jefferys, J. G. (2002). Tetanus toxin induces long-term changes in excitation and inhibition in the rat hippocampal CA1 area. *Neuroscience, 114*(4), 983–994.
Walkowiak, J., Altmann, L., Kramer, U., Sveinsson, K., Turfeld, M., Weishoff-Houben, M., et al. (1998). Cognitive and sensorimotor functions in 6-year-old children in relation to lead and mercury levels: Adjustment for intelligence and contrast sensitivity in computerized testing. *Neurotoxicology and Teratology, 20*(5), 511–521.
Wang, J. D., Jang, C. S., Hwang, Y. H., & Chen, Z. S. (1992). Lead contamination around a kindergarten near a battery recycling plant. *Bulletin of environmental contamination and toxicology, 49*(1), 23–30.
Wang, X. Q., Fang, J., Nunez, A. A., & Clemens, L. G. (2002). Developmental exposure to polychlorinated biphenyls affects sexual behavior of rats. *Physiology and Behavior, 75*(5), 689–696.
Ward, I. L., & Stehm, K. E. (1991). Prenatal stress feminizes juvenile play patterns in male rats. *Physiology and Behavior, 50*(3), 601–605.
Wei, P., Zhang, J., Dowhan, D. H., Han, Y., & Moore, D. D. (2002). Specific and overlapping functions of the nuclear hormone receptors CAR and PXR in xenobiotic response. *The Pharmacogenomics Journal, 2*(2), 117–126.
Weiss, B. (2002). Sexually dimorphic nonreproductive behaviors as indicators of endocrine disruption. *Environmental Health Perspectives, 110*, 387–391.
WHO, (1989). *Levels of PCBs, PCDDs, and PCDFs in breastmilk: Results of WHO-coordinated interlaboratory quality control studies and analytical field studies. Environmental Health Series.* Vol. 34. Copenhagen: FADL.
Widholm, J. J., Clarkson, G. B., Strupp, B. J., Crofton, K. M., Seegal, R. F., & Schantz, S. L. (2001). Spatial reversal learning in Aroclor 1254-exposed rats: Sex-specific deficits in associative ability and inhibitory control. *Toxicology and Applied Pharmacology, 174*(2), 188–198.
Williams, C. L., & Meck, W. H. (1991). The organizational effects of gonadal steroids on sexually dimorphic spatial ability. *Psychoneuroendocrinology, 16*(1–3), 155–176.
Wolff, M. S. (1985). Occupational exposure to polychlorinated biphenyls (PCBs). *Environmental Health Perspectives, 60*, 133–138.
Wolff, M. S., Toniolo, P. G., Lee, E. W., Rivera, M., & Dubin, N. (1993). Blood levels of organochlorine residues and risk of breast cancer. *Journal of the National Cancer Institute, 85*(8), 648–652.
Wood, G. E., & Shors, T. J. (1998). Stress facilitates classical conditioning in males, but impairs classical conditioning in females through activational effects of ovarian hormones. *Proceedings of the National Academy of Sciences of the United States of America, 95*(7), 4066–4071.
Yoshihara, S., Nagata, K., Wada, I., Yoshimura, H., Kuroki, H., & Masuda, Y. (1982). A unique change of steroid metabolism in rat liver microsomes induced with highly toxic polychlorinatedbiphenyl(PCB) and polychlorinated dibenzofuran(PCDF). *Journal of Pharmacobio-Dynamics, 5*(12), 994–1004.
Yu, M. L., Hsu, C. C., Guo, Y. L., Lai, T. J., Chen, S. J., & Luo, J. M. (1994). Disordered behavior in the early-born Taiwan Yucheng children. *Chemosphere, 29*(9–11), 2413–2422.

CHAPTER FOUR

Ovarian Toxicity from Reactive Oxygen Species

Ulrike Luderer[1]
Medicine, Developmental and Cell Biology, and Public Health, University of California Irvine, Irvine, California, USA
[1]Corresponding author: e-mail address: uluderer@uci.edu

Contents

1. Ovarian Follicular Development and Its Hormonal Regulation 100
2. Reactive Oxygen Species and Oxidative Stress 103
3. Hormonal Regulation of and Effects of Depleting or Enhancing Ovarian Antioxidants 104
4. Oxidative Stress Occurs in the Ovarian Follicles When the Normal Hormonal Support for Follicular Survival is Removed 108
5. Effects of Exogenous H_2O_2 on Ovarian Follicles and Granulosa Cells 109
6. Involvement of ROS in Ovarian Toxicity Caused by Chemical Toxicants 109
   6.1 Phthalates 109
   6.2 Methoxychlor 110
   6.3 Polycyclic aromatic hydrocarbons 112
   6.4 Cyclophosphamide 114
   6.5 Chromium 115
   6.6 Menadione 117
7. Involvement of ROS in Ovarian Toxicity Caused by Ionizing Radiation 118
8. Summary and Conclusions 120
References 120

Abstract

Oxidative stress occurs when cellular mechanisms to regulate levels of reactive oxygen species (ROS) are overwhelmed due to overproduction of ROS and/or deficiency of antioxidants. This chapter describes accumulating evidence that oxidative stress is involved in ovarian toxicity caused by diverse stimuli, including environmental toxicants. There is strong evidence that ROS are involved in initiation of apoptosis in antral follicles caused by several chemical and physical agents. Although less attention has been focused on the roles of ROS in primordial and primary follicle death, several studies have shown protective effects of antioxidants and/or evidence of oxidative damage, suggesting that ROS may play a role in these smaller follicles as well. Oxidative damage to lipids in the oocyte has been implicated as a cause of persistently poor oocyte quality after early life exposure to several toxicants. Developing germ cells in the fetal ovary have also been

Vitamins and Hormones, Volume 94
ISSN 0083-6729
http://dx.doi.org/10.1016/B978-0-12-800095-3.00004-3

shown to be sensitive to toxicants and ionizing radiation, which induce oxidative stress. Recent studies have begun to elucidate the mechanisms by which ROS mediate ovarian toxicity.

1. OVARIAN FOLLICULAR DEVELOPMENT AND ITS HORMONAL REGULATION

Ovarian follicles are the functional unit of the mammalian ovary. Follicles consist of the oocyte (germ cell) surrounded by and forming intercellular connections with specialized somatic cells called granulosa cells, which are in turn surrounded by and make connections with specialized somatic cells called theca cells (Fig. 4.1). Follicles progress through various stages of development from primordial to preovulatory/Graafian (Fig. 4.1). Primordial follicles are quiescent, with oocytes arrested in the first meiotic prophase since before birth. Throughout the reproductive life, primordial follicles are continually recruited into the growing pool. When primordial follicles are activated, the oocyte grows and granulosa cells differentiate from a fusiform appearance to a more cuboidal form and proliferate. A follicle with a single layer of cuboidal granulosa cells is called a primary follicle. A follicle with more than one layer of granulosa cells is called a secondary follicle (sometimes referred to as preantral). Eventually, fluid-filled vesicles appear in the granulosa cell layer, forming early antral follicles. The vesicles coalesce to a single fluid-filled antrum. Granulosa cell proliferation then slows and the last stages of follicular growth are mainly due to the expansion of the antrum, eventually forming a preovulatory or Graafian follicle.

Ovarian follicular development and ovulation are regulated by hypothalamic (gonadotropin-releasing hormone, GnRH) and pituitary (luteinizing hormone, LH, and follicle-stimulating hormone, FSH) hormones (Fig. 4.2). GnRH is secreted into the portal circulation to act on the gonadotrope cells in the anterior pituitary gland to stimulate synthesis and secretion of the gonadotropins, LH and FSH. FSH and LH act on their specific receptors in the plasma membranes of granulosa cells and theca cells, respectively, of growing follicles. Follicles are responsive to gonadotropins from the secondary stage on, and preovulatory follicles have an absolute requirement for gonadotropins for survival. Large antral, preovulatory follicles are capable of ovulating in response to a midcycle gonadotropin surge. The ovarian steroids, estradiol (E_2) and progesterone (P), and the peptide hormone, inhibin, are synthesized in the granulosa cells and theca cells. These hormones feed

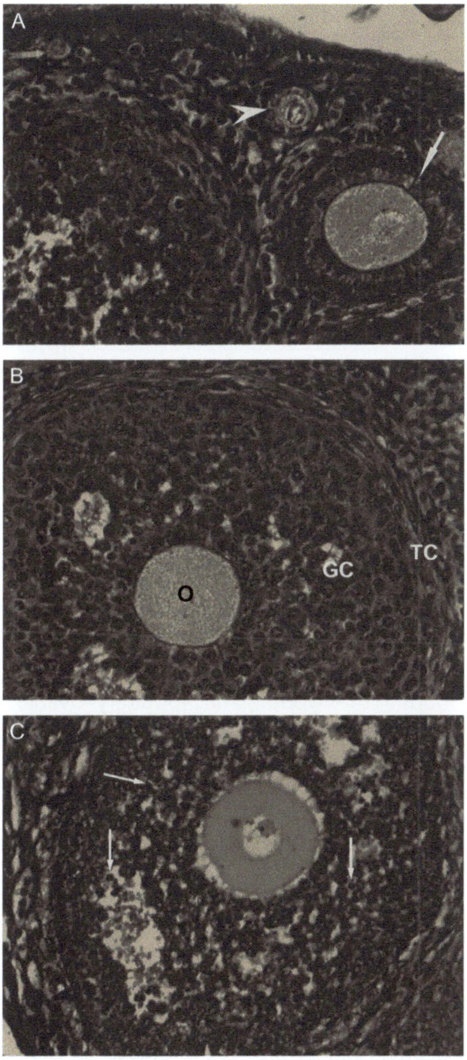

Figure 4.1 Ovarian follicular development. (A) Ovarian follicles progress from the least mature primordial stage (green arrow in A) through primary (yellow arrowhead in A), secondary (yellow arrow in A), antral (B and C), and preovulatory stages. (B) Portion of a healthy small antral follicle with multiple fluid-filled vesicles that have not yet coalesced. Mitotic figures can be seen in the granulosa cell layer. O, oocyte; G, granulosa cells; T, theca cells. (C) Portion of an atretic antral follicle, characterized by pyknotic granulosa cells (arrows) and loss of intercellular connections between oocyte and granulosa cells and among granulosa cells. Images are hematoxylin and periodic acid Schiff-stained sections from mouse ovary. Original magnification 400×. (See color plate.)

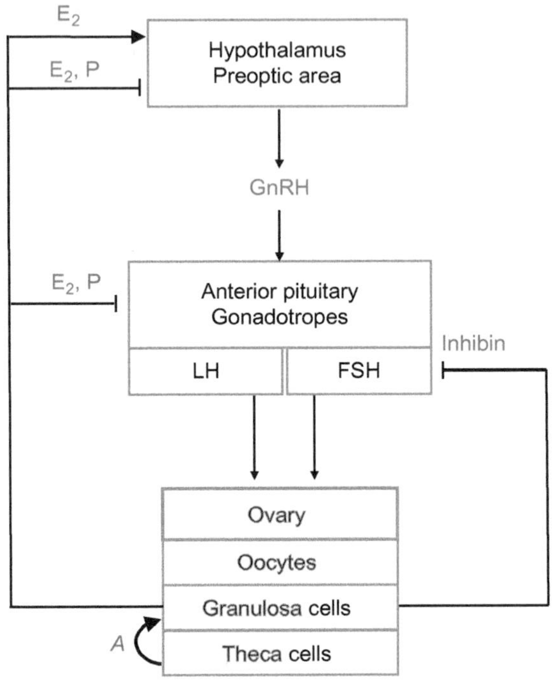

Figure 4.2 Feedback loops in the hypothalamic–pituitary–ovarian axis. Arrows indicate positive feedback/stimulatory effects; blunt ends indicate negative feedback/inhibitory effects. GnRH, gonadotropin-releasing hormone; FSH, follicle-stimulating hormone; LH, luteinizing hormone; A, androgens (androstenedione and testosterone); E_2, estradiol; P, progesterone. GnRH from the hypothalamus stimulates synthesis and secretion of FSH and LH by the anterior pituitary. FSH and LH act on specific membrane receptors in granulosa cells and theca cells of the ovary, stimulating follicular growth and hormone synthesis. The peptide hormone inhibin is synthesized and secreted by granulosa cells and specifically inhibits FSH synthesis and secretion by the pituitary. P is synthesized in granulosa and theca cells, converted to A in theca cells, and A is aromatized to E_2 in granulosa cells. E_2 and P negatively feed back to the hypothalamus and pituitary to suppress GnRH, LH, and FSH. When E_2 levels surpass a threshold, E_2 exerts a positive feedback effect on hypothalamic GnRH, which is the trigger for ovulation.

back to regulate the synthesis and secretion of GnRH, LH, and FSH. The majority of ovarian follicles do not ovulate, but undergo an apoptotic process of degeneration called atresia at the small antral follicle stage (Hirshfield, 1988) (Fig. 4.1).

Stimulation of preovulatory follicle development in rodents via injection of equine chorionic gonadotropin (eCG, also called pregnant mare's serum gonadotropin), which has FSH and LH receptor-binding activity, followed 46–48 h later by an ovulatory dose of human chorionic gonadotropin (hCG), which has only LH receptor-binding activity, is commonly used in experiments assessing the effects of gonadotropin hormones on ovarian gene expression and other endpoints and for generating preovulatory follicles or ovulated oocytes for other studies.

2. REACTIVE OXYGEN SPECIES AND OXIDATIVE STRESS

Reactive oxygen species (ROS) and reactive nitrogen species (RNS) include free radicals such as hydroxyl radical ($OH^•$), superoxide anion radical ($O_2^{-•}$), and nitric oxide ($NO^•$); non-free radical ROS/RNS include hydrogen peroxide (H_2O_2) and peroxynitrite ($ONOO^-$) (Spitz, Azzam, Li, & Gius, 2004) (Fig. 4.3). $O_2^{-•}$ and $OH^•$ are short-lived in biological systems because their unpaired electron makes them highly reactive with cellular macromolecules (Roberts et al., 2009; Roede & Jones, 2010; Wiseman & Halliwell, 1996). H_2O_2 is more long-lived and membrane-permeable and can diffuse from its site of origin within the cells or among cells (Giorgio, Trinei, Migliaccio, & Pelicci, 2007; Spitz et al., 2004). $O_2^{-•}$, H_2O_2, and

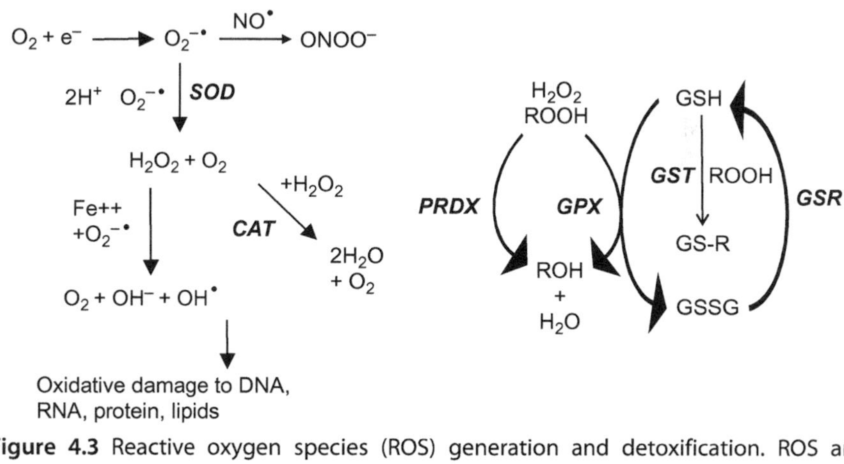

Figure 4.3 Reactive oxygen species (ROS) generation and detoxification. ROS are formed by the sequential addition of electrons to molecular oxygen, forming superoxide anion radical ($O_2^{-•}$), H_2O_2, and hydroxyl radical ($OH^•$). Peroxynitrite ($ONOO^-$) is formed when superoxide anion radical reacts with nitric oxide ($NO^•$). Key antioxidant enzymes (in bold, italicized) and the reactions they catalyze are shown. CAT, catalase; GPX, glutathione peroxidase; GSR, glutathione reductase; GST, glutathione-*S*-transferase; PRDX, peroxiredoxin; SOD, superoxide dismutase. GPXs and GSTs require glutathione (GSH) as a cofactor, and GSH can also scavenge free radicals through direct chemical reactions. GSR reduces the oxidized form of GSH (GSSG, glutathione disulfide). *Modified from Devine et al. (2012).*

$OH^{\bullet}$ are formed by the sequential addition of electrons to molecular oxygen. This occurs in the mitochondria as a result of incomplete reduction of molecular oxygen to water during oxidative phosphorylation; it is estimated that about 0.5% of oxygen consumed by the mitochondria is converted to $O_2^{-\bullet}$ and H_2O_2 (Giorgio et al., 2007). Multiple enzyme systems that generate H_2O_2 exist within cells, including NADPH oxidase and phagocytic oxidases on the cell membranes, peroxisomal oxidases in the peroxisomes, sulfhydryl oxidase in the endoplasmic reticulum, superoxide dismutase 1 (SOD1) and cyclooxygenase in the cytoplasm, and superoxide dismutase 2 (SOD2) and p66shc in the mitochondria (Giorgio et al., 2007). In steroidogenic tissues like the ovary, ROS can be generated as a result of uncoupling of electron transfer from substrate hydroxylation by steroidogenic cytochrome P450 enzymes (Hanukoglu, 2006). ROS are also formed as a result of metabolism of xenobiotics, as will be discussed in detail in the succeeding text.

Many studies in recent years have shown that H_2O_2 and other ROS and RNS function as important signaling molecules within cells (Giorgio et al., 2007). One important mechanism by which this occurs is via oxidation of redox-sensitive cysteine residues in proteins, which reversibly alters protein function (Jones, 2006, 2008). Oxidation and reduction of these residues are regulated by two independent thiol-containing systems, thioredoxins (TXNs) and glutathione (GSH), and its related enzymes, glutathione-*S*-transferases (GSTs), which catalyze glutathionylation of proteins, and glutaredoxins, which catalyze deglutathionylation (Anathy et al., 2012; Jones, 2006, 2008). Ovulation is an example of an ovarian process that is regulated by ROS. ROS levels rise and antioxidant levels fall in response to the preovulatory gonadotropin surges, and treatment with antioxidants inhibits ovulation (Laloraya, Kumar, & Laloraya, 1988; Miyazaki et al., 1991; Sato et al., 1992; Shkolnik et al., 2011). Oxidative stress occurs when the normal cellular redox balance is disturbed, resulting in dysregulation of redox-regulated processes and/or oxidative damage to cellular macromolecules (Jones, 2006, 2008).

3. HORMONAL REGULATION OF AND EFFECTS OF DEPLETING OR ENHANCING OVARIAN ANTIOXIDANTS

Cells possess numerous enzymatic (Fig. 4.3) and nonenzymatic antioxidant systems that function to tightly regulate cellular levels of

ROS/RNS. Deficiency of antioxidant vitamins has profound effects on female fertility. Expression of many ovarian antioxidant genes is regulated by gonadotropin hormones, suggesting that these antioxidants may play important roles in ovarian function. Numerous studies in recent years have examined the biological effects of the deletion of genes encoding antioxidant enzymes and their cofactors, including the effects on ovarian function. These studies demonstrate a role for some but not all antioxidant genes examined in ovarian function.

Cytosolic, mitochondrial, and extracellular SODs (Cu-SOD or SOD1, Mn-SOD or SOD2, and SOD3, respectively) dismutate $O_2^{-\bullet}$ to H_2O_2 and water (Fig. 4.3). *Sod2* and *Sod3* mRNA expression, but not *Sod1* expression, are upregulated in rat ovary by eCG stimulation (Tilly & Tilly, 1995). The eCG-induced increased *Sod2* expression is localized to theca interna cells of growing follicles, and subsequent administration of an ovulatory dose of hCG increases theca cell expression further and upregulates expression in granulosa cells as well (Sasaki et al., 1994). Global deletion of *Sod1* has been reported by two groups using different gene-targeting strategies (Ho et al., 1998; Matzuk, Dionne, Guo, Kumar, & Lebovitz, 1998). Both groups reported that female *Sod1*-null mice were subfertile but reported somewhat different ovarian phenotypes. Matzuk et al. (1998) observed fewer preovulatory follicles and corpora lutea in the ovaries of adult *Sod1*-null females and concluded that *Sod1* deletion adversely affected antral follicle development and ovulation. Ho et al. (1998) reported that *Sod1*-null females had normal ovarian histology and ovulated similar numbers of oocytes during a natural estrous cycle but had smaller litters due to postimplantation embryonic mortality. Another group subsequently reported that female *Sod1*-null mice have decreased serum progesterone levels upon superovulation and during pregnancy and have small corpora lutea with increased numbers of apoptotic cells and fewer blood vessels and demonstrated that embryos null for *Sod1* developed normally when transplanted to wild-type dams (Noda, Ota, Shirasawa, & Shimizu, 2012), suggesting that the postimplantation embryonic mortality observed by Ho et al. may be due to luteal dysfunction. Mice null for copper chaperone of superoxide dismutase, which have decreased ability to incorporate copper into *Sod1*, display a similar ovarian phenotype to that reported by Matzuk et al. (1998) for *Sod1*-null mice, with abnormal antral follicle development and the absence of corpora lutea (Wong et al., 2000). Taken together, the results suggest that *Sod1* is required for normal antral follicle and corpus luteum development. Deletion of *Sod2* results in death before puberty, but transplantation of ovaries from *Sod2*-null females to wild-type recipients results in normal ovarian follicular development, ovulation, and fertility, suggesting that SOD2 is not required for ovarian function (Matzuk et al., 1998).

Glutathione peroxidases (GPXs), catalase, peroxiredoxins (PRDXs), and some GSTs can convert H_2O_2 to water (Fig. 4.3). GPXs utilize the cysteine-containing tripeptide glutathione (GSH, γ-glutamyl cysteinyl glycine) as a cofactor. In the process of reducing peroxides, GSH becomes oxidized to the disulfide form (GSSG), which is reduced back to GSH by the action of glutathione reductase (GSR). GSTs also require GSH as a cofactor, but GSH is covalently linked with the substrate and consumed in these reactions (Hayes & Pulford, 1995). GSH can also scavenge free radicals directly. Ovarian stimulation with eCG does not increase expression of *Gpx1* or catalase in rats (Tilly & Tilly, 1995). Deletion of both of these genes (Ho et al., 1997; Ho, Xiong, Ma, Spector, & Ho, 2004) and inactivating mutations of *Gsr* (Pretsch, 1999; Rogers, Bates, Welty, & Smith, 2006; Rogers et al., 2004) reportedly did not affect fertility in mice, but detailed studies of ovarian effects of deleting these genes have not been conducted. Global deletion of *Gpx4* is embryonic lethal (Yant et al., 2003), but deletion of either the mitochondrial form or the nuclear form alone does not affect female fertility (Conrad et al., 2005; Schneider et al., 2009).

Ovarian stimulation with eCG increases protein expression of the modifier (GCLM) and catalytic (GCLC) subunits of glutamate cysteine ligase (GCL), the rate-limiting enzyme in GSH synthesis, increasing GCL catalytic activity and GSH concentrations in the rat ovary (Aten, Duarte, & Behrman, 1992; Luderer, Kavanagh, White, & Faustman, 2001; Tsai-Turton & Luderer, 2005). Studies in cultured rat antral follicles and granulosa cells show that FSH and estradiol interact to increase mRNA and protein expression of *Gclc* and *Gclm* (Hoang, Nakamura, & Luderer, 2009; Tsai-Turton & Luderer, 2006). Deletion of *Gclc* in mice is embryonic lethal before gestational day 8.5 (Dalton, Dieter, Yang, Shertzer, & Nebert, 2000; Shi et al., 2000). Mice with deletion of *Gclm* survive and reproduce but have low tissue levels of GSH (Giordano et al., 2006; McConnachie et al., 2007; Yang et al., 2002). GSH concentrations in the oocytes of *Gclm*-null mice are less than 20% those of *Gclm*$^{+/+}$ mice, and *Gclm*$^{-/-}$ females have decreased litter sizes due to preimplantation embryonic mortality (Nakamura et al., 2011). *In vivo* fertilization experiments showed that embryos derived from *Gclm*$^{-/-}$ females had decreased rates of formation of the second male pronucleus at 0.5 days post coitum and lower rates of survival to the blastocyst stage (Nakamura et al., 2011). Upon *in vitro* fertilization with wild-type sperm, embryos derived from *Gclm*$^{-/-}$ oocytes progressed to the two-cell stage by 30 h after fertilization, but very few reached the blastocyst stage by 102 h (Nakamura et al., 2011). Together, these results demonstrate that the preimplantation embryonic mortality in *Gclm*$^{-/-}$ females is driven by low GSH concentrations in the oocytes and not by low GSH concentrations in the female reproductive tract.

The enzyme γ-glutamyl transpeptidase-1 (*Ggt1*) is located on plasma membranes in many tissues. It catalyzes the first of two reactions that break down GSH into its three constituent amino acids, enabling them to be taken up by the cell (GSH itself cannot cross cell membranes). Deletion of *Ggt1* shortens lifespan and causes infertility in females, due to the lack of ovarian large antral follicles, corpora lutea, and ovulatory response to exogenous gonadotropins (Kumar et al., 2000; Lieberman et al., 1996; Will et al., 2000). Ovarian GSH concentrations are normal in these mice, but ovarian cysteine concentrations are greatly decreased, and cysteine supplementation completely reverses the ovarian phenotype.

Nonenzymatic antioxidants in the ovary include the vitamins ascorbic acid (vitamin C), vitamin E, and vitamin A. Ascorbic acid directly scavenges free radicals. It is present in ovarian cells at millimolar concentrations and at 50–200 μM in human follicular fluid (Luck, Jeyaseelan, & Scholes, 1995; Zreik, Kodaman, Jones, Olive, & Behrman, 1999). Granulosa cells, theca cells, luteal cells, and oocytes all concentrate ascorbic acid, and its uptake and release from these cells are hormonally regulated (Aten et al., 1992; Luck et al., 1995; Musicki, Kodaman, Aten, & Behrman, 1996; Zreik et al., 1999). Rodents can synthesize ascorbic acid; humans and guinea pigs have an inactive form of the ascorbic acid synthesis gene and therefore have an absolute requirement for it in the diet. In the guinea pig, ascorbic acid depletion causes extensive follicular atresia and ovarian atrophy (Luck et al., 1995). Vitamin E refers to several compounds, chiefly α-, β-, γ-, and δ-tocopherols, which are potent scavengers of peroxyl radicals (Niki & Traber, 2012). Female infertility was one of the first reported effects of vitamin E deficiency, at a time when its molecular identity was unknown (Evans & Bishop, 1922). Initially, infertility was thought to be entirely due to uterine effects, but more recently, ovarian effects of vitamin E deficiency were also reported. Rats fed with a vitamin E-deficient diet beginning before puberty have undetectable serum concentrations of LH, low estradiol levels, absence of the onset of normal estrous cycles, and ovaries with abnormal antral follicles with thickened granulosa cell layers (Das & Chowdhury, 1999).

Ovarian levels of vitamin A increase with eCG stimulation in rats and increase further during luteal regression (Aten et al., 1992). The vitamin A precursor β-carotene and α-tocopherol increase in bovine corpora lutea with increasing progesterone levels (Hanukoglu, 2006). Vitamin A is required for the entry of germ cells into meiosis I, and vitamin A deficiency during prenatal development blocks the entry of ovarian germ cells into meiosis I during fetal life (Li & Clagett-Dame, 2009). This action of vitamin A is mediated by retinoic acid, which is synthesized from retinol in target cells (Duester, 2007). In addition, it was reported nearly a century ago that vitamin A deficiency during adulthood in female rats disrupts normal completion of meiosis II in oocytes and prevents blastogenesis (Evans, 1928).

4. OXIDATIVE STRESS OCCURS IN THE OVARIAN FOLLICLES WHEN THE NORMAL HORMONAL SUPPORT FOR FOLLICULAR SURVIVAL IS REMOVED

Culture of small and large (preovulatory) antral rat follicles without gonadotropin support leads to apoptotic death within 24 h, while FSH suppresses apoptosis (Chun et al., 1994, 1996). The antioxidants SOD, catalase, *N*-acetyl cysteine, and ascorbic acid are all able to inhibit apoptosis in cultured large antral follicles in the absence of FSH (Tilly & Tilly, 1995). ROS levels, measured as increased fluorescence of the probes dichlorofluorescein and dihydrorhodamine, rise when preovulatory follicles are cultured without gonadotropin support before any increase in the markers of apoptosis, and FSH significantly suppresses this rise in ROS and inhibits apoptosis of follicular granulosa cells (Tsai-Turton & Luderer, 2006). Culture of preovulatory follicles without FSH is also associated with a decline in follicular GSH concentrations, whereas culture with FSH stimulates follicular GSH synthesis above initial levels (Tsai-Turton & Luderer, 2006). Biochemical depletion of GSH with buthionine sulfoximine (BSO), a specific inhibitor of GCL, partially and significantly reversed the antiapoptotic effect of FSH, while supplementation with a cell-permeable form of GSH, glutathione ethyl ester, completely prevents the BSO-induced apoptosis (Tsai-Turton & Luderer, 2006). Consistent with the *in vitro* effects of GSH depletion with BSO, *in vivo* treatment of adult female rats with BSO also significantly increases antral and secondary follicle atresia (Lopez & Luderer, 2004). Taken together, these findings strongly support the conclusion that some of the antiapoptotic effects of FSH in antral follicles are mediated by FSH upregulation of antioxidant defenses.

5. EFFECTS OF EXOGENOUS H_2O_2 ON OVARIAN FOLLICLES AND GRANULOSA CELLS

Although endogenous H_2O_2 is an important signaling molecule, high levels of H_2O_2 are toxic to cells. Exogenous H_2O_2 at concentrations ≥ 0.5 mM rapidly induces cytotoxicity in cultured COV434 cells, a human granulosa cell tumor line, which displays many characteristics of normal granulosa cells, such as synthesis of estradiol in the presence of androstenedione and FSH (Cortés-Wanstreet, Giedzinski, Limoli, & Luderer, 2009). Stable overexpression of mouse *Gclm* or *Gclc* in COV434 cells increases cellular GSH concentrations and protects against H_2O_2-induced cytotoxicity (Cortés-Wanstreet et al., 2009). In primary cultures of rat granulosa cells, H_2O_2 dose-dependently inhibits progesterone synthesis via inhibition of steroidogenic acute regulatory (StAR) protein expression (Yu, Lim, Wang, & Wang, 2012). StAR regulates the rate-limiting step in steroid synthesis, the transfer of cholesterol to the inner mitochondrial membrane.

Neonatal rodent ovaries are enriched for primordial follicles, making cultured neonatal ovaries an ideal model system in which to study the effects of toxicants on primordial follicles. In contrast to the adverse effects of H_2O_2 on steroidogenically active granulosa cells, primordial and small primary follicles in cultured neonatal (postnatal day 4) rat ovaries are relatively resistant to H_2O_2 concentrations below 6 mM applied for 8 days (Devine, Perreault, & Luderer, 2012). At 6 mM concentrations, primordial and primary follicles display morphological signs of atresia (Devine et al., 2012).

6. INVOLVEMENT OF ROS IN OVARIAN TOXICITY CAUSED BY CHEMICAL TOXICANTS

6.1. Phthalates

Phthalates are diesters of *o*-phthalic acid with side chains of various lengths, which are commonly used as plasticizers and in other consumer products such as cosmetics. They impart flexibility to plastics in toys, medical devices, vinyl flooring, and food wraps. Phthalate diesters are metabolized to monoesters, which are the toxicologically active metabolites. In adult female rats, di(2-ethylhexyl) phthalate (DEHP) and its monoester metabolite, mono(2-ethylhexyl)phthalate (MEHP), decrease estradiol levels via both intraovarian and extraovarian mechanisms. DEHP and several other phthalates increase the metabolism of estradiol to estrone by inducing hepatic 17β-hydroxysteroid dehydrogenase type IV activity (Lovekamp-Swan & Davis, 2003). In addition, DEHP/MEHP, but not other phthalates, suppresses aromatase mRNA and protein expression, thereby decreasing estradiol secretion in cultured rat granulosa cells (Lovekamp-Swan & Davis, 2003). This effect of MEHP is mediated by activation of the nuclear receptors and transcription factors peroxisome proliferator-activated receptors alpha and gamma (Lovekamp-Swan, Jetten, & Davis, 2003).

Both DEHP and MEHP inhibit the growth of cultured mouse antral follicles via an oxidative stress-dependent mechanism (Wang, Craig, Basavarajappa, Gupta, & Flaws, 2012; Wang, Craig, Basavarajappa, Hafner, & Flaws, 2012). Inhibition of growth is preceded by the upregulation of expression of the proapoptotic *Bax* gene and downregulation of the anti-apoptotic *Bcl2* gene and of several cell cycle regulatory genes (Wang, Craig, Basavarajappa, Gupta, et al., 2012; Wang, Craig, Basavarajappa, Hafner, et al., 2012). Both DEHP and MEHP at concentrations (10 μg/mL and $\geq$1 μg/mL, respectively) that inhibit growth increase follicular ROS production, measured by an assay that utilizes the oxidation-sensitive fluorophore dichlorofluorescein (Wang, Craig, Basavarajappa, Gupta, et al., 2012; Wang, Craig, Basavarajappa, Hafner, et al., 2012). Treatment with the GSH precursor and antioxidant, *N*-acetylcysteine, prevents the DEHP/MEHP-induced growth inhibition and the changes in apoptotic and cell cycle regulatory gene expression (Wang, Craig, Basavarajappa, Gupta, et al., 2012; Wang, Craig, Basavarajappa, Hafner, et al., 2012). These findings strongly support a role for ROS in initiating apoptosis in antral follicles exposed to DEHP/MEHP. It is not known whether cross talk exists between the effects of DEHP/MEHP on estradiol synthesis in granulosa cells and follicle apoptosis; however, this may prove a fruitful avenue for further investigation.

6.2. Methoxychlor

Methoxychlor is an organochlorine insecticide, which was widely used as a less persistent alternative to DDT for many years but which has been banned in the United States since 2002 (http://www.epa.gov/oppsrrd1/REDs/methoxychlor_red.htm). Administration of 32 mg/kg methoxychlor, but not lower doses, for 20 days to adult female mice causes atresia of antral follicles, but not of smaller follicles (Borgeest, Symonds, Mayer, Hoyer, & Flaws, 2002). Treatment regimens that induce antral follicle atresia also increase ovarian H_2O_2 concentrations and ovarian oxidative DNA and protein damage, detected by immunostaining for 8-hydroxy-2′-deoxyguanosine (8-OHdG) and nitrotyrosine, respectively, while decreasing ovarian enzymatic activity and mRNA expression of the antioxidants catalase, GPX, and SOD1 (Gupta, Schuh, Fiskum, & Flaws, 2006). Culture of mouse antral follicles with methoxychlor (1–100 μg/mL) inhibits growth and increases atresia in a concentration- and time-dependent manner (Gupta, Miller, Babus, & Flaws, 2006). There is an initial upregulation of antioxidant gene expression (*Gpx* and catalase) after 48 h of 100 μg/mL methoxychlor treatment, before the onset of atresia, but expression of *Gpx*, catalase, and *Sod1* decreases in all concentration groups by 96 h, when marked atresia is evident (Gupta, Miller, et al., 2006). Cotreatment with *N*-acetylcysteine prevents methoxychlor-induced growth inhibition, atresia, and alterations in antioxidant gene expression (Gupta, Miller, et al., 2006). Together, these findings support a role for oxidative stress in the induction of atresia in antral follicles by methoxychlor.

Although, as noted in the preceding text, methoxychlor does not cause atresia of small follicles in the adult mouse ovary at doses up to 32 mg/kg/day, treatment of neonatal mice with 100 mg/kg/day, but not 50 mg/kg/day, methoxychlor for 7 days decreases the proportion of primordial follicles while increasing proportions of transitional and primary follicles (Sobinoff, Pye, Nixon, Roman, & McLaughlin, 2010). These findings suggest that methoxychlor increases recruitment of primordial follicles into the growing pool, and transcriptomic analysis showed that methoxychlor increases expression of genes in the phosphatidylinositol-3-kinase (PI3K)/Akt pathway and in other signaling pathways that are known to be involved in follicle recruitment and growth (Sobinoff et al., 2010). In addition, the same neonatal treatment regimen with methoxychlor causes dose-dependently decreased *in vitro* sperm binding and sperm fusion to zona pellucida-free oocytes collected after superovulation from 6-week-old mice (Sobinoff et al., 2010). The incubation of superovulated oocytes with the ovotoxic methoxychlor metabolite, 2,2-bis-(*p*-hydroxyphenyl)-1,1,1-trichloroethane, for 2 h increases lipid peroxidation measured by decreased ratio of red/green BODIPY fluorescence (Sobinoff et al., 2010). The latter results suggest that oxidative damage to oocyte plasma membrane lipids due to neonatal exposure to methoxychlor causes permanent decrements in oocyte quality. There is as of yet no direct evidence linking ROS signaling or oxidative stress to increased recruitment of primordial follicles, but culture of neonatal mouse ovaries with methoxychlor for 96 h induces oxidative DNA damage (Sobinoff et al., 2010), and PI3K/Akt signaling pathways are known to respond to and to be modulated by oxidative stress (Sedding, 2008).

6.3. Polycyclic aromatic hydrocarbons

Polycyclic aromatic hydrocarbons (PAHs) are formed during the incomplete combustion of organic materials, such as wood, tobacco, fossil fuels, and foods. They are ubiquitous environmental pollutants to which all Americans are exposed (NHANES, 2009). The parent PAH compounds are relatively nontoxic, but metabolism leads to the formation of DNA-reactive compounds and ROS generation (Winn & Wells, 1997; Xue & Warshawsky, 2005). It has been known for decades that the PAHs benzo[*a*]pyrene (BaP), 9,10-dimethyl-1,2-benzanthracene (DMBA), and 3-methylcholanthrene (3-MC) are potent ovarian toxicants, which dose-dependently destroy primordial and primary follicles in peripubertal mice and rats after single high doses (Mattison, 1979, 1980; Mattison & Thorgeirsson, 1979) or repeated lower doses (Borman, Christian, Sipes, & Hoyer, 2000). Human primordial follicles in ovarian explants placed into mice are also sensitive to depletion by DMBA (Matikainen et al., 2001). Exposure of mice to tobacco smoke, which is rich in PAHs, also depletes primordial follicles (Tuttle, Stampfli, & Foster, 2009), and PAHs in tobacco smoke may be responsible for the earlier onset of menopause in women who smoke (Harlow & Signorello, 2000; Mattison et al., 1989). Very little information is available on the possible roles of ROS in mediating PAH-induced primordial and primary follicle toxicity. One study showed varying effects of *in vivo* tobacco smoke exposure on several markers of oxidative stress; ovarian protein levels of heat shock protein 25 increased, while SOD2 protein levels decreased, but no changes were observed in oxidative protein and DNA damage or GSH concentrations (Gannon, Stämpfli, & Foster, 2012). Another recent study showed that DMBA treatment of neonatal mice (1 mg/kg/day for 7 days) or cultured neonatal mouse ovaries (50 nM) increased activation of primordial follicles (measured by PCNA, phosphorylated Akt immunostaining) while increasing apoptosis in primary and secondary follicles (immunostaining for activated caspases 2 and 3 and TUNEL) (Sobinoff, Mahony, Nixon, Roman, & McLaughlin, 2011). Microarray analysis showed upregulation of methionine metabolism pathway, which was interpreted by the authors as suggesting a role for DMBA-induced oxidative stress in the neonatal ovarian toxicity of DMBA. The same group subsequently reported similar results for the PAHs BaP and 3-MC (Sobinoff, Nixon, Roman, & McLaughlin, 2012; Sobinoff, Pye, Nixon, Roman, & McLaughlin, 2012). In addition, they reported that neonatal treatment with BaP (1.5 or 3.0 mg/kg/day for 7 days) results in increased mitochondrial $O_2^{-\bullet}$ generation measured using the fluorophore MitoSOX, increased lipid peroxidation measured using the fluorophore BODIPY, and decreased *in vitro* sperm binding and sperm fusion in oocytes ovulated at 6 weeks of age (Sobinoff, Pye, et al., 2012).

In addition to destroying primordial and primary follicles, 3-MC also targets secondary follicles, and DMBA also targets antral follicles (Borman et al., 2000; Mattison, 1980). Culture of rat large antral follicles with DMBA concentration-dependently (≥ 1 μM) induces granulosa cell apoptosis, increasing immunostaining for the proapoptotic protein BAX by 24 h and increasing caspase 3 activation and DNA fragmentation by TUNEL staining by 48 h (Tsai-Turton, Nakamura, & Luderer, 2007). Follicular ROS levels, measured by dichlorofluorescein fluorescence, increase by 12 h and remain elevated, and supplementation of GSH protects against DMBA-induced apoptosis, while GSH depletion potentiates DMBA-induced apoptosis (Tsai-Turton, Nakamura, et al., 2007). While these results suggest that the rise in ROS mediates induction of apoptosis by DMBA, the lack of protection against DMBA-induced apoptosis by two other antioxidants, dithiothreitol and butylated hydroxytoluene, suggests that other actions of GSH besides its antioxidant actions may be involved (Tsai-Turton, Nakamura, et al., 2007). Further studies are needed to clarify the role of ROS in DMBA-induced antral follicle toxicity.

The fetal ovary appears to be even more sensitive to PAH ovarian toxicity than the peripubertal ovary. Treatment of pregnant mice by oral gavage with 0, 10, 40, or 160 mg/kg/day BaP from gestational days 7 to 16 dose-dependently decreases fertility of F1 female offspring, with very few follicles observed in the ovaries of mice exposed prenatally to the highest dose (MacKenzie & Angevine, 1981). Support for a role of ROS in mediating BaP fetal ovary toxicity comes from a recent study, which showed that F1 female embryos deficient in GSH synthesis due to deletion of *Gclm* are more sensitive to the transplacental ovarian toxicity of BaP than their wild-type littermates (Lim et al., 2013). F1 female $Gclm^{-/-}$ offspring exposed to 2 or 10 mg/kg/day BaP from gestational days 7 to 16 have greater decrements in fertility and in ovarian follicle numbers compared to vehicle-treated controls of the same genotype than did their $Gclm^{+/+}$ littermates (Lim et al., 2013).

6.4. Cyclophosphamide

Treatment of cancer and autoimmune diseases in women with alkylating antineoplastic drugs often causes temporary amenorrhea or premature ovarian failure, consistent with destruction of large, growing follicles and primordial follicles, respectively (Byrne, 1999; Chemaitilly et al., 2006; Howell & Shalet, 1998; Meirow & Nugent, 2001; Nicosia, Matus-Riley, & Meadows, 1985). Even if menstrual cycles resume after a period of amenorrhea, women may suffer from premature ovarian failure due to partial depletion of the primordial follicle pool.

The anticancer activity of alkylating agents like cyclophosphamide (CP) results from their ability to alkylate DNA of cancer cells; however, DNA damage to nontarget cells is responsible for many of their side effects. CP is metabolically activated by cytochrome P450 enzymes to 4-hydroxycyclophosphamide, which undergoes ring-opening to aldophosphamide, which spontaneously decomposes to phosphoramide mustard (PM) (Chang, Weber, Crespi, & Waxman, 1993; Dirven, van Ommen, & van Bladeren, 1994; Gamcsik, Dolan, Andersson, & Murray, 1999). PM is thought to be the active metabolite in terms of both its anticancer activity and its ovarian toxicity (Gamcsik et al., 1999; Plowchalk & Mattison, 1991). CP destroys follicles at all stages of development in women and in rodent models (Davis & Maronpot, 1996; Jarrell et al., 1987; Kumar, Biggart, McEvoy, & McGeown, 1972; Plowchalk & Mattison, 1991; Shiromizu, Thorgeirsson, & Mattison, 1984; Warne, Fairley, Hobbs, & Martin, 1973). Mice are more sensitive to the destruction of primordial follicles by *in vivo* treatment with CP (Meirow, Lewis, Nugent, & Epstein, 1999; Shiromizu et al., 1984), while rats are more sensitive to the destruction of secondary and antral follicles (Davis & Heindel, 1998). Consistent with these *in vivo* findings, treatment of cultured neonatal mouse and rat ovaries, which are enriched in primordial follicles, with PM concentrations ≥ 3 and 30 μM, respectively, depletes primordial follicles (Desmeules & Devine, 2006; Petrillo, Desmeules, Truong, & Devine, 2011). Caspase activation, a classical marker of apoptosis, is not observed in primordial follicles treated with PM, and inhibition of caspase activation does not protect against primordial follicle depletion (Desmeules & Devine, 2006; Petrillo et al., 2011). Double-stranded DNA breaks are detected by immunostaining for phosphorylated histone H2AFX in primordial follicle oocytes prior to the onset of follicle degeneration at doses that induce follicle degeneration at later time points, consistent with a role for DNA damage in initiating follicular destruction (Petrillo et al., 2011). Although double-stranded DNA breaks can be caused by oxidative DNA damage (Lloyd, Carmichael, & Phillips, 1998), no studies have measured ROS or oxidative damage in primordial follicles exposed to PM.

In contrast to primordial follicles, there is evidence for ROS and caspase activation playing a role in the mechanism of follicular destruction by CP in secondary and antral follicles. A single i.p. dose of ≥ 50 mg/kg CP in normally cycling adult rats significantly increases the percentages of secondary and antral follicles that have apoptotic granulosa cells, as evidenced by TUNEL staining and immunostaining for activated caspases 3 and 9 (Devine et al., 2012; Lopez & Luderer, 2004). COV434 human granulosa cells have been used as a model system in which to study the mechanisms by which CP induces ovarian apoptosis (Tsai-Turton, Luong, et al., 2007). Treatment of COV434 cells with 0, 1, 10, or 50 μM 4-hydroperoxycyclophosphamide (4HC), a preactivated form of CP that decomposes in solution to 4-hydroxycyclophosphamide (Flowers et al., 2000; Gamcsik et al., 1999), causes rapid (within 2 h) concentration-dependent declines in GSH concentrations and increases in ROS assessed by dichlorofluorescein fluorescence (Tsai-Turton, Luong, et al., 2007). These are followed at 12 and 24 h by oxidative DNA damage measured by 8-OHdG immunofluorescence, activation of caspase 3, and DNA fragmentation by TUNEL staining (Tsai-Turton, Luong, et al., 2007). Supplementation with a cell-permeable form of GSH or with the antioxidants ascorbic acid and dithiothreitol is protective against 4HC-induced apoptosis, whereas depletion of GSH with BSO potentiates 4HC-induced apoptosis (Tsai-Turton, Luong, et al., 2007). Together, the available evidence is consistent with an early increase in ROS during CP metabolism initiating apoptosis in the granulosa cells of secondary and antral follicles.

6.5. Chromium

The heavy metal chromium (Cr) is used in numerous industrial processes, including leather tanning, electroplating, wood preservative manufacture, and steel alloy production (Keegan, Learmonth, & Case, 2008). Cr contamination of drinking water from industrial and natural sources is an important exposure route for the general population in parts of the world. Cr exists in several oxidation states. CrVI is a known carcinogen, which is rapidly reduced to CrIII, the most stable oxidation state, in biological systems by ascorbic acid, GSH, and cysteine. However, during reduction, reactive Cr species and ROS are generated (O'Brien, Ceryak, & Patierno, 2003). CrIII is excreted in breast milk, and lactation is thus a source of exposure to the offspring.

Administration of Cr in drinking water causes follicular atresia in adult mice (Murthy, Junaid, & Saxena, 1996). Administration of 200 mg/L potassium dichromate (a CrVI compound) in the drinking water to lactating female rats from the day of parturition until weaning at postnatal day (PND) 21 decreases primordial and primary follicle numbers in F1 female offspring at PNDs 21, 45, and 65 and decreases secondary and antral follicle numbers at PNDs 21 and 45, with recovery by PND 65 (Banu, Samuel, Arosh, Burghardt, & Aruldhas, 2008). Coadministration of 500 mg/L ascorbic acid with Cr prevents the decreases in follicle numbers (Banu et al., 2008). A subsequent dose response study by the same group showed that 50, 100, and 200 mg/L Cr administration dose-dependently increases ovarian follicular atresia and apoptosis over the same age range and that ascorbic acid administered by gavage at 500 mg/kg/day is protective (Stanley et al., 2013). Cr administration also dose-dependently decreases serum estradiol, progesterone, and testosterone concentrations and increases FSH concentrations at all time points in F1 female offspring; ascorbic acid coadministration prevents or mitigates these effects (Banu et al., 2008; Stanley et al., 2013). Cr treatment is associated with increased systemic and ovarian H_2O_2 and lipid hydroperoxide concentrations in F1 female offspring through PND 65, and again, ascorbic acid prevents or mitigates these increases (Stanley et al., 2013). Cr administration dose-dependently decreases plasma and ovarian enzymatic activities of the antioxidant enzymes GPX, GSR, SOD, and catalase and ascorbic acid concentrations, and ascorbic acid supplementation mitigates these effects (Stanley et al., 2013). Similarly, another recent study found that F1 female offspring that were exposed to 200 mg/L Cr in the drinking water from GD9 through PND 65, first via dosing of their mothers and then via direct dosing, had elevated malondialdehyde, an indicator of lipid peroxidation, and H_2O_2 concentrations in the ovaries at various ages from birth until PND 65 compared to controls that received drinking water without Cr (Samuel et al., 2012). Together, these *in vivo* studies are consistent with increased ROS and the resulting oxidative stress mediating the destruction of ovarian follicles and ovarian endocrine dysfunction caused by developmental Cr exposure.

Studies by the same group using cultured primary rat granulosa cells and theca cells or spontaneously immortalized granulosa cells (SIGCs) provide additional insights into the mechanisms of Cr-induced ovarian toxicity. Treatment of cultured rat granulosa cells with 10 μM potassium dichromate for 12 and 24 h induces apoptosis, measured by TUNEL, caspase 3 activation, and cleavage of PARP; treatment with a caspase inhibitor prevents Cr-induced apoptosis (Banu et al., 2011). Induction of apoptosis in granulosa cells appears to be via the mitochondrial pathway, as Cr treatment decreases cellular levels of the antiapoptotic proteins BCL-2 and BCL-XL and increases translocation of the proapoptotic proteins BAX and BAD and of activated p53 to the mitochondria and increases translocation of cytochrome c from the mitochondria to the cytosol (Banu et al., 2011). The same Cr treatment regimen also induces cell cycle arrest and inhibits proliferation of cultured rat granulosa cells (Stanley et al., 2011). All of these effects of Cr in granulosa cell cultures are mitigated by cotreatment with ascorbic acid (Banu et al., 2011; Stanley et al., 2011). More recently, this group showed that treatment of cultured granulosa cells, theca cells, and SIGC with 10 μM potassium dichromate increases H_2O_2 and lipid hydroperoxide concentrations by 12 h, and ascorbic acid prevents this Cr-induced oxidative stress (Stanley et al., 2013). Further, the same Cr treatment decreases ascorbic acid concentrations; mRNA expression of the antioxidant genes *Sod1*, *Sod2*, *catalase*, *Glrx1*, *Gsr*, *Gstm1*, *Gstm2*, *Gsta4*, *Txn1*, *Txn2*, *Txnrd2*, and *Prdx3*; and enzymatic activity of GPX, GSR, and GST in all three cell types by 12 h, and these effects are largely mitigated by ascorbic acid in granulosa cells and SIGC and to a lesser extent in theca cells (Stanley et al., 2013). Together, these results suggest that increased ROS and resultant oxidative stress initiate apoptosis via the mitochondrial pathway in granulosa cells and theca cells upon exposure to Cr.

6.6. Menadione

Menadione or 2-methyl-1,4-naphthoquinone is a vitamin K analog, which can undergo one-electron reduction by enzymes including microsomal NADPH–cytochrome P450 reductase and mitochondrial NADH–ubiquinone oxidoreductase (complex I), resulting in redox cycling, or it can undergo detoxification via two-electron reduction by NAD(P)H–quinone oxidoreductase (Criddle et al., 2006).

In vivo treatment of neonatal mice from PNDs 4 to 10 with 0, 7.5, or 15 mg/kg/day menadione dose-dependently decreased the proportion of primordial follicles and increased the proportions of activating/transitional and primary follicles while decreasing the total number of follicles per section (Sobinoff et al., 2010). Ovaries from the mice treated *in vivo* with menadione and neonatal ovaries cultured with 5 μM menadione showed increased PCNA staining in the granulosa cells and oocytes of primordial follicles, consistent with increased activation of primordial follicles by menadione (Sobinoff et al., 2010). Ovaries cultured with menadione also showed widespread immunostaining for the oxidative DNA lesion, 8-OHdG; widespread TUNEL staining in follicles of all stages; and immunostaining for activated caspase 3 in granulosa cells and caspase 2 in oocytes of primary and secondary follicles. Oocyte quality, measured by *in vitro* sperm binding and sperm fusion to zona pellucida-free oocytes collected at 6 weeks of age from mice treated neonatally with the same regimen of menadione described in the preceding text, was significantly decreased at both menadione doses (Sobinoff et al., 2010). Treatment of cultured superovulated oocytes from 6- to 8-week-old mice with menadione at concentrations from 0 to 25 μM concentration-dependently induced lipid peroxidation in oocytes as measured by BODIPY immunofluorescence (Sobinoff et al., 2010). These results are consistent with the possibilities that menadione-induced oxidative stress initiates apoptosis in ovarian follicles at all stages of development and also increases activation of primordial follicles. In addition, follicles that survive neonatal menadione treatment show persistent abnormalities of oocyte quality, which may be caused by lipid peroxidation of the oocyte plasma membrane.

7. INVOLVEMENT OF ROS IN OVARIAN TOXICITY CAUSED BY IONIZING RADIATION

Women who are treated for cancer with ionizing radiation to the pelvis frequently develop temporary amenorrhea and/or premature ovarian failure, similar to the effects of antineoplastic drugs (Lo Presti, Ruvulo, Gancitano, & Cittadini, 2004; Meirow & Nugent, 2001). Higher radiation doses and older age increase the risk for developing premature ovarian failure. It has been estimated that the dose of radiation required to destroy half of the primordial follicle pool in young women is less than 2 Gray (Wallace, Shalet, Hendry, Morris-Jone, & Gattamaneni, 1989; Wallace, Thomson, & Kelsey, 2003). Ionizing radiation destroys follicles of all developmental stages in women and in rodents (Hanoux, Pairault, Bakalska, Habert, & Livera, 2007; Jarrell et al., 1987; Kim & Lee, 2000; Meirow & Nugent, 2001).

In addition to the direct ionization of DNA, ionizing radiation also ionizes water molecules, resulting in ROS formation, and leads to persistent increases in mitochondrial ROS production (Kim, Fiskum, & Morgan, 2006; Spitz et al., 2004; Wiseman & Halliwell, 1996). Therefore, the toxic effects of ionizing radiation on ovarian follicles may be mediated by ROS. Degeneration of primordial and primary follicles is observed as early as 2 h after gamma irradiation of prepubertal mice with a dose of 8.3 Gray (Kim & Lee, 2000; Lee, Park, Do, Yoon, & Kim, 2000). Pretreatment with 100 μg of the antioxidant melatonin significantly protects against radiation-induced primordial follicle destruction at all time points, while 10 μg is less protective; the beneficial effects of melatonin are less consistent for primary and larger growing follicles (Kim & Lee, 2000). Rapid, sustained increases in ROS occur in human COV434 granulosa cells within 30 min after 1 or 5 Gray gamma irradiation, followed by apoptotic death at 6 h (Cortés-Wanstreet et al., 2009). Stable overexpression of one or both subunits of the rate-limiting enzyme in GSH synthesis, *Gclc* and *Gclm*, increases GSH synthesis, prevents the radiation-induced rise in ROS, and prevents apoptotic death of the cells (Cortés-Wanstreet et al., 2009). Taken together, the available data support a role for ROS in initiating apoptosis in granulosa cells and ovarian follicles following exposure to ionizing radiation, but detailed understanding of the mechanisms awaits further study.

The fetal ovary is also sensitive to the effects of ionizing radiation. Exposure to 1.5 Gray ionizing radiation causes double-stranded DNA breaks, measured using phosphorylated histone H2AFX immunostaining, in oogonia of cultured human fetal ovary pieces (weeks 6–10 of gestation) and GD 12.5 mouse ovary treated *in vivo* or *in vitro* (Guerquin et al., 2009). At 1 h after irradiation, the number of phosphorylated histone H2AFX foci is similar in fetal testes and ovaries, but the number of foci declines more rapidly thereafter in mouse ovaries than in testes, consistent with faster DNA repair in ovaries (Guerquin et al., 2009). Doses $\geq$ 1.5 Gray induce germ cell apoptosis and significantly deplete ovarian germ cells by more than 50% in cultured human and mouse fetal ovaries by 48 h after irradiation by a mechanism that does not involve p53 or p63 (Guerquin et al., 2009). These results contrast with those for fetal testes, where germ cell apoptosis is induced at lower doses and induction of germ cell apoptosis involves p53 activation (Guerquin et al., 2009; Lambrot et al., 2007). As of yet, there is no direct evidence for ROS involvement in the destruction of fetal ovarian germ cells by ionizing radiation exposure. Future studies should examine the effects of ionizing radiation on fetal ovary ROS production and test the protective effects of antioxidants.

8. SUMMARY AND CONCLUSIONS

In recent years, the importance of ROS and oxidative stress in ovarian toxicity by diverse stimuli has been increasingly recognized. There is strong evidence that ROS are involved in the initiation of apoptosis in antral follicles upon gonadotropin hormone withdrawal and exposure to chemicals including phthalates, PAHs, methoxychlor, and CP and ionizing radiation. Although less attention has been focused on the roles of ROS in primordial and primary follicle atresia, several studies have shown protective effects of antioxidants and/or evidence of oxidative damage, suggesting that ROS may play a role in these smaller follicles as well. Oxidative damage to lipids in the oocyte has been implicated as a cause of persistently poor oocyte quality after early life exposure to several toxicants. Developing germ cells in the fetal ovary have also been shown to be sensitive to toxicants and ionizing radiation, which induce oxidative stress. Recent studies have begun to elucidate the mechanisms by which ROS mediate ovarian toxicity. Future studies should test the ability of *in vivo* supplementation with antioxidants to prevent the adverse effects of ovarian toxicants. It will also be important to translate the findings to humans by investigating whether women with polymorphisms in antioxidant genes are at greater risk of ovarian failure or infertility.

REFERENCES

Anathy, V., Roberson, E. C., Guala, A. S., Godburn, K. E., Budd, R. C., & Janssen-Heininger, Y. M. W. (2012). Redox-based regulation of apoptosis: S-glutathionylation as a regulatory mechanism to control cell death. *Antioxidants and Redox Signaling, 16*, 496–505.

Aten, R. F., Duarte, K. M., & Behrman, H. R. (1992). Regulation of ovarian antioxidant vitamins, reduced glutathione, and lipid peroxidation by luteinizing hormone and prostaglandin F_{2alpha}. *Biology of Reproduction, 46*, 401–407.

Banu, S. K., Samuel, J. B., Arosh, J. A., Burghardt, R. C., & Aruldhas, M. M. (2008). Lactational exposure to hexavalent chromium delays puberty by impairing ovarian development, steroidogenesis, and pituitary hormone synthesis in developing Wistar rats. *Toxicology and Applied Pharmacology, 232*, 180–189.

Banu, S. K., Stanley, J. A., Lee, J., Stephen, S. D., Arosh, J. A., Hoyer, P. B., et al. (2011). Hexavalent chromium-induced apoptosis of granulosa cells involves selective sub-cellular translocation of Bcl-2 members, ERK1/2 and p53. *Toxicology and Applied Pharmacology, 251*, 253–266.

Borgeest, C., Symonds, D. A., Mayer, L. P., Hoyer, P. B., & Flaws, J. A. (2002). Methoxychlor may cause ovarian follicular atresia and proliferation of the ovarian surface epithelium in the mouse. *Toxicological Sciences*, *68*, 473–478.

Borman, S. M., Christian, P. J., Sipes, I. G., & Hoyer, P. B. (2000). Ovotoxicity in female Fischer rats and B6 mice induced by low-dose exposure to three polycyclic aromatic hydrocarbons: Comparison through calculation of an ovotoxic index. *Toxicology and Applied Pharmacology*, *167*, 191–198.

Byrne, J. (1999). Long-term genetic and reproductive effects of ionizing radiation and chemotherapeutic agents on cancer patients and their offspring. *Teratology*, *59*, 210–215.

Chang, T. K., Weber, G. F., Crespi, C. L., & Waxman, D. J. (1993). Differential activation of cyclophosphamide and ifosphamide by cytochromes P-450 2B and 3A in human liver microsomes. *Cancer Research*, *53*, 5629–5637.

Chemaitilly, W., Mertens, A. C., Mitby, P., Whitton, J., Stovall, M., Yasui, Y., et al. (2006). Acute ovarian failure in the Childhood Cancer Survivor Study. *Journal of Clinical Endocrinology and Metabolism*, *91*, 1723–1728.

Chun, S.-Y., Billig, H., Tilly, J. L., Furuta, I., Tsafriri, A., & Hsueh, A. J. W. (1994). Gonadotropin suppression of apoptosis in cultured preovulatory follicles: Mediatory role of endogenous insulin-like growth factor I. *Endocrinology*, *135*, 1845–1853.

Chun, S. Y., Eisenhauer, K. M., Minami, S., Billig, H., Perlas, E., & Hsueh, A. J. (1996). Hormonal regulation of apoptosis in early antral follicles: Follicle-stimulating hormone as a major survival factor. *Endocrinology*, *137*, 1447–1456.

Conrad, M., Moreno, S. G., Sinowatz, F., Ursini, F., Kölle, S., Roveri, A., et al. (2005). The nuclear form of phospholipid hydroperoxide glutathione peroxidase is a protein thiol peroxidase contributing to sperm chromatin stability. *Molecular and Cellular Biology*, *25*, 7637–7644.

Cortés-Wanstreet, M. M., Giedzinski, E., Limoli, C. L., & Luderer, U. (2009). Overexpression of glutamate cysteine ligase protects human COV434 granulosa tumor cells against oxidative and γ-radiation-induced cell death. *Mutagenesis*, *24*, 211–224.

Criddle, D. N., Gillies, S., Baumgartner-Wilson, H. K., Jaffar, M., Chinje, E. C., Passmore, S., et al. (2006). Menadione-induced reactive oxygen species generation via redox cycling promotes apoptosis of murine pancreatic acinar cells. *Journal of Biological Chemistry*, *281*, 40485–40492.

Dalton, T. P., Dieter, M. Z., Yang, Y., Shertzer, H. G., & Nebert, D. W. (2000). Knockout of the mouse glutamate cysteine ligase catalytic subunit (Gclc) gene: Embryonic lethal when homozygous, and proposed model for moderate glutathione deficiency when heterozygous. *Biochemical and Biophysical Research Communications*, *279*, 324–329.

Das, P., & Chowdhury, M. (1999). Vitamin E-deficiency induced changes in ovary and uterus. *Molecular and Cellular Biochemistry*, *198*, 151–156.

Davis, B. J., & Heindel, J. J. (1998). Ovarian toxicants: Multiple mechanisms of action. In K. S. Korach (Ed.), *Reproductive and developmental toxicology* (pp. 373–395). New York: Marcel Dekker, Inc.

Davis, B. J., & Maronpot, R. R. (1996). Chemically associated toxicity and carcinogenicity of the ovary. In J. Huff, J. Boyd, & J. C. Barrett (Eds.), *Cellular and molecular mechanisms of hormonal carcinogenesis: Environmental influences* (pp. 285–308). New York: Wiley-Liss.

Desmeules, P., & Devine, P. J. (2006). Characterizing the ovotoxicity of cyclophosphamide metabolites on cultured mouse ovaries. *Toxicological Sciences*, *90*, 500–509.

Devine, P. J., Perreault, S. D., & Luderer, U. (2012). Roles of reactive oxygen species and antioxidants in ovarian toxicity. *Biology of Reproduction*, *86*, 1–10.

Dirven, H. A. A. M., van Ommen, B., & van Bladeren, P. J. (1994). Involvement of human glutathione S-transferase isoenzymes in the conjugation of cyclophosphamide metabolites with glutathione. *Cancer Research*, *54*, 6215–6220.

Duester, G. (2007). Retinoic acid regulation of the somitogenesis clock. *Birth Defects Research Part C: Embryo Today*, *81*, 84–92.

Evans, H. M. (1928). The effects of inadequate vitamin A on the sexual physiology of the female. *Journal of Biological Chemistry, 77*, 651–654.
Evans, H. M., & Bishop, K. S. (1922). On the existence of a hitherto unrecognized dietary factor essential for reproduction. *Science, 56*, 650–651.
Flowers, J., Ludeman, S. M., Gamcsik, M. P., Colvin, O. M., Shao, K.-L., Boal, J. H., et al. (2000). Evidence for a role of chloroethylaziridine in the cytotoxicity of cyclophosphamide. *Cancer Chemotherapy and Pharmacology, 45*, 335–344.
Gamcsik, M. P., Dolan, M. E., Andersson, B. S., & Murray, D. (1999). Mechanisms of resistance to the toxicity of cyclophosphamide. *Current Pharmaceutical Design, 5*, 587–605.
Gannon, A. M., Stämpfli, M. R., & Foster, W. G. (2012). Cigarette smoke exposure leads to follicle loss via an alternative ovarian cell death pathway in a mouse model. *Toxicological Sciences, 125*, 274–284.
Giordano, G., White, C. C., McConnachie, L. A., Fernandez, C., Kavanagh, T. J., & Costa, L. G. (2006). Neurotoxicity of domoic acid in cerebellar granule neurons in a genetic model of glutathione deficiency. *Molecular Pharmacology, 70*, 2116–2126.
Giorgio, M., Trinei, M., Migliaccio, E., & Pelicci, P. G. (2007). Hydrogen peroxide: A metabolic by-product or a common mediator of ageing signals? *Nature Reviews Molecular Cell Biology, 8*, 722–728.
Guerquin, M.-J., Duquenne, C., Coffigny, H., Rouiller-Fabre, V., Lambrot, R., Bakalska, M., et al. (2009). Sex-specific differences in fetal germ cell apoptosis induced by ionizing radiation. *Human Reproduction, 24*, 670–678.
Gupta, R. K., Miller, K. P., Babus, J. K., & Flaws, J. A. (2006). Methoxychlor inhibits growth and induces atresia of antral follicles through an oxidative stress pathway. *Toxicological Sciences, 93*, 382–389.
Gupta, R. K., Schuh, R. A., Fiskum, G., & Flaws, J. A. (2006). Methoxychlor causes mitochondrial dysfunction and oxidative damage in the mouse ovary. *Toxicology and Applied Pharmacology, 216*, 436–445.
Hanoux, V., Pairault, C., Bakalska, M., Habert, R., & Livera, G. (2007). Caspase-2 involvement during ionizing radiation-induced oocyte death in the mouse ovary. *Cell Death and Differentiation, 14*, 671–681.
Hanukoglu, I. (2006). Antioxidant protective mechanisms against reactive oxygen species (ROS) generated by mitochondrial P450 systems in steroidogenic cells. *Drug Metabolism Reviews, 38*, 171–196.
Harlow, B. L., & Signorello, L. B. (2000). Factors associated with early menopause. *Maturitas, 35*, 3–9.
Hayes, J. D., & Pulford, D. J. (1995). The glutathione-*S*-transferase supergene family: Regulation of GST and the contribution of the isoenzymes to cancer chemoprevention and drug resistance. *Critical Reviews in Biochemistry and Molecular Biology, 30*, 445–600.
Hirshfield, A. N. (1988). Size-frequency analysis of atresia in cycling rats. *Biology of Reproduction, 38*, 1181–1188.
Ho, Y.-S., Gargano, M., Cao, J., Bronson, R. T., Heimler, I., & Hutz, R. J. (1998). Reduced fertility in female mice lacking copper-zinc superoxide dismutase. *Journal of Biological Chemistry, 273*, 7765–7769.
Ho, Y.-S., Magnenat, J.-L., Bronson, R. T., Cao, J., Gargano, M., Sugawara, M., et al. (1997). Mice deficient in cellular glutathione peroxidase develop normally and show no increased sensitivity to hyperoxia. *Journal of Biological Chemistry, 272*, 16644–16651.
Ho, Y.-S., Xiong, Y., Ma, W., Spector, A., & Ho, D. S. (2004). Mice lacking catalase develop normally but show differential sensitivity to oxidant tissue injury. *Journal of Biological Chemistry, 279*, 32804–32812.
Hoang, Y. D., Nakamura, B. N., & Luderer, U. (2009). Follicle-stimulating hormone and estradiol interact to stimulate glutathione synthesis in rat ovarian follicles and granulosa cells. *Biology of Reproduction, 81*, 636–646.

Howell, S., & Shalet, S. (1998). Gonadal damage from chemotherapy and radiotherapy. *Endocrinology and Metabolism Clinics of North America, 27*, 927–943.

Jarrell, J., Young Lai, E. V., Barr, R., McMahon, A., Belbeck, L., & O'Connell, G. (1987). Ovarian toxicity of cyclophosphamide alone and in combination with ovarian irradiation in the rat. *Cancer Research, 47*, 2340–2343.

Jones, D. P. (2006). Redefining oxidative stress. *Antioxidants and Redox Signaling, 8*, 1865–1879.

Jones, D. P. (2008). Radical-free biology of oxidative stress. *American Journal of Physiology, 295*, C849–C868.

Keegan, G. M., Learmonth, I. D., & Case, C. P. (2008). A systematic comparison of the actual, potential, and theoretical health effects of cobalt and chromium exposures from industry and surgical implants. *Critical Reviews in Toxicology, 38*, 645–674.

Kim, G. J., Fiskum, G., & Morgan, W. F. (2006). A role for mitochondrial dysfunction in perpetuating radiation-induced genomic instability. *Cancer Research, 66*, 10377–10383.

Kim, J. K., & Lee, C. J. (2000). Effect of exogenous melatonin on the ovarian follicles in gamma-irradiated mouse. *Mutation Research, 449*, 33–39.

Kumar, R., Biggart, J. D., McEvoy, J., & McGeown, M. G. (1972). Cyclophosphamide and reproductive function. *Lancet, 299*(7762), 1212–1214.

Kumar, T. R., Wiseman, A. L., Kala, G., Kala, S. V., Matzuk, M. M., & Lieberman, M. W. (2000). Reproductive defects in Γ-glutamyl transpeptidase deficient mice. *Endocrinology, 141*, 4270–4277.

Laloraya, M., Kumar, P. G., & Laloraya, M. M. (1988). Changes in the levels of superoxide anion radical and superoxide dismutase during the estrous cycle of rattus norvegicus and induction of superoxide dismutase in rat ovary by lutropin. *Biochemical and Biophysical Research Communications, 157*, 146–153.

Lambrot, R., Coffigny, H., Pairault, C., Lécureuil, C., Frydman, R., Habert, R., et al. (2007). High radiosensitivity of germ cells in human male fetus. *Journal of Clinical Endocrinology and Metabolism, 92*, 2632–2639.

Lee, C. J., Park, H. H., Do, B. R., Yoon, Y. D., & Kim, J. K. (2000). Natural and radiation-induced degeneration of the primordial and primary follicles in the mouse ovary. *Animal Reproduction Science, 59*, 109–117.

Li, H., & Clagett-Dame, M. (2009). Vitamin a deficiency blocks the initiation of meiosis of germ cells in the developing rat ovary in vivo. *Biology of Reproduction, 81*, 996–1001.

Lieberman, M. W., Wiseman, A. L., Shi, Z.-Z., Carter, B. Z., Barrios, R., Ou, C.-N., et al. (1996). Growth retardation and cysteine deficiency in γ-glutamyl transpeptidase-deficient mice. *Proceedings of the National Academy of Sciences of the United States of America, 93*, 7923–7926.

Lim, J., Lawson, G. W., Nakamura, B. N., Ortiz, L., Hur, J. A., Kavanagh, T. J., et al. (2013). Glutathione-deficient mice have increased sensitivity to transplacental benzo[a]pyrene-induced premature ovarian failure and ovarian tumorigenesis. *Cancer Research, 73*, 1–10.

Lloyd, D. R., Carmichael, P. L., & Phillips, D. H. (1998). Comparison of the formation of 8-hydroxy-2′-deoxyguanosine and single- and double-strand breaks in DNA mediated by Fenton reactions. *Chemical Research in Toxicology, 11*, 420–427.

Lopez, S. G., & Luderer, U. (2004). Effects of cyclophosphamide and buthionine sulfoximine on ovarian glutathione and apoptosis. *Free Radical Biology and Medicine, 36*, 1366–1377.

Lo Presti, A., Ruvulo, G., Gancitano, R. A., & Cittadini, E. (2004). Ovarian function following radiation and chemotherapy for cancer. *European Journal of Obstetrics, Gynecology, and Reproductive Biology, 113*, S33–S40.

Lovekamp-Swan, T., & Davis, B. J. (2003). Mechanisms of phthalate ester toxicity in the female reproductive system. *Environmental Health Perspectives, 111*, 139–145.

Lovekamp-Swan, T., Jetten, A. M., & Davis, B. J. (2003). Dual activation of PPARα and PPARΓ by mono-(2-ethylhexyl) phthalate in Rat ovarian granulosa cells. *Molecular and Cellular Endocrinology, 201*, 133–141.

Luck, M. R., Jeyaseelan, I., & Scholes, R. A. (1995). Minireview: Ascorbic acid and fertility. *Biology of Reproduction*, *52*, 262–266.

Luderer, U., Kavanagh, T. J., White, C. C., & Faustman, E. M. (2001). Gonadotropin regulation of glutathione synthesis in the rat ovary. *Reproductive Toxicology*, *15*, 495–504.

MacKenzie, K. M., & Angevine, D. M. (1981). Infertility in mice exposed in utero to benzo(a)pyrene. *Biology of Reproduction*, *24*, 183–191.

Matikainen, T., Perez, G. I., Jurisicova, A., Pru, J. K., Schlezinger, J. J., Ryu, H.-Y., et al. (2001). Aromatic hydrocarbon receptor-driven Bax gene expression is required for premature ovarian failure caused by biohazardous environmental chemicals. *Nature Genetics*, *28*, 355–360.

Mattison, D. R. (1979). Difference in sensitivity of rat and mouse primordial oocytes to destruction by polycyclic aromatic hydrocarbons. *Chemico-Biological Interactions*, *28*, 133–137.

Mattison, D. R. (1980). Morphology of oocyte and follicle destruction by polycyclic aromatic hydrocarbons in mice. *Toxicology and Applied Pharmacology*, *53*, 249–259.

Mattison, D. R., Plowchalk, D. R., Meadows, M. J., Miller, M. M., Malek, A., & London, S. (1989). The effect of smoking on oogenesis, fertilization, and implantation. *Seminars in Reproductive Endocrinology*, 7, 291–304.

Mattison, D. R., & Thorgeirsson, S. S. (1979). Ovarian aryl hydrocarbon hydroxylase activity and primordial oocyte toxicity of polycyclic aromatic hydrocarbons in mice. *Cancer Research*, *39*, 3471–3475.

Matzuk, M. M., Dionne, L., Guo, Q., Kumar, T. R., & Lebovitz, R. M. (1998). Ovarian function in superoxide dismutase 1 and 2 knockout mice. *Endocrinology*, *139*, 4008–4011.

McConnachie, L. A., Mohar, I., Hudson, F. N., Ware, C. B., Ladiges, W. C., Fernandez, C., et al. (2007). Glutamate cysteine ligase modifier subunit deficiency and gender as determinants of acetaminophen-induced hepatotoxicity in mice. *Toxicological Sciences*, *99*, 628–636.

Meirow, D., Lewis, H., Nugent, D., & Epstein, M. (1999). Subclinical depletion of primordial follicular reserve in mice treated with cyclophosphamide: Clinical importance and proposed accurate investigative tool. *Human Reproduction*, *14*, 1903–1907.

Meirow, D., & Nugent, D. (2001). The effects of radiotherapy and chemotherapy on female reproduction. *Human Reproduction Update*, 7, 535–543.

Miyazaki, T., Sueoka, K., Dharmarajan, A. M., Atlas, S. J., Bulkley, G. B., & Wallach, E. E. (1991). Effect of inhibition of oxygen free radical on ovulation and progesterone production by the in vitro perfused rabbit ovary. *Journal of Reproduction and Fertility*, *91*, 207–212.

Murthy, R. C., Junaid, M., & Saxena, D. K. (1996). Ovarian dysfunction in mice following chromium (VI) exposure. *Toxicology Letters*, *89*, 147–154.

Musicki, B., Kodaman, P. H., Aten, R. F., & Behrman, H. R. (1996). Endocrine regulation of ascorbic acid transport and secretion in luteal cells. *Biology of Reproduction*, *54*, 399–406.

Nakamura, B. N., Fielder, T. J., Hoang, Y. D., Lim, J., McConnachie, L. A., Kavanagh, T. J., et al. (2011). Lack of maternal glutamate cysteine ligase modifier subunit (*Gclm*) decreases oocyte glutathione concentrations and disrupts preimplantation development in mice. *Endocrinology*, *152*, 2806–2815.

NHANES. (2009). Fourth national report on human exposure to environmental chemicals, Department of Health and Human Services, Centers for Disease Control and Prevention.

Nicosia, S. V., Matus-Riley, M., & Meadows, A. T. (1985). Gonadal effects of cancer therapy in girls. *Cancer*, *55*, 2364–2372.

Niki, E., & Traber, M. G. (2012). A history of vitamin E. *Annals of Nutrition and Metabolism*, *61*, 207–212.

Noda, Y., Ota, K., Shirasawa, T., & Shimizu, T. (2012). Copper/zinc superoxide dismutase insufficiency impairs progesterone secretion and fertility in female mice. *Biology of Reproduction, 86*(16), 1–8.

O'Brien, T. J., Ceryak, S., & Patierno, S. R. (2003). Complexities of chromium carcinogenesis: Role of cellular response, repair, and recovery mechanisms. *Mutation Research, 533*, 3–36.

Petrillo, S. K., Desmeules, P., Truong, T.-Q., & Devine, P. J. (2011). Detection of DNA damage in oocytes of small ovarian follicles following phosphoramide mustard exposures of cultured rodent ovaries *in vitro*. *Toxicology and Applied Pharmacology, 253*, 84–102.

Plowchalk, D. R., & Mattison, D. R. (1991). Phosphoramide mustard is responsible for the ovarian toxicity of cyclophosphamide. *Toxicology and Applied Pharmacology, 107*, 472–481.

Pretsch, W. (1999). Glutathione reductase activity deficiency in homozygous $Gr1^{a1Neu}$ mice does not cause haemolytic anaemia. *Genetics Research, 73*, 1–5.

Roberts, R. A., Laskin, D. L., Smith, C. V., Robertson, F. M., Allen, E. M. G., Doorn, J. A., et al. (2009). Nitrative and oxidative stress in toxicology and disease. *Toxicological Sciences, 112*, 4–16.

Roede, J. R., & Jones, D. P. (2010). Reactive species and mitochondrial dysfunction: Mechanistic significance of 4-hydroxynonenal. *Environmental and Molecular Mutagenesis, 51*, 380–390.

Rogers, L. K., Bates, C. M., Welty, S. E., & Smith, C. V. (2006). Diquat induces renal proximal tubule injury in glutathione reductase-deficient mice. *Toxicology and Applied Pharmacology, 217*, 289–298.

Rogers, L. K., Tamura, T., Rogers, B. J., Welty, S. E., Hansen, T. N., & Smith, C. V. (2004). Analyses of glutathione reductase hypomorphic mice indicate a genetic knockout. *Toxicological Sciences, 82*, 367–373.

Samuel, J. B., Stanley, J. A., Sekar, P., Princess, R. A., Sebastian, M. S., & Aruldhas, M. M. (2012). Persistent hexavalent chromium exposure impaired the pubertal development and ovarian histoarchitecture in Wistar rat offspring. *Environmental Toxicology, 61*, 179–196.

Sasaki, J., Sato, E. F., Nomura, T., Mori, H., Watanabe, S., Kanda, S., et al. (1994). Detection of manganese superoxide dismutase mRNA in the theca interna cells of rat ovary during the ovulatory process by in situ hybridization. *Histochemistry, 102*, 173–176.

Sato, E. F., Kobuchi, H., Edashige, K., Takahashi, M., Yoshioka, T., Utsumi, K., et al. (1992). Dynamic aspects of ovarian superoxide dismutase isozymes during the ovulatory process in the rat. *FEBS Letters, 303*, 121–125.

Schneider, M., Förster, H., Boersma, A., Seiler, A., Wehnes, H., Sinowatz, F., et al. (2009). Mitochondrial glutathione peroxidase 4 disruption causes male infertility. *FASEB Journal, 23*, 3233–3242.

Sedding, D. G. (2008). FoxO transcription factors in oxidative stress response and ageing—A new fork on the way to longevity? *Biological Chemistry, 389*, 279–283.

Shi, Z.-Z., Osei-Frimpong, J., Kala, G., Kala, S. V., Barrios, R. J., Habib, G. M., et al. (2000). Glutathione synthesis is essential for mouse development but not for cell growth in culture. *Proceedings of the National Academy of Sciences of the United States of America, 97*, 5101–5106.

Shiromizu, K., Thorgeirsson, S. S., & Mattison, D. R. (1984). Effect of cyclophosphamide on oocyte and follicle number in Sprague-Dawley rats, C57BL/6N and DBA/2N mice. *Pediatric Pharmacology, 4*, 213–221.

Shkolnik, K., Tadmor, A., Ben-Dor, S., Nevo, N., Galiani, D., & Dekel, N. (2011). Reactive oxygen species are indispensable in ovulation. *Proceedings of the National Academy of Sciences of the United States of America, 108*, 1462–1467.

Sobinoff, A. P., Mahony, M., Nixon, B., Roman, S. D., & McLaughlin, E. A. (2011). Understanding the villain: DMBA-induced preantral ovotoxicity involves selective

follicular destruction and primordial follicle activation through PI3K/Akt and mTOR signaling. *Toxicological Sciences*, *123*, 563–575.
Sobinoff, A. P., Nixon, B., Roman, S. D., & McLaughlin, E. A. (2012). Staying alive: PI3K pathway promotes primordial follicle activation and survival in response to 3MC-induced ovotoxicity. *Toxicological Sciences*, *128*, 258–271.
Sobinoff, A. P., Pye, V., Nixon, B., Roman, S. D., & McLaughlin, E. A. (2010). Adding insult to injury: Effects of xenobiotic-induced preantral ovotoxicity on ovarian development and oocyte fusibility. *Toxicological Sciences*, *118*, 653–666.
Sobinoff, A. P., Pye, V., Nixon, B., Roman, S. D., & McLaughlin, E. A. (2012). Jumping the gun: Smoking constituent BaP causes premature primordial follicle activation and impairs oocyte fusibility through oxidative stress. *Toxicology and Applied Pharmacology*, *260*, 70–80.
Spitz, D. R., Azzam, E. I., Li, J. J., & Gius, D. (2004). Metabolic oxidation/reduction reactions and cellular response to ionizing radiation: A unifying concept in stress response biology. *Cancer and Metastasis Reviews*, *23*, 311–322.
Stanley, J. A., Lee, J., Nithy, T. K., Arosh, J. A., Burghardt, R. C., & Banu, S. K. (2011). Chromium-VI arrests cell cycle and decreases granulosa cell proliferation by down-regulating cyclin-dependent kinases (CDK) and up-regulating CDK-inhibitors. *Reproductive Toxicology*, *32*, 112–123.
Stanley, J. A., Sivakumar, K. K., Nithy, T. K., Arosh, J. A., Hoyer, P. B., Burghardt, R. C., et al. (2013). Postnatal exposure to chromium through mother's milk accelerates follicular atresia in F1 offspring through increased oxidative stress and depletion of antioxidant enzymes. *Free Radical Biology and Medicine*, *61*, 179–196.
Tilly, J. L., & Tilly, K. I. (1995). Inhibitors of oxidative stress mimic the ability of follicle-stimulating hormone to suppress apoptosis in cultured rat ovarian follicles. *Endocrinology*, *136*, 242–252.
Tsai-Turton, M., & Luderer, U. (2005). Gonadotropin regulation of glutamate cysteine ligase catalytic and modifier subunit expression in the rat ovary is subunit and follicle stage-specific. *American Journal of Physiology*, *289*, E391–E402.
Tsai-Turton, M., & Luderer, U. (2006). Opposing effects of glutathione depletion and FSH on reactive oxygen species and apoptosis in cultured preovulatory rat follicles. *Endocrinology*, *147*, 1224–1236.
Tsai-Turton, M., Luong, B. T., Tan, Y., & Luderer, U. (2007). Cyclophosphamide-induced apoptosis in COV434 human granulosa cells involves oxidative stress and glutathione depletion. *Toxicological Sciences*, *98*, 216–230.
Tsai-Turton, M., Nakamura, B. N., & Luderer, U. (2007). Induction of apoptosis by 9,10-dimethyl-1,2-benzanthracene (DMBA) in cultured preovulatory rat follicles is preceded by a rise in reactive oxygen species and is prevented by glutathione. *Biology of Reproduction*, *77*, 442–451.
Tuttle, A. M., Stampfli, M., & Foster, W. G. (2009). Cigarette smoke causes follicle loss in mice ovaries at concentrations representative of human exposure. *Human Reproduction*, *24*, 1452–1459.
Wallace, W. H. B., Shalet, S. M., Hendry, J. H., Morris-Jone, P. H., & Gattamaneni, H. R. (1989). Ovarian failure following abdominal irradiation in childhood: The radiosensitivity of the human oocyte. *British Journal of Radiology*, *62*, 995–998.
Wallace, W. H. B., Thomson, A. B., & Kelsey, T. W. (2003). The radiosensitivity of the human oocyte. *Human Reproduction*, *18*, 117–121.
Wang, W., Craig, Z. R., Basavarajappa, M. S., Gupta, R. K., & Flaws, J. A. (2012). Di(2-ethylhexyl) phthalate inhibits growth of mouse ovarian antral follicles through an oxidative stress pathway. *Toxicology and Applied Pharmacology*, *258*, 288–295.

Wang, W., Craig, Z. R., Basavarajappa, M. S., Hafner, K. S., & Flaws, J. A. (2012). Mono (2-ethylhexyl) phthalate induces oxidative stress and inhibits growth of mouse antral follicles. *Biology of Reproduction, 87*, 152.

Warne, G. L., Fairley, K. F., Hobbs, J. B., & Martin, F. I. R. (1973). Cyclophosphamide-induced ovarian failure. *New England Journal of Medicine, 289*, 1159–1162.

Will, Y., Fishcher, K. A., Horton, R. A., Kaetzel, R. S., Brown, M. K., Hedstrom, O., et al. (2000). Γ-Glutamyltranspeptidase-deficient knockout mice as a model to study the relationship between glutathione status, mitochondrial function, and cellular function. *Hepatology, 32*, 740–749.

Winn, L. M., & Wells, P. G. (1997). Evidence for embryonic prostaglandin H synthase catalyzed bioactivation and reactive oxygen species-mediated oxidation of cellular macromolecules in phenytoin and benzo[a]pyrene teratogenesis. *Free Radical Biology and Medicine, 22*, 607–621.

Wiseman, H., & Halliwell, B. (1996). Damage to DNA by reactive oxygen and nitrogen species: Role in inflammatory disease and progression to cancer. *Biochemistry Journal, 313*, 17–29.

Wong, P. C., Waggoner, D., Subramaniam, J. R., Tessarollo, L., Bartnikas, T. B., Culotta, V. C., et al. (2000). Copper chaperone for superoxide dismutase is essential to activate mammalian Cu/Zn superoxide dismutase. *Proceedings of the National Academy of Sciences of the United States of America, 97*, 2886–2891.

Xue, W., & Warshawsky, D. (2005). Metabolic activation of polycyclic aromatic hydrocarbon and heterocyclic aromatic hydrocarbons and DNA damage: A review. *Toxicology and Applied Pharmacology, 206*, 73–93.

Yang, Y., Dieter, M. Z., Chen, Y., Shertzer, H. G., Nebert, D. W., & Dalton, T. P. (2002). Initial characterization of the glutamate cysteine ligase modifier subunit *Gclm* (-/-) knockout mouse: Novel model system for severely compromised oxidative stress response. *Journal of Biological Chemistry, 277*, 49446–49452.

Yant, L. J., Ran, Q., Rao, L., Van Remmen, H., Shibatani, T., Belter, J. G., et al. (2003). The selenoprotein GPX4 is essential for mouse development and protects from radiation and oxidative damage insults. *Free Radical Biology and Medicine, 34*, 496–502.

Yu, P. L., Lim, T. M., Wang, S. W., & Wang, P. S. (2012). Antisteroidogenic effects of hydrogen peroxide on rat granulosa cells. *Free Radical Research, 46*, 718–725.

Zreik, T. G., Kodaman, P. H., Jones, E. E., Olive, D. L., & Behrman, H. R. (1999). Identification and characterization of an ascorbic acid transporter in human granulosa-lutein cells. *Molecular Human Reproduction, 5*, 299–302.

CHAPTER FIVE

Low-Dose Effects of Hormones and Endocrine Disruptors

Laura N. Vandenberg[1]
Department of Public Health, Division of Environmental Health Sciences, University of Massachusetts - Amherst, Amherst, Massachusetts, USA
[1]Corresponding author: e-mail address: lvandenberg@schoolph.umass.edu

Contents

1. Introduction 130
2. What is Meant by "Low Dose?" 131
3. Hormones Act at Low Doses 133
4. The "Rules" of Hormones are Obeyed by EDCs: Implications for Low-Dose Chemical Exposures 136
5. NTP Panel's Findings on Low-Dose Effects: 2000–2002 138
6. The NTP Panel's Assessment: Low-Dose Effects of Specific Chemicals 140
7. Updates to the NTP Panel Report on Low-Dose Effects 142
8. BPA and the Prostate: A Low-Dose Case Study 143
9. Additional Low-Dose Findings: Evidence from Laboratory Animals and Human Populations 145
10. Traditional Toxicology Studies are Not Designed to Detect Low-Dose Effects 146
11. Low-Dose Effects: Biological Changes are Not Necessarily Adverse 148
12. Real World EDC Exposures: Mixture Effects 150
13. Nonmonotonic Dose Responses 151
14. Conclusions 152
References 153

Abstract

Endogenous hormones have effects on tissue morphology, cell physiology, and behaviors at low doses. In fact, hormones are known to circulate in the part-per-trillion and part-per-billion concentrations, making them highly effective and potent signaling molecules. Many endocrine-disrupting chemicals (EDCs) mimic hormones, yet there is strong debate over whether these chemicals can also have effects at low doses. In the 1990s, scientists proposed the "low-dose hypothesis," which postulated that EDCs affect humans and animals at environmentally relevant doses. This chapter focuses on data that support and refute the low-dose hypothesis. A case study examining the highly controversial example of bisphenol A and its low-dose effects on the prostate is examined through the lens of endocrinology. Finally, the chapter concludes with a discussion of factors that can influence the ability of a study to detect and interpret low-dose effects appropriately.

Vitamins and Hormones, Volume 94
ISSN 0083-6729
http://dx.doi.org/10.1016/B978-0-12-800095-3.00005-5

1. INTRODUCTION

The US Food and Drug Administration (FDA) lists more than 1000 chemicals currently in commerce as having actual or putative endocrine-disrupting properties (FDA, 2010a). These include insecticides, herbicides, plasticizers, industrial chemicals, detergents, preservatives, components in personal care products, flame retardants, and resins. Although different agencies define endocrine-disrupting chemicals (EDCs) in somewhat different ways, one widely accepted definition of these chemicals is "an exogenous agent that interferes with the synthesis, secretion, transport, binding, action, or elimination of natural hormones in the body that are responsible for the maintenance of homeostasis, reproduction, development and/or behavior" (Kavlock et al., 1996).

Human and wildlife exposure to EDCs is thought to be extensive. Biomonitoring studies at the US Centers for Disease Control and Prevention indicate that a large percentage of the general population has detectable levels of a number of these chemicals in their bodies. Examination specifically of pregnant women shows that these individuals have dozens of chemicals, and specifically EDCs, in their bodies at any one time (Woodruff, Zota, & Schwartz, 2011). These types of study are particularly concerning because they provide unequivocal evidence that the fetus is exposed to large numbers of chemicals during gestation (Arbuckle, 2010). Yet, these studies also suggest that humans, including developing fetuses, are typically exposed to low concentrations of these chemicals. It is often argued that the presence of a chemical at detectable levels in the body is not necessarily reason for concern, especially as detection methods improve over time to the point where they can detect chemicals in part-per-trillion (ppt) or part-per-billion (ppb) concentrations. Thus, a major issue that must be addressed in the field of environmental toxicology is whether the presence of these chemicals at low doses indicates the possibility of harm. Additionally, there is always the question of whether effects induced by chemical exposures are adverse. This topic is addressed later in this chapter.

In the 1990s, scientists proposed the "low-dose hypothesis," which postulated that EDCs have effects at low doses, especially on reproductive and developmental end points; that effects observed in animals will occur at doses similar to human exposure levels; and that humans exposed to EDCs will also be affected by low doses. Since that time, work done in laboratories around the world has focused on addressing this hypothesis, and some scientists believe this research has advanced to the point where this concept should no longer be considered a "hypothesis." This chapter will focus on understanding how natural hormones act at low doses and why EDCs are also expected to have effects at low doses. We will then summarize the 2002 National Toxicology Program (NTP) expert panel report on EDCs and low doses and update the low-dose research that has been conducted since that time, with a specific focus on low-dose studies of bisphenol A (BPA), a well-studied EDC. Finally, this chapter will conclude with a discussion of the factors involved in the detection of low-dose effects and a discussion of nonmonotonicity, a related issue that may influence how risk assessments of EDCs are conducted.

2. WHAT IS MEANT BY "LOW DOSE?"

Many of the best links between EDC exposures and adverse health outcomes come from high-dose studies following industrial accidents and pharmaceutical agents with unexpected, adverse health outcomes. The 1976 explosion of a chemical plant in Seveso, Italy, which led to widespread human exposure to large amounts of TCDD, a particularly toxic form of dioxin, and the deposition of this chemical on the land surrounding the chemical plant, is one such example. This industrial accident provided clear evidence that TCDD has endocrine-disrupting properties in humans following high-dose exposures (Eskenazi et al., 2004; Pesatori et al., 2003). Blood samples from exposed children, adolescents, and women collected shortly after the exposure and in follow-up studies correlated serum dioxin levels with adverse outcomes including increased breast cancer risk, abnormal menstrual cycles, and endometriosis (Eskenazi et al., 2007, 2002; Warner et al., 2002). A similar example of a high-dose exposure linked to adverse health outcomes is that of women exposed to the synthetic pharmaceutical estrogen diethylstilbestrol (DES) during gestation (McLachlan, 2001, 2006). These so-called DES daughters have significantly increased rates of uterine, cervical, and vaginal malformations including clear cell adenocarcinoma of the vagina (Herbst, Ulfelder, & Poskanzer, 1971; Mittendorf, 1995) and an increased risk of developing breast cancer after 40 years of age (Palmer et al., 2006). *In utero* DES exposure has also been shown to alter some sexually dimorphic behaviors in women, suggesting that exposures to this pharmaceutical have wider-ranging effects than the initial reports of altered reproductive tract development and fertility (reviewed in Heines, 2002). Finally, additional examples of high doses linked to adverse health outcomes have been reported in workers in certain industries including chemical sprayers and factory workers (Kumar, 2011; Li et al., 2011, 2010; Petrelli, Figa-Talamanca, Lauria, & Mantovani, 2003; Snijder et al., 2012). These studies suggest that occupational exposures to EDCs can be high and that these exposures are concerning for these populations of workers.

In contrast to these high-dose exposures, typical human exposures to EDCs occur at low doses from residues on food, personal care products, household detergents, lawn care products, food packaging, and other sources. Biomonitoring studies of environmentally exposed individuals reveal blood and urine concentrations of EDCs and other chemicals in the ppt and ppb range, although some are found as high as the part-per-million (ppm) range (Barr et al., 2010; Calafat et al., 2007; Calafat, Ye, Wong, Bishop, & Needham, 2010; Calafat, Ye, Wong, Reidy, & Needham, 2008; Lee, Lind, et al., 2011; Lee, Steffes, et al., 2011; Woodruff et al., 2011). Of course, these concentrations refer to the circulating levels of environmental chemicals, or the amount of chemical that is excreted in urine, and alone does not provide information about the actual exposure levels required to produce these circulating concentrations. Taking the blood or urine concentrations and calculating exposure levels requires knowledge about the toxicokinetics of the chemical in question, including whether it bioaccumulates; unfortunately, this information is not available for the vast majority of chemicals.

Thus, an important question remains: when considering a study of environmental chemicals such as EDCs, how can one determine whether the study is examining "low" doses? The term "low dose" is used widely in the field of environmental health science, but there are currently no agreed-upon standards for a low-dose cutoff. In 2002, an expert panel of scientists assembled by the NTP defined a low-dose cutoff as doses in the range of typical human exposures or doses below those tested in traditional toxicological assessments (Melnick et al., 2002). Based on these criteria, any epidemiology study examining environmentally exposed individuals (i.e., anyone other than an occupationally exposed worker) would be defined as a low-dose study. Occupational exposures are often considered "high dose" and thus are examined separately. Others have proposed that low-dose cutoffs should consider toxicokinetic properties of a chemical, and thus, low doses are those administered to an animal that produce blood concentrations of that chemical in the range of what has been measured in the general human population (Brucker-Davis, Thayer, & Colborn, 2001; Vandenberg, Hauser, Marcus, Olea, & Welshons, 2007).

These differing definitions produce quite different cutoffs for the same environmental chemical. For example, the EDC BPA, a synthetic estrogen used in a wide variety of consumer products, has three different cutoff doses based on these three definitions. For human exposure levels, consumer product assessments estimate exposures are in the nanogram or microgram per kilogram range (Lakind & Naiman, 2008). For doses below those tested in traditional toxicology studies, the cutoff dose would be set by the no-observed-adverse-effect level (NOAEL) of 50 mg/kg/day (Welshons et al., 2003). Finally, for doses that produce blood concentrations found in the general population, doses of 100–400 μg/kg/day would be set as the cutoff dose (Taylor et al., 2011; Tharp et al., 2012; Vandenberg et al., 2007). Further, exposure assessments and toxicokinetic studies are not available for the vast majority of chemicals on the market; thus, two of these definitions would require significant increases in available information to establish accurate and appropriate cutoff doses for the majority of chemicals. The lack of a standardized definition for a low-dose cutoff for EDCs and the paucity of data on exposure sources, exposure levels, metabolism, and bioaccumulation for these chemicals contribute to a field with a large number of data gaps that will persist without a significant number of additional studies.

3. HORMONES ACT AT LOW DOSES

Although EDCs by definition can act on any aspect of the hormone signaling process including hormone secretion and transport, many EDCs act by binding to hormone receptors and mimicking or blocking the actions of endogenous hormones. Thus, it has been suggested that our understanding of how EDCs act in the body would be greatly informed by the vast scientific knowledge of natural hormone action from the field of endocrinology (Diamanti-Kandarakis et al., 2009; Myers, vom Saal, et al., 2009; Schug, Janesick, Blumberg, & Heindel, 2011; Zoeller et al., 2012). Understanding low-dose effects from EDC exposures, therefore, would benefit from understanding how hormones act at low doses in the body.

To start, circulating concentrations of hormones are typically in the ppt range for estradiol, testosterone (in adult females), and thyroid hormone and the ppb range for progesterone, testosterone (in adult males), growth hormone, and prolactin (Jones, 1996). Of course, the concentrations of hormones change based on age and physiological status, but the range of concentrations is typically not large. For example, testosterone levels in human male neonates are typically in the range of 0.2–0.5 ng/ml and increase to 4–6 ng/ml in most adult men. Similarly, estradiol concentrations are typically in the range of 50–100 pg/ml in women during the early follicular phase of the menstrual cycle, but raise to 600 pg/ml during the luteal phase, and are even more variable during pregnancy.

Steroid hormones in the blood are distributed into three phases: free, representing the unconjugated, unbound form; bioavailable, representing hormones bound to low-affinity carrier proteins such as albumin; and inactive, representing the form that is bound to high-affinity binding proteins such as sex hormone-binding globulin or alphafetoprotein (Welshons et al., 2003). The "physiologically active" forms of a hormone are those found in the free and bioavailable phases, whereas a hormone bound to high-affinity binding proteins is not available and therefore cannot produce biological effects. In this way, the blood allows for a buffering system of a hormone that is currently available, another portion that is able to be made available quickly, and a backup reserve. When circulating levels of a hormone are corrected for the low fraction of a hormone that is unbound, the free concentrations that produce actual biological effects are therefore much lower than the total.

The potency of hormones and other molecules that signal via receptors is dependent on several factors including affinity of the ligand for the receptor, the number of receptors, the concentration of the hormone, and the developmental stage when exposures occur, among other factors (Barouki, Gluckman, Grandjean, Hanson, & Heindel, 2012; Charlton, 2009; Lees, Cunningham, & Elliott, 2004; Welshons et al., 2003). Thus, although the concentration of circulating hormones is typically very low, each hormone has a high affinity for its receptor, allowing for dozens of signaling molecules to circulate in the body simultaneously yet controlling very specific biological activities. Further, while some hormone receptors are expressed widely throughout the body (i.e., insulin receptors are found in many different cell types), others are expressed in only a select number of cell types (i.e., receptors for thyroid-stimulating hormone (TSH) are concentrated in the thyroid, and binding of TSH triggers the thyroid to release thyroid hormone). Additionally, as discussed earlier, circulating hormone concentrations change based on age, period of development, and even time of day (Son, Chung, & Kim, 2011; Urbanski, 2011). Because the release of one hormone is often controlled by another hormone, that is, the release of thyroid hormone is triggered by binding of TSH, both the frequency and amplitude of the pulsatile release of hormone can modulate the induced response (Gan & Quinton, 2010; Naftolin et al., 2007).

Also important is to consider the relationships between hormone concentration, number of bound receptors, and biological effects. Most hormone receptors are actually unbound—a situation previously termed "the spare receptor hypothesis" (May, Moran, Kimelberg, & Triggle, 1967; Zhu, 1996); less than 10% of hormone receptors are typically bound at any particular time. The relationship between hormone concentration and the percentage of receptors that are bound is nonlinear. Thus, small changes in hormone concentration translate to relatively large changes in the total number of bound receptors (Welshons et al., 2003). Similarly, there is a nonlinear relationship between the total number of bound receptors and the biological effect. Thus, a small increase in the total circulating hormone concentration translates to relatively large increases in the number of bound receptors, which further translates to relatively large increases in the biological effect observed. This is an example of how the effects of a hormone are amplified in a biological system. Additional amplification machinery exists within cells following some hormone signaling events, allowing for small changes in hormone concentration to have large biological effects.

Finally, one cannot discount the influence of the timing of exposures on how some hormone exposures can have large biological effects. For decades, endocrinologists have studied "activational" and "organizational" effects of hormones (Phoenix, Goy, Gerall, & Young, 1959; Schulz, Molenda-Figueira, & Sisk, 2009; Wallen, 2009). Activational effects typically occur in adulthood and are biological changes associated with exposures; once exposures cease, these types of biological effects terminate as well. In contrast, organizational effects are those that occur due to exposures during critical periods of development. Exposures during these vulnerable periods lead to irreversible changes, often in the differentiation of tissues and development of structures and behavioral traits. In this way, these exposures are referred to as "organizational" because they result in the complete reorganization of hormone-sensitive end points.

An excellent example of an activational and organizational effect of a hormone is that of estrogen; during adulthood, women exposed to estrogen will have decreased fertility. In fact, estrogen is a component of many types of prescription birth control pills. Once an adult female stops taking estrogen, her fertility is restored. In contrast, if a woman takes estrogen supplements during pregnancy, there are permanent and grave consequences for her unborn child. Estrogen exposure during fetal development can cause serious malformations of the male reproductive tract and the genitals (Skakkebaek, Rajpert-De Meyts, & Main, 2001). It can also increase a female's risk of developing breast cancer in adulthood (Soto, Vandenberg, Maffini, & Sonnenschein, 2008).

Similarly, low concentrations of circulating thyroid hormone will have effects on an adult including weight gain that will be abrogated somewhat following supplementation with this hormone (Tarim, 2011). In contrast, low concentrations of thyroid hormone during perinatal development will cause irreversible mental retardation (Zoeller & Rovet, 2004). Collectively, our understanding of the effects of exogenous hormone supplementation, or hormone deficits, indicates that there are critical periods in development where concentrations of specific circulating hormones should be extremely low and other periods where other hormones must be present in relatively high concentrations for proper development.

4. THE "RULES" OF HORMONES ARE OBEYED BY EDCs: IMPLICATIONS FOR LOW-DOSE CHEMICAL EXPOSURES

There are five major principles of endocrinology that have been proposed to apply to EDCs: (1) hormones integrate the systems of the body and have roles from conception through aging; (2) hormones act via specific interactions with receptors; (3) hormones act at low doses; (4) the effects of hormones are life stage-dependent; and (5) hormones have nonlinear, and even nonmonotonic, effects. There are several considerations for how these principles relate to EDCs, which will be discussed briefly later.

Principle 1: Hormones integrate the systems of the body and have roles from conception through aging. Because the endocrine system plays an integral role in the health and well-being of individuals from birth until death, disrupting different aspects of the endocrine system is expected to produce disease and other types of dysfunction at various stages of life. Importantly, changes to the endocrine system at one period of life can have effects that manifest decades later (Heindel, 2005, 2008), that is, exposures to estrogens and estrogen mimics in the womb can cause breast cancer four or more decades later (Soto et al., 2008; Trichopoulos, 1990). EDCs can also disrupt body systems beyond the traditional end points associated with the endocrine system (i.e., the reproductive tract, brain, and thyroid) including the cardiovascular system, immune system, and bone, among others (Heindel, 2008; Schug et al., 2011).

At this time, the best studied EDCs are those that mimic certain hormones, block certain hormones, or alter hormone synthesis via enzymatic reactions (Diamanti-Kandarakis et al., 2009; Myers, Zoeller, & vom Saal, 2009; Vandenberg et al., 2012; Zoeller, 2010). Further, most of the EDCs that have been well studied have been characterized to influence the estrogen, androgen (testosterone), and thyroid hormone signaling pathways. Yet, the number of known hormones is much greater, and it has been predicted that there will be EDCs identified that affect these different pathways as well.

Principle 2: Hormones act via specific interactions with receptors. It has been argued that because EDCs that bind to hormone receptors are usually "weaker" ligands than the endogenous hormone, there is no real concern about human and wildlife exposures to these chemicals (Witorsch, 2002a, 2002b). Yet, as discussed earlier, the biological effects of a receptor's ligand cannot be accurately predicted from knowledge only about binding affinity. Instead, other factors including life stage and concentration must be considered.

Principle 3: Hormones act at low doses. Hormones circulate in the ppt and ppb range, and many EDCs circulate in a similar range and are thus expected to have biological effects at these low doses. Yet, while the effects of hormones are held in balance by the innate blood buffering system via the presence of low- and high-affinity binding proteins, many EDCs do not bind to these same proteins; thus, the entirety of the circulating dose of the EDC would be considered "physiologically active" (Dechaud, Ravard, Claustrat, de la Perriere, & Pugeat, 1999; Milligan, Khan, & Nash, 1998; Nagel, vom Saal, & Welshons, 1999; Sheehan & Young, 1979).

Importantly, most EDCs do not exactly replicate the effects of the endogenous hormone because they recruit different cofactors and alter gene expression in ways that differ from the normal signaling processes. Other EDCs can bind to multiple receptors and therefore can induce effects that would be associated with more than one hormone. All of these factors need to be considered when assessing the effects of low doses—or high doses—of EDCs.

Principle 4: The effects of hormones are life stage-dependent. Activational and organizational effects of hormones are well understood; the effects of hormone exposure during adulthood will not predict the effects of the same hormone when exposures occur during critical periods of development (i.e., embryonic and fetal development, neonatal period, and puberty). EDCs have shown similar time-dependent effects. For example, DES produced striking effects in exposed offspring but much less serious effects in exposed mothers (Bern, 1992). Additionally, DES daughters exposed to this pharmaceutical during the first 15 weeks of gestation had the highest incidence of clear cell adenocarcinomas of the vagina and other vaginal and cervical pathologies (Mittendorf, 1995), and further parsing of these exposures indicates the highest risk in women that were exposed during the first 7 weeks of gestation (Hatch et al., 2001). Similarly, in the accidental release of TCDD in the Seveso, Italy, industrial incident, several studies demonstrated that individuals who were either infants or teenagers at the time of the explosion were found to be at greatest risk for developing adult diseases (Medina et al., 2001; Mocarelli et al., 2008; Myers, Zoeller, et al., 2009; Robinson, Karpf, & Kratochwil, 1999). Finally, studies in rodents indicate that relatively large doses of BPA (in the ppm range) are required to induce estrogen-sensitive end points associated with the uterotrophic assay (Markey, Michaelson, Veson, Sonnenschein, & Soto, 2001; Nagel, Hagelbarger, & McDonnell, 2001), but significantly lower doses, in the ppt range, during the fetal period can permanently alter development of the uterus (Markey, Coombs, Sonnenschein, & Soto, 2003; Markey, Wadia, Rubin, Sonnenschein, & Soto, 2005; Schonfelder, Friedrich, Paul, & Chahoud, 2004).

Principle 5: Hormones have nonlinear, and even nonmonotonic, effects. The relationships between hormone concentration, number of bound receptors, and biological effects are nonlinear. In some cases, the relationship between the dose of a hormone and the biological effect can be nonmonotonic, where the slope of the line representing the dose–response curve changes sign (Kohn & Melnick, 2002). Oftentimes, these curves are referred to as U- or inverted U-shaped, or "biphasic," curves because the responses show ascending and descending phases in relation to dose. There are well-established mechanisms for how hormones produce nonmonotonic dose responses; these will be discussed in the last section of this review. Additionally, there are dozens of examples of nonmonotonic dose responses in the EDC literature (Vandenberg et al., 2012). Importantly, the presence of nonlinear and nonmonotonic relationships between dose and effect challenges the way risk assessments are currently performed, where high-dose testing is used to predict the safety of lower doses.

5. NTP PANEL'S FINDINGS ON LOW-DOSE EFFECTS: 2000–2002

In 2000, the US EPA requested that the NTP perform a comprehensive review of the EDC literature to directly address the low-dose hypothesis. At that time, the NTP assembled a panel of experts from government agencies, academia, and industry to review both published and unpublished studies. The NTP defined low-dose effects as "any biological change" occurring in the low-dose range, as defined earlier in this chapter (Melnick et al., 2002). The expert panel was subdivided into five additional groups to specifically examine biological factors and study design, statistics and dose–response modeling, BPA, other environmental estrogens and estradiol, and androgens and antiandrogens. In contrast to other expert panels, the NTP panel examined raw data provided by the original study authors; these data were reanalyzed by statisticians together with answers to a questionnaire that probed the investigator for information related to study design such as the species and strain of animal used, details about animal husbandry, use of positive and negative controls, characterization of the chemicals used, evaluation of the end points assessed, and descriptions of how the data were analyzed.

The panel concluded that several factors had an influence on the ability to detect low-dose effects (Melnick et al., 2002). First, the NTP acknowledged that intrauterine position can influence variability in biological end points due to differential exposure to hormones during fetal development. In fact, fetal male mice produce testosterone starting on gestational day 12, and some of this hormone is transferred passively to neighboring fetuses via the maternal blood supply (Vandenbergh, 2004). Intrauterine position has been demonstrated to influence a large number of physiological, morphological, and behavioral end points including prostate development, mammary gland morphology, responsiveness to testosterone, steroid metabolism, age of pubertal onset, and estrous cycle length, among others (Ryan & Vandenbergh, 2002; Vandenberg, Maffini, Sonnenschein, Rubin, & Soto, 2009; Vandenbergh, 2004). Differences as low as 1 ng/ml testosterone in females and 25 pg/ml estradiol in males have serious effects on a large number of phenotypes (Clark, Crews, & Galef, 1991; Even, Dhar, & vom Saal, 1992; Timms, Peterson, & vom Saal, 2002; Vandenbergh, 2004; vom Saal, 1989; vom Saal & Bronson, 1980; vom Saal et al., 1990). Thus, intrauterine position itself is an incredible, robust example of a low-dose effect.

The NTP panel also noted that strain and species differences can influence the ability to detect low-dose effects of both endogenous hormones and EDCs (Melnick et al., 2002). In particular, they noted that there are specific strains of rat that were selectively bred to produce large litter sizes that are insensitive to estrogens and are therefore inappropriate models to test for low-dose effects. Other analyses have noted the insensitivity of specific rodent strains, even though some studies persist in using them to characterize the effects of EDCs (vom Saal et al., 2010; vom Saal & Hughes, 2005; vom Saal, Richter, Ruhlen, et al., 2005). On a similar note, the NTP panel found that the inclusion of positive controls—and the expected positive results from those controls—was an important factor distinguishing studies that found effects from those that did not. Subsequent analyses of the EDC literature have proposed that the inclusion of a positive control in traditional toxicology studies should be required, particularly when studies conclude "no effect" from an EDC or no evidence of effects at low doses (Vandenberg et al., 2012; vom Saal et al., 2010; vom Saal & Welshons, 2006).

Finally, the NTP noted that factors related to experimental design can strongly influence the ability to detect low-dose effects of EDCs (Melnick et al., 2002). They noted that the phytoestrogen content of the feed used in laboratory animal experiments can mask the effects of EDCs and prevent the detection of low-dose effects, a topic that has been developed further in more recent years (Heindel & vom Saal, 2008; vom Saal, Richter, Mao, & Welshons, 2005). The panel also found that differences in caging, bedding, and housing conditions also influenced whether studies detected low-dose effects (Melnick et al., 2002). Additional studies have reported similar importance for these factors (Howdeshell et al., 2003; Hunt et al., 2003; Myers, vom Saal, et al., 2009).

6. THE NTP PANEL'S ASSESSMENT: LOW-DOSE EFFECTS OF SPECIFIC CHEMICALS

In their assessment of low-dose effects for estradiol and other environmental estrogens, the NTP panel concluded that there was sufficient evidence for low-dose effects for a number of estrogenic chemicals (Melnick et al., 2002). For estradiol, the panel found that there were convincing low-dose effects on changes in serum prolactin, luteinizing hormone, and follicle-stimulating hormone in ovariectomized rats administered doses at or below 3 μg/kg/day. For DES, the panel found convincing evidence for low-dose effects on prostate size in male mice exposed during gestation to doses at or below 20 ng/kg/day. For genistein, a natural estrogen derived from soy, the panel found evidence of low-dose effects on sexual dimorphisms in the brain—specifically in the male brain—and altered tissue organization in the male rat mammary gland, as well as increases in proliferation of immune cells following *in utero* to pubertal exposures via food in at levels of 25 ppm. For methoxychlor, an insecticide, the panel concluded that there was sufficient evidence for low-dose effects on the immune system of rats developmentally exposed via food to 10 ppm. Finally, for nonylphenol, an industrial compound used as a surfactant, the NTP panel found convincing low-dose effects on brain sexual dimorphisms in males, the weight of the thymus, the estrus cycle in female rats, and the proliferation of immune cells following developmental exposures to 25 ppm. Importantly, in making these conclusions, the panelists examined as few as three studies, many of which were not peer-reviewed or published and several of which remain unpublished (NTP, 2001). The panel also reviewed a single rat study of octylphenol, an industrial chemical used in the production of surfactants, and found no evidence of low-dose effects for any end point (Melnick et al., 2002).

In its analysis of anti-androgens, the NTP panel focused on vinclozolin, a fungicide used widely on crops including grapes. The panelists were unable to identify a single study that would qualify as a low dose study; no published experiments existed that had examined vinclozolin at doses below its NOAEL of 1.2 mg/kg/day. For the high dose studies on this chemical, effects on anogenital distance, nipple retention, and reduced prostate weight were observed in male rats administered doses above the NOAEL, and reproductive tract malformations and reduced sperm counts were only observed at the highest doses. The panel also concluded that there were no data to assess the low-dose effects of other anti-androgens including the pharmaceuticals flutamide, finasteride, or Casodex; the insecticides methoxychlor and DDT; the fungicides procymidone and ketoconazole; and the herbicide linuron.

The final chemical examined by the NTP expert panel, and given its own subpanel, was BPA (Melnick et al., 2002). The panelists found that some studies supported low-dose effects of BPA for adult prostate weight and advanced female puberty in animals exposed during early development, as well as low-dose effects on uterine growth and serum prolactin levels in rats. In its assessment, the panel noted that "there is credible evidence that low doses of BPA can cause effects on specific end points. However, due to the inability of other credible studies in several different laboratories to observe low dose effects of BPA, and the consistency of these negative studies, the subpanel is not persuaded that a low dose effect of BPA has been conclusively established as a general or reproducible finding."

Importantly, the panel noted that those studies that included DES as a positive control and found low-dose effects of DES also found low-dose effects of BPA; those studies that included DES but found no evidence of low-dose effects of DES were also unable to find low-dose effects of BPA. Subsequent studies have interpreted these results as evidence that low dose studies of EDCs should prove that the experimental set-up is capable of detecting low-dose effects by showing such effects in animals exposed to an estrogen (DES, 17β-estradiol, ethinyl estradiol) (Vandenberg et al., 2012).

Ultimately, the lack of a consensus on low-dose effects of BPA has contributed to more than a decade of debate on this EDC. Even though more than 90% of low dose studies suggest that BPA causes harm (vom Saal & Hughes, 2005), these conclusions are still considered controversial, largely because there are studies that report no adverse effects of BPA at low doses (Ashby, Tinwell, & Haseman, 1999; Howdeshell et al., 2008; Ryan, Hotchkiss, Crofton, & Gray, 2010; Stump et al., 2010; Tinwell, Haseman, Lefevre, Wallis, & Ashby, 2002; Tyl et al., 2008, 2002).

7. UPDATES TO THE NTP PANEL REPORT ON LOW-DOSE EFFECTS

The NTP panel report on low-dose effects was published in 2002, and included several examples that the panel agreed were strong evidence in favor of reproducible low-dose effects of EDCs including genistein, nonylphenol, and methoxychlor. Thus, it is surprising that some scientists continue to argue that low-dose effects have not been demonstrated (Rhomberg & Goodman, 2012). It is likely that this continued controversy and debate is due to conflicting results about the effects of BPA at low doses; in fact, some of the strongest critics of the low dose data are paid advocates from the polycarbonate and chemical industries, which have vested interests considering the use of BPA polycarbonate plastics and many other consumer products (Burridge, 2008).

BPA has therefore become an interesting case study for the analysis of low-dose effects. As mentioned above, there are a number of studies that have been unable to show low-dose effects; do these studies negate or discount those studies that do show effects at low doses? Certainly, there are some scientists and government agencies that would argue that they do (EFSA, 2006; Goodman et al., 2009). However, in 2007, an expert panel of BPA scientists assembled by NIH found that there was sufficient evidence for low-dose effects on a number of end points including brain development, behaviors, the male reproductive tract, and metabolic machinery (Richter et al., 2007). In 2008, an expert panel assembled by the NTP found that there was sufficient evidence for low-dose effects of BPA on the prostate, the brain, and behavior (Chapin et al., 2008). In 2010, the US FDA released a statement agreeing with the NTP, stating that there was "some concern" for the effect of BPA on the prostate, the brain and behavior (FDA, 2010b). Thus, a careful weight-of-evidence analysis of specific end points provides evidence in favor of low-dose effects and concludes that the positive studies outweigh the studies that are unable to show effects (Vandenberg et al., 2012; Zoeller et al., 2012).

8. BPA AND THE PROSTATE: A LOW-DOSE CASE STUDY

The original study that claimed to demonstrate low-dose effects of BPA reported that fetal exposures to extremely low doses (2 and 20 μg/kg/day administered orally to the dam) increased the weight of the prostate when the male offspring reached several months of age (Nagel et al., 1997). In addition to that original study, several others have reported that low doses of BPA during gestation increase the prostate weight in male offspring in adulthood (Chitra, Latchoumycandane, & Mathur, 2003; Elswick, Welsch, & Janszen, 2000; Gupta, 2000). Other studies have reported effects on tissue organization and protein expression in the prostate following low-dose BPA exposures (Gupta, 2000; Ogura et al., 2007; Ramos et al., 2003, 2001; Timms et al., 2005).

To test the hypothesis that BPA heightens the prostate gland's responsiveness to hormones in adulthood, and therefore that BPA predisposes the prostate to adult cancers, several studies have examined whether low-dose BPA exposures during perinatal development influence the response of adults to a mixture of testosterone and estrogen in adulthood (Ho, Tang, Belmonte de Frausto, & Prins, 2006; Prins, Birch, Tang, & Ho, 2007; Prins, Tang, Belmonte, & Ho, 2008; Prins, Ye, Birch, Ho, & Kannan, 2011). These studies report that males exposed to BPA early in life have an increased incidence of adult-onset prostatic intraepithelial neoplasias. These lesions were not observed in BPA-exposed animals when the hormone cocktail was not administered. Importantly, the mixture of estrogen and testosterone was designed to mimic the hormone changes associated with aging that are believed to accompany the onset of prostate cancer in men. The conclusion from all of these studies taken together is that low doses of BPA during early development (particularly gestational and perinatal exposures) alter development of the prostate in ways that manifest in adulthood, including an altered response to hormones and the development of neoplastic lesions.

In contrast, as mentioned above, a number of studies have shown no effect of BPA on prostate weight (Ashby et al., 1999; Cagen et al., 1999a, 1999b; Ema et al., 2001; Howdeshell et al., 2008; Ichihara et al., 2003; Tinwell et al., 2002; Tyl et al., 2008, 2002). However, analyzing these studies in light of the conclusions from the NTP panel about the importance of appropriate positive controls (Melnick et al., 2002), it is clear that many of these studies are lacking in their experimental design: three failed to include a positive control, so it cannot be determined whether the animals were capable of responding to low doses of any chemical (Ema et al., 2001; Ichihara et al., 2003; Tyl et al., 2002); three used DES as a positive control but found no effect from exposure to this potent xenoestrogen, suggesting that the positive control—and thus the experiment—failed (Ashby et al., 1999; Cagen et al., 1999a, 1999b); one study used 17β-estradiol as a positive control, but administered this estrogen orally which diminishes its biological activity, and reported no effects of this potent hormone on the prostate, also suggesting that the positive control—and thus the experiment—failed (Tyl et al., 2008); and two studies used ethinyl estradiol as a positive control, but only found effects of this chemical at high doses, suggesting that the animal strain used was incapable of responding to low doses (Howdeshell et al., 2008; Tinwell et al., 2002).

Although there continue to be arguments about these data (Tyl, 2009), many studies that reject low-dose effects of BPA on the prostate inaccurately claim that the original results reporting effects of developmental exposure on adult prostate weight have not been replicated. They also suggest that *every* study must find *the same* result for it to be considered reproducible (Kamrin, 2007), an entirely unscientific requirement, especially considering the known role that industries have played in "manufacturing controversy" by publishing poorly designed studies (Michaels, 2005, 2006). The entirety of the data, including those studies that report no low-dose effects, overwhelmingly support a relationship between developmental BPA exposure and altered prostate development, as evidenced by the NIH and NTP expert panel decisions and the FDA's concurrence with them (Chapin et al., 2008; FDA, 2010b; Richter et al., 2007).

9. ADDITIONAL LOW-DOSE FINDINGS: EVIDENCE FROM LABORATORY ANIMALS AND HUMAN POPULATIONS

BPA is one of the best studied EDCs, with thousands of published studies to its credit (vom Saal et al., 2007). This is in striking contrast to the majority of chemicals currently in commerce, which are typically poorly studied at best (Guerrero, 1994). Yet, in spite of this paucity of data, there are additional chemicals that could expand the list of chemicals that act at low doses that was assembled by the NTP. One example is DDT, which has been shown to affect neurobehaviors in laboratory animals following low-dose exposures (Eriksson, Ahlbom, & Fredriksson, 1992; Eriksson, Johansson, Ahlbom, & Fredriksson, 1993; Eriksson, Nilsson-Hakansson, Nordberg, Aspberg, & Fredriksson, 1990; Johansson, Fredriksson, & Eriksson, 1995, 1996; Palanza, Parmigiani, Liu, & vom Saal, 1999; vom Saal et al., 1995). Another is TCDD; several studies show that low doses affect epididymal sperm count, ejaculated sperm number, or sperm morphology and motility in rodents and nonhuman primates (Arima et al., 2009; Bell et al., 2007a, 2007b; Bjerke & Peterson, 1994; Faqi, Dalsenter, Merker, & Chahoud, 1998; Gray, Kelce, Monosson, Ostby, & Birnbaum, 1995; Gray, Ostby, & Kelce, 1997; Jin, Hong, Lee, Kang, & Han, 2010; Loeffler & Peterson, 1999; Mably, Bjerke, Moore, Gendron-Fitzpatrick, & Peterson, 1992; Ohsako et al., 2002; Rebourcet et al., 2010; Simanainen et al., 2004; Sommer, Ippolito, & Peterson, 1996; Wilker, Johnson, & Safe, 1996; Yamano et al., 2009). A relatively large number of studies report low-dose effects of the herbicide atrazine on gonad morphology in amphibians (Carr et al., 2003; Hayes et al., 2002, 2003, 2010, 2006; Hecker et al., 2005; Orton, Carr, & Handy, 2006; Storrs-Mendez & Semlitsch, 2010; Tavera-Mendoza et al., 2002). Finally, a number of studies from multiple species report low-dose effects of tributyltin, a preservative and biocide, on adipogenesis and obesity (Grun et al., 2006; Kirchner, Kieu, Chow, Casey, & Blumberg, 2010; Penza et al., 2011; Zuo et al., 2011). This list is by no means a comprehensive account of all EDCs known to produce low-dose effects, but suggestive that as chemicals are more extensively studied at low doses, more low-dose effects are revealed.

As discussed earlier in this chapter, all human studies of environmental EDC exposures would be classified as low-dose studies. Although it is quite difficult to assign specific mechanisms to the effects of chemicals on human populations, and thus it is difficult to make a conclusive statement that the effects of these chemicals are due to the endocrine disruptive properties, chemicals that are well characterized EDCs have been linked to human diseases and dysfunctions. One such example comes from BPA, which has been repeatedly linked to aspects of metabolic syndrome including diabetes, obesity, liver dysfunction and cardiovascular diseases (Carwile & Michels, 2011; Lang et al., 2008; Melzer et al., 2012; Melzer, Rice, Lewis, Henley, & Galloway, 2010; Wang et al., 2011). Another example comes from persistent organic pollutants and their relationship to similar metabolic end points (Ha, Lee, Son, Park, & Jacobs, 2009; Lee, Lee, Porta, Steffes, & Jacobs, 2007; Lee, Lind, et al., 2011; Lee et al., 2012, 2010; Lee, Steffes, et al., 2011). Additional epidemiology studies indicate that perchlorate, an industrial chemical found in drinking water that reduces thyroid function by inhibiting iodide uptake by the sodium/iodide symporter (Wolff, 1998), disrupts thyroid function in a subset of the human population (Brechner, Parkhurst, Humble, Brown, & Herman, 2000; Crump et al., 2000; Steinmaus, Miller, & Howd, 2007; Steinmaus, Miller, & Smith, 2010). Finally, conclusive data have shown that environmental exposures to PCBs, industrial chemicals that bioaccumulate, affect behaviors in children (reviewed in Boucher, Muckle, & Bastien, 2009; Eubig, Aguiar, & Schantz, 2010); although it is not known whether the effects of PCBs are due to its disruption of thyroid hormone signaling, this is a plausible mechanism for the effects of these chemicals on brain development (Tan & Zoeller, 2007). Because our knowledge of low-dose effects for natural hormones is quite robust and convincing, as the principles of endocrinology are understood and incorporated into toxicology and risk assessment of EDCs, the default assumption is likely to shift, and low-dose effects will be expected, rather than considered an exception, or dismissed outright (Birnbaum, 2012; Myers, Zoeller, et al., 2009; Vandenberg et al., 2012; Zoeller et al., 2012).

10. TRADITIONAL TOXICOLOGY STUDIES ARE NOT DESIGNED TO DETECT LOW-DOSE EFFECTS

The term "guideline study" typically refers to risk assessment studies that meet international guidelines for the study of chemical safety. In most guideline studies, a total of three doses are required, and few studies of EDCs exceed this requirement. Further, high doses must be tested to determine the maximum tolerated intake or maximum tolerated dose; as its name implies, this is a dose that produces biological effects with some toxicity but generally does not produce mortality. Additional doses identify the lowest-observable-adverse-effect level (LOAEL), that is, the lowest dose at which some adverse effects still occur, and the NOAEL, a dose that does not produce adverse effects. Extrapolations are then performed from the NOAEL (or the LOAEL, if a NOAEL is not determined) to calculate a reference dose, which is considered a "safe" dose for humans and wildlife. As noted previously, "these extrapolations use safety factors that acknowledge differences between humans and animals, exposures of vulnerable populations, interspecies variability, and other uncertainty factors. These safety factors are informed guesses, not quantitatively based calculations. Using this traditional way of setting 'safe' doses, the levels declared 'safe' are never in fact tested. Doses in the range of human exposures are therefore also unlikely to be tested" (Vandenberg et al., 2012).

One definition for a "low dose" cutoff proposed by the NTP is any dose below those used in traditional toxicology testing (Melnick et al., 2002). Thus, if a traditional toxicology study tests a particular dose, then lower doses would still need to be tested to reach a "low dose," until the doses reached a level low enough to be relevant for human exposures. There is the added problem from the overall lack of information about all exposure sources, routes, and concentrations for the vast majority of chemicals currently in commerce.

A final issue that should be considered is whether guideline studies test the most appropriate end points to detect low-dose effects (Myers, vom Saal, et al., 2009; Myers, Zoeller, et al., 2009). Guideline compliant reproductive toxicity assays examine end points that are described as "apical" including body weight and food consumption in the dam, timing of gestation, number of pups and uterine implantation sites, sex ratios, weight of organs, and histopathology of reproductive organs (OECD, 1995). Yet, it has been asked whether these assays, and these end points in particular, are sensitive enough to detect low-dose effects and whether they are inordinately affected by experimenter error and large amounts of biological variability (thus precluding the detection of adverse events) and are relevant to human diseases (Myers, Zoeller, et al., 2009; vom Saal & Myers, 2010; Zoeller et al., 2012). For example, does an increase in ovarian weight indicate toxicity, *per se*? Which disease does it map to in the human? If the increase is only seen in the left ovary and not in the right, is this relevant?

If traditional toxicology studies are not designed to detect low-dose effects, what changes are needed to improve these assays? One of the easiest changes that have been proposed is to require toxicology testing to incorporate additional doses that examine concentrations that are relevant to human and wildlife populations. Of course, this requires that these doses be known, which is not trivial for many chemicals on the market and is difficult to predict for new chemicals prior to their use in consumer products. However, acknowledging that many EDCs mimic the actions of hormones, which have biological activity at low doses, requires a similar acknowledgment that low-dose testing capture doses in the ppt and ppb range. Additional suggestions have been made for the incorporation of more sensitive end points such as mammary gland morphology in whole mount preparations, the response of the prostate to endogenous hormones, sensitive behavioral assays that test for sexually dimorphic behaviors, and assays that test cardiovascular and immune function (Heindel, 2008; Rudel, Fenton, Ackerman, Euling, & Makris, 2011; Schug et al., 2011; Vandenberg et al., 2009; Yan et al., 2011). Developing validated assays for these end points that could be added to the traditional end points included in guideline studies would likely take decades, but is an option that should be explored for EDCs.

11. LOW-DOSE EFFECTS: BIOLOGICAL CHANGES ARE NOT NECESSARILY ADVERSE

In the NTP expert panel's assessment (Melnick et al., 2002), the panel chose to define "low-dose effects" as "any biological change" occurring in the low-dose range. The panel specifically noted that "[t]he demonstration that an effect is adverse was not required because in many cases the long-term health consequences of altered endocrine function during development have not been fully characterized." Some scientists have concluded that low-dose effects represent "adaptive" changes, that is, those that are consistent with the maintenance of homeostasis and are therefore not adverse (Rhomberg & Goodman, 2012). However, this presumption has not been adequately tested in experimental studies, and in fact there is sufficient evidence that the embryo and fetus cannot adapt to the excess or insufficient levels of natural hormones (Skakkebaek et al., 2001; Zoeller, 2010).

The question of whether the low-dose effects that have been reported in the EDC literature represent adverse effects hinges on the definition of adverse. The US EPA defines an adverse effect as "a biochemical change, functional impairment, or pathologic lesion that affects the performance of the whole organism, or reduces an organism's ability to respond to an additional environmental challenge" (EPA, 2012). Other risk assessment agencies, including the FDA, have no established definition that they follow for "adverse effects." Further, even working within the constraints of the EPA's definition, it is hard to determine whether the end points assessed in traditional toxicology experiments would be considered adverse, that is, is a change in ovarian weight an adverse effect?

In looking at the kinds of end points that have been observed to be associated with low-dose effects, the end points include alterations in the size of nuclei in the brain, alterations to adult prostate weight, changes to corticosterone levels, altered binding of acetylcholine receptors in the brain, reduced number of ejaculated sperm, altered mammary gland morphology; expression of anxiety-like behaviors, altered release or circulating concentrations of hormones including testosterone and TSH, and abnormal tissue organization in estrogen-sensitive organs such as the prostate, mammary gland, and uterus (reviewed in Vandenberg et al., 2012). Many of these end points would not be considered adverse by traditional toxicologists, but endocrinologists, developmental biologists, and physicians are likely to disagree. Most epidemiology studies focus on end points that are believed to be directly relevant to human diseases (i.e., incidence of diabetes, cryptorchidism, or obesity) although some end points are argued to be irrelevant to human disease (i.e., telomere length and anogenital distance).

A large number of laboratory studies have reported that low-dose EDC exposures during early development alter sexually dimorphic regions of the brain as well as sexually dimorphic behaviors (Adewale, Todd, Mickens, & Patisaul, 2011; Cao, Mickens, McCaffrey, Leyrer, & Patisaul, 2012; Dickerson, Cunningham, Patisaul, Woller, & Gore, 2011; Iwaniuk et al., 2006; Losa et al., 2011; Patisaul, Fortino, & Polston, 2006; Patisaul, Todd, Mickens, & Adewale, 2009; Rubin et al., 2006); sexually dimorphic behaviors are not necessarily those associated with mating and reproduction *per se*, but are instead behaviors that are typically associated with one sex to a larger degree than the other sex. These types of behaviors are important for courting, play, and other types of social interactions (Sakuma, 2009). It is difficult to determine whether changes to these behaviors would be considered "adverse" by a risk assessor, especially considering the role of judgment in risk assessment decisions. However, endocrinologists have concluded that disruptions in these types of behaviors should be considered deleterious and disadvantageous (Gore, 2010).

Similarly, a large number of studies have shown that low doses of BPA alter the response of the mammary gland to carcinogens administered in adulthood, even when the chemical carcinogen is administered at doses that would be considered "subcarcinogenic" (Betancourt, Eltoum, Desmond, Russo, & Lamartiniere, 2010; Durando et al., 2007; Jenkins et al., 2009; Jenkins, Wang, Eltoum, Desmond, & Lamartiniere, 2011; Lamartiniere, Jenkins, Betancourt, Wang, & Russo, 2011; Weber Lozada & Keri, 2011). Clearly, these studies meet the EPA's definition of adverse because they demonstrate that BPA reduces the organism's ability to respond to an additional environmental challenge, the carcinogen. Yet these studies have not led to additional considerations of the reference dose for BPA, set at 50 μg/kg/day, even though doses in this range are sufficient to alter the responsiveness of the mammary gland.

12. REAL WORLD EDC EXPOSURES: MIXTURE EFFECTS

Another factor that should be considered when assessing the low-dose activities of EDCs is the endogenous hormonal environment and the presence of additional toxicants with similar modes of action. In the laboratory, chemical safety screening is performed under incredibly controlled conditions, and exposures are limited—to the best of the experimenter's ability—to the single chemical being tested. Yet, studies suggest that EDC exposures can alter the response of the animal to natural hormones (Munoz-de-Toro et al., 2005; Prins et al., 2007, 2008, 2011; Wadia et al., 2007), suggesting that low-dose effects may only manifest when endogenous hormone levels are controlled.

A number of studies in controlled conditions indicate that cultured cells can have additive and even synergistic responses to mixtures of EDCs, or mixtures of EDCs and natural hormones (Kortenkamp, 2008; Rajapakse, Ong, & Kortenkamp, 2001; Rajapakse, Silva, & Kortenkamp, 2002; Rajapakse, Silva, Scholze, & Kortenkamp, 2004; Silva, Rajapakse, & Kortenkamp, 2002). Some results of these mixtures studies have been referred to as "something from nothing" because xenoestrogens—combined at doses that on their own do not produce measurable effects—produce measurable effects when present together in mixtures (Silva et al., 2002). Further, the xenoestrogen mixtures, together with estradiol, can cause a doubling of the response of the natural hormone (Rajapakse et al., 2002). Thus, these results suggest that the effects of EDCs on human populations could vary significantly depending on the natural endocrine state of the exposed person, plus the presence of other EDCs with similar modes of action. In this way, EDCs may have "low-dose effects" when real-world exposures occur that are not predicted from controlled animal experiments where a single chemical is administered (Kortenkamp, 2006; Kortenkamp, Faust, Scholze, & Backhaus, 2007).

13. NONMONOTONIC DOSE RESPONSES

A similar biological phenomenon, which is often confounded with discussions of low-dose effects, is that of nonmonotonic dose responses. As discussed briefly earlier in this chapter, nonmonotonic dose responses are those where the slope of the line representing the dose response curve changes sign along the range of tested doses (Kohn & Melnick, 2002). In contrast to low-dose effects, which are defined by a cutoff dose that is specific for each chemical, nonmonotonicity can occur anywhere along the dose range. Nonmonotonic dose response curves (NMDRCs) have been observed for more than twenty endogenous hormones in cultured cells, whole organ cultures, laboratory animals, and human populations (Vandenberg et al., 2012). Further, endocrinologists have dissected the mechanisms responsible for these types of curves, including the role of cytotoxicity, receptor downregulation and desensitization, cell and tissue-specific receptors and cofactors, receptor selectivity, receptor competition, negative feedback loops, and complex tissue interactions; many NMDRCs manifest due to overlapping and opposing monotonic curves (i.e., increasing doses of estrogen increase cell proliferation but at high doses, estrogens induce cell death; thus, the overall number of cells has an inverted U-shaped response) (Welshons et al., 2003).

Although NMDRCs are well established and acknowledged in the fields of endocrinology and pharmacology (Arnold, Markham, & Hacker, 1979; Berin, Stein, & Keltz, 2010; Feldberg et al., 1994; Harvey, 1997; McLeod, 2003; Plotkin, Lechner, Jung, & Rosen, 1978; Veldhuis & Santen, 1979; Wallach, 1979), they remain controversial in the field of toxicology, even when the toxicant in question is a hormone mimic (Rhomberg & Goodman, 2012). Yet, similar to what has been reported for endogenous hormones, there are hundreds of examples of NMDRCs for EDCs that have been reported in cultured cells, laboratory animals, and human populations (Vandenberg et al., 2012); in fact, many of the same end points shown to produce NMDRCs following endogenous hormone exposures also produce NMDRCs following EDC exposures. In 2012, the director of the National Institutes of Environmental Health Sciences wrote, "the question is no longer whether nonmonotonic dose responses are 'real' and occur frequently enough to be a concern; clearly these are common phenomena with well-understood mechanisms. Instead, the question is which dose–response shapes should be expected for specific environmental chemicals and under what specific circumstances" (Birnbaum, 2012).

The concept of nonmonotonicity is distinct from low-dose effects, and the mechanisms responsible for these phenomena are distinct as well. However, one aspect that these two occurrences have in common is that they are situations in which safe/reference dose calculations are inappropriate; when low-dose effects or NMDRCs occur, studies cannot test high doses of a chemical and extrapolate those findings to low doses that are expected to be safe. Thus, both low-dose effects and NMDRCs challenge the current ways that chemical risk assessments are conducted.

14. CONCLUSIONS

Since EDCs began to be studied in depth in the 1990s, there has been intense debate over whether the public should be concerned about low-level exposures to these chemicals. The low-dose hypothesis, proposed at that time, has steadily accumulated evidence that EDCs have actions at low doses, and these effects are not necessarily predicted from high-dose toxicology testing. In 2002, the NTP expert panel reported evidence for low-dose effects for a small number of EDCs and estradiol. In 2012, an updated approach identified several dozen additional EDCs with evidence for low-dose effects. Further, epidemiology studies continue to find relationships between EDC exposure levels and diseases in the general public, which has raised concerns because the general public is exposed to a large number of environmental chemicals at low doses.

For decades, hormones have been known to produce striking changes in tissue morphology, physiology, and behaviors at exceedingly low doses. A relatively large body of evidence suggests that EDCs, and in particular those environmental chemicals that mimic endogenous hormones, have similar effects at low doses. Although there is still no consensus about the universality of "low-dose effects" in the toxicology community, the Endocrine Society (Diamanti-Kandarakis et al., 2009; Zoeller et al., 2012) believes not only that there is sufficient evidence in support of this phenomenon but also that it is time for public health agencies to make changes to risk assessment paradigms and give greater consideration to studies that specifically identify low-dose effects when considering risks from chemical exposures.

REFERENCES

Adewale, H. B., Todd, K. L., Mickens, J. A., & Patisaul, H. B. (2011). The impact of neonatal bisphenol-A exposure on sexually dimorphic hypothalamic nuclei in the female rat. *Neurotoxicology, 32*(1), 38–49.

Arbuckle, T. E. (2010). Maternal-infant biomonitoring of environmental chemicals: The epidemiologic challenges. *Birth Defects Research. Part A, Clinical and Molecular Teratology, 88*(10), 931–937.

Arima, A., Kato, H., Ooshima, Y., Tateishi, T., Inoue, A., Muneoka, A., et al. (2009). In utero and lactational exposure to 2,3,7,8-tetrachlorodibenzo-p-dioxin (TCDD) induces a reduction in epididymal and ejaculated sperm number in rhesus monkeys. *Reproductive Toxicology, 28*, 495–502.

Arnold, D. J., Markham, M. J., & Hacker, S. (1979). Tamoxifen flare. *JAMA, 241*(23), 2506.

Ashby, J., Tinwell, H., & Haseman, J. (1999). Lack of effects for low dose levels of bisphenol A and diethylstilbestrol on the prostate gland of CF1 mice exposed in utero. *Regulatory Toxicology and Pharmacology, 30*(2 Pt. 1), 156–166.

Barouki, R., Gluckman, P. D., Grandjean, P., Hanson, M., & Heindel, J. J. (2012). Developmental origins of non-communicable disease: Implications for research and public health. *Environmental Health, 11*, 42.

Barr, D. B., Olsson, A. O., Wong, L. Y., Udunka, S., Baker, S. E., Whitehead, R. D., et al. (2010). Urinary concentrations of metabolites of pyrethroid insecticides in the general U.S. population: National Health and Nutrition Examination Survey 1999–2002. *Environmental Health Perspectives, 118*(6), 742–748.

Bell, D. R., Clode, S., Fan, M. Q., Fernandes, A., Foster, P. M. D., Jiang, T., et al. (2007a). Toxicity of 2,3,7,8-tetrachlorodibenzo-p-dioxin in the developing male Wistar(Han) rat. I: No decrease in epididymal sperm count after a single acute dose. *Toxicological Sciences, 99*(1), 214–223.

Bell, D. R., Clode, S., Fan, M. Q., Fernandes, A., Foster, P. M. D., Jiang, T., et al. (2007b). Toxicity of 2,3,7,8-tetrachlorodibenzo-p-dioxin in the developing male Wistar(Han) rat. II: Chronic dosing causes developmental delay. *Toxicological Sciences, 99*(1), 224–233.

Berin, I., Stein, D. E., & Keltz, M. D. (2010). A comparison of gonadotropin-releasing hormone (GnRH) antagonist and GnRH agonist flare protocols for poor responders undergoing in vitro fertilization. *Fertility and Sterility, 93*(2), 360–363.

Bern, H. A. (1992). The fragile fetus. In T. Colborn, & C. Clement (Eds.), *Chemically-induced alterations in sexual and functional development: The wildlife/human connection* (pp. 9–15). Princeton, NJ: Princeton Scientific Publishing Co., Inc.

Betancourt, A. M., Eltoum, I. A., Desmond, R. A., Russo, J., & Lamartiniere, C. A. (2010). In utero exposure to bisphenol A shifts the window of susceptibility for mammary carcinogenesis in the rat. *Environmental Health Perspectives, 118*(11), 1614–1619.

Birnbaum, L. S. (2012). Environmental chemicals: Evaluating low-dose effects. *Environmental Health Perspectives, 120*(4), A143–A144.

Bjerke, D. L., & Peterson, R. E. (1994). Reproductive toxicity of 2,3,7,8-tetrachlorodibenzo-p-dioxin in male rats: Different effects of in utero versus lactational exposure. *Toxicology and Applied Pharmacology, 127*, 241–249.

Boucher, O., Muckle, G., & Bastien, C. H. (2009). Prenatal exposure to polychlorinated biphenyls: A neuropsychologic analysis. *Environmental Health Perspectives, 117*(1), 7–16.

Brechner, R. J., Parkhurst, G. D., Humble, W. O., Brown, M. B., & Herman, W. H. (2000). Ammonium perchlorate contamination of Colorado River drinking water is associated with abnormal thyroid function in newborns in Arizona. *Journal of Occupational and Environmental Medicine, 42*(8), 777–782.

Brucker-Davis, F., Thayer, K., & Colborn, T. (2001). Significant effects of mild endogenous hormonal changes in humans: Considerations for low-dose testing. *Environmental Health Perspectives, 109*(Suppl. 1), 21–26.

Burridge, E. (2008). Chemical profile: Bisphenol A. *ICIS Chemical Business, 274*(14), 48.

Cagen, S. Z., Waechter, J. M., Jr., Dimond, S. S., Breslin, W. J., Butala, J. H., Jekat, F. W., et al. (1999a). Normal reproductive organ development in CF-1 mice following prenatal exposure to bisphenol A. *Toxicological Sciences, 50*(1), 36–44.

Cagen, S. Z., Waechter, J. M., Jr., Dimond, S. S., Breslin, W. J., Butala, J. H., Jekat, F. W., et al. (1999b). Normal reproductive organ development in Wistar rats exposed to bisphenol A in the drinking water. *Regulatory Toxicology and Pharmacology, 30*(2 Pt. 1), 130–139.

Calafat, A. M., Kuklenyik, Z., Reidy, J. A., Caudill, S. P., Tully, J. S., & Needham, L. L. (2007). Serum concentrations of 11 polyfluoroalkyl compounds in the U.S. population: Data from the national health and nutrition examination survey (NHANES). *Environmental Science & Technology, 41*(7), 2237–2242.

Calafat, A. M., Ye, X., Wong, L. Y., Bishop, A. M., & Needham, L. L. (2010). Urinary concentrations of four parabens in the U.S. population: NHANES 2005–2006. *Environmental Health Perspectives, 118*(5), 679–685.

Calafat, A. M., Ye, X., Wong, L. Y., Reidy, J. A., & Needham, L. L. (2008). Urinary concentrations of triclosan in the U.S. population: 2003–2004. *Environmental Health Perspectives, 116*(3), 303–307.

Cao, J., Mickens, J. A., McCaffrey, K. A., Leyrer, S. M., & Patisaul, H. B. (2012). Neonatal bisphenol A exposure alters sexually dimorphic gene expression in the postnatal rat hypothalamus. *NeuroToxicology, 33*(1), 23–36.

Carr, J. A., Gentles, A., Smith, E. E., Goleman, W. L., Urquidi, L. J., Thuett, K., et al. (2003). Response of larval Xenopus laevis to atrazine: Assessment of growth, metamorphosis, and gonadal and laryngeal morphology. *Environmental Toxicology and Chemistry, 22*(2), 396–405.

Carwile, J. L., & Michels, K. B. (2011). Urinary bisphenol A and obesity: NHANES 2003–2006. *Environmental Research, 111*(6), 825–830.

Chapin, R. E., Adams, J., Boekelheide, K., Gray, L. E. J., Hayward, S. W., Lees, P. S., et al. (2008). NTP-CERHR expert panel report on the reproductive and developmental toxicity of bisphenol A. *Birth Defects Research. Part B, Developmental and Reproductive Toxicology, 83*(3), 157–395.

Charlton, S. J. (2009). Agonist efficacy and receptor desensitization: From partial truths to a fuller picture. *British Journal of Pharmacology, 158*(1), 165–168.

Chitra, K. C., Latchoumycandane, C., & Mathur, P. P. (2003). Induction of oxidative stress by bisphenol A in the epididymal sperm of rats. *Toxicology, 185*(1–2), 119–127.

Clark, M. M., Crews, D., & Galef, B. G. (1991). Concentrations of sex steroid hormones in pregnant and fetal Mongolian gerbils. *Physiology & Behavior, 49*, 239–243.

Crump, C., Michaud, P., Tellez, R., Reyes, C., Gonzalez, G., Montgomery, E. L., et al. (2000). Does perchlorate in drinking water affect thyroid function in newborns or school-age children? *Journal of Occupational and Environmental Medicine, 42*(6), 603–612.

Dechaud, H., Ravard, C., Claustrat, F., de la Perriere, A. B., & Pugeat, M. (1999). Xenoestrogen interaction with human sex hormone-binding globulin (hSHBG). *Steroids, 64*(5), 328–334.

Diamanti-Kandarakis, E., Bourguignon, J. P., Guidice, L. C., Hauser, R., Prins, G. S., Soto, A. M., et al. (2009). Endocrine-disrupting chemical: An Endocrine Society scientific statement. *Endocrine Reviews, 30*, 293–342.

Dickerson, S. M., Cunningham, S. L., Patisaul, H. B., Woller, M. J., & Gore, A. C. (2011). Endocrine disruption of brain sexual differentiation by developmental PCB exposure. *Endocrinology, 152*(2), 581–594.

Durando, M., Kass, L., Piva, J., Sonnenschein, C., Soto, A. M., Luque, E. H., et al. (2007). Prenatal bisphenol A exposure induces preneoplastic lesions in the mammary gland in Wistar rats. *Environmental Health Perspectives*, *115*, 80–86.

EFSA, (2006). Opinion of the Scientific Panel on food additives, flavourings, processing aids and materials in contact with food (AFC) related to 2,2-BIS(4-hydroxyphenyl)propane. *The EFSA Journal*, *428*, 1–75.

Elswick, B. A., Welsch, F., & Janszen, D. B. (2000). Effect of different sampling designs on outcome of endocrine disruptor studies. *Reproductive Toxicology*, *14*(4), 359–367.

Ema, M., Fujii, S., Furukawa, M., Kiguchi, M., Ikka, T., & Harazono, A. (2001). Rat two-generation reproductive toxicity study of bisphenol A. *Reproductive Toxicology*, *15*(5), 505–523.

EPA, (2012). *Integrated Risk Information Systems (IRIS) glossary*. http://www.epa.gov/iris/help_gloss.htm, Accessed 23 August 2012, from.

Eriksson, P., Ahlbom, J., & Fredriksson, A. (1992). Exposure to DDT during a defined period in neonatal life induces permanent changes in brain muscarinic receptors and behaviour in adult mice. *Brain Research*, *582*(2), 277–281.

Eriksson, P., Johansson, U., Ahlbom, J., & Fredriksson, A. (1993). Neonatal exposure to DDT induces increased susceptibility to pyrethroid (bioallethrin) exposure at adult age. Changes in cholinergic muscarinic receptor and behavioural variables. *Toxicology*, *77*(1–2), 21–30.

Eriksson, P., Nilsson-Hakansson, L., Nordberg, A., Aspberg, A., & Fredriksson, A. (1990). Neonatal exposure to DDT and its fatty acid conjugate: Effects on cholinergic and behavioural variables in the adult mouse. *NeuroToxicology*, *11*(2), 345–354.

Eskenazi, B., Mocarelli, P., Warner, M., Needham, L., Patterson, D. G. J., Samuels, S., et al. (2004). Relationship of serum TCDD concentrations and age at exposure of female residents of Seveso, Italy. *Environmental Health Perspectives*, *112*(1), 22–27.

Eskenazi, B., Mocarelli, P., Warner, M., Samuels, S., Vercellini, P., Olive, D., et al. (2007). Serum dioxin concentrations and endometriosis: A cohort study in Seveso, Italy. *Environmental Health Perspectives*, *110*, 629–634.

Eskenazi, B., Warner, M., Mocarelli, P., Samuels, S., Needham, L. L., Patternson, D. G. J., et al. (2002). Serum dioxin concentrations and menstrual cycle characteristics. *American Journal of Epidemiology*, *156*(4), 383–392.

Eubig, P. A., Aguiar, A., & Schantz, S. L. (2010). Lead and PCBs as risk factors for attention deficit/hyperactivity disorder. *Environmental Health Perspectives*, *118*(12), 1654–1667.

Even, M. D., Dhar, M. G., & vom Saal, F. S. (1992). Transport of steroids between fetuses via amniotic fluid in relation to the intrauterine position phenomenon in rats. *Journal of Reproduction and Fertility*, *96*, 709–716.

Faqi, A. S., Dalsenter, P. R., Merker, H.-J., & Chahoud, I. (1998). Reproductive toxicity and tissue concentrations of low doses of 2,3,7,8-tetrachlorodibenzo-p-dioxin in male offspring rats exposed throughout pregnancy and lactation. *Toxicology and Applied Pharmacology*, *150*, 383–392.

FDA U. S., (2010a). *Endocrine disruptor knowledge base*. http://www.fda.gov/ScienceResearch/BioinformaticsTools/EndocrineDisruptorKnowledgebase/default.htm, Accessed 20 August 2012, from.

FDA U. S., (2010b). *Update on bisphenol A for use in food contact applications*. http://www.fda.gov/downloads/NewsEvents/PublicHealthFocus/UCM197778.pdf, Accessed 16 August 2012, from.

Feldberg, D., Farhi, J., Ashkenazi, J., Dicker, D., Shalev, J., & Ben-Rafael, Z. (1994). Minidose gonadotropin-releasing hormone agonist is the treatment of choice in poor responders with high follicle-stimulating hormone levels. *Fertility and Sterility*, *62*(2), 343–346.

Gan, E. H., & Quinton, R. (2010). Physiological significance of the rhythmic secretion of hypothalamic and pituitary hormones. *Progress in Brain Research, 181*, 111–126.
Goodman, J. E., Witorsch, R. J., McConnell, E. E., Sipes, I. G., Slayton, T. M., Yu, C. J., et al. (2009). Weight-of-evidence evaluation of reproductive and developmental effects of low doses of bisphenol A. *Critical Reviews in Toxicology, 39*(1), 1–75.
Gore, A. C. (2010). Neuroendocrine targets of endocrine disruptors. *Hormones (Athens, Greece), 9*(1), 16–27.
Gray, L. E. J., Kelce, W. R., Monosson, E., Ostby, J. S., & Birnbaum, L. S. (1995). Exposure to TCDD during development permanently alters reproductive function in male Long Evans rats and hamsters: Reduced ejaculated and epididymal sperm numbers and sex accessory gland weights in offspring with normal androgenic status. *Toxicology and Applied Pharmacology, 131*, 108–118.
Gray, L. E. J., Ostby, J. S., & Kelce, W. R. (1997). A dose–response analysis of the reproductive effects of a single gestational dose of 2,3,7,8-tetrachlorodibenzo-p-dioxin in male Long Evans hooded rat offspring. *Toxicology and Applied Pharmacology, 146*, 11–20.
Grun, F., Watanabe, H., Zamanian, Z., Maeda, L., Arima, K., Cubacha, R., et al. (2006). Endocrine-disrupting organotin compounds are potent inducers of adipogenesis in vertebrates. *Molecular Endocrinology, 20*(9), 2141–2155.
Guerrero, P. F. (1994). *Toxic substances control act: EPA's limited progress in regulating toxic chemicals. http://archive.gao.gov/t2pbat3/151661.pdf.*
Gupta, C. (2000). Reproductive malformation of the male offspring following maternal exposure to estrogenic chemicals. *Proceedings of the Society for Experimental Biology and Medicine, 224*(2), 61–68.
Ha, M.-H., Lee, D.-H., Son, H.-K., Park, S.-K., & Jacobs, D. R. (2009). Association between serum concentrations of persistent organic pollutants and prevalence of newly diagnosed hypertension: Results from the National Health and Nutrition Examination Survey 1999–2002. *Journal of Human Hypertension, 23*, 274–286.
Harvey, H. A. (1997). Issues concerning the role of chemotherapy and hormonal therapy of bone metastases from breast carcinoma. *Cancer, 80*(8 Suppl.), 1646–1651.
Hatch, E. E., Herbst, A. L., Hoover, R. N., Noller, K. L., Adam, E., Kaufman, R. H., et al. (2001). Incidence of squamous neoplasia of the cervix and vagina in women exposed prenatally to diethylstilbestrol (United States). *Cancer Causes and Control, 12*, 837–845.
Hayes, T. B., Collins, A., Lee, M., Mendoza, M., Noriega, N., Stuart, A. A., et al. (2002). Hermaphroditic, demasculinized frogs after exposure to the herbicide atrazine at low ecologically relevant doses. *Proceedings of the National Academy of Sciences of the United States of America, 99*(8), 5476–5480.
Hayes, T. B., Haston, K., Tsui, M., Hoang, A., Haeffele, C., & Vonk, A. (2003). Atrazine-induced hermaphroditism at 0.1 ppb in American leopard frogs (Rana pipiens): Laboratory and field evidence. *Environmental Health Perspectives, 111*(4), 568–575.
Hayes, T. B., Khoury, V., Narayan, A., Nazir, M., Park, A., Brown, T., et al. (2010). Atrazine induces complete feminization and chemical castration in male African clawed frogs (Xenopus laevis). *Proceedings of the National Academy of Sciences of the United States of America, 107*(10), 4612–4617.
Hayes, T. B., Stuart, A. A., Mendoza, M., Collins, A., Noriega, N., Vonk, A., et al. (2006). Characterization of atrazine-induced gonadal malformations in African clawed frogs (Xenopus laevis) and comparisons with effects of an androgen antagonist (Cyproterone Acetate) and exogenous estrogen (17b-Estradiol): Support for the demasculinization/feminization hypothesis. *Environmental Health Perspectives, 114*(Suppl. 1), 134–141.
Hecker, M., Kim, W. J., Park, J. W., Murphy, M. B., Villeneuve, D., Coady, K. K., et al. (2005). Plasma concentrations of estradiol and testosterone, gonadal aromatase activity

and ultrastructure of the testis in Xenopus laevis exposed to estradiol or atrazine. *Aquatic Toxicology*, *72*(4), 383–396.

Heindel, J. J. (2005). The fetal basis of adult disease: Role of environmental exposures—Introduction. *Birth Defects Research. Part A, Clinical and Molecular Teratology*, *73*(3), 131–132.

Heindel, J. J. (2008). Animal models for probing the developmental basis of disease and dysfunction paradigm. *Basic & Clinical Pharmacology & Toxicology*, *102*(2), 76–81.

Heindel, J. J., & vom Saal, F. S. (2008). Meeting report: Batch-to-batch variability in estrogenic activity in commercial animal diets—Importance and approaches for laboratory animal research. *Environmental Health Perspectives*, *116*(3), 389–393.

Heines, M. (2002). Sexual differentiation of human brain and behavior. In D. W. Pfaff, A. P. Arnold, A. M. Etgen, S. E. Fahrbach, & R. T. Rubin (Eds.), *Hormones, brain and behavior* (pp. 425–485). San Diego, CA: Academic Press.

Herbst, A. L., Ulfelder, H., & Poskanzer, D. C. (1971). Adenocarcinoma of the vagina. Association of maternal stilbestrol therapy with tumor appearance in young women. *New England Journal of Medicine*, *284*(15), 878–881.

Ho, S. M., Tang, W. Y., Belmonte de Frausto, J., & Prins, G. S. (2006). Developmental exposure to estradiol and bisphenol A increases susceptibility to prostate carcinogenesis and epigenetically regulates phosphodiesterase type 4 variant 4. *Cancer Research*, *66*(11), 5624–5632.

Howdeshell, K. L., Furr, J., Lambright, C. R., Wilson, V. S., Ryan, B. C., & Gray, L. E., Jr. (2008). Gestational and lactational exposure to ethinyl estradiol, but not bisphenol A, decreases androgen-dependent reproductive organ weights and epididymal sperm abundance in the male long evans hooded rat. *Toxicological Sciences*, *102*(2), 371–382.

Howdeshell, K. L., Peterman, P. H., Judy, B. M., Taylor, J. A., Orazio, C. E., Ruhlen, R. L., et al. (2003). Bisphenol A is released from polycarbonate animal cages into water at room temperature. *Environmental Health Perspectives*, *111*(9), 1180–1187.

Hunt, P. A., Koehler, K. E., Susiarjo, M., Hodges, C. A., Ilagan, A., Voigt, R. C., et al. (2003). Bisphenol a exposure causes meiotic aneuploidy in the female mouse. *Current Biology*, *13*(7), 546–553.

Ichihara, T., Yoshino, H., Imai, N., Tsutsumi, T., Kawabe, M., Tamano, S., et al. (2003). Lack of carcinogenic risk in the prostate with transplacental and lactational exposure to bisphenol A in rats. *The Journal of Toxicological Sciences*, *28*(3), 165–171.

Iwaniuk, A. N., Koperski, D. T., Cheng, K. M., Elliott, J. E., Smith, L. K., Wilson, L. K., et al. (2006). The effects of environmental exposure to DDT on the brain of a songbird: Changes in structures associated with mating and song. *Behavioural Brain Research*, *173*(1), 1–10.

Jenkins, S., Raghuraman, N., Eltoum, I., Carpenter, M., Russo, J., & Lamartiniere, C. A. (2009). Oral exposure to bisphenol A increases dimethylbenzanthracene-induced mammary cancer in rats. *Environmental Health Perspectives*, *117*(6), 910–915.

Jenkins, S., Wang, J., Eltoum, I., Desmond, R., & Lamartiniere, C. A. (2011). Chronic oral exposure to bisphenol A results in a non-monotonic dose response in mammary carcinogenesis and metastasis in MMTV-erbB2 mice. *Environmental Health Perspectives*, *119*(11), 1604–1609.

Jin, M. H., Hong, C. H., Lee, H. Y., Kang, H. J., & Han, S. W. (2010). Toxic effects of lactational exposure to 2,3,7,8-tetrachlorodibenzo-p-dioxin (TCDD) on development of male reproductive system: Involvement of antioxidants, oxidants, and p53 protein. *Environmental Toxicology*, *25*, 1–8.

Johansson, U., Fredriksson, A., & Eriksson, P. (1995). Bioallethrin causes permanent changes in behavioural and muscarinic acetylcholine receptor variables in adult mice exposed neonatally to DDT. *European Journal of Pharmacology*, *293*(2), 159–166.

Johansson, U., Fredriksson, A., & Eriksson, P. (1996). Low-dose effects of paraoxon in adult mice exposed neonatally to DDT: Changes in behavioural and cholinergic receptor variables. *Environmental Toxicology and Pharmacology, 2*(4), 307–314.

Jones, K. A. (1996). Summation of basic endocrine data. In G. H. Gass, & H. M. Kaplan (Eds.), Handbook of endocrinology: Vol. I. (pp. 1–42) (2nd ed). New York, NY: CRC Press.

Kamrin, M. A. (2007). The "low dose" hypothesis: Validity and implications for human risk. *International Journal of Toxicology, 26*(1), 13–23.

Kavlock, R. J., Daston, G. P., DeRosa, C., Fenner-Crisp, P., Gray, L. E., Kaattari, S., et al. (1996). Research needs for the risk assessment of health and environmental effects of endocrine disruptors: A report of the U.S. EPA-sponsored workshop. *Environmental Health Perspectives, 104*(Suppl. 4), 715–740.

Kirchner, S., Kieu, T., Chow, C., Casey, S., & Blumberg, B. (2010). Prenatal exposure to the environmental obesogen tributyltin predisposes multipotent stem cells to become adipocytes. *Molecular Endocrinology, 24*(3), 526–539.

Kohn, M. C., & Melnick, R. L. (2002). Biochemical origins of the non-monotonic receptor-mediated dose–response. *Journal of Molecular Endocrinology, 29*, 113–123.

Kortenkamp, A. (2006). Breast cancer, oestrogens and environmental pollutants: A re-evaluation from a mixture perspective. *International Journal of Andrology, 29*, 193–198.

Kortenkamp, A. (2008). Low dose mixture effects of endocrine disrupters: Implications for risk assessment and epidemiology. *International Journal of Andrology, 31*(2), 233–240.

Kortenkamp, A., Faust, M., Scholze, M., & Backhaus, T. (2007). Low-level exposure to multiple chemicals: Reason for human health concerns? *Environmental Health Perspectives, 115*(Suppl. 1), 106–114.

Kumar, S. (2011). Occupational, environmental and lifestyle factors associated with spontaneous abortion. *Reproductive Sciences, 18*(10), 915–930.

Lakind, J. S., & Naiman, D. Q. (2008). Bisphenol A (BPA) daily intakes in the United States: Estimates from the 2003–2004 NHANES urinary BPA data. *Journal of Exposure Analysis and Environmental Epidemiology, 18*(6), 608–615.

Lamartiniere, C. A., Jenkins, S., Betancourt, A. M., Wang, J., & Russo, J. (2011). Exposure to the endocrine disruptor bisphenol A alters susceptibility for mammary cancer. *Hormone Molecular Biology and Clinical Investigation, 5*(2), 45–52.

Lang, I. A., Galloway, T. S., Scarlett, A., Henley, W. E., Depledge, M., Wallace, R. B., et al. (2008). Association of urinary bisphenol A concentration with medical disorders and laboratory abnormalities in adults. *JAMA, 300*(11), 1303–1310.

Lee, D.-H., Lee, I. K., Porta, M., Steffes, M., & Jacobs, D. R. (2007). Relationship between serum concentrations of persistent organic pollutants and the prevalence of metabolic syndrome among non-diabetic adults: Results from the National Health and Nutrition Examination Survey 1999–2002. *Diabetologia, 50*, 1841–1851.

Lee, D. H., Lind, P. M., Jacobs, D. R., Jr., Salihovic, S., van Bavel, B., & Lind, L. (2011). Polychlorinated biphenyls and organochlorine pesticides in plasma predict development of type 2 diabetes in the elderly: The prospective investigation of the vasculature in Uppsala Seniors (PIVUS) study. *Diabetes Care, 34*(8), 1778–1784.

Lee, D. H., Lind, L., Jacobs, D. R., Jr., Salihovic, S., van Bavel, B., & Lind, P. M. (2012). Associations of persistent organic pollutants with abdominal obesity in the elderly: The Prospective Investigation of the Vasculature in Uppsala Seniors (PIVUS) study. *Environmental International, 40*, 170–178.

Lee, D.-H., Steffes, M. W., Sjodin, A., Jones, R. S., Needham, L. L., & Jacobs, D. R. (2010). Low dose of some persistent organic pollutants predicts type 2 diabetes: A nested case-control study. *Environmental Health Perspectives, 118*, 1235–1242.

Lee, D.-H., Steffes, M. W., Sjodin, A., Jones, R. S., Needham, L. L., & Jacobs, D. R. (2011). Low dose organochlorine pesticides and polychlorinated biphenyls predict obesity, dyslipidemia, and insulin resistance among people free of diabetes. *PLoS One*, *6*(1), e15977.

Lees, P., Cunningham, F. M., & Elliott, J. (2004). Principles of pharmacodynamics and their applications in veterinary pharmacology. *Journal of Veterinary Pharmacology and Therapeutics*, *27*(6), 397–414.

Li, D. K., Zhou, Z., Miao, M., He, Y., Wang, J., Ferber, J., et al. (2011). Urine bisphenol-A (BPA) level in relation to semen quality. *Fertility and Sterility*, *95*, 625–630.

Li, D., Zhou, Z., Qing, D., He, Y., Wu, T., Miao, M., et al. (2010). Occupational exposure to bisphenol-A (BPA) and the risk of self-reported male sexual dysfunction. *Human Reproduction*, *25*(2), 519–527.

Loeffler, I. K., & Peterson, R. E. (1999). Interactive effects of TCDD and p, p′-DDE on male reproductive tract development in in utero and lactationally exposed rats. *Toxicology and Applied Pharmacology*, *154*, 28–39.

Losa, S. M., Todd, K. L., Sullivan, A. W., Cao, J., Mickens, J. A., & Patisaul, H. B. (2011). Neonatal exposure to genistein adversely impacts the ontogeny of hypothalamic kisspeptin signaling pathways and ovarian development in the peripubertal female rat. *Reproductive Toxicology*, *31*(3), 280–289.

Mably, T. A., Bjerke, D. L., Moore, R. W., Gendron-Fitzpatrick, A., & Peterson, R. E. (1992). In utero and lactational exposure of male rats to 2,3,7,8-tetrachlorodibenzo-p-dioxin. 3. Effects on spermatogenesis and reproductive capability. *Toxicology and Applied Pharmacology*, *114*(1), 118–126.

Markey, C. M., Coombs, M. A., Sonnenschein, C., & Soto, A. M. (2003). Mammalian development in a changing environment: Exposure to endocrine disruptors reveals the developmental plasticity of steroid-hormone target organs. *Evolution and Development*, *5*(1), 67–75.

Markey, C. M., Michaelson, C. L., Veson, E. C., Sonnenschein, C., & Soto, A. M. (2001). The mouse uterotrophic assay: A reevaluation of its validity in assessing the estrogenicity of bisphenol A. *Environmental Health Perspectives*, *109*(1), 55–60.

Markey, C. M., Wadia, P. R., Rubin, B. S., Sonnenschein, C., & Soto, A. M. (2005). Long-term effects of fetal exposure to low doses of the xenoestrogen bisphenol-A in the female mouse genital tract. *Biology of Reproduction*, *72*(6), 1344–1351.

May, M., Moran, J. F., Kimelberg, H., & Triggle, D. J. (1967). Studies on the noradrenaline alpha-receptor. II. Analysis of the "spare-receptor" hypothesis and estimation of the concentration of alpha-receptors in rabbit aorta. *Molecular Pharmacology*, *3*(1), 28–36.

McLachlan, J. A. (2001). Environmental signaling: What embryos and evolution teach us about endocrine disrupting chemicals. *Endocrine Reviews*, *22*(3), 319–341.

McLachlan, J. A. (2006). Commentary: Prenatal exposure to diethylstilbestrol (DES): A continuing story. *International Journal of Epidemiology*, *35*(4), 868–870.

McLeod, D. G. (2003). Hormonal therapy: Historical perspective to future directions. *Urology*, *61*(2 Suppl. 1), 3–7.

Medina, D., Sivaraman, L., Hilsenbeck, S. G., Conneely, O. M., Ginger, M., Rosen, J. M., et al. (2001). Mechanisms of hormonal prevention of breast cancer. *Annals of the New York Academy of Sciences*, *952*, 23–35.

Melnick, R., Lucier, G., Wolfe, M., Hall, R., Stancel, G., Prins, G., et al. (2002). Summary of the National Toxicology Program's report of the endocrine disruptors low-dose peer review. *Environmental Health Perspectives*, *110*(4), 427–431.

Melzer, D., Osborne, N. J., Henley, W. E., Cipelli, R., Young, A., Money, C., et al. (2012). Urinary bisphenol A concentration and risk of future coronary artery disease in apparently healthy men and women. *Circulation*, *125*(12), 1482–1490.

Melzer, D., Rice, N. E., Lewis, C., Henley, W. E., & Galloway, T. S. (2010). Association of urinary bisphenol A concentration with heart disease: Evidence from NHANES 2003/06. *PLoS ONE*, *5*(1), e8673.

Michaels, D. (2005). Doubt is their product. *Scientific American*, *292*(6), 96–101.

Michaels, D. (2006). Manufactured uncertainty: Protecting public health in the age of contested science and product defense. *Annals of the New York Academy of Sciences*, *1076*, 149–162.

Milligan, S. R., Khan, O., & Nash, M. (1998). Competitive binding of xenobiotic oestrogens to rat alpha-fetoprotein and to sex steroid binding proteins in human and rainbow trout (Oncorhynchus mykiss) plasma. *General and Comparative Endocrinology*, *112*(1), 89–95.

Mittendorf, R. (1995). Teratogen update: Carcinogenesis and teratogenesis associated with exposure to diethylstilbestrol (DES) in utero. *Teratology*, *51*, 435–445.

Mocarelli, P., Gerthoux, P. M., Patterson, D. G. J., Milani, S., Limonta, G., Bertona, M., et al. (2008). Dioxin exposure, from infancy through puberty, produces endocrine disruption and affects human semen quality. *Environmental Health Perspectives*, *116*, 70–77.

Munoz-de-Toro, M., Markey, C. M., Wadia, P. R., Luque, E. H., Rubin, B. S., Sonnenschein, C., et al. (2005). Perinatal exposure to bisphenol-A alters peripubertal mammary gland development in mice. *Endocrinology*, *146*(9), 4138–4147.

Myers, J. P., vom Saal, F. S., Akingbemi, B. T., Arizono, K., Belcher, S., Colborn, T., et al. (2009). Why public health agencies cannot depend upon 'Good Laboratory Practices' as a criterion for selecting data: The case of bisphenol-A. *Environmental Health Perspectives*, *117*(3), 309–315.

Myers, J. P., Zoeller, R. T., & vom Saal, F. S. (2009). A clash of old and new scientific concepts in toxicity, with important implications for public health. *Environmental Health Perspectives*, *117*(11), 1652–1655.

Naftolin, F., Garcia-Segura, L. M., Horvath, T. L., Zsarnovszky, A., Demir, N., Fadiel, A., et al. (2007). Estrogen-induced hypothalamic synaptic plasticity and pituitary sensitization in the control of the estrogen-induced gonadotrophin surge. *Reproductive Sciences*, *14*(2), 101–116.

Nagel, S. C., Hagelbarger, J. L., & McDonnell, D. P. (2001). Development of an ER action indicator mouse for the study of estrogens, selective ER modulators (SERMs), and xenobiotics. *Endocrinology*, *142*(11), 4721–4728.

Nagel, S. C., vom Saal, F. S., Thayer, K. A., Dhar, M. G., Boechler, M., & Welshons, W. V. (1997). Relative binding affinity-serum modified access (RBA-SMA) assay predicts the relative in vivo bioactivity of the xenoestrogens bisphenol A and octylphenol. *Environmental Health Perspectives*, *105*(1), 70–76.

Nagel, S. C., vom Saal, F. S., & Welshons, W. V. (1999). Developmental effects of estrogenic chemicals are predicted by an in vitro assay incorporating modification of cell uptake by serum. *Journal of Steroid Biochemistry and Molecular Biology*, *69*(1–6), 343–357.

NTP, (2001). *National toxicology program's report of the endocrine disruptors low dose peer review.* http://ntp.niehs.nih.gov/ntp/htdocs/liason/LowDosePeerFinalRpt.pdf.

OECD, (1995). *OECD guideline for testing of chemicals: Reproductive/Developmental toxicity screening test.* http://iccvam.niehs.nih.gov/SuppDocs/FedDocs/OECD/OECD_GL421.pdf.

Ogura, Y., Ishii, K., Kanda, H., Kanai, M., Arima, K., Wang, Y., et al. (2007). Bisphenol A induces permanent squamous change in mouse prostatic epithelium. *Differentiation*, *75*(8), 745–756.

Ohsako, S., Miyabara, Y., Sakaue, M., Ishimura, R., Kakeyama, M., Izumi, H., et al. (2002). Developmental stage-specific effects of perinatal 2,3,7,8-tetrachlorodibenzo-p-dioxin exposure on reproductive organs of male rat offspring. *Toxicological Sciences*, *66*, 283–292.

Orton, F., Carr, J. A., & Handy, R. D. (2006). Effects of nitrate and atrazine on larval development and sexual differentiation in the northern leopard frog Rana pipiens. *Environmental Toxicology and Chemistry*, *25*(1), 65–71.

Palanza, P., Parmigiani, S., Liu, H., & vom Saal, F. S. (1999). Prenatal exposure to low doses of the estrogenic chemicals diethylstilbestrol and o, p′-DDT alters aggressive behavior of male and female house mice. *Pharmacology, Biochemistry, and Behavior, 64*(4), 665–672.

Palmer, J. R., Wise, L. A., Hatch, E. E., Troisi, R., Titus-Ernstoff, L., Strohsnitter, W., et al. (2006). Prenatal diethylstilbestrol exposure and risk of breast cancer. *Cancer Epidemiology, Biomarkers & Prevention, 15*(8), 1509–1514.

Patisaul, H. B., Fortino, A. E., & Polston, E. K. (2006). Neonatal genistein or bisphenol-A exposure alters sexual differentiation of the AVPV. *Neurotoxicology and Teratology, 28*, 111–118.

Patisaul, H. B., Todd, K. L., Mickens, J. A., & Adewale, H. B. (2009). Impact of neonatal exposure to the ERalpha agonist PPT, bisphenol-A or phytoestrogens on hypothalamic kisspeptin fiber density in male and female rats. *NeuroToxicology, 30*(3), 350–357.

Penza, M., Jeremic, M., Marrazzo, E., Maggi, A., Ciana, P., Rando, G., et al. (2011). The environmental chemical tributyltin chloride (TBT) shows both estrogenic and adipogenic activities in mice which might depend on the exposure dose. *Toxicology and Applied Pharmacology, 255*(1), 65–75.

Pesatori, A. C., Consonni, D., Bachetti, S., Zocchetti, C., Bonzini, M., Baccarelli, A., et al. (2003). Short- and long-term morbidity and mortality in the population exposed to dioxin after the "Seveso accident" *Industrial Health, 41*(3), 127–138.

Petrelli, G., Figa-Talamanca, I., Lauria, L., & Mantovani, A. (2003). Spontaneous abortion in spouses of greenhouse workers exposed to pesticides. *Environmental Health and Preventive Medicine, 8*(3), 77–81.

Phoenix, C. H., Goy, R. W., Gerall, A. A., & Young, W. C. (1959). Organizing action of prenatally administered testosterone propionate on the tissues mediating mating behavior in the female guinea pig. *Endocrinology, 65*, 369–382.

Plotkin, D., Lechner, J. J., Jung, W. E., & Rosen, P. J. (1978). Tamoxifen flare in advanced breast cancer. *JAMA, 240*(24), 2644–2646.

Prins, G. S., Birch, L., Tang, W. Y., & Ho, S. M. (2007). Developmental estrogen exposures predispose to prostate carcinogenesis with aging. *Reproductive Toxicology, 23*(3), 374–382.

Prins, G. S., Tang, W. Y., Belmonte, J., & Ho, S. M. (2008). Perinatal exposure to oestradiol and bisphenol A alters the prostate epigenome and increases susceptibility to carcinogenesis. *Basic & Clinical Pharmacology & Toxicology, 102*(2), 134–138.

Prins, G. S., Ye, S. H., Birch, L., Ho, S.-M., & Kannan, K. (2011). Serum bisphenol A pharmacokinetics and prostate neoplastic responses following oral and subcutaneous exposures in neonatal Sprague–Dawley rats. *Reproductive Toxicology, 31*(1), 1–9.

Rajapakse, N., Ong, D., & Kortenkamp, A. (2001). Defining the impact of weakly estrogenic chemicals on the action of steroidal estrogens. *Toxicological Sciences, 60*(2), 296–304.

Rajapakse, N., Silva, E., & Kortenkamp, A. (2002). Combining xenoestrogens at levels below individual no-observed-effect concentrations dramatically enhances steroid hormone activity. *Environmental Health Perspectives, 110*, 917–921.

Rajapakse, N., Silva, E., Scholze, M., & Kortenkamp, A. (2004). Deviation from additivity with estrogenic mixtures containing 4-nonylphenol and 4-tert-octylphenol detected in the E-SCREEN assay. *Environmental Science & Technology, 38*(23), 6343–6352.

Ramos, J. G., Varayoud, J., Kass, L., Rodrigues, H., Costabel, L., Munoz-de-Toro, M., et al. (2003). Bisphenol A induces both transient and permanent histofunctional alterations of the hypothalamic-pituitary-gonadal axis in prenatally exposed male rats. *Endocrinology, 144*(7), 3206–3215.

Ramos, J. G., Varayoud, J., Sonnenschein, C., Soto, A. M., Munoz-de-Toro, M., & Luque, E. H. (2001). Prenatal exposure to low doses of bisphenol A alters the periductal stroma and glandular cell function in the rat ventral prostate. *Biology of Reproduction, 65*, 1271–1277.

Rebourcet, D., Odet, F., Verot, A., Combe, E., Meugnier, E., Pesenti, S., et al. (2010). The effects of an in utero exposure to 2,3,7,8-tetrachlorodibenzo-p-dioxin on male reproductive function: Identification of Ccl5 as a potential marker. *International Journal of Andrology*, *33*, 413–424.

Rhomberg, L. R., & Goodman, J. E. (2012). Low-dose effects and nonmonotonic dose-responses of endocrine disrupting chemicals: Has the case been made? *Regulatory Toxicology and Pharmacology*, *64*(1), 130–133.

Richter, C., Birnbaum, L. S., Farabollini, F., Newbold, R. R., Rubin, B. S., Talsness, C. E., et al. (2007). In vivo effects of bisphenol A in laboratory rodent studies. *Reproductive Toxicology*, *24*(2), 199–224.

Robinson, G. W., Karpf, A. B. C., & Kratochwil, K. (1999). Regulation of mammary gland development by tissue interaction. *Journal of Mammary Gland Biology and Neoplasia*, *4*, 9–19.

Rubin, B. S., Lenkowski, J. R., Schaeberle, C. M., Vandenberg, L. N., Ronsheim, P. M., & Soto, A. M. (2006). Evidence of altered brain sexual differentiation in mice exposed perinatally to low, environmentally relevant levels of bisphenol A. *Endocrinology*, *147*(8), 3681–3691.

Rudel, R. A., Fenton, S. E., Ackerman, J. M., Euling, S. Y., & Makris, S. L. (2011). Environmental exposures and mammary gland development: State of the science, public health implications, and research recommendations. *Environmental Health Perspectives*, *119*(8), 1053–1061.

Ryan, B. C., Hotchkiss, A. K., Crofton, K. M., & Gray, L. E., Jr. (2010). In utero and lactational exposure to bisphenol A, in contrast to ethinyl estradiol, does not alter sexually dimorphic behavior, puberty, fertility, and anatomy of female LE rats. *Toxicological Sciences*, *114*(1), 133–148.

Ryan, B. C., & Vandenbergh, J. G. (2002). Intrauterine position effects. *Neuroscience and Biobehavioral Reviews*, *26*, 665–678.

Sakuma, Y. (2009). Gonadal steroid action and brain sex differentiation in the rat. *Journal of Neuroendocrinology*, *21*(4), 410–414.

Schonfelder, G., Friedrich, K., Paul, M., & Chahoud, I. (2004). Developmental effects of prenatal exposure to bisphenol A on the uterus of rat offspring. *Neoplasia*, *6*, 584–594.

Schug, T. T., Janesick, A., Blumberg, B., & Heindel, J. J. (2011). Endocrine disrupting chemicals and disease susceptibility. *The Journal of Steroid Biochemistry and Molecular Biology*, *127*(3–5), 204–215.

Schulz, K. M., Molenda-Figueira, H. A., & Sisk, C. L. (2009). Back to the future: The organizational-activational hypothesis adapted to puberty and adolescence. *Hormones and Behavior*, *55*, 597–604.

Sheehan, D. M., & Young, M. (1979). Diethylstilbestrol and estradiol binding to serum albumin and pregnancy plasma of rat and human. *Endocrinology*, *104*(5), 1442–1446.

Silva, E., Rajapakse, N., & Kortenkamp, A. (2002). Something from "nothing"—Eight weak estrogenic chemicals combined at concentrations below NOECs produce significant mixture effects. *Environmental Science & Technology*, *36*, 1751–1756.

Simanainen, U., Haavisto, T., Tuomisto, J. T., Paranko, J., Toppari, J., Tuomisto, J., et al. (2004). Pattern of male reproductive system effects after in utero and lactational 2,3,7,8-tetrachlorodibenzo-p-dioxin (TCDD) exposure in three differentially TCDD-sensitive rat lines. *Toxicological Sciences*, *80*, 101–108.

Skakkebaek, N. E., Rajpert-De Meyts, E., & Main, K. M. (2001). Testicular dysgenesis syndrome: An increasingly common developmental disorder with environmental aspects. *Human Reproduction*, *16*(5), 972–978.

Snijder, C. A., Roeleveld, N., Te Velde, E., Steegers, E. A., Raat, H., Hofman, A., et al. (2012). Occupational exposure to chemicals and fetal growth: The Generation R Study. *Human Reproduction*, *27*(3), 910–920.

Sommer, R. J., Ippolito, D. L., & Peterson, R. E. (1996). In utero and lactational exposure of the male Holtzman rat to 2,3,7,8-tetrachlorodibenzo-p-dioxin: Decreased epididymal and ejaculated sperm numbers without alterations in sperm transit rate. *Toxicology and Applied Pharmacology*, *140*, 146–153.

Son, G. H., Chung, S., & Kim, K. (2011). The adrenal peripheral clock: Glucocorticoid and the circadian timing system. *Frontiers in Neuroendocrinology*, *32*(4), 451–465.

Soto, A. M., Vandenberg, L. N., Maffini, M. V., & Sonnenschein, C. (2008). Does breast cancer start in the womb? *Basic and Clinical Pharmacology and Toxicology*, *102*(2), 125–133.

Steinmaus, C., Miller, M. D., & Howd, R. (2007). Impact of smoking and thiocyanate on perchlorate and thyroid hormone associations in the 2001–2002 national health and nutrition examination survey. *Environmental Health Perspectives*, *115*(9), 1333–1338.

Steinmaus, C., Miller, M. D., & Smith, A. H. (2010). Perchlorate in drinking water during pregnancy and neonatal thyroid hormone levels in California. *Journal of Occupational and Environmental Medicine*, *52*(12), 1217–1524.

Storrs-Mendez, S. I., & Semlitsch, R. D. (2010). Intersex gonads in frogs: Understanding the time course of natural development and role of endocrine disruptors. *Journal of Experimental Zoology. Part B, Molecular and Developmental Evolution*, *314*(1), 57–66.

Stump, D. G., Beck, M. J., Radovsky, A., Garman, R. H., Freshwater, L. L., Sheets, L. P., et al. (2010). Developmental neurotoxicity study of dietary bisphenol A in Sprague–Dawley rats. *Toxicological Sciences*, *115*(1), 167–182.

Tan, S. W., & Zoeller, R. T. (2007). Integrating basic research on thyroid hormone action into screening and testing programs for thyroid disruptors. *Critical Reviews in Toxicology*, *37*(1–2), 5–10.

Tarim, O. (2011). Thyroid hormones and growth in health and disease. *Journal of Clinical Research in Pediatric Endocrinology*, *3*(2), 51–55.

Tavera-Mendoza, L., Ruby, S., Brousseau, P., Fournier, M., Cyr, D., & Marcogliese, D. (2002). Response of the amphibian tadpole (Xenopus laevis) to atrazine during sexual differentiation of the testis. *Environmental Toxicology and Chemistry*, *21*(3), 527–531.

Taylor, J. A., vom Saal, F. S., Welshons, W. V., Drury, B., Rottinghaus, G., Hunt, P. A., et al. (2011). Similarity of bisphenol A pharmacokinetics in rhesus monkeys and mice: Relevance for human exposure. *Environmental Health Perspectives*, *119*(4), 422–430.

Tharp, A. P., Maffini, M. V., Hunt, P. A., Vandevoort, C. A., Sonnenschein, C., & Soto, A. M. (2012). Bisphenol A alters the development of the rhesus monkey mammary gland. *Proceedings of the National Academy of Sciences of the United States of America*, *109*(21), 8190–8195.

Timms, B. G., Howdeshell, K. L., Barton, L., Bradley, S., Richter, C. A., & vom Saal, F. S. (2005). Estrogenic chemicals in plastic and oral contraceptives disrupt development of the fetal mouse prostate and urethra. *Proceedings of the National Academy of Sciences of the United States of America*, *102*, 7014–7019.

Timms, B. G., Peterson, R. E., & vom Saal, F. S. (2002). 2,3,7,8-tetrachlorodibenzo-p-dioxin interacts with endogenous estradiol to disrupt prostate gland morphogenesis in male rat fetuses. *Toxicological Sciences*, *67*, 264–274.

Tinwell, H., Haseman, J., Lefevre, P. A., Wallis, N., & Ashby, J. (2002). Normal sexual development of two strains of rat exposed in utero to low doses of bisphenol A. *Toxicological Sciences*, *68*(2), 339–348.

Trichopoulos, D. (1990). Is breast cancer initiated *in utero*? *Epidemiology*, *1*, 95–96.

Tyl, R. W. (2009). Basic exploratory research versus guideline-compliant studies used for hazard evaluation and risk assessment: Bisphenol A as a case study. *Environmental Health Perspectives*, *117*(111), 1644–1651.

Tyl, R. W., Myers, C. B., Marr, M. C., Sloan, C. S., Castillo, N. P., Veselica, M. M., et al. (2008). Two-generation reproductive toxicity study of dietary bisphenol A in CD-1 (Swiss) mice. *Toxicological Sciences*, *104*(2), 362–384.

Tyl, R. W., Myers, C. B., Marr, M. C., Thomas, B. F., Keimowitz, A. R., Brine, D. R., et al. (2002). Three-generation reproductive toxicity study of dietary bisphenol A in CD Sprague–Dawley rats. *Toxicological Sciences*, *68*(1), 121–146.

Urbanski, H. F. (2011). Role of circadian neuroendocrine rhythms in the control of behavior and physiology. *Neuroendocrinology*, *93*(4), 211–222.

Vandenberg, L. N., Colborn, T., Hayes, T. B., Heindel, J. J., Jacobs, D. R., Lee, D.-H., et al. (2012). Hormones and endocrine disrupting chemicals: Low dose effects and non-monotonic dose responses. *Endocrine Reviews*, *33*(3), 378–455.

Vandenberg, L. N., Hauser, R., Marcus, M., Olea, N., & Welshons, W. V. (2007). Human exposure to bisphenol A (BPA). *Reproductive Toxicology*, *24*(2), 139–177.

Vandenberg, L. N., Maffini, M. V., Sonnenschein, C., Rubin, B. S., & Soto, A. M. (2009). Bisphenol-A and the great divide: A review of controversies in the field of endocrine disruption. *Endocrine Reviews*, *30*(1), 75–95.

Vandenbergh, J. G. (2004). Animal models and studies of in utero endocrine disruptor effects. *ILAR Journal*, *45*, 438–442.

Veldhuis, J. D., & Santen, R. J. (1979). Tamoxifen flare. *JAMA*, *241*(23), 2506–2507.

vom Saal, F. S. (1989). Sexual differentiation in litter-bearing mammals: Influence of sex of adjacent fetuses in utero. *Journal of Animal Science*, *67*, 1824–1840.

vom Saal, F. S., Akingbemi, B. T., Belcher, S. M., Birnbaum, L. S., Crain, D. A., Eriksen, M., et al. (2007). Chapel Hill bisphenol A expert panel consensus statement: Integration of mechanisms, effects in animals and potential to impact human health at current levels of exposure. *Reproductive Toxicology*, *24*(2), 131–138.

vom Saal, F. S., Akingbemi, B. T., Belcher, S. M., Crain, D. A., Crews, D., Guidice, L. C., et al. (2010). Flawed experimental design reveals the need for guidelines requiring appropriate positive controls in endocrine disruption research. *Toxicological Sciences*, *115*(2), 612–613.

vom Saal, F. S., & Bronson, F. H. (1980). Sexual characteristics of adult female mice are correlated with their blood testosterone levels during prenatal development. *Science*, *208*, 597–599.

vom Saal, F. S., & Hughes, C. (2005). An extensive new literature concerning low-dose effects of bisphenol A shows the need for a new risk assessment. *Environmental Health Perspectives*, *113*, 926–933.

vom Saal, F. S., & Myers, J. P. (2010). Good laboratory practices are not synonymous with good scientific practices, accurate reporting, or valid data. *Environmental Health Perspectives*, *118*(2), A60.

vom Saal, F. S., Nagel, S. C., Palanza, P., Boechler, M., Parmigiani, S., & Welshons, W. V. (1995). Estrogenic pesticides: Binding relative to estradiol in MCF-7 cells and effects of exposure during fetal life on subsequent territorial behaviour in male mice. *Toxicology Letters*, 77(1–3), 343–350.

vom Saal, F. S., Quadagno, D. M., Even, M. D., Keisler, L. W., Keisler, D. H., & Khan, S. (1990). Paradoxical effects of maternal stress on fetal steroids and postnatal reproductive traits in female mice from different intrauterine positions. *Biology of Reproduction*, *43*(5), 751–761.

vom Saal, F. S., Richter, C. A., Mao, J., & Welshons, W. V. (2005). Commercial animal feed: Variability in estrogenic activity and effects on body weight in mice. *Birth Defects Research, Part A: Clinical and Molecular Teratology*, *73*(7), 474–475.

vom Saal, F. S., Richter, C. A., Ruhlen, R. R., Nagel, S. C., Timms, B. G., & Welshons, W. V. (2005). The importance of appropriate controls, animal feed, and animal models in interpreting results from low-dose studies of bisphenol A. *Birth Defects Research, Part A: Clinical and Molecular Teratology*, *73*, 140–145.

vom Saal, F. S., & Welshons, W. V. (2006). Large effects from small exposures. II. The importance of positive controls in low-dose research on bisphenol A. *Environmental Research*, *100*, 50–76.

Wadia, P. R., Vandenberg, L. N., Schaeberle, C. M., Rubin, B. S., Sonnenschein, C., & Soto, A. M. (2007). Perinatal bisphenol A exposure increases estrogen sensitivity of the mammary gland in diverse mouse strains. *Environmental Health Perspectives, 115*(4), 592–598.

Wallach, H. W. (1979). Tamoxifen flare. *JAMA, 242*(1), 27.

Wallen, K. (2009). The organizational hypothesis: Reflections on the 50th anniversary of the publication of Phoenix, Goy, Gerall, and Young (1959). *Hormones and Behavior, 55*(5), 561–565.

Wang, T., Li, M., Chen, B., Xu, M., Xu, Y., Huang, Y., et al. (2011). Urinary bisphenol A (BPA) concentration associates with obesity and insulin resistance. *The Journal of Clinical Endocrinology Metabolism, 97*, E223–E227.

Warner, M., Eskenazi, B., Mocarelli, P., Gerthoux, P. M., Samuels, S., Needham, L., et al. (2002). Serum dioxin concentrations and breast cancer risk in the Seveso Women's Health Study. *Environmental Health Perspectives, 110*, 625–628.

Weber Lozada, K., & Keri, R. A. (2011). Bisphenol A increases mammary cancer risk in two distinct mouse models of breast cancer. *Biology of Reproduction, 85*, 490–497.

Welshons, W. V., Thayer, K. A., Judy, B. M., Taylor, J. A., Curran, E. M., & vom Saal, F. S. (2003). Large effects from small exposures: I. Mechanisms for endocrine-disrupting chemicals with estrogenic activity. *Environmental Health Perspectives, 111*, 994–1006.

Wilker, C., Johnson, L., & Safe, S. (1996). Effects of developmental exposure to indole-3-carbinol or 2,3,7,8-tetrachlorodibenzo-p-dioxin on reproductive potential of male rat offspring. *Toxicology and Applied Pharmacology, 141*, 68–75.

Witorsch, R. J. (2002a). Endocrine disruptors: Can biological effects and environmental risks be predicted? *Regulatory Toxicology and Pharmacology, 36*(1), 118–130.

Witorsch, R. J. (2002b). Low-dose in utero effects of xenoestrogens in mice and their relevance to humans: An analytical review of the literature. *Food and Chemical Toxicology, 40*(7), 905–912.

Wolff, J. (1998). Perchlorate and the thyroid gland. *Pharmacological Reviews, 50*(1), 89–105.

Woodruff, T. J., Zota, A. R., & Schwartz, J. M. (2011). Environmental chemicals in pregnant women in the US: NHANES 2003–2004. *Environmental Health Perspectives, 119*(6), 878–885.

Yamano, Y., Asano, A., Ohta, M., Hirata, S., Shoda, T., & Ohyama, K. (2009). Expression of rat sperm flagellum-movement associated protein genes under 2,3,7,8-tetrachlorodibenzo-p-dioxin treatment. *Bioscience, Biotechnology, and Biochemistry, 73*(4), 946–949.

Yan, S., Chen, Y., Dong, M., Song, W., Belcher, S. M., & Wang, H. S. (2011). Bisphenol A and 17beta-estradiol promote arrhythmia in the female heart via alteration of calcium handling. *PLoS ONE, 6*(9), e25455.

Zhu, B. T. (1996). Rational design of receptor partial agonists and possible mechanisms of receptor partial activation: A theory. *Journal of Theoretical Biology, 181*(3), 273–291.

Zoeller, R. T. (2010). Environmental chemicals targeting thyroid. *Hormones, 9*(1), 28–40.

Zoeller, R. T., Brown, T. R., Doan, L. L., Gore, A. C., Skakkebaek, N. E., Soto, A. M., et al. (2012). Endocrine-disrupting chemicals and public health protection: A statement of principles from the Endocrine Society. *Endocrinology, 153*, 4097–4110.

Zoeller, R. T., & Rovet, J. (2004). Timing of thyroid hormone action in the developing brain: Clinical observations and experimental findings. *Journal of Neuroendocrinology, 16*(10), 809–818.

Zuo, Z., Chen, S., Wu, T., Zhang, J., Su, Y., Chen, Y., et al. (2011). Tributyltin causes obesity and hepatic steatosis in male mice. *Environmental Toxicology, 26*(1), 79–85.

CHAPTER SIX

Contamination from Endocrine Disrupters of the General Population at Low and High Concentrations

Miquel Porta[*,†,‡,§,1], **José Pumarega**[*,‡], **Magda Gasull**[*,‡], **Tomàs Lopez**[*,†,‡]
[*]Unit of Clinical and Molecular Epidemiology of Cancer, Hospital del Mar Institute of Medical Research—IMIM, Barcelona, Catalonia, Spain
[†]School of Medicine, Universitat Autònoma de Barcelona, Barcelona, Spain
[‡]CIBER en Epidemiología y Salud Pública (CIBERESP), Spain
[§]Gillings School of Global Public Health, University of North Carolina at Chapel Hill, Chapel Hill, North Carolina, USA
[1]Corresponding author: e-mail address: mporta@imim.es

Contents

1. Introduction 168
   1.1 Human contamination and endocrine disrupting chemicals 168
   1.2 Human exposure to and contamination from POPs 170
   1.3 Mixtures of endocrine disrupters 171
   1.4 New indicator: Number of chemicals detected at high concentrations 172
2. How to Implement the Indicator? An Example 172
   2.1 Definitions of the cutoff point 172
   2.2 Study population 173
   2.3 Analytical chemical methods 174
3. Results of the Implementation of the Indicator 175
4. Discussion 183
   4.1 Study conclusions 187
   4.2 General conclusions and proposals for future work 187
References 189

Abstract

Analyses of the concentrations of a given environmental compound usually show that most citizens have much lower concentrations than a certain minority, whose members have high body concentrations. Surveys of human exposure to chemicals do not usually integrate the number of chemical compounds detected per person and the concentration of each compound. This leaves untested relevant exposure situations, for example, whether individuals with low concentrations of some compounds have high concentrations of the other compounds. On scientific grounds, it is puzzling that this possibility,

Vitamins and Hormones, Volume 94
ISSN 0083-6729
http://dx.doi.org/10.1016/B978-0-12-800095-3.00006-7

arithmetically and conceptually rather simple, has seldom if ever been tested in studies based on a representative sample of the general population. A study based on a representative sample of the general population of Catalonia (Spain) (Porta, Pumarega, & Gasull, 2012), which integrated the number of compounds detected per person and the concentration of each compound, found that more than half of the population had concentrations in the top quartile of 1 or more of the 19 persistent toxic substances (PTS) (pesticides and polychlorinated biphenyls) analyzed. Significant subgroups of the population accumulated PTS mixtures at high concentrations. For instance, 48% of women 60–74 years had concentrations of 6 or more PTS in the top quartile; half of the entire population had levels of 1–5 PTS above 500 ng/g, and less than 4% of citizens had all PTS in the lowest quartile. Thus, PTS concentrations appear low in most of the population only when each individual compound is looked at separately. It is not accurate to state that most of the population has low concentrations of PTS. The assessment of mixture effects must address the fact that most individuals are contaminated by PTS mixtures made of compounds at both low and high concentrations.

1. INTRODUCTION

1.1. Human contamination and endocrine disrupting chemicals

Human biomonitoring studies in Europe, North America, and elsewhere have repeatedly revealed that humans are usually contaminated with a variety of persistent organic pollutants (POPs), other endocrine disrupting chemicals (EDCs), and other environmental chemical agents (DHHS, 2009; Health Canada, 2010; Patterson et al., 2009; Porta et al., 2008; Thornton, McCally, & Houlihan, 2002). Such contaminants bioaccumulate and build up in the food chain over time and, once ingested, persist for a long time, usually in body fat or bound (attached) to blood proteins. For example, over 25 years since the pesticide dichlorodiphenyltrichloroethane (DDT) was banned in Spain, *p,p′*-DDT was detected in 88% of the general population (specifically, in a representative sample of 919 citizens of Catalonia) (Porta et al., 2010). Similarly, in a statistically representative sampling of the US population conducted during 2003 and 2004, *p,p′*-DDT was detected in 74% of citizens (Patterson et al., 2009), despite the fact that DDT was banned in the United States in the 1970s. During recent decades, other EDCs have also been shown to be ubiquitous contaminants in humans (DHHS, 2009; Health Canada, 2010; Patterson et al., 2009; Porta et al., 2008; Thornton et al., 2002; Weinhold, 2003).

For ethical and practical reasons, all scientific studies on human chemical contamination focus on a limited number of compounds; therefore, it is not possible to state firmly how many chemicals humans are exposed to and accumulate during lifetime. This knowledge gap is surprising, and it hampers risk assessment. The number of chemicals to which humans are exposed to and that we accumulate during lifetime is of particular relevance given the increasing health risks that we assume with exposure to an increasing number of contaminants and the plausible or well-established chemical interactions when the number and variety of compounds are high (Kortenkamp et al., 2009; NRC, 2008; Patterson et al., 2009; Porta, 2012; Porta & Zumeta, 2002; Porta et al., 2008, 2010). Some studies provide an illustration of the extent of the problem. For example, the US Fourth National Report on Human Exposure to Environmental Chemicals has documented contamination from a large number of compounds in representative samples of the US general population, including pregnant women (DHHS, 2009; Woodruff, Zota, & Schwartz, 2011).

Compared with high-dose exposure to a few selected chemicals in occupational settings, background exposure in the general population is characterized by low-dose and long-term—mostly, lifetime—exposure to a complex mixture of various chemical agents. In our daily lives, most of us are usually exposed to dozens among tens of thousands of chemicals. On the European market, there are now over 150,000 chemical substances (ECA, 2012), and approximately 12,000 new substances are added daily to the American Chemical Society's CAS registry (ASHG et al., 2011; CAS Registry, 2012); although only a fraction of these chemicals are introduced into the environment, comprehensive databases on human exposure to many of such chemicals are lacking.

Some of the relevant chemicals that populations accumulate are EDCs. Sometimes also called hormone-disrupting chemicals or endocrine-active compounds (EACs)—EDCs are exogenous substances that mimic hormones in the endocrine system or disrupt in some way the normal physiological function of endogenous hormones (Alonso-Magdalena, Quesada, & Nadal, 2011; Diamanti-Kandarakis et al., 2009; Olea & Fernandez, 2007; Soto & Sonnenschein, 2011; Stein, 2012; Vandenberg et al., 2012). They encompass a wide variety of chemicals, including compounds used in plastics (e.g., certain phthalates and bisphenol A (BPA)), cosmetics and other consumer products (e.g., some parabens and UV filters), pesticides (e.g., vinclozolin, prochloraz, DDE, and tributyltin), and other industrial by-products and pollutants (e.g., dioxins and polychlorinated biphenyls,

PCBs) (Tickner, 2011). Some EDCs—including some pesticides and industrial chemicals—have long contaminated animal and human food chains. In the majority of the general population, exposure occurs largely through dietary intake (Institute of Medicine, 2003; UNEP, 2002). Numerous studies have monitored the presence of some EDCs in many types of foods, including fish, dairy products, meat, fruits, and vegetables. The results of these and other studies indicate that in many populations, meat, fish, and dairy products are often important contributors to total dietary intake of EDCs (Gasull, Bosch de Basea, Puigdomènech, Pumarega, & Porta, 2011; Institute of Medicine, 2003; Schafer & Kegley, 2002). Exposure may also occur through cosmetics and other consumer products (Diamanti-Kandarakis et al., 2009; Soto & Sonnenschein, 2011).

EDCs can act via a variety of biological and physiological mechanisms, including binding or blocking receptors or altering hormone synthesis and metabolism (Diamanti-Kandarakis et al., 2009). The lists of EDCs and information about some screening and testing initiatives to identify chemicals with such properties can be found on websites as

http://www.epa.gov/scipoly/oscpendo/index.htm

http://ec.europa.eu/environment/chemicals/endocrine/strategy/substances_en.htm

Although some natural products—as plant constituents—are also EDCs, this report focuses on man-made chemicals and specifically on POPs, whose endocrine disrupting properties are well established and whose presence in human societies became generalized after World War II.

1.2. Human exposure to and contamination from POPs

POPs comprise a large variety of toxic substances such as hexachlorobenzene (HCB), hexachlorocyclohexanes (HCHs), dioxins, DDT and its metabolites (notably, dichlorodiphenyldichloroethylene, DDE), and PCBs. POPs are highly lipophilic and resistant to degradation; they thus accumulate in adipose tissue and in organs such as the liver, brain, or pancreas (WHO, 2003). Many human populations are exposed to POP mixtures over the life course (Luzardo et al., 2009; Woodruff et al., 2011). A variety of studies have shown that POPs may adversely influence health and well-being: they are endocrine disrupters, and they contribute to cause infertility, birth defects, learning disabilities, several cancers, Alzheimer's and Parkinson's disease, and other neurological, gynecological, and immunological disorders (Alonso-Magdalena et al., 2011; Casals-Casas & Desvergne, 2011;

Diamanti-Kandarakis et al., 2009; Kaiser, 2005; La Merrill & Birnbaum, 2011; Schug, 2011; Soto & Sonnenschein, 2011; UNEP, 2002; Vandenberg et al., 2012). Moreover, several POPs—at low doses, similar to current exposure levels in postindustrial populations—have been shown to increase the risk of type 2 diabetes (Gasull et al., 2012; Porta & Lee, 2012; Wu et al., 2012). Scientific evidence on such effects is sometimes neglected or downplayed in the biomedical literature. Such toxic exposures may also partly explain important disease–disease associations, for example, between some cancers and obesity, diabetes, and cardiovascular, autoimmune, or inflammatory disorders (Gasull et al., 2012; Porta, 2012; Porta & Lee, 2012; Porta et al., 2009, Wu et al., 2012).

Many POPs have long been targeted for elimination or reduction. Legal instruments as the Stockholm Convention encourage countries to integrate population-based surveillance of POP levels in humans within their health monitoring systems (Porta & Zumeta, 2002; UNEP, 2002). POP monitoring programs are useful for exposure assessment, to analyze trends and patterns of contamination and to evaluate the effectiveness of policies aimed at decreasing exposure. However, worldwide, comprehensive monitoring of human contamination by POPs is scarce, fragmented, and heterogeneous. Methodological characteristics of studies vary largely, including selection of participants, sociodemographic information, chemical and statistical methods, and frameworks for interpretation of results (Haines et al., 2011; Porta et al., 2008, 2009).

1.3. Mixtures of endocrine disrupters

Studies monitoring human exposure to POPs and other environmental chemical agents have traditionally addressed with difficulties the well-known fact that populations are contaminated by mixtures of chemicals at very different concentrations; in particular, analyses of the population distribution of the concentrations of a given compound usually show that most citizens have much lower concentrations than a certain minority (DHHS, 2009; Health Canada, 2010; NRC, 2006; Patterson et al., 2009; Porta et al., 2008, 2010; Thornton et al., 2002). It is indeed important to assess the full population distribution of the concentrations of environmental chemicals and, as also recommended by the National Research Council, the number of chemicals detected per person (NRC, 2006). Yet, biomonitoring studies commonly report separately the number of compounds detected per person (if at all) and the concentration of each individual compound (DHHS, 2009; Health Canada, 2010; Patterson et al., 2009; Porta et al., 2008, 2010; Thornton et al., 2002;Woodruff et al., 2011). Reasonably, the emphasis is usually on the latter: the number of compounds detected per person may be misleading, since it does not account for the corresponding concentrations, among other reasons. Yet, the analysis of the concentrations chemical by chemical does not tackle adequately the accumulation of multiple chemicals (Gladen, Doucet, & Hansen, 2003; Kortenkamp et al., 2009; Porta, 2012; Porta et al., 2008; Porta, Gasull, & Pumarega, 2012). Combination effects may result from pollutants, each of which produces small effects, if they are present in sufficiently large numbers. The existence of mixture effects (e.g., additive, synergistic, and antagonistic) depends on the number of contaminants in the mixture, their respective concentrations, and the concentration–response curves. Two crucial factors for combination effects to occur are the number of chemicals and their concentrations (Kortenkamp et al., 2009; NRC, 2008).

1.4. New indicator: Number of chemicals detected at high concentrations

Population surveys of human exposure to chemicals have not attempted to arithmetically integrate the number of compounds detected per person and the concentration of each compound. Therefore, we developed and implemented a new indicator, the "number of chemicals detected at high concentrations." This parameter clearly shows that in populations, some people have low levels of certain compounds and also have high concentrations of other compounds detected; consequently, individuals with high concentrations of certain compounds have low levels of other compounds detected. And the other hand, this indicator shows that not all individuals who have high/low concentrations of certain compounds have high/low concentrations of the other compounds detected, respectively.

2. HOW TO IMPLEMENT THE INDICATOR? AN EXAMPLE

2.1. Definitions of the cutoff point

We created the variable "number of POPs at high concentrations" as follows: For each subject, we added the number of POPs whose serum concentrations were equal to or greater than a selected cutoff point. To be conservative, we included only the eight POPs that had been detected (each) in >85% of the study subjects to generate the variable "number of chemicals detected at high concentrations." We used two types of definitions of "high concentrations" based on two types of cutoff points:

a. Compound- and population-specific percentiles, based on the POP distributions previously published (Porta et al., 2010): for the main statistical analyses, the main cutoff point selected was percentile 75 (the upper quartile).

b. A particular serum concentration, applied to all compounds (e.g., 250, 500 ng/g): such level can be considered high in different populations (e.g., the 95th percentile for a prevalent compound in the US general population).

2.2. Study population

We implemented the indicator of the number of POPs at high concentrations in a sample of the population of Catalonia, specifically, in participants of the Catalan Health Interview Survey (CHIS) at 2002 (Porta et al., 2009, 2010).

Briefly, participants in the CHIS aged 18–74 years old were offered to take part in a health examination, which included a physical exam, a supplementary interview, and the collection of urine and blood samples (DSGC, 2004). A total of 1374 individuals—who gave specific written informed consent—participated during 2002 in the health examination. Trained nurses recorded the weight and height, and the corresponding body mass index (BMI) was computed (Porta et al., 2010). Participants were asked to fast for 12 h before blood extraction. The blood sample was drawn by venipuncture, kept refrigerated, and centrifuged within 4 h; the separated serum was first stored frozen at −20 °C to determine immunological, biochemical, and nutritional parameters. Once these initial analyses were completed, the remaining serum was kept frozen at −80 °C until 2006, when POP concentrations began to be analyzed. Information on blood lipids and $\geq$1 mL of serum (for organochlorine analyses) was available from 919 participants. There were no significant differences between these 919 subjects and the remaining participants in the health examination with respect to age, sex, BMI, and education (Porta et al., 2010). Sociodemographic variables (sex, age, educational level, occupational social class, and birthplace) were obtained from the CHIS interview. The lower educational category of subjects without formal studies included the illiterate. The occupational social class was based on Goldthorpe's scheme (Porta et al., 2009); the class was hence assigned through the current or last occupation of the head of the household, whom in 46.3% of the cases was the participant himself or herself. The classification includes five well-established main social groups: I, managers of companies with ≥10 employees, senior technical staff, and free professionals; II, managers of companies with <10 employees and intermediate occupations; III, administrative personnel and financial management supporting professionals, self-employed professionals, supervisors of manual workers, and other skilled nonmanual workers; IV, skilled and partly skilled manual workers; and V, unskilled manual workers.

2.3. Analytical chemical methods

We analyzed the following POPs in serum: *o,p′*-DDT; *p,p′*-DDT; *o,p′*-DDE; *p,p′*-DDE; *o,p′*-DDD; *p,p′*-DDD; PCBs 28, 52, 101, 118, 138, 153, and 180; PeCB; HCB; α-HCH; β-HCH; γ-HCH; and δ-HCH (Porta et al., 2009). 10 mL screw-capped Pyrex centrifuge tubes capped with Teflon septa were used to keep and digest the samples. 25 mL of the surrogate solution (0.36 mg/L of tetrabromobenzene and 0.52 mg/L of PCB 209) was added to 1 mL aliquots of serum in the same Pyrex centrifuge tubes where the samples were stored. Acid digestion of the mixture was performed by the addition of 3 mL of hexane and 2 mL of concentrated sulfuric acid. Gas chromatography analyses were performed with an Agilent Technologies model GC-6890N provided with an electron capture detection and a 60 m, 0.25 mm i.d. DB-5 column (film thickness 0.25 μm). Analyses were carried out in the Department of Environmental Chemistry (IIQAB-CSIC) in Barcelona, Spain. Limits of detection and quantification ranged from 0.0023 ng/mL and 0.0069 ng/mL, respectively, for PCB 101 to 0.0235 ng/mL and 0.0706 ng/mL, respectively, for γ-HCH; they were 0.0156 ng/mL and 0.0468 ng/mL for *p,p′*-DDE, 0.0135 ng/mL and 0.0406 ng/mL for PCB 138, and 0.0111 ng/mL and 0.0334 ng/mL for HCB (Porta et al., 2009). When a sample had a concentration of a compound below the detection threshold, it was assigned the midvalue of this limit; when a POP was detected but under the quantification threshold, the midvalue between detection and quantification limits was used (Porta et al., 2009, 2010). Eight of the 19 POPs analyzed were detected (each) in >85% of subjects: four organochlorine pesticides or related compounds (*p,p′*-DDT, *p,p′*-DDE, HCB, and β-HCH) and four PCBs (congeners 118, 138, 153, and 180). Thus, these 8 are the most common or prevalent

POPs, while the other 11 are the least prevalent POPs; the percentage of detection for the 11 compounds ranged between 12% and 64%. Therefore, all 19 POPs were detected in the study sample; the smallest number of POPs detected in one person was 3, and the largest was 19. Total cholesterol and triglyceride levels were determined enzymatically, using serum obtained in the health examination (DSGC, 2004). Total serum lipids (TLs) were calculated by the standard formula 2, based on total cholesterol and triglycerides (Bernert, Turner, Patterson & Needham, 2007). POP concentrations were individually corrected for TL by dividing the crude serum POP concentration by TL.

3. RESULTS OF THE IMPLEMENTATION OF THE INDICATOR

In Catalonia, 73% of the population accumulates 10 or more POPs (of only the 19 analyzed) (Porta et al., 2009, 2010); this percentage was 79.9% in participants with high concentrations of at least one of the most prevalent POPs (80.2% in men and 79.4% in women) and 63.3% in subjects without any of such POPs at high concentrations (63.3% in men and 63.2% in women) (Porta, Pumarega, et al., 2012). In general, the percentage of participants with $\geq$1 of the most prevalent POPs in the upper quartile was greater in subjects with a higher number of compounds detected, but the relationship was not linear: 31% of subjects in whom 7 compounds were detected had at least one of the eight most prevalent POPs in the top quartile; the corresponding percentages among subjects with 10, 13, 14, and 16 compounds detected were 54%, 77%, 64%, and 70%, respectively (Porta, Pumarega, et al., 2012). Among men, the corresponding percentages were 20%, 48.9%, 76.3%, 64.3%, and 58.8% (see Fig. 6.1). Among women, the corresponding percentages were 36.8%, 57.8%, 76.9%, 63.5%, and 75.8% (see Fig. 6.2).

Over 58% of the 919 participants had concentrations of $\geq$1 of the eight most prevalent POPs equal to or greater than percentile 75, while 43.7% had $\geq$2 POPs, and 33.9% had $\geq$3 POPs in such top quartile (36.7% of women and 30.3% of men) (see Fig. 6.3). One in five subjects had concentrations of two PCBs in the upper quartile; for example, 21.9% of participants had both PCB 138 and PCB 153 in their respective upper quartiles. Simultaneous high concentrations of PCBs 138, 153, and 180 (i.e., all three congeners in their respective upper quartile) were observed in 18.4% of subjects and of p,p'-DDE, HCB, and β-HCH in 13.4%. There was substantial mixture

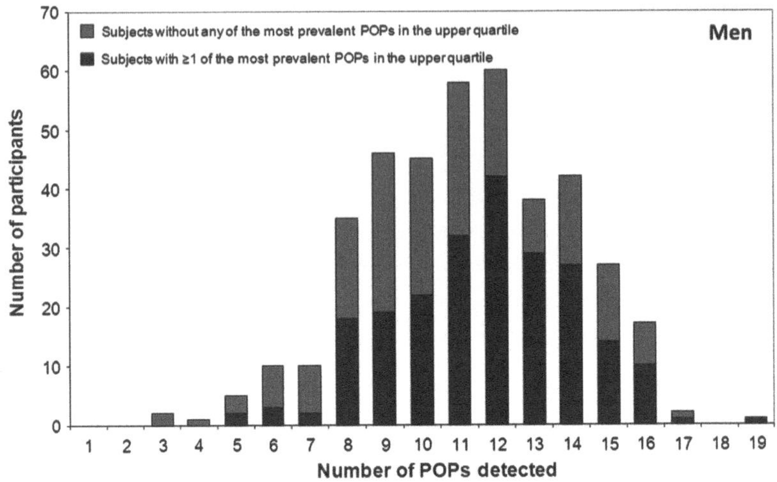

Figure 6.1 Distribution of the number of POPs detected in men with or without any of the eight most prevalent POPs in the upper quartile.

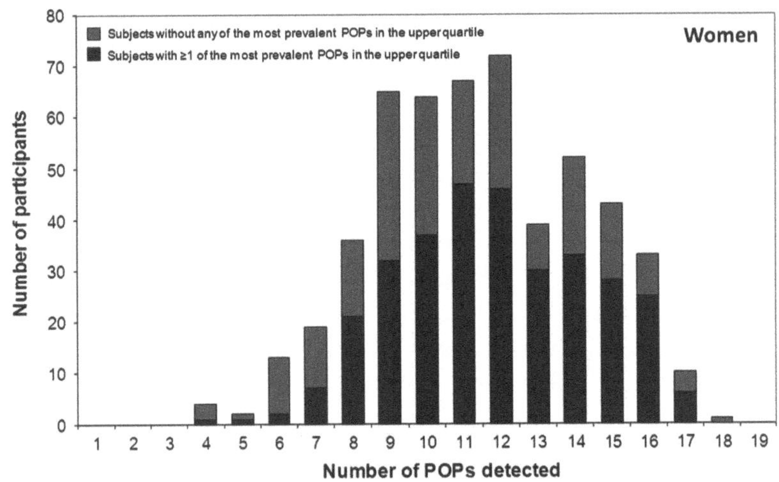

Figure 6.2 Distribution of the number of POPs detected in women with or without any of the eight most prevalent POPs in the upper quartile.

of the two chemical classes at high concentrations: 74.1% of subjects with concentrations of ≥ 1 of the four PCBs in the upper quartile also had ≥ 1 of the four pesticides in the upper quartile, and 58.2% of subjects with concentrations of ≥ 1 of the four pesticides in the upper quartile also had ≥ 1 of the four PCBs in the upper quartile.

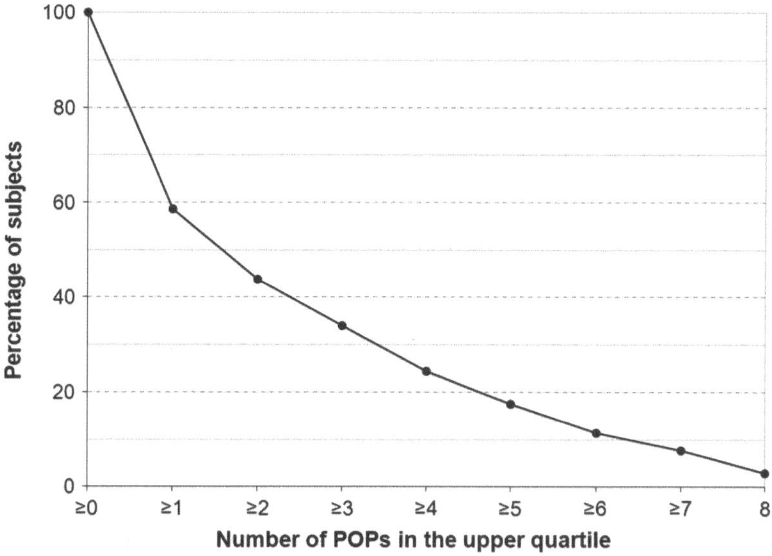

Figure 6.3 Cumulative percentage of subjects with serum concentrations of the eight most prevalent POPs in the upper quartile.

The proportion of women, subjects over 44 years old, and obese individuals was higher in participants with concentrations of ≥ 1 of the eight most prevalent POPs in the upper quartile than in participants without any of such compounds at high concentrations.

Of the subjects with high concentrations of ≥ 1 of the most prevalent POPs, 25% had only one POP at high concentrations, while 30% had 5 or more POPs at such levels (Porta, Pumarega, et al., 2012). There were significant differences in the number of the most prevalent POPs with high concentrations by sex, age, BMI, and occupational social class. 78.5% of women with high concentrations of at least one of the most common POPs had ≥ 2 compounds at high concentrations, whereas for men, this percentage was 69.4%. The number of POPs at high concentrations showed a positive linear relation with age and with BMI. Among subjects with high concentrations of ≥ 1 of the most prevalent POPs, 66.1% of subjects with normal weight, 76.3% of subjects overweight, and 83.2% of obese subjects had ≥ 2 POPs with concentrations in the upper quartile. 7.5% of subjects of the less affluent occupational social class (V) had all eight most prevalent POPs at high concentrations, while none of the participants of the most affluent class (I) had all such POPs at high levels.

Significant differences in the number of most prevalent POPs at high concentrations were also found for parity, educational level, birthplace, and area of residence.

The 11 least prevalent POPs also commonly contaminated subjects with high levels of the 8 most prevalent POPs: as compared to participants without any of the 8 most prevalent POPs at high concentrations, participants with high concentrations of ≥ 1 of the 8 most prevalent POPs also had higher percentages of detection of 9 of the 11 least prevalent POPs. 74.9% of subjects with high concentrations of ≥ 1 of the most prevalent POPs had between 1 and 6 of the least prevalent POPs detected; and 15.6% had 7 or more. *o,p′*-DDT was detected in 65.2% of participants who also had simultaneous high concentrations of PCBs 138 and 153 and in 73.8% of participants with simultaneous high concentrations of both HCB and β-HCH. When we considered all 19 POPs analyzed in the study, the corresponding percentages increased to 89.4% and to 80.6%, respectively.

The proportion of subjects with concentrations of ≥ 1 of the eight most common POPs in the top quartile increased from over 20% among the 18–29 years old, to over 60% and 80% for men and women 45–59 years old, respectively, and to over 80% among 60–74-year-old subjects (Porta, Pumarega, et al., 2012). The largest differences between women and men were seen in the oldest group, in which 95% of women had high concentrations of ≥ 1 of the most prevalent POPs, and 48.4% had high concentrations of ≥ 6 of such POPs; the corresponding percentages for men were 85% and 25%, respectively (see Fig. 6.4). 55.8% of women 60–74 years old had high concentrations of *p,p′*-DDE, HCB, and β-HCH simultaneously and 53.7% of PCB 118, HCB, and β-HCH.

Figure 6.5 shows the number of POPs with concentrations in the upper quartile by BMI and sex groups. The proportion of subjects with concentrations of ≥ 1 of the eight most common POPs in the top quartile increased from over 45% among the normal-weight individuals, to over 56% and 70% for men and women overweight, respectively, and to over 65% and 80% among obese subjects. The largest differences between women and men were seen in the obese group (BMI ≥ 30 kg/m^2), in which 84% of women had high concentrations of ≥ 1 of the most prevalent POPs, and 29% had high concentrations of ≥ 6 of such POPs; the corresponding percentages for men were 66% and 14%, respectively (see Fig. 6.5).

Over 30% of subjects had concentrations in the top decile of 1–5 of the eight most prevalent POPs; half of the population has levels of 1–5 POPs

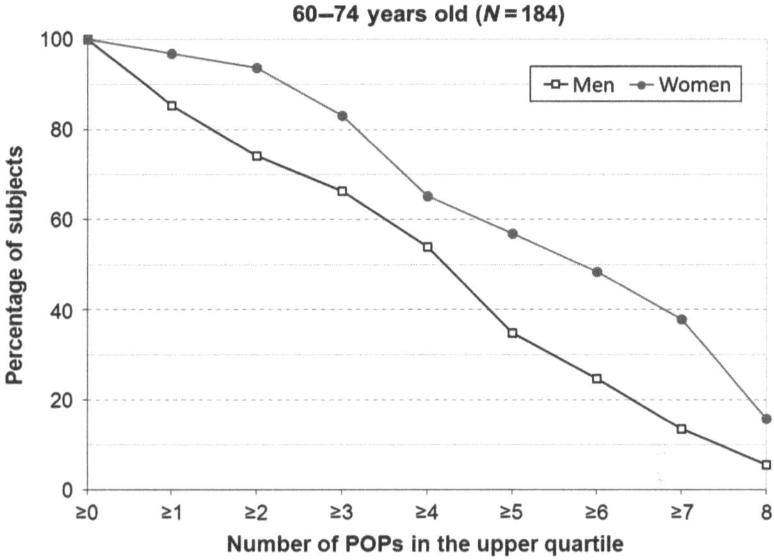

Figure 6.4 Cumulative percentage of subjects 60–74 years old with serum concentrations of the eight most prevalent POPs in the upper quartile, by sex.

>500 ng/g; among women 60–74 years old (a subgroup with an obviously high incidence and prevalence of morbidity), 83% have concentrations of ≥3 POPs in the top quartile, and 48% have concentrations of ≥6 POPs in the top quartile. Over 20% of participants had concentrations of ≥1 POPs in the top quartile and simultaneously concentrations of ≥1 POPs in the lowest quartile. This "discordance" was inversely associated to BMI: participants with a lower BMI were more likely to have POPs in the upper and lower quartiles simultaneously; subjects with higher BMI tended to have concentrations of virtually all POPs in the upper and middle quartiles. We next considered the 13 POPs that had been detected in >25% of subjects (the eight most prevalent POPs and *o,p'*-DDT, *o,p'*-DDD, *p,p'*-DDD, δ-HCH, and γ-HCH): 82.9% of the participants had concentrations of ≥1 of these POPs in the upper quartile, and 68.2% had ≥2. Less than 4% of the Catalan population has concentrations of all the eight most common POPs in the lowest quartile (Porta et al., 2010; Porta, Pumarega, et al., 2012). Hence, it is not accurate to state that most of the population has low concentrations of POPs: contamination from selected toxic chemicals is common at high and low concentrations (Porta, Pumarega, et al., 2012).

Although a positive association between the number of POPs detected and the number of common POPs at high concentrations could be expected, the

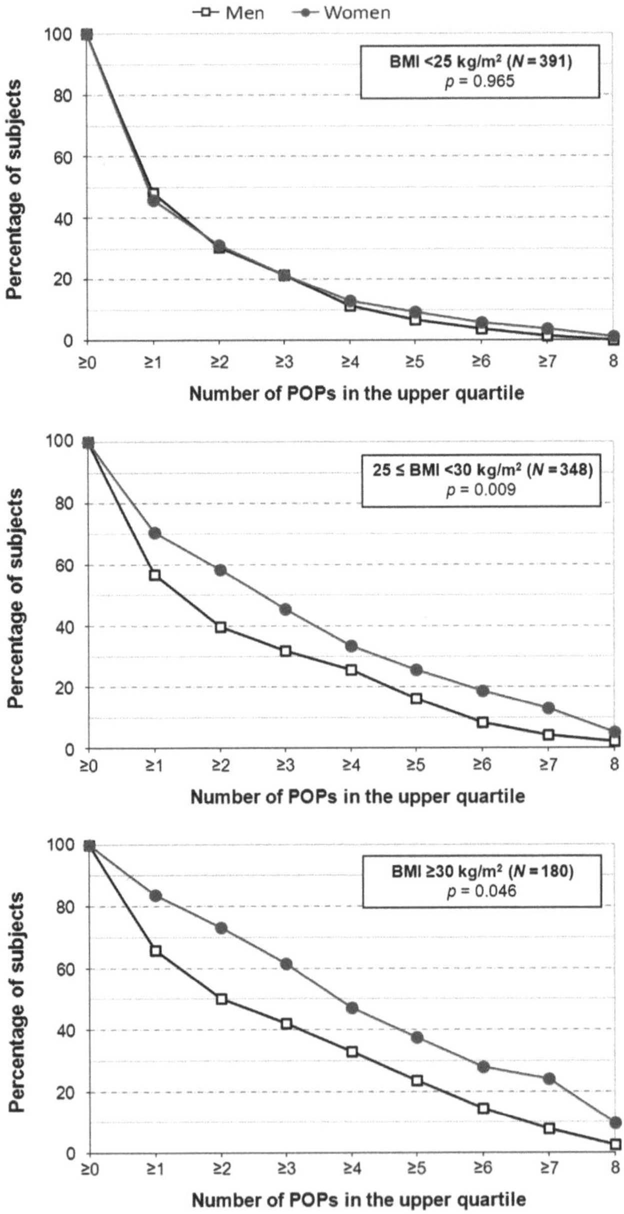

Figure 6.5 Cumulative percentage of subjects with serum concentrations of the eight most prevalent POPs in the upper quartile, by BMI and sex.

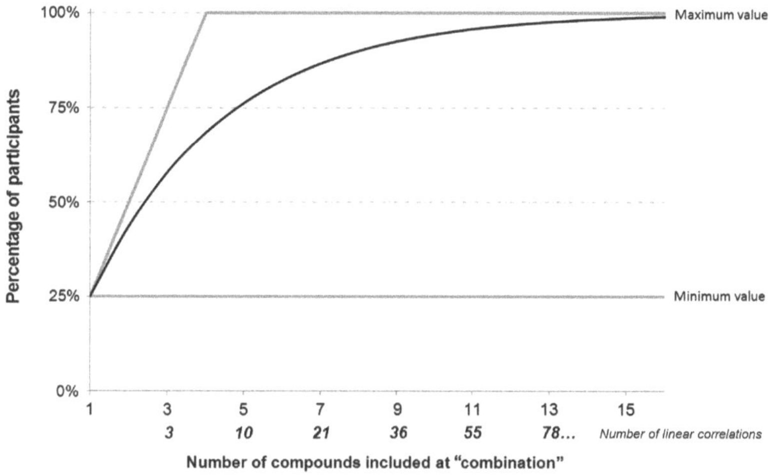

Figure 6.6 Percentage of participants with ≥1 of POPs analyzed in the top quartile for each number of compounds analyzed if all POPs were completely uncorrelated with the other POPs.

association was moderate in strength and not linear. The percentage of subjects with ≥1 of the POPs at high concentrations was higher when the POPs considered were poorly correlated with each other than when the POPs were highly correlated. The minimum value of the percentage of participants with ≥1 of the eight most prevalent POPs in the upper quartile will always be 25%, while the maximum value depends on the number of compounds considered (see Fig. 6.6). The percentage will be higher when the POPs considered are poorly correlated with each other than when the POPs are highly correlated. Thus, if two compounds are completely uncorrelated ($\rho = 0$), about 50% of participants will have one or both POPs in the upper quartile. By contrast, if the two compounds are completely correlated ($\rho = 1$), 25% of subjects will have ≥2 of the POPs in the upper quartile. When ≥4 POPs are considered, the percentage will be near 100% only if the compounds are highly uncorrelated. In the figure, the black line represents the proportion of participants with ≥1 concentrations of POPs in the upper quartile if these POPs are completely uncorrelated. Values close to this line indicate that the POPs are poorly correlated, and values above this line indicate that POPs are negatively correlated. In the expanded figure published by Porta et al. 2012 (Supplementary material), which includes the results of CHIS, the black point is the percentage of participants in our study with ≥1 of the POPs in the upper quartile (58.5%), and green and blue lines are two alternative combinations of POPs to get to eight POPs. The green line is the way to the black point when POPs are poorly correlated, and the blue line is the path when the

POPs are highly correlated. For example, the green line started with the two compounds less correlated and the following compound added is the compound less correlated with these two compounds of the other six we have, and so on. Thus, when four POPs were considered (six correlations), the percentage of participants with ≥1 of the POPs in the upper quartile was 53.3% if the compounds were poorly correlated and 38.2% when they were highly correlated. When six POPs were considered (15 correlations), the percentages were 58.0% and 50.9%, respectively.

The number of POPs at high concentrations was related to variables that are often associated with concentrations of POPs when each compound is analyzed separately (sex, age, and BMI). The indicators presented may complement other estimates of POP body burden in biomonitoring surveys (DHHS, 2009; Health Canada, 2010; NRC, 2006; Patterson et al., 2009; Porta et al., 2008, 2010; Thornton et al., 2002).

The upper quartile or 75th percentile is not a universal cutoff point to define high concentrations of POPs in humans: choices depend on context and purpose. The primary definition of "high concentration" (percentile 75) was compound-specific and internal or specific to the study population. The number of compounds analyzed also determines the results. Instead of observing the 8 most prevalent POPs, observe the 11 most prevalent POPs (detected in >50% of participants) and the results are quite different (see Fig. 6.7).

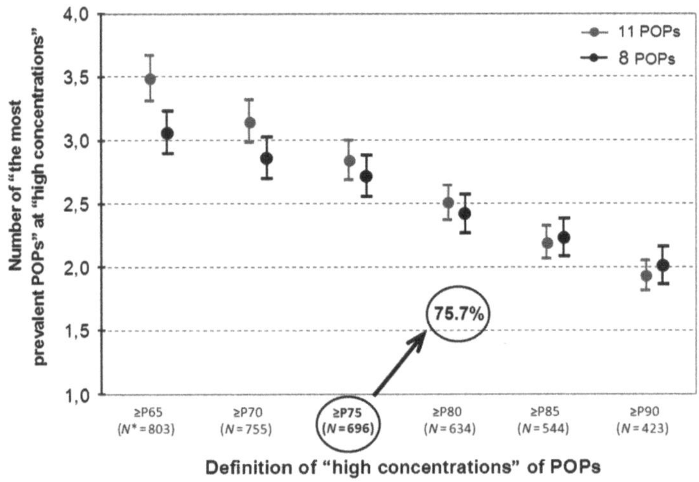

Figure 6.7 Geometric mean and 95% CI for the number of the most prevalent POPs at "high concentrations," according to different definitions of "high concentrations." *N=number of participants with ≥1 of the *eleven* most prevalent POPs at "high concentrations," according to each definition.

If we use a different cutoff percentage to the 75th percentile, the number of participants with "high concentrations" is also different. In Fig. 6.7, we can see that being more conservative, choosing less POPs and cutting points higher than the 75th percentile, the number of compounds to high doses is very similar; for example, to 85th percentile, the average number of compounds at "high concentrations" per participant would be 2.2 or 2.3, depending if 8 or 11 compounds are used (see Fig. 6.7).

We also used definitions of "high concentration" independent of the study population; thus, for instance, half of participants had concentrations of 1–5 POPs greater than 500 ng/g (Porta, Pumarega et al., 2012). Some of our cutoff points were similar to US reference values as percentile 95 (P95) of β-HCH and PCB 153 or percentile 75 (P75) of *p,p′*-DDE. P75 of the eight most prevalent POPs at Catalonia were between 2 and 20 times higher than the corresponding P75 in the US Fourth National Report (see Tables 6.1 and 6.2) (DHHS, 2009; Patterson et al., 2009). Therefore, concentrations that we qualified as "high" were indeed rather high as compared with concentrations in the United States. They also are high compared with population-based studies in Canada (Health Canada, 2010), New Zealand (Bates, Buckland, Garrett, Caudill, & Ellis, 2005), and other countries that report blood levels corrected by lipids (Porta et al., 2008) (see Tables 6.1 and 6.2).

4. DISCUSSION

In Catalonia, 73% of the population accumulates 10 or more POPs (of only 19 analyzed); 34% of citizens have concentrations in the top quartile of ≥3 of the 8 most frequent POPs; over 30% of the population has concentrations in the top decile of 1–5 of the 8 most prevalent POPs; half of the population has levels of 1–5 POPs >500 ng/g; among women 60–74 years old (a subgroup with an obviously high incidence and prevalence of morbidity), 83% have concentrations of ≥3 POPs in the top quartile, and 48% have concentrations of ≥6 POPs in the top quartile; less than 4% of the Catalan population has concentrations of all the 8 most common POPs in the lowest quartile (Porta et al., 2010; Porta, Pumarega, et al., 2012). Hence, it is not accurate to state that most of the population has low concentrations of POPs: contamination from selected toxic chemicals is common at high and low concentrations (Porta, Pumarega, et al., 2012).

Few studies based on representative samples of the general population have assessed a large number of compounds—up to 91 in Canada (Health

Table 6.1 Concentrations of P50 (median), P75 (highest quartile), and P95 (highest 5%) in several population-based studies

	Catalonia (Porta et al., 2010)			The United States (fouth report) (DHHS, 2009)			Canada (Health Canada, 2010)			New Zealand (Bates et al., 2004)	
Compound	**P50**	**P75**	**P95**	**P50**	**P75**	**P95**	**P50**	**P75**	**P95**	**P50**	**Maximum value**
p,p′-DDT	29.3	56.4	131	<LOD	<LOD	19.5	<LOD	<LOD	16	—	49.2
p,p′-DDE	399	833	2481	203	509	1860	127	285	1077	919	2780
PCB 118	22.8	38.0	82.4	5.19	10.4	31.3	4	8	20	—	10.0
PCB 138	69.5	113	209	15.1[a]	30.5[a]	75.3[a]	10	19	45	15.6[a]	36.2[a]
PCB 153	100	153	294	20.8	43.3	97.1	19	36	86	24.6	49.9
PCB 180	77.3	116	197	18.0	37.1	81.5	16	32	77	20.0	44.6
HCB	159	358	894	14.9	19.0	28.9	9	14	27	—	53.6
β-HCH	91.9	201	519	<LOD	14.1	56.5	5	10	90	10.7	73.1

Units: ng/g lipid.
[a]PCB 138 and 158. US fourth report *p,p′*-DDT and β-HCH LOD = 7.8 ng/g lipid.

Table 6.2 Concentrations of P50 (median), P75 (highest quartile), and P95 (highest 5%) in several population-based studies

	Catalonia (Porta et al., 2010)			The United States (fourth report) (DHHS, 2009)			Canada (Health Canada, 2010)			Germany (GerS III) (Umweltbundesamt, 1985–2006)	
Compound	**P50**	**P75**	**P95**	**P50**	**P75**	**P95**	**P50**	**P75**	**P95**	**P50**	**P95**
p,p′-DDT	0.179	0.337	0.828	<LOD	<LOD	0.128	<LOD	<LOD	0.09	–	–
p,p′-DDE	2.227	5.227	14.01	1.26	3.16	12.1	0.75	1.77	6.51	1.54	8.74
PCB 118	0.128	0.241	0.557	0.032	0.066	0.216	0.03	0.05	0.12	–	–
PCB 138	0.414	0.670	1.327	0.095	0.206[a]	0.477[a]	0.06	0.12	0.28	0.48	1.35
PCB 153	0.594	0.933	1.921	0.135	0.283	0.624	0.12	0.22	0.54	0.72	2.16
PCB 180	0.462	0.695	1.325	0.114	0.246	0.534	0.10	0.20	0.49	0.48	1.51
HCB	0.916	2.196	5.951	0.090	0.120	0.186	0.06	0.09	0.17	0.43	4.46
β-HCH	0.538	1.311	3.535	<LOD	0.092	0.372	0.03	0.06	0.54	<0.1	0.49

Units: ng/mL serum.
[a]PCB 138 and 158. US fourth report *p,p′*-DDT LOD = 0.0246 ng/mL serum. Canada *p,p′*-DDT LOD = 0.05 ng/mL serum.

Canada, 2010) and 212 in the US Fourth National Report on Human Exposure to Environmental Chemicals (DHHS, 2009). However, for ethical and logistic reasons, not all compounds were studied in the same individuals, a fact that, as we previously mentioned, hampers inferences that are highly relevant for human risk assessment.

The information available on different studies and sets of compounds and individuals could be pooled to model the distribution of the number of contaminants and chemical classes that commonly contaminate individuals at different concentrations (Porta, Gasull, et al., 2012). However, at present, the full range of POP concentrations is often overlooked, and little attention is paid to the characteristics of the distribution of the concentrations (Porta, 2004; Porta et al., 2008, 2010). Also, national studies monitoring human exposure to POPs do not usually include data on parity and breastfeeding (Dewailly et al., 1996; Tajimi, Watanabe, Oki, Ojima, & Nakamura, 2004). Another example of a variable that is not usually collected in population biomonitoring studies is weight change, which may alter blood lipid levels and bias estimates of exposure to lipophilic compounds like POPs and other EDCs (Porta, López, et al., 2012).

In Catalonia, we studied 19 organochlorines, a number of compounds similar to other initial surveys in representative samples of a general population; for example, 27 compounds were included in the first US National Report on Human Exposure to Environmental Chemicals (NRC, 2006; Porta et al., 2008). Surveys have not yet estimated a common range of chemicals that humans may accumulate over the life course. Case series (Watson, 2005; Weinhold, 2003) provides anecdotal evidence. In 155 volunteers from the United Kingdom, the median and highest number of chemicals found were 27 and 49, respectively (out of 78 substances analyzed) (WWF, 2003). A study of 541 pregnant women from Spain detected $\geq$8 POPs per person (out of 16 analyzed) in 43% of women; the median was 7 compounds detected per woman (Llop et al., 2010). In a US nationally representative assessment of 268 pregnant women's exposure to 163 chemicals, essentially all women were contaminated by $\geq$43 different chemicals; the median number of organochlorine pesticides detected was 6 (out of 13 analyzed); across chemical classes, the median number ranged from 8 (out of 17 chemical analytes) to 50 (out of 71 chemical analytes) (Woodruff et al., 2011). In brief, studies suggest that citizens of the post-industrial economies may often accumulate mixtures of 50, 70, or even more toxic agents (Watson, 2005; Weinhold, 2003; Woodruff et al., 2011; WWF, 2003).

To our knowledge, the findings summarized in this chapter on the mixtures of POPs in a general population have not been reported before. Our methods and findings do not assume or imply that compounds will cause adverse health effects when present above a given absolute concentration or percentile. Nor do they mean that effects at low doses are irrelevant: several environmental chemicals have been shown to increase risk at low concentrations (Alonso-Magdalena et al., 2011; Casals-Casas & Desvergne, 2011; Diamanti-Kandarakis et al., 2009; Henkler & Luch, 2011; Hernández, van Steeg, Luijten, & van Benthem, 2009; Kortenkamp et al., 2009; Myers, Zoeller, & vom Saal, 2009; NRC, 2008; Vandenberg et al., 2012).

Nevertheless, our primary targets were not etiologic and mechanistic studies, but biomonitoring studies (NRC, 2006). Although we simply added the number of POPs at high concentrations, the present results do not suggest whether dose addition, independent action, or some other method is the most appropriate for cumulative risk assessment (NRC, 2008); empirical uses of the study indicators in a variety of populations will clarify these issues.

4.1. Study conclusions

More than half of the study population had concentrations in the top quartile of ≥ 1 of the eight most commonly detected POPs, 34% had ≥ 3 such compounds in their respective top dose quartiles and 32% ≥ 1 POPs in the top decile. Less than 4% of subjects had concentrations of all eight POPs in the lowest quartile. Significant subgroups of the general population accumulate POP mixtures at high concentrations. It is misleading to state that most of the population has low concentrations of POPs and other EDCs. POP concentrations appear low in most of the population only when each individual compound is looked at separately. Based on our methods and findings, studies could analyze more systematically the number and type of compounds detected at high concentrations, integrate these indicators with traditional measures of exposure, and analyze the characteristics and causes of the mixtures of contaminants at high concentrations, their coexistence with mixtures at low concentrations, and their joint health effects.

4.2. General conclusions and proposals for future work

The available evidence indicates that most countries are not assessing comprehensively

a. what chemical mixtures the general population is significantly exposed to in critical periods of life,
b. how many POPS and other EDCs humans accumulate during the life course at low and high concentrations, and
c. the number of chemicals whose continued presence in the human body is most relevant to analyze (Porta et al., 2008; Porta, Gasull, et al., 2012; Porta, Pumarega, et al., 2012).

It is thus not accurate to state that most of the population has low concentrations of EDCs: contamination is common at high and low concentrations throughout the life course (Porta, Pumarega, et al., 2012).

In summary,

a. we know quite a lot about the generalized human contamination by environmental chemical agents (a statement that is fully compatible with the assessment that most countries lack the necessary monitoring systems) (Porta et al., 2008);
b. we also know quite a lot about the toxic effects of environmental pollutants (a statement that is fully compatible with the proposal that we need both more research and more energetic policies to decrease human contamination by such pollutants); and
c. we know too little about the causes and the etiopathogenesis of the most prevalent diseases, and we will continue to miss the relevant causes and mechanisms if we neglect toxic chemicals.

Or we may put it this way: when we do not integrate biomarkers of internal dose of environmental pollutants in our research on the etiopathogenesis of human diseases of complex etiology,

1. we are trying to study "something" that hardly exists (fully uncontaminated human beings);
2. our causal inferences are less likely to be relevant for human health; and
3. we are likely to miss causes and mechanisms of the processes that we aim to study (e.g., causes of changes in gene expression, of accumulation of genetic defects, and of alterations in metabolic functions). Knowledge on the joint effects of "chemical cocktails" during the life course ought to be used more often when building causal scenarios that aim at being relevant for human health.

We may suggest that medicine—and a few other biomedical and public health sciences—should more often consider integrating biomarkers of internal dose of EDCs and other environmental chemical pollutants in their approaches to the etiology and prevention of human diseases. In the future, when we neglect less the generalized human contamination by endocrine disrupters and their toxic effects, we will expand mechanistic knowledge, and we shall also increase the effectiveness of interventions and policies that enable the primary prevention of diseases that globally cause a huge economic burden and, most importantly, a huge amount of preventable human suffering.

REFERENCES

Alonso-Magdalena, P., Quesada, I., & Nadal, A. (2011). Endocrine disruptors in the etiology of type-2 diabetes. *Nature Reviews Endocrinology*, *7*, 346–353.

ASHG (American Society of Human Genetics), American Society for Reproductive Medicine, Endocrine Society, Genetics Society of America, Society for Developmental Biology, Society for Pediatric Urology, et al. (2011). Assessing chemical risk: Societies offer expertise. *Science*, *331*, 1136.

Bates, M. N., Buckland, S. J., Garrett, N., Caudill, S. P., & Ellis, H. (2005). Methodological aspects of a national population-based study of persistent organochlorine compounds in serum. *Chemosphere*, *58*, 943–951.

Bates, M., Buckland, S., Garrett, N., Ellis, H., Needham, L. L., Patterson, D. G., Jr., et al. (2004). Persistent organochlorines in the serum of the non-occupationally exposed New Zealand population. *Chemosphere*, *54*, 1431–1443.

Bernert, J. T., Turner, W. E., Patterson, D. G., Jr., & Needham, L. L. (2007). Calculation of serum "total lipid" concentrations for the adjustment of persistent organohalogen toxicant measurements in human samples. *Chemosphere*, *68*, 824–831.

Casals-Casas, C., & Desvergne, B. (2011). Endocrine disruptors: From endocrine to metabolic disruption. *Annual Review of Physiology*, *73*, 135–162.

CAS Registry. *Chemical abstracts service (a division of the American Chemical Society)*. Available from, http://www.cas.org/expertise/cascontent/registry/regsys.html, Accessed 04 December 2012.

Dewailly, E., Ayotte, P., Laliberté, C., Weber, J. P., Gingras, S., & Nantel, J. (1996). Polychlorinated biphenyl (PCB) and dichlorodiphenyl dichloroethylene (DDE) concentrations in the breast milk of women in Quebec. *American Journal of Public Health*, *86*, 1241–1246.

DHHS (Department of Health and Human Services), (2009). *Fourth national report on human exposure to environmental chemicals*. Atlanta: Centers for Disease Control and Prevention.Available from, http://www.cdc.gov/exposurereport/index.html, Accessed 4 December 2012.

Diamanti-Kandarakis, E., Bourguignon, J. P., Giudice, L. C., Hauser, R., Prins, G. S., Soto, A. M., et al. (2009). Endocrine-disrupting chemicals: An Endocrine Society scientific statement. *Endocrine Reviews*, *30*, 293–342.

DSGC (Departament de Salut de la Generalitat de Catalunya), (2004). *Examen de salut a la població de Catalunya de 18 a 74 anys*. Available from, http://www.gencat.net/salut/depsalut/pdf/exsalcat.pdf2004, Accessed 4 December 2012.

ECA (European Chemicals Agency), (2012). http://echa.europa.eu/home_en.asp, Accessed 4 December 2012.

Gasull, M., Bosch de Basea, M., Puigdomènech, E., Pumarega, J., & Porta, M. (2011). Empirical analyses of the influence of diet on human concentrations of persistent organic pollutants: A systematic review of all studies conducted in Spain. *Environment International*, *37*, 1226–1235.

Gasull, M., Pumarega, J., Téllez-Plaza, M., Castell, C., Tresserras, R., Lee, D. H., et al. (2012). Blood concentrations of persistent organic pollutants and prediabetes and diabetes in the general population of Catalonia. *Environmental Science and Technology*, *46*, 7799–7810.

Gladen, B. C., Doucet, J., & Hansen, L. G. (2003). Assessing human polychlorinated biphenyl contamination for epidemiologic studies: Lessons from patterns of congener concentrations in Canadians in 1992. *Environmental Health Perspectives*, *111*, 437–443.

Haines, D. A., Arbuckle, T. E., Lye, E., Legrand, M., Fisher, M., Langlois, R., et al. (2011). Reporting results of human biomonitoring of environmental chemicals to study participants: A comparison of approaches followed in two Canadian studies. *Journal of Epidemiology and Community Health*, *65*, 191–198.

Health Canada (2010). *Report on human biomonitoring of environmental chemicals in Canada. Results of the Canadian Health Measures Survey Cycle 1 (2007–2009)*. Ottawa, Ontario: Health Canada., Available from, http://www.healthcanada.gc.ca, Accessed 4 December 2012.

Henkler, F., & Luch, A. (2011). Adverse health effects of environmental chemical agents through non-genotoxic mechanisms. *Journal of Epidemiology and Community Health*, *65*, 1–3.

Hernández, L., van Steeg, H., Luijten, M., & van Benthem, J. (2009). Mechanisms of non-genotoxic carcinogens and importance of a weight of evidence approach. *Mutation Research*, *682*, 94–109.

Institute of Medicine (2003). *Dioxins and dioxin-like compounds in the food supply. Strategies to decrease exposure*. Washington, DC: The National Academies Press.

Kaiser, J. (2005). Endocrine disrupters trigger fertility problems in multiple generations. *Science*, *308*, 1391–1392.

Kortenkamp, A., Backhaus, T., & Faust, M. (2009). *State of the art report on mixture toxicity. Final report to the environment directorate general of the European Commission. Study contract No. 070307/2007/485103/ETU/D.1*. Available from, http://ec.europa.eu/environment/chemicals/pdf/report_Mixture%20toxicity.pdf, Accessed 4 December 2012. Brussels: 22 December 2009 (released 9 February 2010).

La Merrill, M., & Birnbaum, L. S. (2011). Childhood obesity and environmental chemicals. *The Mount Sinai Journal of Medicine*, *78*, 22–48.

Llop, S., Ballester, F., Vizcaino, E., Murcia, M., Lopez-Espinosa, M. J., Rebagliato, M., et al. (2010). Concentrations and determinants of organochlorine levels among pregnant women in Eastern Spain. *The Science of the Total Environment*, *408*, 5758–5767.

Luzardo, O. P., Mahtani, V., Troyano, J. M., Alvarez de la Rosa, M., Padilla-Pérez, A. I., & Zumbado, M. (2009). Determinants of organochlorine levels detectable in the amniotic fluid of women from Tenerife Island (Canary Islands, Spain). *Environmental Research*, *109*, 607–613.

Myers, J. P., Zoeller, R. T., & vom Saal, F. S. (2009). A clash of old and new scientific concepts in toxicity, with important implication for public health. *Environmental Health Perspectives*, *117*, 1652–1655.

NRC (National Research Council) (2006). *Human biomonitoring for environmental chemicals*. Washington, DC: The National Academies Press. Available from, http://www.nap.edu/catalog/11700.html, Accessed 4 December 2012. Committee on Human Biomonitoring for Environmental Toxicants.

NRC (National Research Council) (2008). *Phthalates and cumulative risk assessment. The tasks ahead*. Washington, DC: The National Academies Press. Available from, http://www.nap.edu/catalog/12528.html, Accessed 4 December 2012. Committee on the Health Risks of Phthalates.

Olea, N., & Fernandez, M. (2007). Endocrine disruption. *Journal of Epidemiology and Community Health*, *61*, 372–373.

Patterson, D. G., Jr., Wong, L. Y., Turner, W. E., Caudill, S. P., Dipietro, E. S., McClure, P. C., et al. (2009). Levels in the U.S. population of those persistent organic pollutants (2003–2004) included in the Stockholm Convention or in other long range transboundary air pollution agreements. *Environmental Science and Technology*, *43*, 1211–1218.

Porta, M. (2004). Persistent toxic substances: Exposed individuals and exposed populations. *Journal of Epidemiology and Community Health*, *58*, 534–535.

Porta, M. (2012). Human contamination by environmental chemical pollutants: Can we assess it more properly? *Preventive Medicine*, *55*, 560–562.

Porta, M., Gasull, M., Puigdomènech, E., Garí, M., Bosch de Basea, M., Guillén, M., et al. (2010). Distribution of blood concentrations of persistent organic pollutants in a representative sample of the population of Catalonia. *Environment International*, *36*, 655–664.

Porta, M., Gasull, M., & Pumarega, J. (2012). A step towards more comprehensive analyses of lifecourse effects of mixtures of environmental factors. *International Journal of Epidemiology*, *41*, 843–846.

Porta, M., & Lee, D.-H. (2012). *Review of the science linking chemical exposures to the human risk of obesity and diabetesA CHEM Trust, UK report.* Available from, http://www.chemtrust.org.uk/documents/CHEM%20Trust%20Obesity%20&%20Diabetes%20Full%20Report.pdf, Accessed 4 December 2012.

Porta, M., López, T., Gasull, M., Rodríguez-Sanz, M., Garí, M., Pumarega, J., et al. (2012). Distribution of blood concentrations of persistent organic pollutants in a representative sample of the population of Barcelona in 2006, and comparison with levels in 2002. *The Science of the Total Environment*, *423*, 151–161.

Porta, M., Puigdomènech, E., Ballester, F., Selva, J., Ribas-Fitó, N., Llop, S., et al. (2008). Monitoring concentrations of persistent organic pollutants in the general population: The international experience. *Environment International*, *34*, 546–561.

Porta, M., Pumarega, J., & Gasull, M. (2012). Number of persistent organic pollutants detected at high concentrations in a general population. *Environment International*, *44*, 106–111.

Porta, M., & Zumeta, E. (2002). Implementing the Stockholm treaty on POPs. *Occupational and Environmental Medicine*, *59*, 651–652.

Porta, M., Puigdomènech, E., Gasull, M., Bosch de Basea, M., Garí, M., & Grimalt, J. O. (2009). *Distribució de les concentracions sèriques de compostos orgànics persistents (COPs) en una mostra representativa de la població general de Catalunya.* Barcelona: Departament de Salut, Generalitat de Catalunya. Available from, http://www.imim.es/media/upload//arxius/porta/COPs%2004.pdf, Accessed 4 December 2012.

Schafer, K. S., & Kegley, S. E. (2002). Persistent toxic chemicals in the US food supply. *Journal of Epidemiology and Community Health*, *56*, 813–817.

Schug, T. (2011). *NTP workshop investigates links between chemicals and obesity.* Available from, http://www.niehs.nih.gov/news/newsletter/2011/february/science-ntp-workshop, Accessed 4 December 2012.

Soto, A., & Sonnenschein, C. (2011). Environmental causes of cancer: Endocrine disruptors as carcinogens. *Nature Reviews Endocrinology*, *6*, 363–370.

Stein, R. A. (2012). Epigenetics and environmental exposures. *Journal of Epidemiology and Community Health*, *66*, 8–13.

Tajimi, M., Watanabe, M., Oki, I., Ojima, T., & Nakamura, Y. (2004). PCDDs, PCdfs and Co-PCBs in human breast milk samples collected in Tokyo, Japan. *Acta Paediatrica*, *93*, 1098–1102.

Thornton, J. W., McCally, M., & Houlihan, J. (2002). Biomonitoring of industrial pollutants: Health and policy implications of the chemical body burden. *Public Health Reports*, *117*, 315–323.

Tickner, J. A. (2011). Science of problems, science of solutions or both? A case example of bisphenol A. *Journal of Epidemiology and Community Health*, *65*, 649–650.

Umweltbundesamt. German Environmental Survey (GerES) (1985–2006) http://www.umweltbundesamt.de/en/topics/health/assessing-environmentally-related-health-risks/german-environmental-surveys.

UNEP (United Nations Environment Programme) (2002). *Chemicals. Regionally-based assessment of persistent toxic substances, Mediterranean regional report.* Châtelaine, Sweden: UNEP Chemicals.Available from, http://www.chem.unep.ch, Accessed 4 December 2012.

Vandenberg, L. N., Colborn, T., Hayes, T. B., Heindel, J. J., Jacobs, D. R., Jr., Lee, D. H., et al. (2012). Hormones and endocrine-disrupting chemicals: Low-dose effects and nonmonotonic doses responses. *Endocrine Reviews, 33*, 378–455.

Watson, G. (2005). *Generations X. Results of WWF's European family biomonitoring survey. WWF DetoX campaign.* Brussels: World Wildlife Fund (WWF). Available from, http://www.panda.org/downloads/toxics/generationsx.pdf, Accessed 4 December 2012.

Weinhold, B. (2003). Body of evidence. *Environmental Health Perspectives, 111*, A394–A399.

WHO (World Health Organization) (2003). *Health risks of persistent organic pollutants from long-range transboundary air pollution.* Copenhagen, Denmark: Regional Office for Europe of the World Health Organization.

Woodruff, T. J., Zota, A. R., & Schwartz, J. M. (2011). Environmental chemicals in pregnant women in the US: NHANES 2003–2004. *Environmental Health Perspectives, 119*, 878–885.

Wu, H., Bertrand, K. A., Choi, A. L., Hu, F. B., Laden, F., Grandjean, P., et al. (2012). Persistent organic pollutants and type 2 diabetes: A prospective analysis in the nurses' health study and meta-analysis. *Environmental Health Perspectives, 121*, 153–161.

WWF (World Wildlife Fund) (2003). *ContamiNation. The results of WWF's national biomonitoring survey 2003.* Godalming, Surrey: World Wildlife Fund (WWF). Available from, http://www.wwf.org.uk/filelibrary/pdf/biomonitoringresults.pdf, Accessed 4 December 2012.

CHAPTER SEVEN

Reproductive Toxicities of Methoxychlor Based on Estrogenic Properties of the Compound and Its Estrogenic Metabolite, Hydroxyphenyltrichloroethane

Hiroaki Aoyama*^,1, Robert E. Chapin†
*Toxicology Division, Institute of Environmental Toxicology, Joso, Ibaraki, Japan
†Developmental and Reproductive Toxicology, Drug Safety R&D, Pfizer, Inc., Groton, Connecticut, USA
[1]Corresponding author: e-mail address: aoyama@iet.or.jp

Contents

1. Introduction 194
2. Estrogenicity of Methoxychlor and Its Active Metabolite, HPTE 195
   2.1 *In vitro* screening assays 195
   2.2 *In vivo* screening assays 198
3. Reproductive and Developmental Toxicities of Methoxychlor 199
   3.1 Effects on female reproductive organs 199
   3.2 Effects on male reproductive organs 202
   3.3 Effects on endogenous hormone levels 203
   3.4 Effects on fertility and fetal development 205
4. Conclusion 206
Acknowledgment 207
References 207

Abstract

Methoxychlor is an organochlorine pesticide having a weak estrogenicity, which is estimated to be approximately 1000- to 14,000-fold less potent to a natural ligand, 17β-estradiol. However, its active metabolite, hydroxyphenyltrichloroethane, has much more potent estrogenic activity and probably acts in the target organs of animals exposed to methoxychlor at least 100 times stronger than the parent compound. A variety of *in vivo* reproductive toxicity studies have shown that treatment with methoxychlor exerts typical endocrine-disrupting effects manifest as estrogenic effects, such as formation of cystic ovaries resulting in ovulation failures, uterine hypertrophy, hormonal imbalances, atrophy of male sexual organs, and deteriorations of sperm

Vitamins and Hormones, Volume 94
ISSN 0083-6729
http://dx.doi.org/10.1016/B978-0-12-800095-3.00007-9

production in rats and/or mice, through which it causes serious reproductive damages in both sexes of animals at sufficient dose levels. However, methoxychlor is not teratogenic. The no-observed-adverse-effect level of methoxychlor among reliable experimental animal studies in terms of the reproductive toxicity is 10 ppm (equivalent to 0.600 mg/kg/day) in a two-generation reproduction toxicity study.

1. INTRODUCTION

Methoxychlor, 1,1,1-trichloro-2,2-bis(4-methoxyphenyl)ethane (CAS number 72-43-5), is one of the organochlorine pesticides (Fig. 7.1), which was first synthesized in 1893 (Agency for Toxic Substances and Disease Registry, 2002). The commercial production of methoxychlor was first reported in 1946, and the compound was first registered in 1948 as a less persistent alternative pesticide of DDT in the United States (Agency for Toxic Substances and Disease Registry, 2002; United States Environmental Protection Agency, 2004). Since then, methoxychlor has been used widely in North America against pests such as houseflies, mosquitoes, cockroaches, and various arthropods commonly found on field crops, vegetables, and fruits (Agency for Toxic Substances and Disease Registry, 2002). However, the registration was canceled in 2003 in the United States mainly due to endocrine disrupting effects of the compound and/or its estrogenic active metabolite, hydroxyphenyltrichloroethane (HPTE, Fig. 7.1; United States Environmental Protection Agency, 2004). Recent monitoring reports revealed that only a trace amount of methoxychlor was detected in a sample of animal feed in 2007 fiscal year (United States Food and Drug Administration, 2008).

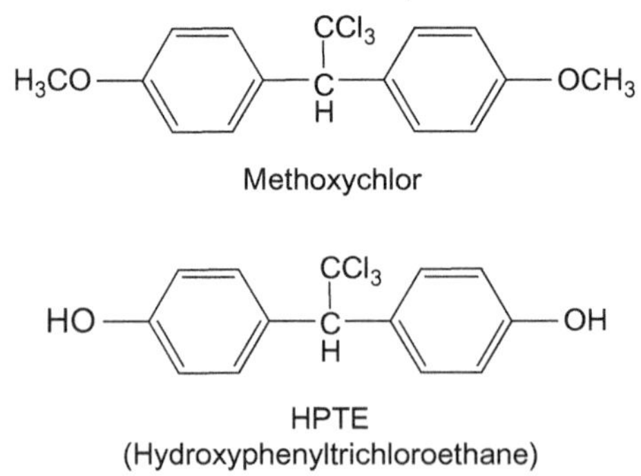

Figure 7.1 Structures of methoxychlor and its estrogenic metabolite, HPTE (hydroxyphenyltrichloroethane)

Methoxychlor has been studied so extensively for its toxicological features, including acute, subchronic and chronic toxicities, carcinogenicity, reproductive and developmental toxicities, and developmental neuro- and immunotoxicities, as well as its estrogenic activities, which has become the prototypical estrogenic reference chemical. In fact, it has been used for validating the sensitivity and/or accuracy of several bioassays including both *in vitro* and *in vivo* screening assays for detecting estrogenic activities such as a reporter gene assay and a uterotrophic assay in rats and/or mice, as well as *in vivo* definitive studies such as a two-generation reproduction toxicity study for predicting toxicological effects based on estrogenic properties. This chapter intends to summarize briefly the available information on estrogenic properties and the consequent reproductive toxicities of methoxychlor at sufficient exposure levels based on the rodent studies for risk assessment of human health. Effects of methoxychlor on domestic and/or wild animals including birds, reptiles, amphibians, and fishes are out of the focus in this manuscript, although impacts on these animals can be significant. Readers who are interested in these issues are referred to other excellent reviews (Craig, Wang, & Flaws, 2011; Cummings, 1997; Eroschenko, Amstislavsky, Schwabel, & Ingermann, 2002; Ottinger et al., 2005; Padmanabhan, Sarma, Savabieasfahani, Steckler, & Veiga-Lopez, 2010; Sweeney, 2002; Tiemann, 2008).

2. ESTROGENICITY OF METHOXYCHLOR AND ITS ACTIVE METABOLITE, HPTE

2.1. *In vitro* screening assays

Methoxychlor has been shown to be able to bind to human estrogen receptor alpha (ER-α) by a classical receptor binding assay, but the affinity to the receptor is very weak (Bolger, Wiese, Ervin, Nestich, & Checovich, 1998; Kuiper et al., 1997) or sometimes less than the detectable limit (Kuiper et al., 1998). We have confirmed, using recombinant human ER-α, that methoxychlor weakly competes with fluorescent nonsteroidal estrogen (FES 1) at 10^{-6} M or higher concentrations (Fig. 7.2A, Unpublished observation). The estrogenic activities of methoxychlor through ER-α seem to be slightly more potent in the reporter gene assays regardless of utilized cell lines, where human HepG 2 cells, Eker rat leiomyoma-derived ELT 3 cells, or CHO-K cells derived from Chinese hamster were transiently transfected human ER-α expression plasmid with a reporter gene (Gaido et al., 2000; Hodges, Bergerson, Hunter, & Walker, 2000; Kojima, Katsura, Takeuchi, Niiyama, & Kobayashi, 2004). Based on these results, methoxychlor is

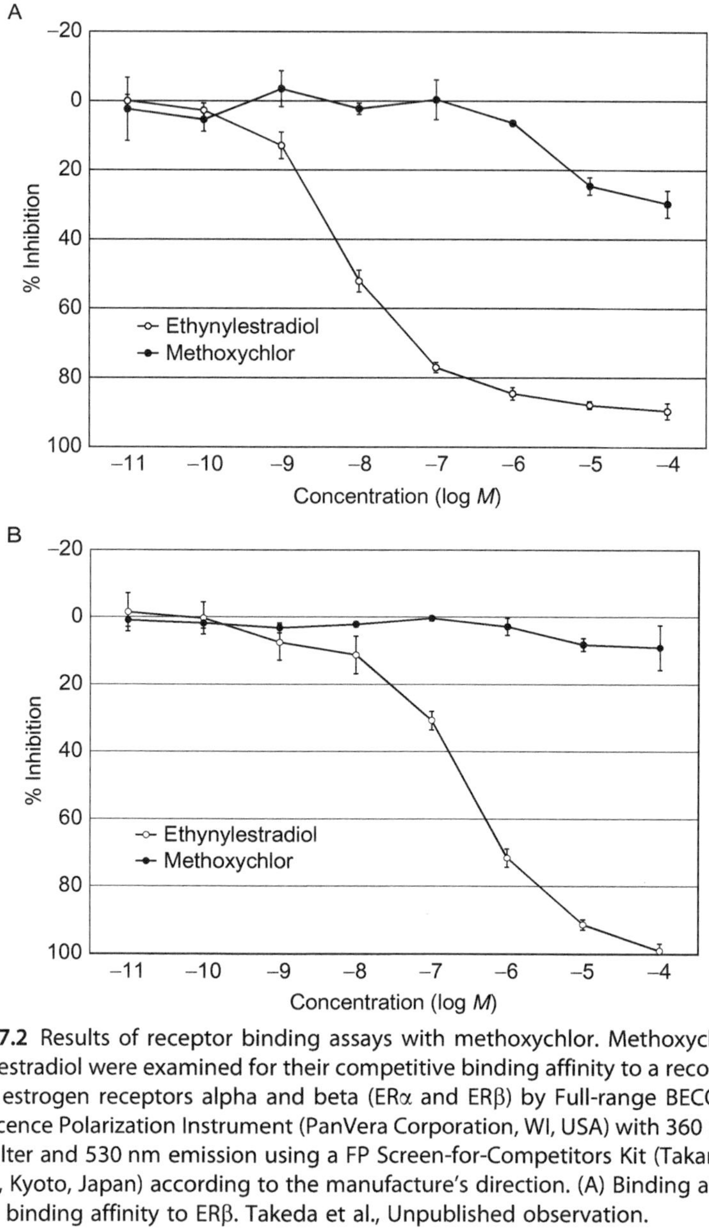

Figure 7.2 Results of receptor binding assays with methoxychlor. Methoxychlor and ethynylestradiol were examined for their competitive binding affinity to a recombinant human estrogen receptors alpha and beta (ERα and ERβ) by Full-range BECON 2000 Fluorescence Polarization Instrument (PanVera Corporation, WI, USA) with 360 nm excitation filter and 530 nm emission using a FP Screen-for-Competitors Kit (Takara Shuzo Co. Ltd., Kyoto, Japan) according to the manufacture's direction. (A) Binding affinity to ERα; (B) binding affinity to ERβ. Takeda et al., Unpublished observation.

estimated to have approximately 1000- to 14,000-fold lower binding affinity to human ER-α compared to the natural ligand, 17β-estradiol (Bolger et al., 1998; Kuiper et al., 1997, 1998).

Methoxychlor binds much less avidly to ER-β than to ER-α and seems to be traceable or negligible in our experimental conditions (Fig. 7.2B,

Unpublished observation). Similar results were obtained in other studies: methoxychlor showed lower relative transactivation activity through ER-β when compared to that through ER-α (Kuiper et al., 1998) or showed no overt affinity to ER-β (Kojima et al., 2004).

Methoxychlor can stimulate ER-positive cancer cell lines such as MCF-7 cells derived from human mammary cancer and/or cause upregulation of typical estrogen-responsive genes in these cells, although binding affinities to ERs are not so potent (Andersen et al., 1999; Lee et al., 2012; Okubo, Yokoyama, Kano, Soya, & Kano, 2004). Hodges et al. (2000) reported similar results: methoxychlor induced both the growth of cells and expression of progesterone receptor mRNA dose-dependently in ER-positive ELT-3 cells derived from Eker rat leiomyoma. Our unpublished observations also revealed weak estrogenic effects of methoxychlor, in which the compound stimulated the growth of MCF-7 cells at and above 10^{-6} M (Fig. 7.3). The cell-stimulating effect of methoxychlor is

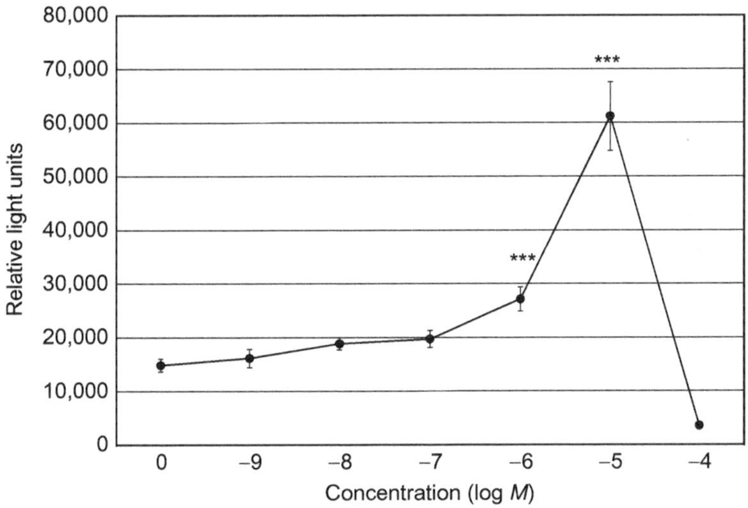

Figure 7.3 Results of an E-screening assay with methoxychlor. MCF-7 cells, 1×10^4 cells/well, were incubated in Dulbecco's Modified Eagle Medium (D-MEM) supplemented by L-glutamine (4 mM), 5% charcoal stripped human serum and antibiotic (penicillin and streptomycin at final concentrations of 100 IU/mL and 100 μg/mL, respectively) together with various concentrations of methoxychlor on Falcon 24-well plate (Becton, Dickinson and Company, NJ, USA). Cells were harvested after 6 days of treatment and their ATP concentrations were measured for evaluating cell growth by Lumitester C-100LU (Kikkoman Corporation, Chiba, Japan) with a luciferine–luciferase agent (Lucifel 250, Kikkoman) according to the manufacture's direction. Note that methoxychlor stimulated cell growth (increased ATP contents) at high concentrations. ***, significantly different form control at $p < 0.001$. Matsumoto et al., Unpublished observation.

thought to be ER-mediated since cotreatment with ICI 182,720, a synthetic antiestrogen, clearly blocked the effect (Okubo et al., 2004).

Several *in vitro* experiments have demonstrated that a metabolite of methoxychlor, HPTE, has much more potent estrogenic properties than methoxychlor (Bolger et al., 1998; Gaido et al., 1999, 2000; Hodges et al., 2000; Shelby, Newbold, Tully, Chae, & Davis, 1996). The relative estrogenic activity of HPTE to ERs is estimated to be at least 100 times greater than methoxychlor (Bolger et al., 1998; Hodges et al., 2000; Shelby et al., 1996). Interestingly, HPTE is a clear agonist for ER-α regardless of the experimental condition while also acting as an antagonist with both human and rat ERβ against 17β-estradiol with a minimal agonistic activity (Gaido et al., 1999, 2000).

In addition to estrogenic and/or antiestrogenic properties, methoxychlor and HPTE have been reported to weakly bind to androgen receptor to cause antiandrogenic effects (Gaido et al., 2000; Kojima et al., 2004; Tamura et al., 2006). These observations demonstrate the complexity and difficulty in accurately determining the underlying mechanism(s) of action of methoxychlor in the many *in vivo* studies.

2.2. *In vivo* screening assays

One of the simplest and most reliable *in vivo* screening assays to examine the estrogenic properties of xenobiotics is a uterotrophic assay in rats and/or mice, in which ovariectomized adult females or juvenile females were treated with chemicals of interest for several days to measure wet and/or blotted uterine weights as the most sensitive markers of estrogenic responses (Kanno et al., 2001; Owens & Koeter, 2003). Additional endpoints include epithelial cell heights and cell proliferation rates in the uterus and vagina, as well as uterine and vaginal histology (Kanno et al., 2001).

Overt estrogenic effects of methoxychlor were repeatedly observed at relatively high-dose levels in 3-day uterotrophic assays in rats and mice regardless of the administration routes (Kanno et al., 2003; Laws, Carey, Ferrell, Bodman, & Cooper, 2000; Shelby et al., 1996; Shin et al., 2007). However, the majority of these assays with juvenile female rats failed to find a significant increase in uterine weights at or less than 50 mg/kg/day when methoxychlor was injected subcutaneously, although the effects were evident when the same dose levels were administered orally (Kanno et al., 2003; Laws et al., 2000; Shin et al., 2007). We have confirmed the similar tendency in a 3-day uterotrophic assay with ovariectomized adult female rats, in which oral gavage but not subcutaneous injection of methoxychlor caused significant increases in wet uterine weights at dose levels of 100 and

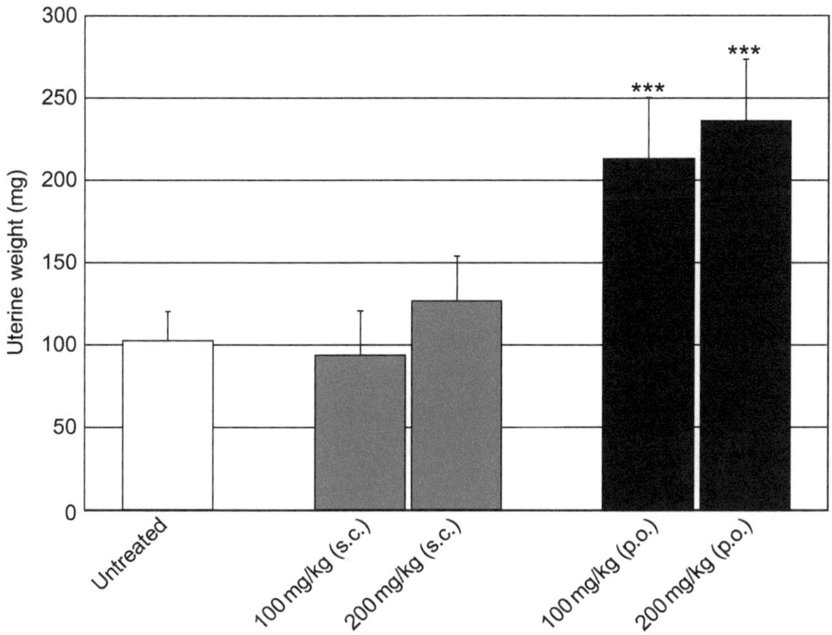

Figure 7.4 Wet uterine weights (mean ± SD) of ovariectomized Wistar rats (6/group) treated subcutaneously (s.c.) or orally (p.o.) with methoxychlor for three consecutive days. Note that methoxychlor exerted overt uterotrophic effects when it was administered orally. ***, significantly different form control (untreated) at $p < 0.001$. Aoyama et al., Unpublished observation.

200 mg/kg/day (Fig. 7.4, Unpublished observation). Interestingly, serum concentrations of methoxychlor in juvenile female rats treated subcutaneously were two- to threefold higher than those treated orally (Shin et al., 2007). As several *in vitro* studies have demonstrated that a metabolite of methoxychlor, HPTE, has much more potent estrogenic activity than its parent compound (Bolger et al., 1998; Hodges et al., 2000; Shelby et al., 1996), the observations suggest that orally administered methoxychlor was metabolized to HPTE in the liver sooner than what was subcutaneously injected, which in turn induced clearer uterine responses.

3. REPRODUCTIVE AND DEVELOPMENTAL TOXICITIES OF METHOXYCHLOR

3.1. Effects on female reproductive organs

Many *in vivo* studies have shown that the main target organs of methoxychlor are the ovary, uterus, and vagina in rodent females. Among them, the ovary was most conspicuously affected in a variety of studies regardless of the timing and length of treatment period, as well as the administration route (Aoyama et al., 2012; Armenti, Zama, Passantino, & Uzumcu, 2008; Chapin et al., 1997; Eroschenko, Abuel-Atta, & Grober, 1995; Gray et al., 1989; Martinez & Swartz, 1991; Masutomi et al., 2003; Quignot et al., 2012; Uzumcu, Kuhn, Marano, Armenti, & Passantino, 2006; Walters, Rourke, & Eroschenko, 1993; You et al., 2002). A possible unifying explanation to explain these results is that chronic exposures to methoxychlor at sufficient dose levels may provide an estrogenic stimulus to the hypothalamus–pituitary–gonad feedback system that would block the proestrus LH surge and the FSH surge on estrus day. This would lead to ovulation failures and an increased number of large antral and/or cystic follicles without formation of corpora lutea in the ovary to keep a serum progesterone level significantly low.

Oral treatment of young adult female rats for 2 weeks with methoxychlor at a dose level of 200 mg/kg/day significantly reduced ovary weights and induced a significant decrease in number of corpora lutea (Quignot et al., 2012). Similar effects were seen in young adult female mice where oral treatment with methoxychlor at dose levels of 2.5 or 5.0 mg/mouse/day, which were equivalent to 100 or 200 mg/kg/day, caused a significant decrease in ovary weights and a significant increase in the number of atretic large follicles (Martinez & Swartz, 1991). Oral or intraperitoneal treatment of female rats and mice during the gestational, perinatal, early postnatal and/or juvenile periods, as well as two successive generations, at and above 50 mg/kg/day or dietary concentration of 500 ppm or more (equivalent to 43.5 mg/kg/day) repeatedly demonstrated significant decreases in absolute and/or relative weights of the ovary accompanied by histopathologic abnormalities in adult females (Aoyama et al., 2012; Armenti et al., 2008; Chapin et al., 1997; Eroschenko et al., 1995; Gray et al., 1989; Masutomi et al., 2003; You et al., 2002).

Typical histopathologic features of the ovaries in methoxychlor-treated females included an increased number of large antral and/or cystic follicles that were often accompanied by numerous small developing follicles and fewer corpora lutea, suggesting a lack of normal ovulation (Aoyama et al., 2012; Armenti et al., 2008; Chapin et al., 1997; Eroschenko et al., 1995; Martinez & Swartz, 1991; You et al., 2002). Daily subcutaneous injection of methoxychlor during the early postnatal period (postnatal days 3–10) also reduced ovary size and inhibited folliculogenesis in prepubertal weanlings (Uzumcu et al., 2006). Aoyama et al. (2012) reported that histopathologic damage in the ovaries such as formation of cystic follicles and loss of corpora lutea was more prominent in F1 females than in parental females, suggesting that fetuses, neonates, and/or juveniles are more susceptible than adults to methoxychlor or HPTE.

The uterus is also a target organ of methoxychlor. Neonatal mice treated with 0.05, 0.5, or 1.0 mg/mouse/day of methoxychlor intraperitoneally for 14 days exhibited significant and dose-dependent increases in uterine weights and epithelial cell heights at postnatal day 15 (Walters et al., 1993). A significant and dose-dependent increase in uterine weights was also noted in 25-day-old weanlings of a two-generation reproduction study in rats at 500 ppm (equivalent to 43.5 mg/kg/day) and higher exposure levels (Aoyama et al., 2012). However, the effect was much less clear when the uteruses of parental females were weighed on the day of proestrus after weaning of their pups. You et al. (2002) reported that treatment of pregnant dams with methoxychlor (800 ppm in feed) increased the mean uterine weights of their offspring at postnatal day 21. Perinatal and juvenile exposure of methoxychlor at 150 mg/kg/day induced epithelial hyperplasia of the uterus in 42-day-old female rats (Chapin et al., 1997).

Methoxychlor accelerated vaginal opening (sexual maturation) of female juveniles and/or weanlings (Chapin et al., 1997; Gray et al., 1989; Masutomi et al., 2003; Walters et al., 1993; You et al., 2002). The lowest effective dose for this parameter was 5 mg/kg/day in rats when they were orally exposed to methoxychlor during the perinatal and juvenile period (Chapin et al., 1997). Interestingly, dietary exposure to methoxychlor at 24 or 240 ppm from gestation day 10 to lactation day 15 (calculated to be equivalent to approximately 2 and 20 mg/kg/day, respectively) did not accelerate vaginal opening of F1 female weanlings (Masutomi et al., 2003), while oral gavage treatment of dams with methoxychlor at 25 mg/kg/day did accelerate it even when the treatment of dams ended at lactation day 15 (Gray et al., 1989).

Vaginal cytology revealed that mean estrous cycle lengths in methoxychlor-treated females were significantly prolonged in rats and mice (Aoyama et al., 2012; Armenti et al., 2008; Chapin et al., 1997; Eroschenko et al., 1995; Gray et al., 1989; Martinez & Swartz, 1991; Quignot et al., 2012; You et al., 2002). This is due to an increase in the days of estrous and/or an induction of persistent estrus where vaginal lavage is filled with cornified epithelial cells (Armenti et al., 2008; Chapin et al., 1997; Eroschenko et al., 1995; Gray et al., 1989; You et al., 2002). Martinez and Swartz (1991) reported that daily oral treatments of young adult female mice with methoxychlor at dose levels of

1.25 mg/mouse (equivalent to 50 mg/kg/day) or more caused persistent vaginal estrus dose-dependently within 8 days.

3.2. Effects on male reproductive organs

Oral treatment of young adult male rats with 200 mg/kg/day of methoxychlor for 2 weeks caused significant reductions in both absolute and relative weights of the testis, epididymis, seminal vesicles, and prostate (Quignot et al., 2012). Perinatal and juvenile oral exposures to methoxychlor at 50 or 150 mg/kg/day from gestation day 14 to postnatal day 42 also induced significant reductions in absolute and/or relative weights of the testis, epididymis, seminal vesicles, and prostate in 6-week-old males (Chapin et al., 1997). The preputial separation of these males was delayed by approximately 8 and 34 days, respectively. Similar results were obtained by Gray et al. (1989), where significant reductions in absolute weights of the testis, seminal vesicles and/or cauda epididymis, and delayed preputial separation were evident at and above 50 mg/kg/day when male rats were orally treated with various doses of methoxychlor from postnatal day 21 to the day of necropsy between 77 and 100 days of age.

Effects on male reproductive organ weights seem less obvious when methoxychlor was exposed via the diet. In a two-generation reproduction study in rats, for example, only the seminal vesicles and prostate showed a significant reduction in both absolute and relative weights at 1500 ppm (equivalent to 96.0 mg/kg/day), while relative weights of the testis and epididymis in these males significantly exceeded the control values due to markedly lowered body weights, although absolute weights of these organs were significantly lowered (Aoyama et al., 2012). The preputial separation was significantly delayed in males of the 500 and 1500 ppm groups in this study, but the difference from control was only 4.5 days even at the highest dose level. You et al. (2002) also reported that dietary exposure to methoxychlor at 800 ppm in a one-generation reproduction study induced a significant weight reduction in the testis and epididymis but not in the ventral prostate, although preputial separation of these males was delayed by 2.4 days. In addition, intraperitoneal injection of methoxychlor to pregnant rats during gestation days 7–15 induced a decrease in the area of seminiferous cords and an increase in the interstitial area in male fetuses on gestation day 16 at a dose level of 50 mg/kg/day (Cupp et al., 2003). However, reproductive organ weights were comparable to those of the controls up to the highest dose level of 150 mg/kg/day when these were determined at postnatal day 60.

Methoxychlor significantly suppressed sperm production and/or number of sperms in the testis and/or epididymis. Dietary exposure of male rats induced a significant reduction in both testicular spermatid head counts and cauda epididymal sperm number in males of both F0 and F1 generations at a dose level of 1500 ppm (equivalent to 96.0 mg/kg/day) in a two-generation reproduction toxicity study (Aoyama et al., 2012). However, when expressed as per gram organ weights, these were comparable to control values, as were epididymal sperm motility and % normal sperm. This lack of change in sperm(atids) per gram suggests that the organs were smaller, but germ cell density was not reduced. In contrast to the dietary exposure study, effects on sperm production were prominent in oral gavage studies. For example, gavage of young adult rats for two weeks with methoxychlor at 200 mg/kg/day caused significant reduction in numbers of sperms per gram testis and per gram epididymis, as well as a significant decrease of daily sperm production in the testis (Quignot et al., 2012). Gray et al. (1989) also reported that cauda epididymal sperm count was significantly decreased in the treated males at 12 weeks of age when 25 mg/kg/day of methoxychlor was orally gavaged to these rats from postnatal day 21 to the day of necropsy.

Chapin and colleagues closely examined the effects of methoxychlor on the testis and spermatogenesis by perinatal and juvenile treatment studies, in which methoxychlor was gavaged at 5, 50, or 150 mg/kg/day from gestation day 14 to postnatal day 42 (Chapin et al., 1997; Johnson, Staub, Silge, Harris, & Chapin, 2002; Staub, Hardy, Chapin, Harris, & Johnson, 2002). Based on this study, they concluded that a dose-dependent reduction in numbers of epididymal spermatozoa and testicular spermatids, which was evident in the higher two dose groups (Chapin et al., 1997), was correlated to reduced numbers of Sertoli cells, spermatogonia, and spermatids per testis (Johnson et al., 2002; Staub et al., 2002). Staub et al. (2002) also reported that the ratio of spermatid number per spermatogonia was increased significantly in methoxychlor-treated males, perhaps in an attempt to compensate for the reduction in number of spermatogonia.

3.3. Effects on endogenous hormone levels

As might be expected from a compound with estrogenic activity, hormonal imbalance was induced by methoxychlor in several studies in rats but the measures varied widely. Gray et al. (1989) reported that continuous oral treatment with methoxychlor from postnatal day 21 to the day of necropsy at dose levels of 100 and 200 mg/kg/day caused a significant decrease in serum testosterone level in male rats at the age of 77–80 days but the effect disappeared in 97- to 100-day-old males. FSH and LH levels were unchanged in both cohorts. Similar results were obtained by Quignot et al. (2012), in which oral gavage of young male rats for 2 weeks caused only a slight and statistically insignificant decrease in serum testosterone level accompanied by significant elevation of E_2 level at a dose of 200 mg/kg/day. FSH and LH were also unchanged in this study. Methoxychlor also induced no hormonal change in male rats up to the highest concentration of 1500 ppm in a two-generation reproduction study, where serum concentrations of FSH, LH, testosterone, and dihydrotestosterone in F0 males were measured (Aoyama et al., 2012). Contrary to these study results, dietary exposure of dams to methoxychlor during the perinatal period are reported to decrease serum FSH level of male offspring dose-dependently at and above 24 ppm and to suppress LH level at 1200 ppm, although the serum concentration of testosterone was unchanged (Suzuki, Lee, Chiba, Yonezawa, & Nishihara, 2004). The discrepancy among these study results still remains to be understood.

Effects of methoxychlor treatment on female hormone levels are also complicated. When serum was collected from proestrus females whose litter sizes were lower than those in the control group in a two-generation reproduction study with methoxychlor, serum E_2 was significantly decreased at and above 500 ppm (equivalent to 43.5 mg/kg/day), while concentrations of FSH, LH, and progesterone in these females were unchanged up to the highest concentration (Aoyama et al., 2012). This can be interpreted that estrogenic stimuli of methoxychlor and/or HPTE may substitute for estrogen to decrease the endogenous E_2 level.

On the other hand, fertile females in the 5 mg/kg/day group and infertile females in the 50 mg/kg/day group at estrus or estrus-like stage in a perinatal and juvenile exposure study exhibited dose-dependent decreases in serum FSH level accompanied by significantly increased E_2/progesterone ratio due to a decrease in progesterone level (Chapin et al., 1997). In that study, FSH level of proestrus females whose fertility remained almost normal in the 5 mg/kg/day group was comparable to that in the control group. Suzuki et al. (2004) reported that the LH surge of female rats in the evening of proestrus was significantly attenuated by perinatal dietary exposure to methoxychlor at dose levels of 24 ppm and above. A significant decrease in serum LH level, but not FSH and E_2, was also seen in diestrus young adult female rats gavaged with methoxychlor for 2 weeks (Quignot et al., 2012). The likely cause of such alterations is based on the estrogenic activity of methoxychlor and/or HPTE to the brain, as described previously.

3.4. Effects on fertility and fetal development

Chronic and/or transgenerational exposures to methoxychlor have been reported to induce serious reproductive toxicities in rats. When female rats were gavaged with methoxychlor from 21 days of age to the termination of study, their fertilities were dose-dependently reduced: that is, most females in the 200 mg/kg/day group copulated with males but none of them became pregnant even when they were mated with untreated males, and 50% of females paired with untreated males in the 100 mg/kg/day group became pregnant but still showed significantly decreased litter sizes (Gray et al., 1989). All females in the 25 and 50 mg/kg/day groups had normal fertility. Fertilities of males were thought to be unaffected even in the highest dose group because all the males were fertile when mated with untreated females and there was no reduction in the number of implants in paired females. In this study, animal growth was retarded significantly at 100 and 200 mg/kg/day.

A perinatal and juvenile oral gavage study revealed more potent reproductive toxicity of methoxychlor, in which only 3 of 15 females in the 50 mg/kg/day group gave birth when they were mated with untreated proven males, while none of 15 females in the 150 mg/kg/day group was fertile (Chapin et al., 1997). Males in the 150 mg/kg/day group were also severely affected in this study, where the majority of males did not mate with untreated females. Systemic toxicities such as lowered body weights and/or body weight gains were evident only in animals of both sexes at 150 mg/kg/day. These results demonstrate that developmental and/or neonatal exposures increase the sensitivity to methoxychlor in terms of the reproductive toxicities.

Dietary exposure to methoxychlor seems to cause milder reproductive effects than oral gavage exposure. In a two-generation reproduction study (Aoyama et al., 2012), at dietary concentrations up to 1500 ppm, mating indices of both males and females in all treated groups were comparable to those in the control group in both F0 and F1 generations, yet the numbers of implants and newborns were decreased dose-dependently in the 500 and 1500 ppm groups (equivalent to 43.5 and 122 mg/kg/day, respectively, for females). In this study, more than 50% (12/22) of copulated F1 females were nonpregnant in the 1500 ppm group. However, males in the 1500 ppm group (equivalent to 96.0 mg/kg/day for males) that failed to produce offspring at the first mating trial with females of the same group did inseminate untreated females, suggesting that male fertility was unaffected. Systemic toxicities such as significantly lowered body weights, body weight gains, and food consumption were evident at 500 ppm and above.

Methoxychlor induced uterine decidualization when administered to ovariectomized female rats at dose levels of 5–100 mg/kg/day together with an appropriate amount of progesterone (Cummings, 1993). The effects of methoxychlor at 75 and 100 mg/kg/day were similar to that of estrone (0.004 mg/kg/day), but the decidualization response decreased at 500 mg/kg/day. Cummings and colleagues also reported that oral treatment of pregnant rats with methoxychlor during gestation days 1–3 accelerated embryo transport from the oviduct to the uterus at 100–500 mg/kg/day dose-dependently (Cummings & Perreault, 1990), while dosing during gestation days 1–8 or 4–8 increased resorptions up to 100% (Cummings & Gray, 1989; Cummings & Laskey, 1993).

Subcutaneous injection of methoxychlor at a dose level of 0.5 mg/mouse/day (equivalent to 16.5 mg/kg/day) during gestation days 2–4 suppressed embryonic development to blastocyst, decreased embryonic cell numbers, and caused abnormal blastocyst formation in mice (Amstislavsky, Kizilova, & Eroschenko, 2003). However, methoxychlor was not structurally teratogenic in rats when administered orally during gestation days 6–19, although it suppressed fetal growth at the highest dose level of 150 mg/kg/day (Shimizu et al., 2001).

4. CONCLUSION

Studies have clearly shown that the estrogenic pesticide methoxychlor exerts typical endocrine disrupting effects such as formation of cystic ovaries resulting in ovulation failures, uterine hypertrophy, hormonal imbalances, atrophy of male sexual organs, and deterioration of sperm production in rats and/or mice, through which it causes serious reproductive damage in both sexes of animals at sufficient dose levels. The adverse effects are observed at lower doses in females than in males. It is also obvious that developmental and neonatal exposures to methoxychlor induce more serious reproductive damage than postweaning exposures. However, methoxychlor does not produce structural malformations. The no-observed-adverse-effect level of methoxychlor among reliable experimental animal studies in terms of the reproductive toxicity is 10 ppm (equivalent to 0.600 mg/kg/day) in a two-generation reproduction toxicity study (Aoyama et al., 2012).

ACKNOWLEDGMENT

The authors express their thanks to Drs. Makio Takeda, Kyomu Matsumoto, and Kazutoshi Ohyama at the Institute of Environmental Toxicology for their excellent assistance in conducting screening assays and/or providing the figures.

REFERENCES

Agency for Toxic Substances and Disease Registry (2002). *Toxicological profile for methoxychlor*. Atlanta, GA: Public Health Service, U.S. Department of Health and Human Services.

Amstislavsky, S. Y., Kizilova, E. A., & Eroschenko, V. P. (2003). Preimplantation mouse embryo development as a target of the pesticide methoxychlor. *Reproductive Toxicology (Elmsford, N.Y.)*, *17*, 79–86.

Andersen, H. R., Andersson, A. M., Arnold, S. F., Autrup, H., Barfoed, M., Beresford, N. A., et al. (1999). Comparison of short-term estrogenicity tests for identification of hormone-disrupting chemicals. *Environmental Health Perspectives*, *107*(Suppl. 1), 89–108.

Aoyama, H., Hojo, H., Takahashi, K. L., Shimizu-Endo, N., Araki, M., Takeuchi-Kashimoto, Y., et al. (2012). Two-generation reproduction toxicity study in rats with methoxychlor. *Congenital Anomalies*, *52*, 28–41.

Armenti, A. E., Zama, A. M., Passantino, L., & Uzumcu, M. (2008). Developmental methoxychlor exposure affects multiple reproductive parameters and ovarian folliculogenesis and gene expression in adult rats. *Toxicology and Applied Pharmacology*, *233*, 286–296.

Bolger, R., Wiese, T. E., Ervin, K., Nestich, S., & Checovich, W. (1998). Rapid screening of environmental chemicals for estrogen receptor binding capacity. *Environmental Health Perspectives*, *106*, 551–557.

Chapin, R. E., Harris, M. W., Davis, B. J., Ward, S. M., Wilson, R. E., Mauney, M. A., et al. (1997). The effects of perinatal/juvenile methoxychlor exposure on adult rat nervous, immune, and reproductive system function. *Fundamental and Applied Toxicology: Official Journal of the Society of Toxicology*, *40*, 138–157.

Craig, Z. R., Wang, W., & Flaws, J. A. (2011). Endocrine-disrupting chemicals in ovarian function: Effects on steroidogenesis, metabolism and nuclear receptor signaling. *Reproduction (Cambridge, England)*, *142*, 633–646.

Cummings, A. M. (1993). Replacement of estrogen by methoxychlor in the artificially-induced decidual cell response in the rat. *Life Sciences*, *52*, 347–352.

Cummings, A. M. (1997). Methoxychlor as a model for environmental estrogens. *Critical Reviews in Toxicology*, *27*, 367–379.

Cummings, A. M., & Gray, L. E., Jr. (1989). Antifertility effect of methoxychlor in female rats: Dose- and time-dependent blockade of pregnancy. *Toxicology and Applied Pharmacology*, *97*, 454–462.

Cummings, A. M., & Laskey, J. (1993). Effect of methoxychlor on ovarian steroidogenesis: Role in early pregnancy loss. *Reproductive Toxicology (Elmsford, N.Y.)*, *7*, 17–23.

Cummings, A. M., & Perreault, S. D. (1990). Methoxychlor accelerates embryo transport through the rat reproductive tract. *Toxicology and Applied Pharmacology*, *102*, 110–116.

Cupp, A. S., Uzumcu, M., Suzuki, H., Dirks, K., Phillips, B., & Skinner, M. K. (2003). Effect of transient embryonic in vivo exposure to the endocrine disruptor methoxychlor on embryonic and postnatal testis development. *Journal of Andrology*, *24*, 736–745.

Eroschenko, V. P., Abuel-Atta, A. A., & Grober, M. S. (1995). Neonatal exposures to technical methoxychlor alters ovaries in adult mice. *Reproductive Toxicology (Elmsford, N.Y.)*, *9*, 379–387.

Eroschenko, V. P., Amstislavsky, S. Y., Schwabel, H., & Ingermann, R. L. (2002). Altered behaviors in male mice, male quail, and salamander larvae following early exposures to the estrogenic pesticide methoxychlor. *Neurotoxicology and Teratology, 24*, 29–36.

Gaido, K. W., Leonard, L. S., Maness, S. C., Hall, J. M., McDonnell, D. P., Saville, B., et al. (1999). Differential interaction of the methoxychlor metabolite 2,2-bis-(p-hydroxyphenyl)-1,1,1-trichloroethane with estrogen receptors alpha and beta. *Endocrinology, 140*, 5746–5753.

Gaido, K. W., Maness, S. C., McDonnell, D. P., Dehal, S. S., Kupfer, D., & Safe, S. (2000). Interaction of methoxychlor and related compounds with estrogen receptor alpha and beta, and androgen receptor: Structure-activity studies. *Molecular Pharmacology, 58*, 852–858.

Gray, L. E., Jr., Ostby, J., Ferrell, J., Rehnberg, G., Linder, R., Cooper, R., et al. (1989). A dose-response analysis of methoxychlor-induced alterations of reproductive development and function in the rat. *Fundamental and Applied Toxicology: Official Journal of the Society of Toxicology, 12*, 92–108.

Hodges, L. C., Bergerson, J. S., Hunter, D. S., & Walker, C. L. (2000). Estrogenic effects of organochlorine pesticides on uterine leiomyoma cells in vitro. *Toxicological Sciences: An Official Journal of the Society of Toxicology, 54*, 355–364.

Johnson, L., Staub, C., Silge, R. L., Harris, M. W., & Chapin, R. E. (2002). The pesticide methoxychlor given orally during the perinatal/juvenile period, reduced the spermatogenic potential of males as adults by reducing their Sertoli cell number. *Reproduction, Nutrition, Development, 42*, 573–580.

Kanno, J., Onyon, L., Haseman, J., Fenner-Crisp, P., Ashby, J., & Owens, W. (2001). The OECD program to validate the rat uterotrophic bioassay to screen compounds for in vivo estrogenic responses: Phase 1. *Environmental Health Perspectives, 109*, 785–794.

Kanno, J., Onyon, L., Peddada, S., Ashby, J., Jacob, E., & Owens, W. (2003). The OECD program to validate the rat uterotrophic bioassay. Phase 2: Dose-response studies. *Environmental Health Perspectives, 111*, 1530–1549.

Kojima, H., Katsura, E., Takeuchi, S., Niiyama, K., & Kobayashi, K. (2004). Screening for estrogen and androgen receptor activities in 200 pesticides by in vitro reporter gene assays using Chinese hamster ovary cells. *Environmental Health Perspectives, 112*, 524–531.

Kuiper, G. G., Carlsson, B., Grandien, K., Enmark, E., Haggblad, J., Nilsson, S., et al. (1997). Comparison of the ligand binding specificity and transcript tissue distribution of estrogen receptors alpha and beta. *Endocrinology, 138*, 863–870.

Kuiper, G. G., Lemmen, J. G., Carlsson, B., Corton, J. C., Safe, S. H., van der Saag, P. T., et al. (1998). Interaction of estrogenic chemicals and phytoestrogens with estrogen receptor beta. *Endocrinology, 139*, 4252–4263.

Laws, S. C., Carey, S. A., Ferrell, J. M., Bodman, G. J., & Cooper, R. L. (2000). Estrogenic activity of octylphenol, nonylphenol, bisphenol A and methoxychlor in rats. *Toxicological Sciences: An Official Journal of the Society of Toxicology, 54*, 154–167.

Lee, H. R., Hwang, K. A., Park, M. A., Yi, B. R., Jeung, E. B., & Choi, K. C. (2012). Treatment with bisphenol A and methoxychlor results in the growth of human breast cancer cells and alteration of the expression of cell cycle-related genes, cyclin D1 and p21, via an estrogen receptor-dependent signaling pathway. *International Journal of Molecular Medicine, 29*, 883–890.

Martinez, E. M., & Swartz, W. J. (1991). Effects of methoxychlor on the reproductive system of the adult female mouse. 1. Gross and histologic observations. *Reproductive Toxicology (Elmsford, N.Y.), 5*, 139–147.

Masutomi, N., Shibutani, M., Takagi, H., Uneyama, C., Takahashi, N., & Hirose, M. (2003). Impact of dietary exposure to methoxychlor, genistein, or diisononyl phthalate during the perinatal period on the development of the rat endocrine/reproductive systems in later life. *Toxicology, 192*, 149–170.

Okubo, T., Yokoyama, Y., Kano, K., Soya, Y., & Kano, I. (2004). Estimation of estrogenic and antiestrogenic activities of selected pesticides by MCF-7 cell proliferation assay. *Archives of Environmental Contamination and Toxicology, 46*, 445–453.

Ottinger, M. A., Quinn, M. J., Jr., Lavoie, E., Abdelnabi, M. A., Thompson, N., Hazelton, J. L., et al. (2005). Consequences of endocrine disrupting chemicals on reproductive endocrine function in birds: Establishing reliable end points of exposure. *Domestic Animal Endocrinology, 29*, 411–419.

Owens, W., & Koeter, H. B. (2003). The OECD program to validate the rat uterotrophic bioassay: An overview. *Environmental Health Perspectives, 111*, 1527–1529.

Padmanabhan, V., Sarma, H. N., Savabieasfahani, M., Steckler, T. L., & Veiga-Lopez, A. (2010). Developmental reprogramming of reproductive and metabolic dysfunction in sheep: Native steroids vs. environmental steroid receptor modulators. *International Journal of Andrology, 33*, 394–404.

Quignot, N., Arnaud, M., Robidel, F., Lecomte, A., Tournier, M., Cren-Olive, C., et al. (2012). Characterization of endocrine-disrupting chemicals based on hormonal balance disruption in male and female adult rats. *Reproductive Toxicology (Elmsford, N.Y.), 33*, 339–352.

Shelby, M. D., Newbold, R. R., Tully, D. B., Chae, K., & Davis, V. L. (1996). Assessing environmental chemicals for estrogenicity using a combination of in vitro and in vivo assays. *Environmental Health Perspectives, 104*, 1296–1300.

Shimizu, N., Aoyama, H., Hojo, H., Takahashi, K. L., Kikuta, M., Kushida, H., et al. (2001). Prenatal developmental toxicity studies of 1,1,1-trichloro-2,2-bis(4-methoxyphenyl) ethane (methoxychlor) in rats and rabbits. *Congenital Anomalies, 41*, 329–337.

Shin, J. H., Moon, H. J., Kang, I. H., Kim, T. S., Lee, S. J., Oh, J. Y., et al. (2007). Calbindin-D9k mRNA expression in the rat uterus following exposure to methoxychlor: A comparison of oral and subcutaneous exposure. *The Journal of Reproduction and Development, 53*, 179–188.

Staub, C., Hardy, V. B., Chapin, R. E., Harris, M. W., & Johnson, L. (2002). The hidden effect of estrogenic/antiandrogenic methoxychlor on spermatogenesis. *Toxicology and Applied Pharmacology, 180*, 129–135.

Suzuki, M., Lee, H. C., Chiba, S., Yonezawa, T., & Nishihara, M. (2004). Effects of methoxychlor exposure during perinatal period on reproductive function after maturation in rats. *The Journal of Reproduction and Development, 50*, 455–461.

Sweeney, T. (2002). Is exposure to endocrine disrupting compounds during fetal/post-natal development affecting the reproductive potential of farm animals? *Domestic Animal Endocrinology, 23*, 203–209.

Tamura, H., Ishimoto, Y., Fujikawa, T., Aoyama, H., Yoshikawa, H., & Akamatsu, M. (2006). Structural basis for androgen receptor agonists and antagonists: Interaction of SPEED 98-listed chemicals and related compounds with the androgen receptor based on an in vitro reporter gene assay and 3D-QSAR. *Bioorganic & Medicinal Chemistry, 14*, 7160–7174.

Tiemann, U. (2008). In vivo and in vitro effects of the organochlorine pesticides DDT, TCPM, methoxychlor, and lindane on the female reproductive tract of mammals: A review. *Reproductive Toxicology (Elmsford, N.Y.), 25*, 316–326.

United States Environmental Protection Agency, (2004). *Methoxychlor registration eligibility decision (RED)*. Washington, DC: United States Environmental Protection Agency.

United States Food and Drug Administration, (2008). *FDA pesticide program residue monitoring: 1993–2007, residue monitoring report*. Washington, DC: United States Food and Drug Administration, US Department of Health & Human Services.

Uzumcu, M., Kuhn, P. E., Marano, J. E., Armenti, A. E., & Passantino, L. (2006). Early postnatal methoxychlor exposure inhibits folliculogenesis and stimulates anti-Mullerian hormone production in the rat ovary. *The Journal of Endocrinology, 191*, 549–558.

Walters, L. M., Rourke, A. W., & Eroschenko, V. P. (1993). Purified methoxychlor stimulates the reproductive tract in immature female mice. *Reproductive Toxicology (Elmsford, N.Y.)*, 7, 599–606.

You, L., Casanova, M., Bartolucci, E. J., Fryczynski, M. W., Dorman, D. C., Everitt, J. I., et al. (2002). Combined effects of dietary phytoestrogen and synthetic endocrine-active compound on reproductive development in Sprague-Dawley rats: Genistein and methoxychlor. *Toxicological Sciences: An Official Journal of the Society of Toxicology, 66*, 91–104.

CHAPTER EIGHT

Epigenetic Effects of Methoxychlor and Vinclozolin on Male Gametes

Ariane Paoloni-Giacobino[1]

Department of Genetic Medicine and Development, University of Geneva Medical School, Geneva, Switzerland

Swiss Center for Applied Human Toxicology, University of Geneva Medical School, Geneva, Switzerland

[1]Corresponding author: e-mail address: ariane.giacobino@unige.ch

Contents

1. Introduction 212
2. Epigenetics 213
3. Imprinting 213
4. Environmental Changes Affect Imprinting 215
5. Imprinting Defects and Male Infertility 215
6. Endocrine Disruptors and Male Infertility 216
   6.1 Effects of vinclozolin on imprinting and fertility 217
   6.2 Effects of methoxychlor on imprinting and fertility 219
   6.3 CpG-specific effects of methoxychlor 221
7. Conclusion and Perspectives 223

References 224

Abstract

Imprinting is an epigenetic form of gene regulation that mediates a parent-of-origin-dependent expression of the alleles of a number of genes. Imprinting, which occurs at specific sites within or surrounding the gene, called differentially methylated domains, consists in a methylation of CpGs. The appropriate transmission of genomics imprints is essential for the control of embryonic development and fetal growth. A number of endocrine disruptors (EDs) affect male reproductive tract development and spermatogenesis. It was postulated that the genetic effects of EDs might be induced by alterations in gene imprinting. We tested two EDs: methoxychlor and vinclozolin. Their administration during gestation induced in the offspring a decrease in sperm counts and significant modifications in the methylation pattern of a selection of paternally and maternally expressed canonical imprinted genes. The observation that imprinting was largely untouched in somatic cells suggests that EDs exert their damaging effects via the process of reprogramming that is unique to gamete development. Interestingly, the effects were transgenerational, although disappearing gradually from F1 to F3. A systematic analysis showed a heterogeneity in the CpG sensitivity to EDs.

Vitamins and Hormones, Volume 94
ISSN 0083-6729
http://dx.doi.org/10.1016/B978-0-12-800095-3.00008-0

We propose that the deleterious effects of EDs on the male reproductive system are mediated by imprinting defects in the sperm. The reported effects of EDs on human male spermatogenesis might be mediated by analogous imprinting alterations.

1. INTRODUCTION

Our view of genetics has been based on DNA and changes in its nucleotidic sequence for many years. Most efforts were concentrated on understanding how phenotypes, or diseases, are linked to DNA mutations or variants transmitted through generations. Epigenetics is defined as the study of changes in gene expression that occur without an underlying change in the DNA nucleotidic sequence. This new field is changing the way we think about transmission. An important feature of epigenetics is its response to changes in the environment. This response is now seen as very important for the expression of specific phenotypes and for their potential transmission. Nutritional factors, exposure to toxics, and even human interactions have been demonstrated to induce epigenetic changes. We can now understand genetics as based on genotypes, epigenotypes, phenotypes, and epiphenotypes.

We can imagine how the field of toxicology may be affected by epigenetic studies. The diseases for which epidemiology is reporting alarming increases over the last decades, such as specific types of cancer, urogenital malformations, or infertility in males, might be demonstrated in the future as directly linked to exposure to specific chemicals. Among the latter, compounds with endocrine-disrupting properties are the objects of deep interrogations and worries. They have a well-known capacity of affecting hormone-sensitive systems in numerous living organisms and in humans, and recent findings show that they are ubiquitously present in the environment and might cause epigenetic changes.

We therefore became interested in analyzing the possible induction, by specific endocrine disruptors (EDs) of epigenetic defects, and to look at possibly correlated epiphenotypes. In particular, vinclozolin (VCZ) and methoxychlor (MXC), two compounds with different endocrine-disrupting properties, were investigated for such putative effects, through the use of a mouse model. Spermatogenesis seems to be particularly sensitive to environmental changes, and we therefore focused on possible spermatogenic impairment after exposure to VCZ and MXC.

2. EPIGENETICS

Different types of epigenetic modifications, affecting the structure of chromatin, can reversibly modulate gene expression. Among them are histone acetylation or phosphorylation, RNA-mediated gene silencing, and DNA methylation, the latter being probably the best characterized to date. These mechanisms seem complementary to each other and are essential for tissue development and for the regulation of various cellular processes. DNA methylation corresponds to the covalent addition of a methyl group to the carbon-5 of a cytosine, within a CpG dinucleotide (Smallwood & Kelsey, 2012). Clusters of CpGs, known as CpG islands, range in length from 200 bp to 5 kb (Tang & Ho, 2007). Three different genomic regions seem to be the possible targets of environmentally induced epigenetic methylation changes. Approximately 70% of CpG islands are located in the promoter region of genes and the remaining 30% in the transposable elements adjacent to the so-called imprinted genes displaying differentially methylated regions (Jirtle & Skinner, 2007).

Epigenetic changes are essential for integrating signals from the environment and subsequently modulating gene expression in a beneficial manner, at the level of the organism. However, it is easily understandable that these processes can also be dysregulated. The degree of the dysregulation depends on the environmental factor or on the amount or time of exposure. Indeed, a change in DNA methylation can result in an inappropriate silencing of the corresponding gene or in a dysregulation of the expression of a specific cluster of genes.

3. IMPRINTING

Imprinting is a form of gene regulation, defined as the marking of the parental alleles of a diploid organism with regards to their parental origin. A small subset of autosomal genes is subject to imprinting. Imprinting is controlled by DNA methylation in such a way that the methylated allele is silenced and the nonmethylated allele expressed. There is therefore a monoallelic expression of the imprinted gene, one of the alleles being silenced, while the other one from the other parent is expressed.

It is estimated that the total number of imprinted genes in the human/mouse genomes ranges between 100 and 600 (Lucifero, Chaillet, & Trasler, 2004; Luedi, Hartemink, & Jirtle, 2005).

Most imprinted genes are physically grouped on chromosomal regions in the so-called clusters, of approximately 1 Mb in size. These clusters contain maternally and paternally imprinted genes. More than 80% of known imprinted genes are clustered into 16 genomic regions that contain two or more genes (Barlow, 2011). Several clusters show considerable tissue-specific and developmental regulation of their imprinted gene expression (Sasaki et al., 1992). For some of the clusters, imprinting control elements have been identified, which are involved in the regulation of the expression of the genes within the cluster. Imprinted genes are characterized by specific sites called differentially methylated domains (DMD). These are generally 1–5 kb in size (Reinhart, Eljanne, & Chaillet, 2002). Gametic DMDs refer to DMDs displaying differential methylation between the sperm and the oocyte. Within a DMD, one parental allele is methylated on all/most of CpG dinucleotides and the other is unmethylated on all/most CpGs. Outside the DMDs, the same levels of methylation are found on both alleles.

During germ cell differentiation and maturation, gametic DNA methylation marks of imprinted genes are reprogrammed. From observations in mouse embryos, it was described that, at the time of migration of primordial germ cells into the genital ridge, preexisting methylation marks were erased and that this might be an active process (Hajkova et al., 2002). After sex determination of the embryo, and during germ cell differentiation into oocytes or sperm, methylation marks are reestablished (Reik, Dean, & Walter, 2001). The remethylation dynamic in the gametic DMDs at different stages of gametogenesis has been defined. Paternal imprints were found to be established in diploid gonocytes before the onset of meiosis, whereas maternal imprints were found to be established in growing oocytes arrested in the diplotene stage of meiosis (Lucifero, Mertineit, Clarke, Bestor, & Trasler, 2002). This process is highly complex and tightly regulated. It should prevent the genetic transmission of the epigenetic modifications having occurred during life in the parental genomes. However, some paternal or maternal methylation marks escape reprogramming and are still found in the germline, transmitted, through fertilization, to the zygote and maintained throughout embryonic development. Of importance, the gametic DMDs escape the global genome-wide epigenetic reprogramming occurring in preimplantation embryos (Sasaki & Matsui, 2008).

Establishment and maintenance of DNA methylation are performed by a family of so-called DNA methyl transferases (DNMTs) (Bird, 2002). Targeted deletion of specific DNMT genes in mice has shown that some members of the DNMT family (in particular DNMT1, 3a, and L) are involved in the control of methylation at imprinted loci (Holmes & Soloway, 2006).

4. ENVIRONMENTAL CHANGES AFFECT IMPRINTING

Imprinted genes, playing a critical role in early growth and development, are particularly sensitive to the environment during prenatal life or early childhood. Furthermore, imprinting reprogramming in germ cells, occurring mostly *in utero*, may be the target of dysregulations with consequences on the next generation.

Numerous studies have explored the safety of assisted reproductive technologies by testing the possible effects of the *in vitro* procedures on the embryo gene imprinting in mice. Several reports have described that *in vitro*-cultured embryos may display imprinting pattern changes (Calle et al., 2012). Some culture media were shown to have effects on the methylation and expression of genes in the embryos and, after implantation, in extraembryonic tissues (Mann et al., 2004; Shi & Haaf, 2002). By analyzing different culture media commercialized for embryo culture, it was reported that they all induced imprinted methylation loss, as compared to *in vivo*-derived embryos (Market-Velker, Fernandes, & Mann, 2010).

Nutritional changes during pregnancy were also found to affect the methylation of imprinted genes in mice (Radford et al., 2012) and in humans. A famous example is the Hunger Winter Family Study showing that prenatal exposure to famine was associated with increased neonatal adiposity and poor health of the offspring with some indication of an epigenetic change at the imprinted gene *IGF2* (Heijmans et al., 2008).

The idea that the prenatal and early-life environment may affect imprinted genes and be responsible of the development of human diseases is now emerging more and more, with additional hypothesis linking pathologies such as intrauterine growth retardation or preeclampsia to imprinted gene dysregulation (Lim & Ferguson-Smith, 2010).

5. IMPRINTING DEFECTS AND MALE INFERTILITY

Imprinting defects have been identified in various groups of infertile men. Houshdaran et al. (2007) demonstrated that poor semen parameters were linked with increased DNA methylation at several imprinted loci, possibly due to a defect in erasure and/or methylation during imprinting reprogramming in the male germline. Kobayashi et al. (2007) examined the methylation pattern of seven imprinted genes, in a cohort of infertile men. They reported that 14.4% of the patients studied exhibited an abnormal paternal imprinting and 20.6% an abnormal maternal imprinting, whereas global DNA methylation was normal, suggesting that abnormalities were specific to imprinted loci. Poplinski, Tüttelmann, Kanber, Horsthemke, and Gromoll (2009) compared the methylation status of the *H19/IGF2* imprinting control region 1 (ICR1) and of *Peg1/Mest* imprinted locus in men with idiopathic infertility compared to healthy donor. Normozoospermic men displayed high methylation at the *H19/IGF2* ICR1 locus and low methylation at the *Peg1/Mest* locus, while the opposite was found in men with low sperm concentration. Similarly, Boissonnas et al. (2010) found that many patients with teratozoospermia and oligoasthenoteratozoospermia exhibited hypomethylation at variable CpG islands of the *H19* imprinted locus.

6. ENDOCRINE DISRUPTORS AND MALE INFERTILITY

In the past century, a decline in sperm counts has been documented in young healthy men of industrialized countries, which could be responsible for the currently observed decline in fertility rates (Carlsen, Giwercman, Keiding, & Skakkebaek, 1992; Roeleveld & Bretveld, 2008). A causative link between male infertility and exposure to various deleterious agents was suggested (Anderson, 2005). Environmental factors such as radioactivity, chemicals, and toxins have shown a potential for inducing epigenetic defects (Anway, Cupp, Uzumcu, & Skinner, 2005). EDs are molecules that can mimic estrogens, antiestrogens, or antiandrogens. They are used as pesticides and fungicides, and their release in the environment is considered potentially hazardous to human development and/or reproduction. EDs may specifically affect reproductive pathways through modulation of the DNA methylation pattern and consequent changes in gene expression. In an exposed pregnant mother, *in utero* effects on the early embryo germline epigenetic reprogramming may induce an abnormal phenotype, such as infertility, in the offspring (Skinner, 2007). Studies performed in humans reported that exposure to pesticides may decrease spermatogenesis and male fertility (Roeleveld & Bretveld, 2008). Furthermore, a significant association was found between organochlorine concentrations in the semen of male volunteers and sperm quality (Pant et al., 2007).

6.1. Effects of vinclozolin on imprinting and fertility

VCZ (3-(3,5-dichlorophenyl)-5methyl-5-vinyl-1,3-oxazolidine-2,4-dione), a fungicide used to treat fruits and vegetables, was found to exert significant antiandrogenic effects. When administered to pregnant female mice during the period of fetal gonadal sex determination, that is, from days 13 to 17 of pregnancy (Buckley, Willingham, Agras, & Baskin, 2006), VCZ was found to affect the offspring. It virilized females, feminized males, and increased the expression of progesterone receptors in both genders (Buckley et al., 2006). VCZ administration during pregnancy also induced decreases in the anogenital distance and in the prostate weight as well hypospadias (Buckley et al., 2006; Elzeinova, Novakova, Buckiova, Kubatova, & Peknicova, 2008; Shimamura et al., 2002). Eventually, VCZ affected spermatogenesis, inducing decreases in sperm number and motility, sperm head abnormalities, and apoptosis in the seminiferous tubules germ cells (Anway et al., 2005; Anway, Leathers, & Skinner, 2006; Anway, Rekow, & Skinner, 2008; Buckley et al., 2006; Shimamura et al., 2002; Elzeinova et al., 2008). In contrast, two other studies performed using the same protocol, that is, VCZ administration to pregnant female rats during the gestational period of gonadal sex determination, failed to demonstrate any change in spermatogenesis. The reason for this discrepancy has not been identified (Inawaka et al., 2009; Schneider, Kaufmann, Buesen, & van Ravenzwaay, 2008).

It is generally admitted that, due to the mechanisms of erasure and reprogramming, abnormal epigenetic states are not transmitted to the next generation. An intriguing feature of VCZ is that the effects on male genital tract and spermatogenesis were found to be transgenerational, extending from F1 to F4 (Anway et al., 2005, 2006, 2008). An outcross of the female offspring of a VCZ-exposed female with a wild-type male had no phenotype, suggesting that the male germline is responsible for the transmission of the phenotype (Anway et al., 2006).

In the mouse studies in which a transgenerational effect of VCZ was observed, the possibility of an epigenetic effect of the ED on the male germline was investigated. A methylation-sensitive restriction enzyme study revealed altered methylation patterns on various DNA fragments, called "imprinted-like gene/DNA sequences" in the F1–F3 offspring sperm (Anway et al., 2005). However, these studies were only preliminary, and it is still not known if these DNA fragments are or not associated with genes exhibiting imprinted (i.e., monoallelic and parent-of-origin-dependent) expression.

In a recent study (Stouder & Paoloni-Giacobino, 2010), the possible deleterious effects of VCZ administration in mice from days 10 to 18 of pregnancy on imprinted genes were analyzed. The study was performed by testing possible methylation defects in the DMDs of two paternally (*H19* and GTL2) and three maternally (PEG1, SNRPN and PEG3) imprinted genes in the sperm as well as in the tail, liver, and skeletal muscle DNAs of the male offspring over three generations.

VCZ was shown to affect the imprinting status of the two paternally (*H19* and GTL2) and of the three maternally (PEG1, SNRPN and PEG3) imprinted genes in the sperm of the offspring. These data corroborate the finding by Anway et al. (2005) who showed that VCZ administration to pregnant female mice altered the methylation patterns on "imprinted-like gene/DNA sequences" in the sperm of the offspring (Anway et al., 2005) and extend it to well-characterized imprinted genes. Outcross experiments, showing no phenotype in the sperm of the F2 offspring, confirmed the results of Anway et al. (2006), suggesting that the male germline is responsible for the transmission of the phenotype. In a previous study, addressing the possible effect on imprinted genes of superovulation, we had observed, in the sperm of superovulated female offspring, methylation disturbances that affected both paternally and maternally methylated genes in 75% or more of the F1 offspring (Stouder, Deutsch, & Paoloni-Giacobino, 2009). The effects of VCZ, described by Stouder and Paoloni-Giacobino (2010), are more marked and affect 100% of the F1 offspring.

In the study of Stouder and Paoloni-Giacobino (2010), the effects of VCZ in the sperm were found to be transgenerational but had disappeared in F3, for three out of five imprinted genes. The possible mechanism of this resistance to reprogramming is not known. One hypothesis is that it is due to modified expressions of genes coding for proteins involved in the epigenetic reprogramming, like DNMTs, that are involved in resetting of the imprints. The partial disappearance of the effects of VCZ in F3 suggests that the resistance to reprogramming is reversible and little by little eroded by the successive reprogramming periods occurring during each gestation.

Furthermore, a decrease in sperm count that might be a consequence of the sperm imprinting errors was observed in the F1 offspring of VCZ-administered female mice (Stouder & Paoloni-Giacobino, 2010).

This same study (Stouder & Paoloni-Giacobino, 2010) showed, in the somatic cells, two different types of changes depending whether F1 or F2/F3 generations are considered. In the F1 offspring, the methylation pattern of Snrpn was altered in all somatic cells studied, that is, those of the tail, liver, and muscle. The occurrence of this alteration in F1 shows that it is not mediated by the germline. It might be the result of a direct toxic effect of VCZ on somatic cells. The reason why this effect targets *Snrpn* is unknown. The direct alteration of somatic cells was not transmitted to the next generations in the tail and in the liver. In the F2, an alteration in the methylation pattern of Peg3 was observed in the somatic cells of the tail, liver, and skeletal muscle. In the F3, interestingly, this alteration was still observed in the tail and liver. The reason why this effect targets *Peg3* is unknown. The latter gene encodes a zinc-finger protein that is ubiquitously expressed, although at the highest mRNA levels in the placenta, uterus, ovary, testis, and brain (Hiby et al., 2001). The high conservation of Peg3 protein between mice and humans suggests that it is critical for cellular function. *Peg3*$^{+/-}$ mice demonstrated an impaired maternal behavior (Li et al., 1999), an impaired olfactory processing (Swaney, Curley, Champagne, & Keverne, 2007), a lower growth rate, a delayed puberty, and a tendency to become obese (Curley et al., 2005). The deficits observed in *Peg3*$^{+/-}$ mice might be explained by an increased postnatal apoptosis in the neuroanatomical structures that support reproductive behavior and metabolic homoeostasis (Broad, Curley, & Keverne, 2009). Therefore, prenatal exposure to VCZ might affect, in addition to sperm concentration, reproductive behavior and energy balance in the offspring. The effects observed in somatic cells of F2 and F3 offspring are probably transmitted through the germline. We therefore deal with a phenomenon that mimics a DNA mutation, with the important difference, however, that it seems to be reversible.

The observation that VCZ administration to pregnant female mice induces transgenerational alterations in the imprinted status of five canonical paternally and maternally imprinted genes in the sperm of the offspring that are paralleled by a decrease in the sperm concentration (Stouder & Paoloni-Giacobino, 2010) proposes a mechanism for the previously observed effects of VCZ on the rodent reproductive system (Anway et al., 2005, 2006, 2008; Buckley et al., 2006; Elzeinova et al., 2008; Shimamura et al., 2002).

6.2. Effects of methoxychlor on imprinting and fertility

MXC, an ED used as a pesticide, is a synthetic organochlorine derived from DDT [1,1,1-trichloro-2,2-bis(4-methoxyphenyl)ethane], possessing estrogenic, antiestrogenic, and antiandrogenic activities (Alworth et al., 2002; Cummings, 1997; Gaido et al., 2000).

MXC administration in adult male rats has been found to induce abnormalities in the male reproductive tract, affecting testes, prostate, and seminal vesicle development as well as spermatogenesis (Okazaki et al., 2001). MXC was also found to induce an oxidative stress in the testes that has been proposed as a mechanism for its toxicity in this tissue (Vaithinathan, Saradha, & Mathur, 2009).

MXC administration in early pregnancy or during the perinatal and neonatal periods has been found to result in adult-onset abnormalities in both female and male animals. In female rodents, MXC induced reductions in the pregnancy outcome (Swartz & Eroschenko, 1998), in ovarian functions, and in ovulatory rates (Eroschenko, Abuel-Atta, & Grober, 1995; Eroschenko, Swartz, & Ford, 1997) that could be attributed to a possible dysfunction of the hypothalamic–pituitary–ovarian axis. MXC was also found to induce a decrease in the ovarian estrogen receptor beta expression (Armenti, Zama, Passantino, & Uzumcu, 2008). In male rodents, MXC induced a decrease in sexual arousal (Eroschenko, Amstislavsky, Schwabel, & Ingermann, 2002), an increase in sexual maturation (Amstislavsky, Kizilova, Golubitsa, Vasilkova, & Eroschenko, 2004), a decrease in the circulating testosterone level (Amstislavsky et al., 2006), and decreases in testis weight, Sertoli cell number, and spermatogenesis potential (Staub, Hardy, Chapin, Harris, & Johnson, 2002).

MXC, like VCZ, might act by altering the epigenetic programming of the genome. The perinatal exposure to MXC has, indeed, been shown to cause a hypermethylation of the ERb promoter and of 10 other genes in the ovary (Zama & Uzumcu, 2009).

In a recent study (Stouder & Paoloni-Giacobino, 2011), we analyzed the possible direct effects of MXC administration in adult male mice and the possible indirect effects in mice, from days 10 to 18 of pregnancy, on imprinted genes by testing possible methylation defects in the DMDs of two paternally (*H19* and GTL2) and three maternally (PEG+, SNRPN and PEG3) imprinted genes in the sperm as well as in the tail, liver, and skeletal muscle DNAs of the male offspring over three generations.

In adult mice, MXC administration for 8 days did not affect sperm concentration but modified the methylation pattern of four out of the five paternally and maternally imprinted genes tested in the sperm. It is noteworthy that MXC affected specifically the imprinted genes of the germline, leaving untouched those of somatic cells (tail, liver, and skeletal muscle) (Stouder & Paoloni-Giacobino, 2011). MXC administration in adult male rats has been found to induce a decrease in the number of sperm cells in the caudal epididymis (Okazaki et al., 2001).

In pregnant mice, MXC administration during the gestational period of gonadal sex determination decreased the sperm concentration and affected the imprinting status of the two paternally and three maternally imprinted genes tested in the germline of the F1 offspring. The somatic cell (tail, liver, and skeletal muscle) imprinting status was not modified. Since MXC affected only the sperm cells, we can consider that it exerts its damaging effects via the process of reprogramming that is unique to gamete development (Stouder et al., 2009; Stouder & Paoloni-Giacobino, 2011).

The observation that the administration of MXC exerts more toxic effects on sperm imprinting in the embryo than in the adult (Stouder & Paoloni-Giacobino, 2011) might suggest that the imprinting reestablishment occurring after puberty in the last stages of gametogenesis (Lee et al., 2002; Li, Lees-Murdock, Xu, & Walsh, 2004) is less sensitive to the damaging effects of MXC than that occurring during embryogenesis.

The effects of MXC, like those of VCZ, were found to be transgenerational but had already disappeared for one out of five imprinted genes in F2 and totally in F3.

The discrepancy observed between the effects of VCZ and MXC, on the methylation status of sperm imprinted genes, which persisted in the F2 offspring, and the effect of VCZ and MXC on the sperm count, which had already disappeared in the F2 offspring (Stouder & Paoloni-Giacobino, 2011), does not necessarily mean that the decrease in the sperm count observed in the F1 offspring is not related to the changes in the methylation status imprinted genes of the sperm. It suggests that a certain threshold of imprinting unbalance has to be reached to translate into a detectable decrease in spermatogenesis.

A synopsis of the reproductive effects of VCZ and MXC is shown in Table 8.1.

6.3. CpG-specific effects of methoxychlor

A systematic analysis at the CpG level should allow a better understanding of the mechanism of the deleterious effects of MXC. This was done in the study of Stouder and Paoloni-Giacobino (2011), and the results revealed a heterogeneity in, first, the CpG sensitivity to MXC and, second, the CpG resistance to reprogramming. Indeed, first, in F1 offspring sperm, a few CpGs resisted to the MXC in the paternally methylated, whereas 100

Table 8.1 Statistical significance of the methylation changes observed for the different genes, in three generations, for vinclozolin and methoxychlor exposures

VCZ dose: 50 mg/kg/day; period of exposure: D10–18

	Sperm DNA methylation					
	H19	**GTL2/PEG3**	**PEG+/MEST**	**SNRPN**	**PEG3**	**Sperm concentration**
F1	$p<0.001$	$p<0.001$	$p<0.001$	$p<0.001$	$p<0.001$	$p<0.005$
F2	$p<0.001$	$p<0.001$	$p<0.001$	$p<0.001$	$p<0.001$	*
F3	$p<0.001$	*	*	*	$p<0.01$	Not explored

MXC dose: 10 mg/kg/day; period of exposure: D10–18

	Sperm DNA methylation					
	H19	**GTL2/MEG3**	**PEG1/MEST**	**SNRPN**	**PEG3**	**Sperm concentration**
F1	$p<0.001$	$p<0.001$	$p<0.001$	$p<0.001$	$p<0.001$	$p<0.005$
F2	$p<0.01$	$p<0.001$	$p<0.001$	$p<0.001$	*	*
F3	*	*	*	*	*	Not explored

Statistical significance of the methylation changes observed for the different genes tested, in all three generations, as compared to control mice. VCZ, vinclozolin; MXC, methoxychlor. Statistical significance of the sperm concentration changes, as compared to control mice. *, No significant change.

% of the CpGs were affected by the latter in the maternally methylated gene DMDs. This observation suggests that the methylation process in the paternally methylated genes is less sensitive to MXC than the inhibition of remethylation in the maternally methylated genes. Furthermore, the CpGs resisting to MXC in the sperm of adult versus embryo MXC-exposed mice were different. Second, in F2 offspring sperm, if the paternally methylated genes were considered, it could be seen that most of the CpGs of the H19 (four out of five) and a minority of the CpGs of GTL2 (4 out of 15) resisted to reprogramming. If the maternally methylated genes were considered, all the CpGs of Peg1, most of the CpGs of Snrpn (three out of four), and a minority of the CpGs of PEG3 (two out of six) resisted to reprogramming. Therefore, the dichotomy observed between paternally and maternally methylated genes in the sensitivity to MXC is not observed when the resistance to reprogramming is considered, suggesting a different mechanism for the latter. Li et al. (2004) had shown that a relatively high level of methylation was retained in GTL2 and H19 of e12.5 germ cells when the methylation of other imprinted genes was totally removed. It could, therefore, be proposed that a resistance to reprogramming occurs when the erasure step of reprogramming is incomplete. Our results, obtained on a different genetic background, showing that most of the CpGs of the H19 but a minority of the CpGs of GTL2 resisted to reprogramming are not in line with this hypothesis. It has been postulated that, in male and female germ cells, epigenetic marks other than DNA methylation, perhaps those based on histone modifications, are not removed during reprogramming, allowing parental alleles to remember their origin (Arnaud, 2010; Lucifero et al., 2004; Morgan, Santos, Green, Dean, & Reik, 2005). If MXC affects histones, it might create an epigenetic mark that, by resisting to reprogramming, might explain why its effects for some CpGs are transgenerational. The GTL2 DMD of the silent paternal allele is hypoacetylated on H3 and H4, while the DLK1 DMD of the active maternal allele is highly acetylated on both histones, indicating that both histone acetylation and DNA methylation are involved in maintaining the imprinting of GTL2-DLK1 genes (Carr, Yevtodiyenko, Schmidt, & Schmidt, 2007). It would be interesting to study possible effects of MXC on H3 and H4. The heterogeneity of the responses to MXC of the various CpGs tested suggests that, in addition to DNA methylation, MXC might affect specific DNMTs or histone marks.

7. CONCLUSION AND PERSPECTIVES

The interest in the effects of environmental pollutants on imprinted gene methylation patterns and on the reproductive tract is relatively recent, and a review like this one shows how much still needs to be done in this field.

I would like to focus on two major domains that need to be explored to make gene methylation studies more interpretable.

First, the mechanisms involved in the control of DNA methylation at the DMDs of imprinted genes should be actively investigated. In the studies of Stouder and Paoloni-Giacobino (2011) and Stouder and Paoloni-Giacobino (2010), VCZ and MXC were found to affect all imprinted genes studied in the sperm. This apparent lack of specificity was not observed at the level of individual CpGs of the DMDs. Indeed, MXC affected some but not all CpGs and the pattern was different whether the exposure occurred *in utero* or in adulthood. Furthermore, an inter-CpG heterogeneity was observed in the resistance to reprogramming. These observations imply a very complex mechanism of DNA methylation/demethylation control at the CpG level. The factors that attracting a specific member of the DNMT family to a specific CpG imply, in particular, the DNA sequence, the local arrangement of the CpGs, and the chromatin structure, that is, the local arrangement of the histone marks and *trans*-acting proteins or RNAs. These factors would change during development and during the process of reprogramming.

Second, the possible causal relationship, after exposure to a pollutant, between an observed change in the methylation pattern of imprinted genes in sperm and a phenotype, like hypospermia/oligospermia is difficult to demonstrate. Targeted gene deletion models should be created showing, for instance, that the abolition of the methylation change induced by a pollutant erases the reproductive phenotype. Until the precise mechanism of DNA methylation control is elucidated, it will not be possible to create such animal models.

The challenge is therefore great in the type of studies described in this chapter but the task is important: understanding epigenetic implication in the possible disturbances of the reproductive system.

REFERENCES

Alworth, L. C., Howdeshell, K. L., Ruhlen, R. L., Day, J. K., Lubahn, D. B., Huang, T. H., et al. (2002). Uterine responsiveness to estradiol and DNA methylation are altered by fetal exposure to diethylstilbestrol and methoxychlor in CD-1 mice: Effects of low versus high doses. *Toxicology and Applied Pharmacology, 183*, 10–22.

Amstislavsky, S. Y., Amstislavskaya, T. G., Amstislavsky, V. S., Tibeikina, M. A., Osipov, K. V., & Eroschenko, V. P. (2006). Reproductive abnormalities in adult male mice following preimplantation exposures to estradiol or pesticide methoxychlor. *Reproductive Toxicology, 21*, 154–159.

Amstislavsky, S. Y., Kizilova, E. A., Golubitsa, A. N., Vasilkova, A. A., & Eroschenko, V. P. (2004). Preimplantation exposures of murine embryos to estradiol or methoxychlor change postnatal development. *Reproductive Toxicology, 18*, 103–108.

Anderson, D. (2005). Male-mediated developmental toxicity. *Toxicology and Applied Pharmacology, 207*, 506–513.

Anway, M. D., Cupp, A. S., Uzumcu, M., & Skinner, M. K. (2005). Epigenetic transgenerational actions of endocrine disruptors and male fertility. *Science, 308*, 1466–1469.

Anway, M. D., Leathers, C., & Skinner, M. K. (2006). Endocrine disruptor vinclozolin induced epigenetic transgenerational adult-onset disease. *Endocrinology, 147*, 5515–5523.

Anway, M. D., Rekow, S. S., & Skinner, M. K. (2008). Comparative anti-androgenic actions of vinclozolin and flutamide on transgenerational adult onset disease and spermatogenesis. *Reproductive Toxicology, 26*, 100–106.

Armenti, A. E., Zama, A. M., Passantino, L., & Uzumcu, M. (2008). Developmental methoxychlor exposure affects multiple reproductive parameters and ovarian folliculogenesis and gene expression in adult rats. *Toxicology and Applied Pharmacology, 233*, 286–296.

Arnaud, P. (2010). Genomic imprinting in germ cells: Imprints are under control. *Reproduction, 140*, 411–423.

Barlow, D. P. (2011). Genomic imprinting: A mammalian epigenetic discovery model. *Annual Review of Genetics, 45*, 379–403.

Bird, A. (2002). DNA methylation patterns and epigenetic memory. *Genes and Development, 16*, 6–21.

Boissonnas, C. C., Abdalaoui, H. E., Haelewyn, V., Fauque, P., Dupont, J. M., Gut, I., et al. (2010). Specific epigenetic alterations of IGF2-H19 locus in spermatozoa from infertile men. *European Journal of Human Genetics, 18*, 73–80.

Broad, K. D., Curley, J. P., & Keverne, E. B. (2009). Increased apoptosis during neonatal brain development underlies the adult behavioral deficits seen in mice lacking a functional paternally expressed gene 3 (Peg3). *Developmental Neurobiology, 69*, 314–325.

Buckley, J., Willingham, E., Agras, K., & Baskin, L. S. (2006). Embryonic exposure to the fungicide vinclozolin causes virilization of females and alteration of progesterone receptor expression in vivo: An experimental study in mice. *Environmental Health, 21*, 4.

Calle, A., Fernandez-Gonzalez, R., Ramos-Ibeas, P., Laguna-Barraza, R., Perez-Cerezales, S., Bermejo-Alvarez, P., et al. (2012). Long-term and transgenerational effects of in vitro culture on mouse embryos. *Theriogenology, 77*, 785–793.

Carlsen, E., Giwercman, A., Keiding, N., & Skakkebaek, N. E. (1992). Evidence for decreasing quality of semen during past 50 years. *British Medical Journal, 305*, 609–613.

Carr, M. S., Yevtodiyenko, A., Schmidt, C. L., & Schmidt, J. V. (2007). Allele-specific histone modifications regulate expression of the Dlk1-Gtl2 imprinted domain. *Genomics, 89*, 280–290.

Cummings, A. M. (1997). Methoxychlor as a model for environmental estrogens. *Critical Reviews in Toxicology, 27*, 367–379.

Curley, J. P., Pinnock, S. B., Dickson, S. L., Thresher, R., Miyoshi, N., Surani, M. A., et al. (2005). Increased body fat in mice with a targeted mutation of the paternally expressed imprinted gene Peg3. *The FASEB Journal, 19*, 1302–1304.

Elzeinova, F., Novakova, V., Buckiova, D., Kubatova, A., & Peknicova, J. (2008). Effect of low dose of vinclozolin on reproductive tract development and sperm parameters in CD1 outbred mice. *Reproductive Toxicology, 26*, 231–238.

Eroschenko, V. P., Abuel-Atta, A. A., & Grober, M. S. (1995). Neonatal exposures to technical methoxychlor alters ovaries in adult mice. *Reproductive Toxicology, 9*, 379–387.

Eroschenko, V. P., Amstislavsky, S. Y., Schwabel, H., & Ingermann, R. L. (2002). Altered behaviors in male mice, male quail, and salamander larvae following early exposures to the estrogenic pesticide methoxychlor. *Neurotoxicology and Teratology, 24*, 29–36.

Eroschenko, V. P., Swartz, W. J., & Ford, L. C. (1997). Decreased superovulation in adult mice following neonatal exposures to technical methoxychlor. *Reproductive Toxicology, 11*, 807–814.

Gaido, K. W., Maness, S. C., McDonnell, D. P., Dehal, S. S., Kupfer, D., & Safe, S. (2000). Interaction of methoxychlor and related compounds with estrogen receptor alpha and beta, and androgen receptor: Structure-activity studies. *Molecular Pharmacology, 58*, 852–858.

Hajkova, P., Erhardt, S., Lane, N., Haaf, T., El-Maarri, O., Reik, W., et al. (2002). Epigenetic reprogramming in mouse primordial germ cells. *Mechanisms of Development, 117*, 15–23.

Heijmans, B. T., Tobi, E. W., Stein, A. D., Putter, H., Blauw, G. J., Susser, E. S., et al. (2008). Persistent epigenetic differences associated with prenatal exposure to famine in humans. *Proceedings of the National Academy of Sciences of the United States of America, 105*, 17046–17049.

Hiby, S. E., Lough, M., Keverne, E. B., Surani, M. A., Loke, Y. W., & King, A. (2001). Paternal monoallelic expression of PEG3 in the human placenta. *Human Molecular Genetics, 10*, 1093–1100.

Holmes, R., & Soloway, P. D. (2006). Regulation of imprinted DNA methylation. *Cytogenetic and Genome Research, 113*, 122–129.

Houshdaran, S., Cortessis, V. K., Siegmund, K., Yang, A., Laird, P. W., & Skolt, R. Z. (2007). Widespread epigenetic abnormalities suggest a broad DNA methylation erasure defect in abnormal human sperm. *PLoS One*, *2*, e1289.

Inawaka, K., Kawabe, M., Takahashi, S., Doi, Y., Tomigahara, Y., Tarui, H., et al. (2009). Maternal exposure to anti-androgenic compounds, vinclozolin, flutamide and procymidone, has no effects on spermatogenesis and DNA methylation in male rats of subsequent generations. *Toxicology and Applied Pharmacology*, *237*, 178–187.

Jirtle, R. L., & Skinner, M. K. (2007). Environmental epigenomics and disease susceptibility. *Nature Reviews Genetics*, *8*, 253–262.

Kobayashi, H., Sato, A., Otsu, E., Hiura, H., Tomatsu, C., Utsunomiya, T., et al. (2007). Aberrant DNA methylation of imprinted loci in sperm from oligospermic patients. *Human Molecular Genetics*, *16*, 2542–2551.

Lee, J., Inoue, K., Ono, R., Ogonuki, N., Kohda, T., Kaneko-Ishino, T., et al. (2002). Erasing genomic imprinting memory in mouse clone embryos produced from day 11.5 primordial germ cells. *Development*, *129*, 1807–1817.

Li, L., Keverne, E. B., Aparicio, S. A., Ishino, F., Barton, S. C., & Surani, M. A. (1999). Regulation of maternal behavior and offspring growth by paternally expressed Peg3. *Science*, *284*(5412), 330–333.

Li, J. Y., Lees-Murdock, D. J., Xu, G. L., & Walsh, C. P. (2004). Timing of establishment of paternal methylation imprints in the mouse. *Genomics*, *84*, 952–960.

Lim, A. L., & Ferguson-Smith, A. C. (2010). Genomic imprinting effects in a compromised in utero environment: Implications for a healthy pregnancy. *Seminars in Cell and Developmental Biology*, *21*, 201–208.

Lucifero, D., Chaillet, J. R., & Trasler, J. M. (2004). Potential significance of genomic imprinting defects for reproduction and assisted reproductive technology. *Human Reproduction Update*, *10*, 3–18.

Lucifero, D., Mertineit, C., Clarke, H. J., Bestor, T. H., & Trasler, J. M. (2002). Methylation dynamics of imprinted genes in mouse germ cells. *Genomics*, *79*, 530–538.

Luedi, P. P., Hartemink, A. J., & Jirtle, R. L. (2005). Genome-wide prediction of imprinted murine genes. *Genome Research*, *15*, 875–884.

Mann, M. R., Lee, S. S., Doherty, A. S., Verona, R. I., Nolen, L. D., Schultz, R. M., et al. (2004). Selective loss of imprinting in the placenta following preimplantation development in culture. *Development*, *131*, 3727–3735.

Market-Velker, B. A., Fernandes, A. D., & Mann, M. R. (2010). Side-by-side comparison of five commercial media systems in a mouse model: Suboptimal in vitro culture interferes with imprint maintenance. *Biology of Reproduction*, *83*, 938–950.

Morgan, H. D., Santos, F., Green, K., Dean, W., & Reik, W. (2005). Epigenetic reprogramming in mammals. *Human Molecular Genetics*, *14*, R47–R58.

Okazaki, K., Okazaki, S., Nishimura, S., Nakamura, H., Kitamura, Y., Hatayama, K., et al. (2001). A repeated 28-day oral dose toxicity study of methoxychlor in rats, based on the 'enhanced OECD test guideline 407' for screening endocrine-disrupting chemicals. *Archives of Toxicology*, *75*, 513–521.

Pant, N., Kumar, R., Mathur, N., Srivastava, S. P., Saxena, D. K., & Gujrati, V. R. (2007). Chlorinated pesticide concentration in semen of fertile and infertile men and correlation with sperm quality. *Environmental Toxicology and Pharmacology*, *23*, 135–139.

Poplinski, A., Tüttelmann, F., Kanber, D., Horsthemke, B., & Gromoll, J. (2009). Idiopathic male infertility is strongly associated with aberrant methylation of MEST and IGF2/H19 ICR1. *International Journal of Andrology*, *33*, 642–649.

Radford, E. J., Isganaitis, E., Jimenez-Chillaron, J., Schroeder, J., Molla, M., Andrews, S., et al. (2012). An unbiased assessment of the role of imprinted genes in an intergenerational model of developmental programming. *PLoS Genetics*, *8*, e1002605.

Reik, W., Dean, W., & Walter, J. (2001). Epigenetic reprogramming in mammalian development. *Science, 293*, 1089–1093.

Reinhart, B., Eljanne, M., & Chaillet, J. R. (2002). Shared role for differentially methylated domains of imprinted genes. *Molecular and Cellular Biology, 22*, 2089–2098.

Roeleveld, N., & Bretveld, R. (2008). The impact of pesticides on male fertility. *Current Opinion in Obstetrics and Gynecology, 20*, 229–233.

Sasaki, H., Jones, P. A., Chaillet, J. R., Ferguson-Smith, A. C., Barton, S. C., Reik, W., et al. (1992). Parental imprinting: Potentially active chromatin of the repressed maternal allele of the mouse insulin-like growth factor II (*Igf2*) gene. *Genes and Development, 6*, 1843–1856.

Sasaki, H., & Matsui, Y. (2008). Epigenetic events in mammalian germ-cell development: Reprogramming and beyond. *Nature Reviews Genetics, 9*, 129–140.

Schneider, S., Kaufmann, W., Buesen, R., & van Ravenzwaay, B. (2008). Vinclozolin—The lack of a transgenerational effect after oral maternal exposure during organogenesis. *Reproductive Toxicology, 25*, 352–360.

Shi, W., & Haaf, T. (2002). Aberrant methylation patterns at the two-cell stage as an indicator of early developmental failure. *Molecular Reproduction and Development, 63*, 329–334.

Shimamura, M., Kodaira, K., Kenichi, H., Ishimoto, Y., Tamura, H., & Iguchi, T. (2002). Comparison of antiandrogenic activities of vinclozolin and D, L-camphorquinone in androgen receptor gene transcription assay in vitro and mouse in utero exposure assay in vivo. *Toxicology, 174*, 97–107.

Skinner, M. K. (2007). Endocrine disruptors and epigenetic transgenerational disease etiology. *Pediatric Research, 61*, 48R–50R.

Smallwood, S. A., & Kelsey, G. (2012). De novo DNA methylation: A germ cell perspective. *Trends in Genetics, 28*, 33–42.

Staub, C., Hardy, V. B., Chapin, R. E., Harris, M. W., & Johnson, L. (2002). The hidden effect of estrogenic/antiandrogenic methoxychlor on spermatogenesis. *Toxicology and Applied Pharmacology, 180*, 129–135.

Stouder, C., Deutsch, S., & Paoloni-Giacobino, A. (2009). Superovulation in mice alters the methylation pattern of imprinted genes in the sperm of the offspring. *Reproductive Toxicology, 28*, 536–541.

Stouder, C., & Paoloni-Giacobino, A. (2010). Transgenerational effects of the endocrine disruptor vinclozolin on the methylation pattern of imprinted genes in the mouse sperm. *Reproduction, 139*, 373–379.

Stouder, C., & Paoloni-Giacobino, A. (2011). Specific transgenerational imprinting effects of the endocrine disruptor methoxychlor on male gametes. *Reproduction, 141*, 207–216.

Swaney, W. T., Curley, J. P., Champagne, F. A., & Keverne, E. B. (2007). Genomic imprinting mediates sexual experience-dependent olfactory learning in male mice. *Proceedings of the National Academy of Sciences of the United States of America, 104*, 6084–6089.

Swartz, W. J., & Eroschenko, V. P. (1998). Neonatal exposure to technical methoxychlor alters pregnancy outcome in female mice. *Reproductive Toxicology, 12*, 565–573.

Tang, W. Y., & Ho, S. M. (2007). Epigenetic reprogramming and imprinting in origins of disease. *Reviews in Endocrine and Metabolic Disorders, 8*, 173–182.

Vaithinathan, S., Saradha, B., & Mathur, P. P. (2009). Methoxychlor-induced alteration in the levels of HSP70 and clusterin is accompanied with oxidative stress in adult rat testis. *Journal of Biochemical and Molecular Toxicology, 23*, 29–35.

Zama, A. M., & Uzumcu, M. (2009). Fetal and neonatal exposure to the endocrine disruptor methoxychlor causes epigenetic alterations in adult ovarian genes. *Endocrinology, 150*, 4681–4691.

CHAPTER NINE

Nuclear Receptor Profiling of Bisphenol-A and Its Halogenated Analogues

Vanessa Delfosse[*,†,‡], **Marina Grimaldi**[§,¶,**,††], **Albane le Maire**[*,†,‡], **William Bourguet**[*,†,‡,1], **Patrick Balaguer**[§,¶,**,††,1]

[*]Centre de Biochimie Structurale, Institut National de la Santé et de la Recherche Médicale U1054, Montpellier, France
[†]Centre National de la Recherche Scientifique, Unité Mixte de Recherche 5048,
[‡]Universités Montpellier 1 and 2, Montpellier, France
[§]Institut de Recherche en Cancérologie de Montpellier,Montpellier, France
[¶]Institut National de la Santé et de la Recherche Médicale U896, Montpellier, France
[**]Institut régional du Cancer de Montpellier, Montpellier, France
[††]Universités Montpellier 1, Montpellier, France
[1]Corresponding authors: e-mail address: bourguet@cbs.cnrs.fr; patrick.balaguer@icm.unicancer.fr

Contents

1. Introduction 230
2. Estrogen Receptors 232
   2.1 ERs activity of bisphenols 233
   2.2 Structures of BP-bound ERs 233
3. Estrogen-Related Receptor γ 236
   3.1 ERRγ activity of bisphenols 237
   3.2 Structural basis of BPs interaction with ERRγ 237
4. Androgen Receptor 239
   4.1 AR activity of bisphenols 239
5. Peroxysome Proliferator-Activated Receptor γ 240
   5.1 PPARγ activity of bisphenols 240
   5.2 Structural basis of halogenated bisphenols action on PPARγ 241
6. Thyroid Receptors 243
   6.1 TR activity of bisphenols 243
7. Pregnane X Receptor 243
   7.1 Pregnane X activity of bisphenols 244
8. Conclusions 245
Acknowledgments 245
References 246

Abstract

Bisphenol-A (BPA) is one of the highest-volume chemicals produced worldwide and the widespread exposure of individuals to BPA is suspected to affect a variety of

Vitamins and Hormones, Volume 94
ISSN 0083-6729
http://dx.doi.org/10.1016/B978-0-12-800095-3.00009-2

physiological functions, including reproduction, development, and metabolism. Its estrogenic activity has been well documented in the last 15 years. In addition to estrogen receptors, BPA has been also shown to bind to and activate the estrogen-related receptor γ and pregnane X receptor and inhibit the androgen receptor. Halogenated BPAs were also shown to activate the peroxisome proliferator-activated receptor γ and inhibit thyroid hormone receptors. In this chapter, we review recent studies shedding light on the structural and molecular mechanisms by which BPA and its halogenated derivatives interfere with nuclear hormone receptor signaling. These data provide guidelines for the development of safer substitutes devoid of hormonal activity and may help environmental risk assessment.

1. INTRODUCTION

Human nuclear hormone receptors (NHRs) are a family of 48 transcription factors, many of which have been shown to be activated by ligands. NHRs regulate cognate gene networks involved in key physiological functions such as cell growth and differentiation, development, homeostasis, or metabolism (Germain, Staels, Dacquet, Spedding, & Laudet, 2006; Gronemeyer, Gustafsson, & Laudet, 2004). As a consequence, inappropriate exposure to environmental pollutants often leads to proliferative, reproductive, and metabolic diseases, including hormonal cancers, infertility, obesity, or diabetes. NHRs are modular proteins composed of several domains, most notably an N-terminal domain, which harbors a ligand-independent activation function (AF-1), a central DNA-binding domain (DBD), and a C-terminal ligand-binding domain (LBD) hosting a ligand-dependent transcriptional activation function (AF-2) (Gronemeyer et al., 2004). In the absence of the cognate ligand, some NHRs are located in the nucleus, bind to the DNA response elements of their target genes, and recruit corepressors, while others are located in the cytoplasm in an inactive complex with chaperones. Ligand binding induces major structural alterations of the receptor LBDs, leading to (1) destabilization of corepressor or chaperone interfaces, (2) exposure of nuclear localization signals to allow nuclear translocation and DNA binding of cytoplasmic receptors, and (3) recruitment of coactivators triggering gene transcription through chromatin remodeling and activation of the general transcription machinery. The crystal structures of many NHR LBDs have been determined, revealing a conserved core of 12 α-helices (H1–H12) and a short two-stranded antiparallel β-sheet (S1 and S2) arranged into a three-layered sandwich fold. This arrangement generates a mostly hydrophobic cavity in the lower half of the domain, which can accommodate the cognate ligand. In all hormone-bound LBD structures, the ligand-binding pocket (LBP) is sealed by helix H12. This conformation is specifically induced by the binding of hormones or synthetic agonists and is referred to as the "active conformation" because it allows the dissociation of corepressors and favors the recruitment of transcriptional coactivators (Bourguet, Germain, & Gronemeyer, 2000; Pike, 2006; Renaud & Moras, 2000). It is noteworthy that this conformational state can also be achieved by some constitutively active orphan receptors for which no natural ligand has been identified. In this active form, helices H3, H4, and H12 define a hydrophobic binding groove for short LxxLL helical motifs (L stands for leucine and x for any amino acid) found within coactivators. In contrast to agonist binding, interaction with antagonists prevents the correct positioning of helix H12, thus avoiding association with the LxxLL motifs of coactivators (Bourguet et al., 2000; Pike, 2006; Renaud & Moras, 2000). The LBD also contributes to the modulation of the N-terminal AF-1 through interdomain cross talk so that both AF-1 and AF-2 domains can recruit a range of coregulatory proteins and act individually or in a synergistic manner (Benecke, Chambon, & Gronemeyer, 2000; Bommer, Benecke, Gronemeyer, & Rochette-Egly, 2002; Wilson, 2011). The precise structural basis of this interdomain communication is unknown, as no 3D structure of an entire NR has been obtained.

Bisphenol-A (BPA) is one of the highest-volume chemicals produced worldwide, with over 6 billion pounds produced each year. BPA enters into the composition of polycarbonate plastic, epoxy resins used in metallic food cans, dentistry sealants, and thermal paper (Vandenberg, Maffini, Sonnenschein, Rubin, & Soto, 2009).

Halogenated derivatives of BPA, which feature bromine or chlorine substituents on the phenolic rings, are used as flame retardants. Tetrabromobisphenol-A (TBBPA) is mainly used as a flame retardant to protect computer motherboards and other electronic equipment. Its production is currently estimated around 200,000 tons/year, and its presence has been reported in the environment (de Wit, Herzke, & Vorkamp, 2010) and in wildlife (Darnerud, 2003). Tetrachlorobisphenol-A (TCBPA) has also been reported to be used as a flame retardant but in much lower quantities than TBBPA (<10,000 tons/year) (Chu, Haffner, & Letcher, 2005). The presence of TCBPA and that of lower chlorinated analogues (monoCBPA, diCBPA, and triCBPA) in environmental samples has been unequivocally demonstrated (Fukazawa, Hoshino, Shiozawa, Matsushita, & Terao, 2001; Gallart-Ayala, Nunez, Moyano, &

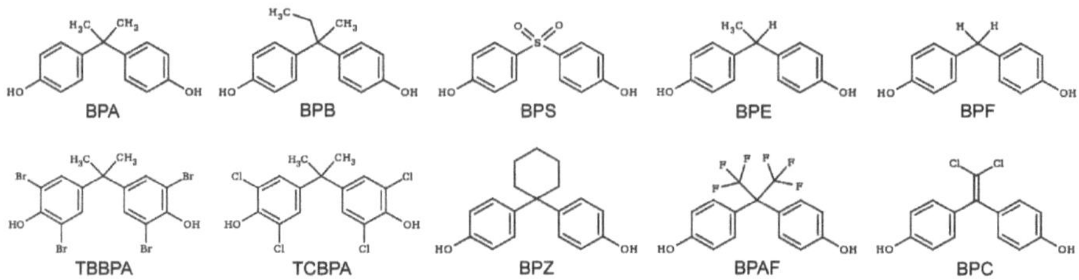

Figure 9.1 Chemical structures of some bisphenols described in this study.

Galceran, 2010; Liu, Zhao, Quan, Zhang, & Chen, 2009). Contrary to TBBPA, and given the low levels of production of TCBPA, the origin of most chlorinated BPA in the environment is more likely the chlorination of BPA than the dechlorination of TCBPA (Fig. 9.1).

BPA or its halogenated derivatives have been shown to target several NHRs including the estrogen receptors (ERα and β), the androgen receptor (AR), the estrogen-related receptor γ (ERRγ), the thyroid hormone (TH) receptors (TRα and β), the pregnane X receptor (PXR), and the peroxisome proliferator-activated receptors (PPARα, γ, and δ). The crystal structures of ERα and ERRγ in complex with BPA and of PPARγ bound to TBBPA or TCBPA have been reported recently. Here, we review recent studies showing the ways in which BPA and halogenated BPAs bind to and activate NHRs.

2. ESTROGEN RECEPTORS

ERα and ERβ are receptors for the sex hormone, 17β-estradiol (E_2), which play important roles in the growth and maintenance of a diverse range of tissues such as the mammary gland, uterus, bones, or the cardiovascular system. Both ERs are widely distributed throughout the body, displaying distinct but overlapping expression patterns in a variety of tissues (Couse & Korach, 1999). ERα is expressed primarily in the uterus, liver, kidney, and heart, whereas ERβ is expressed primarily in the ovary, prostate, lung, gastrointestinal tract, bladder, and hematopoietic and central nervous systems (Kuiper et al., 1997). However, ERα and ERβ are coexpressed in a number of tissues including the mammary gland, thyroid, adrenal, bones, and some regions of the brain. Although ERα and ERβ share similar mechanisms of action, several differences in the transcriptional abilities of each receptor and distinct phenotypes between gene-null animals have been identified, suggesting that these receptors may regulate distinct cellular pathways (Couse & Korach, 1999; Curtis et al., 1996).

2.1. ERs activity of bisphenols

BPA is considered as a weak environmental estrogen because of its relatively low affinity for the nuclear ERs compared with estradiol (10,000–100,000-fold lower affinity) (Delfosse et al., 2012; Kitamura et al., 2005; Paris et al., 2002). Several studies indicated that BPA is a partial agonist (Gould et al., 1998; Routledge, White, Parker, & Sumpter, 2000). In a recent work, we have confirmed that BPA is a selective estrogen receptor modulator that functions in a cell-selective manner (Delfosse et al., 2012). Our data reveal that BPA activity relies mostly on the AF-1 and depends on the cellular context. In this study, we compared BPA with different bisphenols for their affinity and activity using HeLa ERα and ERβ reporter cell lines. For ERα and ERβ affinity, the ranking order was BPC > BPAF > BPB > BPA > BPE > BPF > BPS. For activity, the ranking order is almost the same for ERα and ERβ. It is BPF = BPE = BPS > BPA > BPC = BPAF = BPB, BPC being less active on ERβ than ERα. The potency likely originates from the differential synergy between AF-1 and AF-2 and this synergism is probably more important in the HeLa cellular context for ERβ than for ERα.

In two other studies (Riu, Grimaldi, et al., 2011; Riu, le Maire, et al., 2011), we have characterized the estrogenic activity of TBBPA and TCBPA together with lower halogenated BPA. For brominated analogues, the ranking order of estrogenic potency on ERα and ERβ was monoBBPA > diBBPA > triBBPA, while TBBPA showed no estrogenic activity at all. Chlorinated BPA analogues are at least as potent agonists as BPA for ERα as already published by other groups (Mutou, Ibuki, Terao, Kojima, & Goto, 2006; Takemura et al., 2005). Contrary to brominated BPA, the halogenation degree of chlorinated bisphenols did not decrease their ER potency. Likely due to the lower LBP size of ERβ compared to ERα, chlorinated analogues with the lowest molecular weight (mono- and diCBPA) exhibited the highest agonistic activity on ERβ.

2.2. Structures of BP-bound ERs

Structures of the complexes between ERα and BPA, BPAF, and BPC were recently reported (Delfosse et al., 2012) and their comparison with that of the E_2- and the OHT-bound ERα allowed the description of the binding mode of these BPs and the explanation of their different activities and binding affinities. The structures with BPA, BPAF, and TCBPA display the canonical active conformation with H12 capping the LBP and the

LxxLL-containing coactivator peptide bound to the AF-2 surface (Fig. 9.2A). The structure with BPC displays an antagonist conformation similar to that observed in the OHT-bound structure (PDB code 3ERT) with H12 occupying the coactivator-binding groove (Fig. 9.2A). The structures also reveal two divergent binding mechanisms of BPs. BPA adopts a binding mode reminiscent of that used by E_2 with the two phenol groups hydrogen-bonded to three polar residues located at the two ends of the pocket, namely, H524 (H11) on one side and E353 (H3) and R394 (H5) on the other side (Fig. 9.2B and C). The remaining contacts involve van der Waals interactions. In contrast, BPC is positioned in the pocket so as to draw the phenol ring B into an alternate position as compared with that of the corresponding ring in BPA and TCBPA. A rotation by 180° around the main axis of phenol ring A orients ring B toward H12 (Fig. 9.2D). Finally, in the BPAF complex, each subunit of the ERα homodimer contains one BPAF molecule with the "BPA-like" or "BPC-like" positioning. The different activities of BPs could be attributed to the destabilization of the AF-2 surface as many of the previously recognized ligand–H11-stabilizing interactions observed in the E_2-bound structure are altered in the bisphenol-containing complexes (Bruning et al., 2010; Delfosse et al., 2012; Nettles et al., 2008). One of the key differences resides in the differential interaction of the various ligands with L525. In the E_2-bound structure, E_2 imposes a conformation of this leucine that strengthens a network of van der Waals interactions involving T347, L525, and L536 (Fig. 9.2A). This cluster of interactions is of utmost importance because it holds together helices H3, H11, and the loop preceding H12, thereby stabilizing the AF-2 surface. In the structure with BPA (Fig. 9.2B), the stabilizing interaction between the bisphenol and L525 is absent. This renders L525 more dynamic so that its side chain adopts different conformations in the two subunits of the homodimer. The situation is even worse in the structure with BPC where the side chain of T347 rotates by 180° to form a hydrogen bond with the hydroxyl moiety from the phenol ring B of BPC (Fig. 9.2D). This loss of stabilizing contacts provoked by bisphenols renders the lower part of the ERα LBP more dynamic. Indeed, this portion of LBDs has been previously shown to have some of the characteristics of a molten globule and a large part of the agonistic properties of a ligand relies in its capacity to stabilize this region encompassing the H3/H11 docking surface for H12 in the active conformation (Gee & Katzenellenbogen, 2001; Nagy & Schwabe, 2004). The complete disruption of the hydrophobic cluster by BPC probably accounts for the marked antagonistic character of this

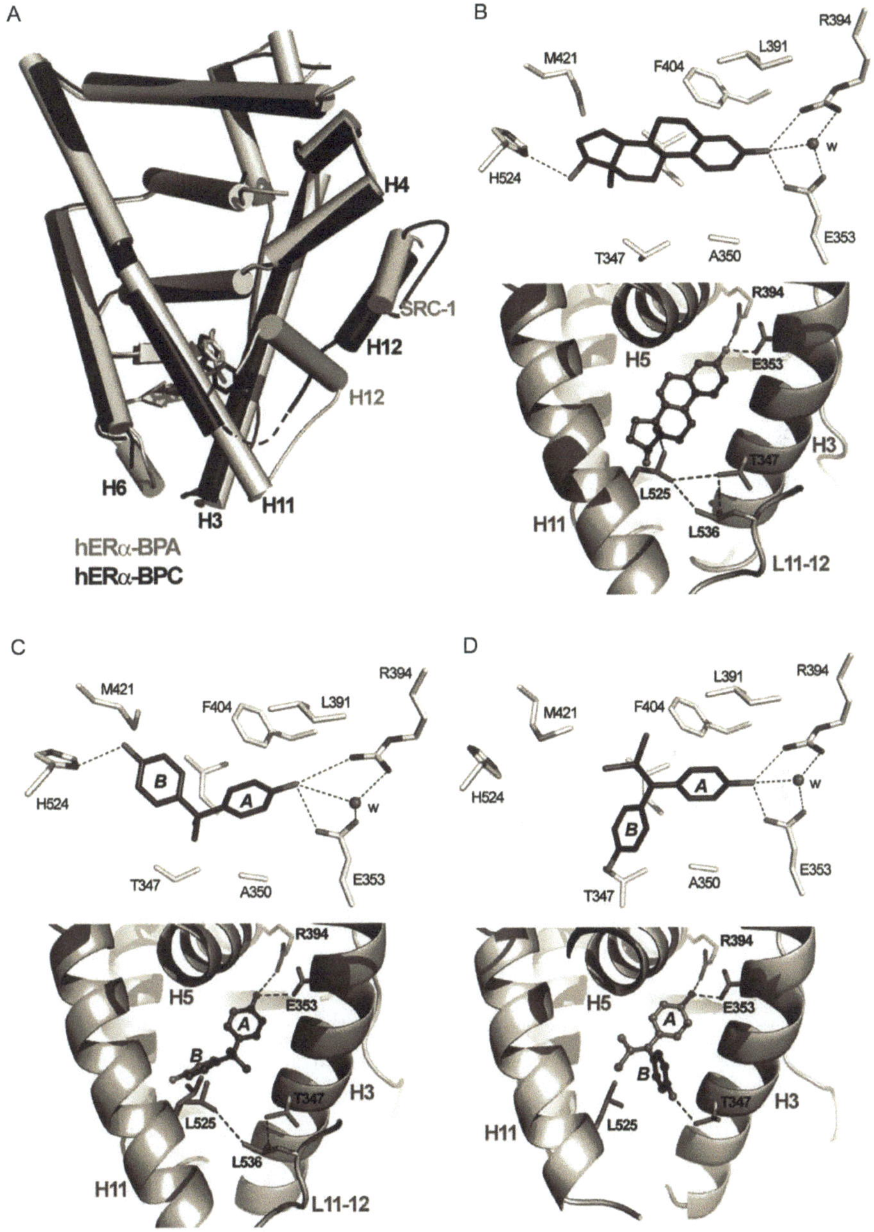

Figure 9.2 Two different binding modes of BPs. (A) The whole structure of the ERα LBD in complex with SRC-1 coactivator peptide and BPA (gray) superimposed on that of ERα LBD bound to BPC (black). The dashed line denotes residues not visible in the electron density map. Interaction networks of E_2 (B), BPA (C), and BPC (D) with ligand-binding pocket residues in ERα. Hydrogen bonds are indicated by dashed lines.
(Continued)

bisphenol. Modeling studies indicated similar binding modes in ERβ (Delfosse et al., 2012).

3. ESTROGEN-RELATED RECEPTOR γ

ERRγ is a member of the ERR subfamily of orphan receptors, which are closely related to ERs (Giguere, 2002) The ERR family includes three members, ERRα, ERRβ, and ERRγ. The three receptors are very similar, with 90% sequence identity in the DBD and more than 60% in the LBD.

ERRγ is expressed in a tissue-restricted manner, for example, very strongly in the mammalian brain during development and then in the brain, lung, and many others tissues during adulthood. In terms of structure, ERRγ is very close to ERs. Sequence alignment reveals a 60% identity in the DBD regions and a moderate similarity (<35%) of the LBDs, consistent with the incapacity of ERRγ to bind E_2 (Horard & Vanacker, 2003). Nevertheless, it has been demonstrated that ERRγ can interfere with estrogen signaling (Giguere, 2002). Indeed, ERs and ERRγ recognize the same DNA-binding elements, share common target genes, and are coexpressed in many tissues (Lu, Kiriyama, Lee, & Giguere, 2001; Vanacker, Pettersson, Gustafsson, & Laudet, 1999).

Exogenous overexpression of ERRγ in prostate cancer cell line results in inhibition of proliferation (Yu, Wang, Ng, Chen, & Chan, 2007). Furthermore, treatment with an ERRβ/γ agonist has been shown to promote this antiproliferative effect, consistent with ERRγ being a favorable prognosis factor (Ariazi & Jordan, 2006). Additionally, several lines of evidence suggest that ERRs play a central role in regulating energy metabolism. Genetic studies in mice reveal that their presence is essential for the generation of energy and related tissue-specific functions, and functional genomics/proteomics studies have associated ERRγ with the control of vast metabolic gene networks, in particular those involved in mitochondrial biogenesis and function (Giguere, 2008). The rise in the incidence of metabolic syndromes correlates with the rise in the use and distribution of industrial chemicals that may play a role in generation of obesity (Baillie-Hamilton, 2002), suggesting that

Figure 9.2—Cont'd For clarity, not all the protein–ligand interactions are depicted. Figures (B–D) also depict the interaction of the various ligands with L525. (B) E_2 strengthens a van der Waals interaction network involving T347 (H3), L525 (H11), and L536 (L11–12). (C) Due to a lack of contact with BPA, L525 is not stabilized and adopts two different conformations. (D) In the BPC-bound ERα structure, T347 rotates by 180° to form a hydrogen bond with the bisphenol, resulting in the disruption of the hydrophobic network.

EDCs and ERRγ may be linked to this epidemic crisis. To date, the ERRγ have not been shown to interact with any physiologically relevant small molecules, suggesting that these receptors manifest constitutive activity (Greschik et al., 2002; Li, Ma, & Wang, 2010), and, indeed, crystallographic analyses of ERRγ indicated that these receptors adopt the transcriptionally active conformation in the absence of any ligand (Greschik et al., 2002).

3.1. ERRγ activity of bisphenols

Compounds screening for activity on ERRγ have identified diethylstilbestrol and 4-hydroxytamoxifen as inverse agonists and BPA as agonist for ERRγ (Coward, Lee, Hull, & Lehmann, 2001; Okada et al., 2008; Tremblay et al., 2001). Among bisphenols, BPA, BPE, and BPB have been found to have the highest affinity for ERRγ (Li, Ma, & Wang, 2010; Okada et al., 2008). Interestingly, these two studies have enabled to discriminate between ERα- and ERRγ-selective agonists. BPA could be considered as a pan agonist for ERα. BPAF and BPC could be considered as ERα-selective agonists and BPE and BPF as ERRγ-selective agonists. It is not surprising that these ligands can be used as tools to determine the respective roles of ERα and ERRγ in cells or organs coexpressing these two receptors.

3.2. Structural basis of BPs interaction with ERRγ

Although a natural ligand remains to be found for ERRγ, several synthetic ligands have been identified for this receptor (Li, Ma, & Wang, 2010; Okada et al., 2008). All display a conserved phenol ring such as BPs. The structure of ERRγ in complex with BPA and BPZ has been solved, revealing an overall protein conformation indistinguishable from that of the unliganded receptor (Abad et al., 2008; Matsushima et al., 2007, 2008) (Fig. 9.3A). A close look at the LBP shows that, as previously anticipated, one of the two phenol-hydroxyl groups of BPA and BPZ forms hydrogen bonds with residues E275 (H3) and R316 (H5), while the second is hydrogen-bonded to N346 in H7 (Fig. 9.3B). A hydrogen bond between Y326 and N346 holds N346 in position to interact with the second phenol group of BPs. Interestingly, this asparagine residue is not conserved in ERRα and ERRβ, thus accounting for the specific ERRγ–BP interaction. Moreover, comparison of ERRγ and ERRα LBPs reveals a much smaller cavity for the latter (Kallen et al., 2004). The replacement of two alanine residues (A272 and A431) in ERRγ by a phenylalanine (F328) and a valine (V491) in ERRα accounts for this size reduction and further explains why BPA does not bind to the latter. BP binding provokes

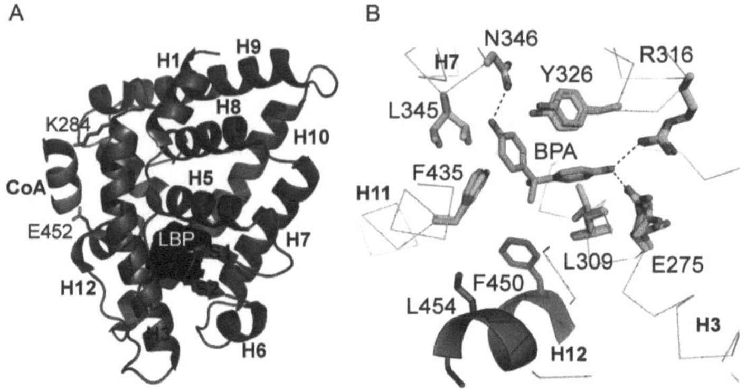

Figure 9.3 Structural determinants of BP recognition by ERRs. (A) Overall structure of unliganded ERRγ LBD (PDB code 1KV6) in cartoon representation. The unoccupied LBP is highlighted in black and CoA stands for coactivator-derived peptide. (B) Superposition of ERRγ LBPs in absence of ligand (light gray, PDB code 1KV6) and in complex with BPA (dark gray, PDB code 2E2R). Residues involved in BPA binding are colored in dark gray and equivalent residues in the unliganded receptor are colored in light gray.

only minimal LBP rearrangements (Fig. 9.3B). E275, which appears disordered in the unliganded structure, adopts a unique conformation to make a hydrogen bond with one OH group of BPs, and the side chain of L345 moves away from the pocket upon BP binding to open up the cavity and make room for the second phenol group of BPs. In summary, ERRγ possesses a LBP to which BPs can bind with high affinity and specificity while preserving the constitutively active conformation of the receptor. The limited impact of BPA binding on receptor structure is consistent with the fact that this ligand does not enhance or disrupt coactivator binding and thus appears as functionally silent ligand (Abad et al., 2008; Matsushima et al., 2007). Thus, the classical mechanism of NHR activation involving the relocalization and stabilization of helix H12 in the active conformation does not explain how ERRγ could mediate the estrogenic effects of BPs. Rather, thermal stability studies revealed that BPA binding leads to global thermodynamic stabilization of ERRγ LBD, a phenomenon that could increase steady-state levels of the receptor and impact both its cellular half-life and biological activity (Abad et al., 2008; Matsushima et al., 2007; Wang et al., 2006). A recent modeling study indicated that in ERRγ, all bisphenols adopt the agonist BPA-like position observed in ERα due to the hydrogen bond with N346 from helix H7. This *in silico* result correlates both with functional data showing that bisphenols are ERRγ activators (Delfosse et al., 2012) and the crystal structure of ERRγ in complex with BPA (Abad et al., 2008; Matsushima et al., 2007).

4. ANDROGEN RECEPTOR

AR plays crucial role in the regulation of target gene expression in physiological processes like development and differentiation of the male embryo and spermatogenesis initiation and maintenance, as well as neuroendocrine system functioning (Matsumoto et al., 2012). The central role of AR has been verified by AR-deficient mice (AR-KO) and by hereditary disorders of androgen insensitivity syndrome in human males. AR-KO mice display an array of phenotypes involving several organs and cell types. Reproductive tract and gonadal development and sexual behavior are severely impacted. In humans, AR mutations cause abnormalities from mild virilization defects to complete male-to-female sex reversal. These mutations lead to either complete or partial androgen insensitivity syndromes (McPhaul, 1999; Quigley et al., 1995). In the absence of ligands, AR is localized essentially in the cytoplasm. Binding to androgens enables HSP dissociation and AR translocation to the nucleus. The AR LBD strongly contributes to the modulation of the N-terminal AF-1 through ligand-induced interdomain association. Furthermore, in AR, it appears that AF-1 predominates over AF-2 (He, Kemppainen, & Wilson, 2000).

Androgens are thus male sex hormones that are critical for the development and maintenance of the male reproductive system. The plasma androgen/estrogen ratio during fetal life creates a male-versus-female hormonal milieu (McLachlan & Newbold, 1987). This delicate balance could be disrupted by environmental antiandrogens or estrogens and lead to hermaphroditism.

Finally, prostate development and prostate cancer are also critically dependent on androgens (McCarthy, 2011). Current therapies of prostate cancers are primarily based on androgen antagonists that interact with AR and completely or partially block the hormone-responsive pathways.

4.1. AR activity of bisphenols

BPA is considered a weak environmental antiandrogen because of its relatively low affinity for AR (Li, Ma, & Wang, 2010; Paris et al., 2002; Stroheker, Picard, Lhuguenot, Canivenc-Lavier, & Chagnon, 2004). In a recent work, we have confirmed these results (Delfosse et al., 2012). In this study, we compared BPA with different bisphenols for their antiandrogenic activity using an AR reporter cell line. The ranking order was BPC $\gg$ BPAF $>$ BPA $=$ BPB $=$ BPE $>$ BPF $>$ BPS. It is noteworthy that

BPC has the same potency than the vinclozolin metabolite M2, which is the most potent xenoantiandrogen (Kelce, Lambright, Gray, & Roberts, 1997; Paris et al., 2002).

As it was observed for estrogenic activity, TCBPA was able to inhibit AR activity, while TBBPA was not (Li, Ma, & Wang, 2010) (P. Balaguer, unpublished data). Interestingly, lower halogenated analogues were also AR inhibitors, mono- and dibromo and chloro-BPA being the most potent (P. Balaguer, unpublished data). Interestingly, in a recent modeling study, all bisphenols appeared to bind to AR exclusively in the antagonist BPC-like orientation, in agreement with the observation that these compounds act as AR antagonists. This orientation appears to be stabilized by formation of a hydrogen bond between one hydroxyl group of the ligand and N705, a polar residue specific of AR (Delfosse et al., 2012).

5. PEROXYSOME PROLIFERATOR-ACTIVATED RECEPTOR γ

PPARs are involved in the regulation of glucose, lipid, and cholesterol metabolism in response to fatty acids and their derivatives, eicosanoids, and drugs used in the treatment of hyperlipidemia and diabetes. The PPAR subfamily contains three members known as PPARα, PPARβ, and PPARγ. Each PPAR subtype shows a distinct tissue distribution and ligand preference.

PPARγ is highly expressed in adipose tissue and is a central regulator of lipid storage and adipocyte gene expression and differentiation (Tontonoz, Hu, & Spiegelman, 1995) and is involved in various pathophysiological disorders, including metabolic disease, insulin resistance, and diabetes (Rosen & Spiegelman, 2001). PPARγ is the target for antidiabetic agents of the thiazolidinedione class, which includes troglitazone, pioglitazone, and rosiglitazone.

The LBD of PPARγ is rather large and the diversity of ligands that can be accommodated within its pocket, mainly presented by lipid derivatives, may contribute to the large array of roles that have been assigned to PPARγ.

5.1. PPARγ activity of bisphenols

There is consistency between the large PPARγ LBP and the capacity to bind various compounds. Several reports have showed PPARγ activation by environmental pollutants such as organotins used as agricultural fungicides and antifouling agents in ship paints, phthalates, and perfluorooctane-based chemicals found in industrial surfactants (Bility et al., 2004; Grun et al., 2006; Takacs & Abbott, 2007). In two recent studies (Riu, Grimaldi, et al., 2011; Riu, le Maire, et al., 2011), we investigated the capability of the flame retardants TBBPA and TCBPA, of their biotransformation products, and of their lower-molecular-weight analogues formed in the environment to activate PPARγ. The activity of the different compounds was studied using reporter cell lines expressing PPARs. None of the compounds tested significantly impacted PPARα or PPARδ activity. In contrast, both TBBPA and TCBPA were capable of activating partially PPARγ, despite being approximately 100-fold less potent (EC_{50} values in the μM range) than the reference pharmaceutical compound rosiglitazone (EC_{50} values in the 10 nM range). We also demonstrated that TBBPA and TCBPA are human, zebrafish, and *Xenopus* PPARγ ligands, while rosiglitazone does not bind zebrafish PPARγ. This work also provides evidence that activation of PPARγ depends on the halogenation degree of BPA analogues. The bulkier the halogenated BPA analogues, the greater their capability to activate PPARγ. In addition, using PPARγ-based affinity column and crystallographic analysis, we clearly demonstrated that the sulfation pathway, usually considered as a detoxification process, leads for TBBPA and TCBPA, to the formation of sulfate conjugates, which possess a residual PPARγ-binding activity (Riu, le Maire, et al, 2011).

5.2. Structural basis of halogenated bisphenols action on PPARγ

Despite the fact that the halogenated bisphenols are structurally unrelated to known PPARγ ligands, the crystal structures of TBBPA and TCBPA bound to the PPARγ LBD (Fig. 9.4A) revealed the canonical tertiary fold of agonist-bound NHR LBDs (Bourguet et al., 2000; Riu, Grimaldi, et al., 2011). The TBBPA and TCBPA complex structures are indistinguishable with an rmsd value of 0.29 Å for superimposed alpha carbons and nearly identical to that of PPARγ in complex with the agonist rosiglitazone (Nolte et al., 1998) with an rmsd value of 0.62 Å. PPARγ displays a large LBP that extends from the C-terminal helix H12 to the β-sheet S1/S2 so that halogenated BPA occupies a small portion of the LBP. Whereas rosiglitazone occupies a region of the LBP spanning from H11/H12 to the β-sheet S1/S2, TBBPA and TCBPA occupy only the region between H3 and the β-sheet S1/S2, with one of its phenol cycle nestled between H3 and the β-sheet (Fig. 9.4B). In contrast with rosiglitazone, a consequence of their smaller size is that halogenated BPA do not interact directly with H12. A close look at the LBP shows that the phenol groups of

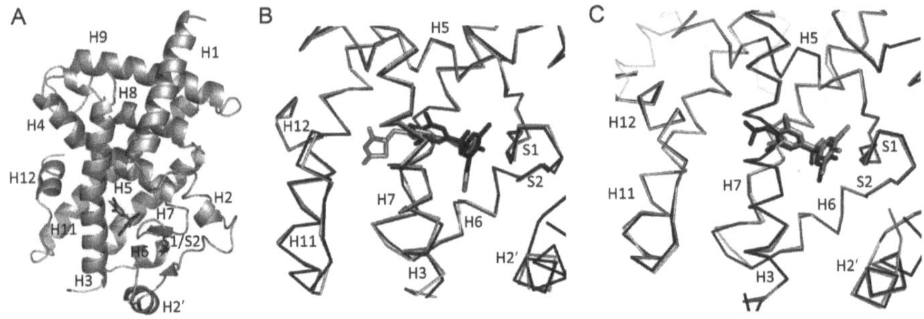

Figure 9.4 Crystal structures of PPARγ LBD in complex with TBBPA and TBBPA-sulfate. (A) Overall structure of the TBBPA-bound PPARγ LBD. The polypeptide backbone is illustrated as a gray ribbon and TBBPA is shown in stick representation. (B) Superimposition of the cocrystal structure of TBBPA-bound PPARγ LBD (in black) on the structure with rosiglitazone (gray, PDB code 2PRG). (C) Superimposition of the cocrystal structure of PPARγ LBD bound to TBBPA-sulfate (black) on the structure with TBBPA (gray). Rosiglitazone, TBBPA, and TBBPA-sulfate are shown in stick representation.

the BPA derivatives are involved in hydrogen bonds with S342 (β-sheet S1/S2) on one side and Y473 from H12 through a water-mediated hydrogen bond network on the other side. TBBPA and TCBPA contain four halogen atoms that contribute to ligand binding through van der Waals interactions. Additional interactions involving the ligand backbone are also observed. Interestingly, comparison of human, mouse, and zebrafish PPARγ sequences reveals several residue differences that could explain the differential ligand specificity of the various species. In particular, the replacement of human PPARγ G284 and C285 by larger serine and tyrosine residues in zebrafish PPARγ provides a rationale for the weak binding affinity of rosiglitazone for this receptor as compared to that observed for the human homolog. In contrast, the different binding mode of halogenated compounds allows both human PPARγ and zebrafish PPARγ to accommodate TBBPA and TCBPA. The structure of PPARγ LBD bound to the metabolite TBBPA-sulfate has been also solved (Riu, le Maire, et al., 2011). Overall, the structure of PPARγ LBD is identical when bound to TBBPA or TBBPA-sulfate, with an rmsd value of 0.24 Å for superimposed alpha carbons (Fig. 9.4C). The ligand is positioned almost identical to that of TBBPA, the sulfate group pointing toward H11/H12. Interestingly, accommodation of the sulfate group by PPARγ does not require any conformational change of the surrounding residue side chains. In this orientation, the sulfate moiety fills a portion of the LBP occupied by water molecules in the TBBPA structure and is potentially involved in hydrogen bonds with Y327, K367, H449, Q286, and S289. The presence of a conserved water molecule mediates the indirect interaction between TBBPA-sulfate and PPARγ helix H12. Overall, the crystallographic data validate the notion that this TBBPA metabolite is a PPARγ ligand with partial agonistic profile.

6. THYROID RECEPTORS

THs are essential for the normal development, growth, and metabolism of all vertebrates (Zoeller et al., 2002), playing a major role in neurogenesis and brain function at all stages of development (Bernal, 2007). They are produced by the thyroid. THs, namely, tetraiodothyronine (thyroxine or T4) and triiodothyronine (T3), are the principal representative of circulating THs. In target cells, T4 is converted in T3, which is the most active TH. Moreover, THs are key developmental and differentiation hormones in all organs of the body, including the central nervous system and the skeleton. In amphibians, THs peak at birth and parallel metamorphosis that is totally dependent upon T3 (Leloup, 1977). The functions of THs are mediated by several isoforms of nuclear thyroid receptors, TRα and TRβ. The tissue distributions of TRs are relatively ubiquitous and the expression of these proteins begins early in development (Zoeller et al., 2002).

6.1. TR activity of bisphenols

Several articles report *in vitro* studies, revealing that BPA and its halogenated derivatives can alter thyroid hormone action by inhibiting T3 binding to and activation of TRs in the 1–10 μM concentration range (Freitas et al., 2011; Moriyama et al., 2002; Sun et al., 2009). Halogenated BPAs share more structural similarities with TH than BPA, which could explain why in certain studies, TBBPA and TCBPA were found active at lower concentrations than BPA (Fini et al., 2012). Halogenated BPAs were also shown to bind to transthyretin, the carrier protein for T4 (Meerts et al., 2000), and their *in vivo* effects on thyroid signaling have been often observed in amphibians (Fini et al., 2007; Jagnytsch, Opitz, Lutz, & Kloas, 2006; Shi et al., 2010; Veldhoen, Boggs, Walzak, & Helbing, 2006).

7. PREGNANE X RECEPTOR

PXR is a broad-specificity sensor playing a critical role in the regulation of phase I (CYP), phase II (conjugating), and phase III (ABC family transporters) detoxifying enzymes, coordinately regulating steroid, drug, and xenobiotic clearance in the liver and intestine (Orans, Teotico, & Redinbo, 2005). Activated PXR binds to gene promoters as a heterodimer with RXR and induces the expression of target genes such as CYP3Aand CYP2B6. This receptor plays a prominent role as protector of the endocrine system from chemical perturbation by sensing increases in the concentration of a multitude of EDCs and inducing detoxification pathways to prevent other NHRs from interactions with these chemicals.

Activation of PXR can be positive, as it accelerates the detoxification process and consequently the elimination of xenobiotics. In contrast, the premature metabolism of active compounds such as hormones or drugs means that target responses will not be activated and can lead to harmful effects or adverse interactions. The metabolism of inactive compounds can also lead to the synthesis of active metabolites, such as the transformation of methoxychlor by CYP2C11, a PXR-induced enzyme, into HPTE, a compound sharing structural similarity with BPA (Mikamo, Harada, Nishikawa, & Nishihara, 2003).

Overall, it is difficult to conclude whether the xenobiotic activation of PXR is predominantly negative or positive, but clearly, PXR plays an essential role in endocrine disruption (di Masi, Marinis, Ascenzi, & Marino, 2009).

7.1. Pregnane X activity of bisphenols

Unlike most NHRs that tend to be specialized to bind few ligands with structural homologies, PXR is able to bind a large number of structurally diverse ligands with a wide range of affinities. Human PXR binds a multitude of drugs such as the antibiotic rifampicin, the anticancer taxol, the anticholesterol SR12813, the barbituric phenobarbital, and the St. John's wort antidepressor hyperforin, recently reviewed in di Masi et al. (2009). Furthermore, numerous studies have focused on its ability to bind environmental compounds, such as pesticides (Lemaire et al., 2006), polychlorinated biphenyls (Jacobs, Nolan, & Hood, 2005; Tabb et al., 2004), brominated flame retardants (Pacyniak et al., 2007), antimicrobial triclosan (Jacobs et al., 2005), or natural and synthetic estrogens (Jacobs et al., 2005; Mnif et al., 2007; Xue et al., 2007) and, among them, BPA in the 1–10 μM concentration range (Jacobs et al., 2005; Mnif et al., 2007; Sui et al., 2012; Takeshita et al., 2001; Xue et al., 2007). Interestingly, Sui et al. (2012) found that BPA activated human PXR but not mouse PXR. Furthermore, they also showed that two other bisphenols, BPB and BPAF, are active on human PXR.

8. CONCLUSIONS

Exposure to BPA is highly suspected to cause adverse effects in humans, but controversy remains about its mechanism of action and low-dose effects. Though ERα and ERβ are primary targets of BPA, alterations of other signaling pathways are probably implicated in the endocrine-disruptive effects of bisphenols. In particular, other members of the NHR family, including AR, ERRγ, PPARγ, TRs, and PXR, have been shown to correspond to secondary targets of bisphenols and crystallographic and modeling studies have provided structural insights as to how BPA and congeners interact with these NHRs. In addition, recent studies have revealed additional BPA targets through which bisphenols can stimulate rapid cellular responses at very low concentrations. These include the membrane-associated ERα and ERβ (Alonso-Magdalena et al., 2012) and the G protein-coupled receptor 30 (Chevalier, Bouskine, & Fenichel, 2012). These two types of receptors are capable of mediating the nongenomic effects of estrogens and xenoestrogens (reviewed in Wetherill et al., 2007) and it is now widely accepted that BPA not only has the efficacy of estradiol but is also equally potent regarding several of its effects (Alonso-Magdalena et al., 2012; Chevalier et al., 2012; Wetherill et al., 2007). Thus is conceivable that BPA could act in a synergistic way through simultaneous action on various nuclear- and membrane-associated receptors. Moreover, most of our current knowledge of BPA action is based on single molecule exposure in model systems *in vitro* or *in vivo*. These efforts have therefore taken little account of a more realistic situation in which humans are chronically exposed to low doses of multiple EDCs, which very likely act also in a synergistic manner.

Both biological and structural data on EDC interactions with nuclear and membrane receptors, in addition to enable a better understanding of EDC activities, will provide guidelines for the development of safer substitutes devoid of hormonal activity and may help environmental risk assessment. Alternatively, they will have potential applications in drug discovery by revealing unforeseen binding mechanisms.

ACKNOWLEDGMENTS

This work was supported by Programme National de Recherche sur les Perturbateurs Endocriniens (P. B.), Agence Nationale de Recherches Contaminants, Ecosystèmes, Santé Project "BISCOT" 2010 Contaminants et Environnements: Métrologie, Santé, Adaptabilité, Comportements et Usages 004 02 (to P. B. and W. B.), and Programme Environnement Cancer Project "SynerPXR" 2012 (to P. B. and W. B.).

REFERENCES

Abad, M. C., Askari, H., O'Neill, J., Klinger, A. L., Milligan, C., Lewandowski, F., et al. (2008). Structural determination of estrogen-related receptor gamma in the presence of phenol derivative compounds. *The Journal of Steroid Biochemistry and Molecular Biology, 108*, 44–54.

Alonso-Magdalena, P., Ropero, A. B., Soriano, S., Garcia-Arevalo, M., Ripoll, C., Fuentes, E., et al. (2012). Bisphenol-A acts as a potent estrogen via non-classical estrogen triggered pathways. *Molecular and Cellular Endocrinology, 355*, 201–207.

Ariazi, E. A., & Jordan, V. C. (2006). Estrogen-related receptors as emerging targets in cancer and metabolic disorders. *Current Topics in Medicinal Chemistry, 6*, 203–215.

Baillie-Hamilton, P. F. (2002). Chemical toxins: A hypothesis to explain the global obesity epidemic. *Journal of Alternative and Complementary Medicine, 8*, 185–192.

Benecke, A., Chambon, P., & Gronemeyer, H. (2000). Synergy between estrogen receptor alpha activation functions AF1 and AF2 mediated by transcription intermediary factor TIF2. *EMBO Reports, 1*, 151–157.

Bernal, J. (2007). Thyroid hormone receptors in brain development and function. *Nature Clinical Practice Endocrinology and Metabolism, 3*, 249–259.

Bility, M. T., Thompson, J. T., McKee, R. H., David, R. M., Butala, J. H., Vanden Heuvel, J. P., et al. (2004). Activation of mouse and human peroxisome proliferator-activated receptors (PPARs) by phthalate monoesters. *Toxicological Sciences, 82*, 170–182.

Bommer, M., Benecke, A., Gronemeyer, H., & Rochette-Egly, C. (2002). TIF2 mediates the synergy between RARalpha 1 activation functions AF-1 and AF-2. *The Journal of Biological Chemistry, 277*, 37961–37966.

Bourguet, W., Germain, P., & Gronemeyer, H. (2000). Nuclear receptor ligand-binding domains: Three-dimensional structures, molecular interactions and pharmacological implications. *Trends in Pharmacological Sciences, 21*, 381–388.

Bruning, J. B., Parent, A. A., Gil, G., Zhao, M., Nowak, J., Pace, M. C., et al. (2010). Coupling of receptor conformation and ligand orientation determine graded activity. *Nature Chemical Biology, 6*, 837–843.

Chevalier, N., Bouskine, A., & Fenichel, P. (2012). Bisphenol A promotes testicular seminoma cell proliferation through GPER/GPR30. *International Journal of Cancer, 130*, 241–242.

Chu, S., Haffner, G. D., & Letcher, R. J. (2005). Simultaneous determination of tetrabromobisphenol A, tetrachlorobisphenol A, bisphenol A and other halogenated analogues in sediment and sludge by high performance liquid chromatography-electrospray tandem mass spectrometry. *Journal of Chromatography A, 1097*, 25–32.

Couse, J. F., & Korach, K. S. (1999). Estrogen receptor null mice: What have we learned and where will they lead us? *Endocrine Reviews, 20*, 358–417.

Coward, P., Lee, D., Hull, M. V., & Lehmann, J. M. (2001). 4-Hydroxytamoxifen binds to and deactivates the estrogen-related receptor gamma. *Proceedings of the National Academy of Sciences of the United States of America, 98*, 8880–8884.

Curtis, S. W., Washburn, T., Sewall, C., DiAugustine, R., Lindzey, J., Couse, J. F., et al. (1996). Physiological coupling of growth factor and steroid receptor signaling pathways: Estrogen receptor knockout mice lack estrogen-like response to epidermal growth factor. *Proceedings of the National Academy of Sciences of the United States of America, 93*, 12626–12630.

Darnerud, P. O. (2003). Toxic effects of brominated flame retardants in man and in wildlife. *Environment International, 29*, 841–853.

de Wit, C. A., Herzke, D., & Vorkamp, K. (2010). Brominated flame retardants in the Arctic environment-trends and new candidates. *The Science of the Total Environment, 408*, 2885–2918.

Delfosse, V., Grimaldi, M., Pons, J.-L., Boulahtouf, A., le Maire, A., Cavailles, V., et al. (2012). Structural and mechanistic insights into bisphenols action provide guidelines for risk assessment and discovery of bisphenol A substitutes. *Proceedings of the National Academy of Sciences of the United States of America, 109*, 14930–14935.

di Masi, A., Marinis, E. D., Ascenzi, P., & Marino, M. (2009). Nuclear receptors CAR and PXR: Molecular, functional, and biomedical aspects. *Molecular Aspects of Medicine, 30*, 297–343.

Fini, J., Le Mevel, S., Turque, N., Palmier, K., Zalko, D., Cravedi, J., et al. (2007). An in vivo multiwell-based fluorescent screen for monitoring vertebrate thyroid hormone disruption. *Environmental Science and Technology, 41*, 5908–5914.

Fini, J. B., Riu, A., Debrauwer, L., Hillenweck, A., Le Mevel, S., Chevolleau, S., et al. (2012). Parallel biotransformation of tetrabromobisphenol A in Xenopus laevis and mammals: Xenopus as a model for endocrine perturbation studies. *Toxicological Sciences, 125*, 359–367.

Freitas, J., Cano, P., Craig-Veit, C., Goodson, M. L., Furlow, J. D., & Murk, A. J. (2011). Detection of thyroid hormone receptor disruptors by a novel stable in vitro reporter gene assay. *Toxicology In Vitro, 25*, 257–266.

Fukazawa, H., Hoshino, K., Shiozawa, T., Matsushita, H., & Terao, Y. (2001). Identification and quantification of chlorinated bisphenol A in wastewater from wastepaper recycling plants. *Chemosphere, 44*, 973–979.

Gallart-Ayala, H., Nunez, O., Moyano, E., & Galceran, M. T. (2010). Field-amplified sample injection-micellar electrokinetic capillary chromatography for the analysis of bisphenol A, bisphenol F, and their diglycidyl ethers and derivatives in canned soft drinks. *Electrophoresis, 31*, 1550–1559.

Gee, A. C., & Katzenellenbogen, J. A. (2001). Probing conformational changes in the estrogen receptor: Evidence for a partially unfolded intermediate facilitating ligand binding and release. *Molecular Endocrinology, 15*, 421–428.

Germain, P., Staels, B., Dacquet, C., Spedding, M., & Laudet, V. (2006). Overview of nomenclature of nuclear receptors. *Pharmacological Reviews, 58*, 685–704.

Giguere, V. (2002). To ERR in the estrogen pathway. *Trends in Endocrinology and Metabolism, 13*, 220–225.

Giguere, V. (2008). Transcriptional control of energy homeostasis by the estrogen-related receptors. *Endocrine Reviews, 29*, 677–696.

Gould, J. C., Leonard, L. S., Maness, S. C., Wagner, B. L., Conner, K., Zacharewski, T., et al. (1998). Bisphenol A interacts with the estrogen receptor alpha in a distinct manner from estradiol. *Molecular and Cellular Endocrinology, 142*, 203–214.

Greschik, H., Wurtz, J. M., Sanglier, S., Bourguet, W., van Dorsselaer, A., Moras, D., et al. (2002). Structural and functional evidence for ligand-independent transcriptional activation by the estrogen-related receptor 3. *Molecular Cell, 9*, 303–313.

Gronemeyer, H., Gustafsson, J. A., & Laudet, V. (2004). Principles for modulation of the nuclear receptor superfamily. *Nature Reviews Drug Discovery, 3*, 950–964.

Grun, F., Watanabe, H., Zamanian, Z., Maeda, L., Arima, K., Cubacha, R., et al. (2006). Endocrine-disrupting organotin compounds are potent inducers of adipogenesis in vertebrates. *Molecular Endocrinology, 20*, 2141–2155.

He, B., Kemppainen, J. A., & Wilson, E. M. (2000). FXXLF and WXXLF sequences mediate the NH2-terminal interaction with the ligand binding domain of the androgen receptor. *The Journal of Biological Chemistry, 275*, 22986–22994.

Horard, B., & Vanacker, J. M. (2003). Estrogen receptor-related receptors: Orphan receptors desperately seeking a ligand. *Journal of Molecular Endocrinology, 31*, 349–357.

Jacobs, M. N., Nolan, G. T., & Hood, S. R. (2005). Lignans, bacteriocides and organochlorine compounds activate the human pregnane X receptor (PXR). *Toxicology and Applied Pharmacology, 209*, 123–133.

Jagnytsch, O., Opitz, R., Lutz, I., & Kloas, W. (2006). Effects of tetrabromobisphenol A on larval development and thyroid hormone-regulated biomarkers of the amphibian Xenopus laevis. *Environmental Research, 101*, 340–348.

Kallen, J., Schlaeppi, J. M., Bitsch, F., Filipuzzi, I., Schilb, A., Riou, V., et al. (2004). Evidence for ligand-independent transcriptional activation of the human estrogen-related receptor alpha (ERRalpha): Crystal structure of ERRalpha ligand binding domain in complex with peroxisome proliferator-activated receptor coactivator-1alpha. *The Journal of Biological Chemistry, 279*, 49330–49337.

Kelce, W. R., Lambright, C. R., Gray, L. E., Jr., & Roberts, K. P. (1997). Vinclozolin and p, p'-DDE alter androgen-dependent gene expression: In vivo confirmation of an androgen receptor-mediated mechanism. *Toxicology and Applied Pharmacology, 142*, 192–200.

Kitamura, S., Kato, T., Iida, M., Jinno, N., Suzuki, T., Ohta, S., et al. (2005). Anti-thyroid hormonal activity of tetrabromobisphenol A, a flame retardant, and related compounds: Affinity to the mammalian thyroid hormone receptor, and effect on tadpole metamorphosis. *Life Sciences, 76*, 1589–1601.

Kuiper, G. G., Carlsson, B., Grandien, K., Enmark, E., Haggblad, J., Nilsson, S., et al. (1997). Comparison of the ligand binding specificity and transcript tissue distribution of estrogen receptors alpha and beta. *Endocrinology, 138*, 863–870.

Leloup, Buscaglia (1977). La triiodothyronine, hormone de la métamorphose des amphibiens. *Comptes rendus hebdomadaires des scéances de l'académie des sciences Série D, 284*, 2261–2263.

Lemaire, G., Mnif, W., Pascussi, J. M., Pillon, A., Rabenoelina, F., Fenet, H., et al. (2006). Identification of new human pregnane X receptor ligands among pesticides using a stable reporter cell system. *Toxicological Sciences, 91*, 501–509.

Li, J., Ma, M., & Wang, Z. (2010). In vitro profiling of endocrine disrupting effects of phenols. *Toxicology In Vitro, 24*, 201–207.

Liu, H., Zhao, H., Quan, X., Zhang, Y., & Chen, S. (2009). Formation of chlorinated intermediate from bisphenol A in surface saline water under simulated solar light irradiation. *Environmental Science and Technology, 43*, 7712–7717.

Lu, D., Kiriyama, Y., Lee, K. Y., & Giguere, V. (2001). Transcriptional regulation of the estrogen-inducible pS2 breast cancer marker gene by the ERR family of orphan nuclear receptors. *Cancer Research, 61*, 6755–6761.

Matsumoto, T., Sakari, M., Okada, M., Yokoyama, A., Takahashi, S., Kouzmenko, A., et al. (2012). The androgen receptor in health and disease. *Annual Review of Physiology, 75*, 201–224.

Matsushima, A., Kakuta, Y., Teramoto, T., Koshiba, T., Liu, X., Okada, H., et al. (2007). Structural evidence for endocrine disruptor bisphenol A binding to human nuclear receptor ERR gamma. *Journal of Biochemistry, 142*, 517–524.

Matsushima, A., Teramoto, T., Okada, H., Liu, X., Tokunaga, T., Kakuta, Y., et al. (2008). ERRgamma tethers strongly bisphenol A and 4-alpha-cumylphenol in an induced-fit manner. *Biochemical and Biophysical Research Communications, 373*, 408–413.

McCarthy, N. (2011). Prostate cancer: Studying the classics. *Nature Reviews Cancer, 11*, 386.

McLachlan, J. A., & Newbold, R. R. (1987). Estrogens and development. *Environmental Health Perspectives, 75*, 25–27.

McPhaul, M. J. (1999). Molecular defects of the androgen receptor. *The Journal of Steroid Biochemistry and Molecular Biology, 69*, 315–322.

Meerts, I. A., van Zanden, J. J., Luijks, E. A., van Leeuwen-Bol, I., Marsh, G., Jakobsson, E., et al. (2000). Potent competitive interactions of some brominated flame retardants and related compounds with human transthyretin in vitro. *Toxicological Sciences, 56*, 95–104.

Mikamo, E., Harada, S., Nishikawa, J., & Nishihara, T. (2003). Endocrine disruptors induce cytochrome P450 by affecting transcriptional regulation via pregnane X receptor. *Toxicology and Applied Pharmacology, 193*, 66–72.

Mnif, W., Pascussi, J. M., Pillon, A., Escande, A., Bartegi, A., Nicolas, J. C., et al. (2007). Estrogens and antiestrogens activate hPXR. *Toxicology Letters, 170*, 19–29.

Moriyama, K., Tagami, T., Akamizu, T., Usui, T., Saijo, M., Kanamoto, N., et al. (2002). Thyroid hormone action is disrupted by bisphenol A as an antagonist. *The Journal of Clinical Endocrinology and Metabolism, 87*, 5185–5190.

Mutou, Y., Ibuki, Y., Terao, Y., Kojima, S., & Goto, R. (2006). Change of estrogenic activity and release of chloride ion in chlorinated bisphenol A after exposure to ultraviolet B. *Biological and Pharmaceutical Bulletin, 29*, 2116–2119.

Nagy, L., & Schwabe, J. W. (2004). Mechanism of the nuclear receptor molecular switch. *Trends in Biochemical Sciences, 29*, 317–324.

Nettles, K. W., Bruning, J. B., Gil, G., Nowak, J., Sharma, S. K., Hahm, J. B., et al. (2008). NFkappaB selectivity of estrogen receptor ligands revealed by comparative crystallographic analyses. *Nature Chemical Biology, 4*, 241–247.

Nolte, R. T., Wisely, G. B., Westin, S., Cobb, J. E., Lambert, M. H., Kurokawa, R., et al. (1998). Ligand binding and co-activator assembly of the peroxisome proliferator-activated receptor-[gamma]. *Nature, 395*, 137–143.

Okada, H., Tokunaga, T., Liu, X., Takayanagi, S., Matsushima, A., & Shimohigashi, Y. (2008). Direct evidence revealing structural elements essential for the high binding ability of bisphenol A to human estrogen-related receptor-gamma. *Environmental Health Perspectives, 116*, 32–38.

Orans, J., Teotico, D. G., & Redinbo, M. R. (2005). The nuclear xenobiotic receptor pregnane X receptor: Recent insights and new challenges. *Molecular Endocrinology, 19*, 2891–2900.

Pacyniak, E. K., Cheng, X., Cunningham, M. L., Crofton, K., Klaassen, C. D., & Guo, G. L. (2007). The flame retardants, polybrominated diphenyl ethers, are pregnane X receptor activators. *Toxicological Sciences, 97*, 94–102.

Paris, F., Balaguer, P., Terouanne, B., Servant, N., Lacoste, C., Cravedi, J. P., et al. (2002). Phenylphenols, biphenols, bisphenol-A and 4-tert-octylphenol exhibit alpha and beta estrogen activities and antiandrogen activity in reporter cell lines. *Molecular and Cellular Endocrinology, 193*, 43–49.

Pike, A. C. (2006). Lessons learnt from structural studies of the oestrogen receptor. *Best Practice and Research Clinical Endocrinology and Metabolism, 20*, 1–14.

Quigley, C. A., De Bellis, A., Marschke, K. B., el-Awady, M. K., Wilson, E. M., & French, F. S. (1995). Androgen receptor defects: Historical, clinical, and molecular perspectives. *Endocrine Reviews, 16*, 271–321.

Renaud, J. P., & Moras, D. (2000). Structural studies on nuclear receptors. *Cellular and Molecular Life Sciences, 57*, 1748–1769.

Riu, A., Grimaldi, M., le Maire, A., Bey, G., Phillips, K., Boulahtouf, A., et al. (2011). Peroxisome proliferator-activated receptor gamma is a target for halogenated analogs of bisphenol A. *Environmental Health Perspectives, 119*, 1227–1232.

Riu, A., le Maire, A., Grimaldi, M., Audebert, M., Hillenweck, A., Bourguet, W., et al. (2011). Characterization of novel ligands of ERalpha, Erbeta, and PPARgamma: The case of halogenated bisphenol A and their conjugated metabolites. *Toxicological Sciences, 122*, 372–382.

Rosen, E. D., & Spiegelman, B. M. (2001). PPARgamma: A nuclear regulator of metabolism, differentiation, and cell growth. *The Journal of Biological Chemistry, 276*, 37731–37734.

Routledge, E. J., White, R., Parker, M. G., & Sumpter, J. P. (2000). Differential effects of xenoestrogens on coactivator recruitment by estrogen receptor (ER) alpha and ERbeta. *The Journal of Biological Chemistry, 275*, 35986–35993.

Shi, H., Qian, L., Guo, S., Zhang, X., Liu, J., & Cao, Q. (2010). Teratogenic effects of tetrabromobisphenol A on Xenopus tropicalis embryos. *Comparative Biochemistry and Physiology Toxicology and Pharmacology, 152*, 62–68.

Stroheker, T., Picard, K., Lhuguenot, J. C., Canivenc-Lavier, M. C., & Chagnon, M. C. (2004). Steroid activities comparison of natural and food wrap compounds in human breast cancer cell lines. *Food and Chemical Toxicology, 42*, 887–897.

Sui, Y., Ai, N., Park, S. H., Rios-Pilier, J., Perkins, J. T., Welsh, W. J., et al. (2012). Bisphenol A and its analogues activate human pregnane X receptor. *Environmental Health Perspectives, 120*, 399–405.

Sun, H., Shen, O.-X., Wang, X.-R., Zhou, L., Zhen, S. Q., & Zhen, X. D. (2009). Anti-thyroid hormone activity of bisphenol A, tetrabromobisphenol A and tetrachlorobisphenol A in an improved reporter gene assay. *Toxicology In Vitro, 23*, 950–954.

Tabb, M. M., Kholodovych, V., Grun, F., Zhou, C., Welsh, W. J., & Blumberg, B. (2004). Highly chlorinated PCBs inhibit the human xenobiotic response mediated by the steroid and xenobiotic receptor (SXR). *Environmental Health Perspectives, 112*, 163–169.

Takacs, M. L., & Abbott, B. D. (2007). Activation of mouse and human peroxisome proliferator-activated receptors (alpha, beta/delta, gamma) by perfluorooctanoic 'acid and perfluorooctane sulfonate. *Toxicological Sciences, 95*, 108–117.

Takemura, H., Ma, J., Sayama, K., Terao, Y., Zhu, B. T., & Shimoi, K. (2005). In vitro and in vivo estrogenic activity of chlorinated derivatives of bisphenol A. *Toxicology, 207*, 215–221.

Takeshita, A., Koibuchi, N., Oka, J., Taguchi, M., Shishiba, Y., & Ozawa, Y. (2001). Bisphenol-A, an environmental estrogen, activates the human orphan nuclear receptor, steroid and xenobiotic receptor-mediated transcription. *European Journal of Endocrinology, 145*, 513–517.

Tontonoz, P., Hu, E., & Spiegelman, B. M. (1995). Regulation of adipocyte gene expression and differentiation by peroxisome proliferator activated receptor gamma. *Current Opinion in Genetics and Development, 5*, 571–576.

Tremblay, G. B., Kunath, T., Bergeron, D., Lapointe, L., Champigny, C., Bader, J. A., et al. (2001). Diethylstilbestrol regulates trophoblast stem cell differentiation as a ligand of orphan nuclear receptor ERR beta. *Genes and Development, 15*, 833–838.

Vanacker, J. M., Pettersson, K., Gustafsson, J. A., & Laudet, V. (1999). Transcriptional targets shared by estrogen receptor- related receptors (ERRs) and estrogen receptor (ER) alpha, but not by ERbeta. *The EMBO Journal, 18*, 4270–4279.

Vandenberg, L. N., Maffini, M. V., Sonnenschein, C., Rubin, B. S., & Soto, A. M. (2009). Bisphenol-A and the great divide: A review of controversies in the field of endocrine disruption. *Endocrine Reviews, 30*, 75–95.

Veldhoen, N., Boggs, A., Walzak, K., & Helbing, C. C. (2006). Exposure to tetrabromobisphenol-A alters TH-associated gene expression and tadpole metamorphosis in the Pacific tree frog Pseudacris regilla. *Aquatic Toxicology, 78*, 292–302.

Wang, L., Zuercher, W. J., Consler, T. G., Lambert, M. H., Miller, A. B., Orband-Miller, L. A., et al. (2006). X-ray crystal structures of the estrogen-related receptor-gamma ligand binding domain in three functional states reveal the molecular basis of small molecule regulation. *The Journal of Biological Chemistry, 281*, 37773–37781.

Wetherill, Y. B., Akingbemi, B. T., Kanno, J., McLachlan, J. A., Nadal, A., Sonnenschein, C., et al. (2007). In vitro molecular mechanisms of bisphenol A action. *Reproductive Toxicology, 24*, 178–198.

Wilson, E. M. (2011). Analysis of interdomain interactions of the androgen receptor. *Methods in Molecular Biology, 776*, 113–129.

Xue, Y., Moore, L. B., Orans, J., Peng, L., Bencharit, S., Kliewer, S. A., et al. (2007). Crystal structure of the pregnane X receptor-estradiol complex provides insights into endobiotic recognition. *Molecular Endocrinology, 21*, 1028–1038.

Yu, S., Wang, X., Ng, C. F., Chen, S., & Chan, F. L. (2007). ERRgamma suppresses cell proliferation and tumor growth of androgen-sensitive and androgen-insensitive prostate cancer cells and its implication as a therapeutic target for prostate cancer. *Cancer Research*, *67*, 4904–4914.

Zoeller, T. R., Dowling, A. L., Herzig, C. T., Iannacone, E. A., Gauger, K. J., & Bansal, R. (2002). Thyroid hormone, brain development, and the environment. *Environmental Health Perspectives*, *110*(Suppl. 3), 355–361.

CHAPTER TEN

Long-Lasting Effects of Neonatal Bisphenol A Exposure on the Implantation Process

Jorgelina Varayoud, Jorge G. Ramos, Mónica Muñoz-de-Toro, Enrique H. Luque[1]
Laboratorio de Endocrinología y Tumores Hormonodependientes, School of Biochemistry and Biological Sciences, Universidad Nacional del Litoral, Santa Fe, Argentina
[1]Corresponding author: e-mail address: eluque@fbcb.unl.edu.ar

Contents

1. Introduction 254
2. Uterine Implantation of the Embryo 255
   2.1 Implantation-associated gene expression 256
   2.2 Ovarian steroids and their nuclear receptors 257
   2.3 Cell proliferation in the stroma and the endothelium 258
3. Endocrine Disruptors and the Developmental Programming Hypothesis 259
   3.1 BPA effects on reproductive performance 261
   3.2 BPA alters endocrine signaling in the preimplantation uterus 262
   3.3 BPA and the expression of implantation-associated genes 263
   3.4 Early postnatal BPA exposure impairs the uterine response to ovarian steroids in the adult 264
4. Endocrine Disruption and Female Fertility 269
5. Conclusions 270
Acknowledgments 270
References 270

Abstract

Successful implantation is the result of complex molecular interactions between the hormonally primed uterus and a mature blastocyst. This very carefully synchronized interplay of hormonal signals and feedback loops is potentially vulnerable to chemicals such as endocrine disruptors that may disrupt endocrine signaling. Bisphenol A (BPA) is one of the highest-volume chemicals produced worldwide. This chapter describes the effects of brief postnatal exposure to BPA on female reproductive performance and specifically on the uterine adaptations during the preimplantation period. We propose that an early alteration in *Hoxa10* gene expression affects the functional differentiation of the preimplantation uterus as part of an altered endocrine signal transduction pathway. These molecular alterations could explain, at least in part,

Vitamins and Hormones, Volume 94
ISSN 0083-6729
http://dx.doi.org/10.1016/B978-0-12-800095-3.00010-9

the adverse effects of BPA on uterine implantation. Exposure to endocrine disruptors, such as BPA, could contribute to the impaired female fertility noted over the past decades.

1. INTRODUCTION

During the past several decades, infertility rates and early pregnancy loss have increased worldwide and currently affect 10–15% of couples in the United States and other developed countries (Hayashi, Saitou, & Yamanaka, 2012). An important determinant of reduced fertility is failed implantation, which is thought to account for 50–70% of preclinical pregnancy losses in humans (Macklon et al., 2002; Norwitz, Schust, & Fisher, 2001). Although both the society and families have benefited from advancements in the field of assisted reproductive technology (ART), the overall success rate of ART still remains low. In the United States, 1% of births can currently be attributed to ART (Ola & Li, 2006). Many of the unsuccessful ART pregnancies can likely be attributed to the transfer of embryos into a nonreceptive uterus. In fact, recurrent implantation failure is considered to be an important limiting factor in the establishment of pregnancy by either ART or natural means (Norwitz et al., 2001).

Successful implantation is the result of complex molecular interactions between the hormonally primed uterus and a mature blastocyst. This very carefully synchronized interplay of hormonal signals and feedback loops is potentially vulnerable to chemicals such as endocrine disruptors that may disrupt endocrine signaling (Crain et al., 2008; Varayoud et al., 2011). Although many losses involve genetic abnormalities, there is often no known cause. Hormonal factors, endometrial or uterine gland changes, cytokines, and growth factors, among others, are part of the complex process that leads to implantation and the early stages of placental development (Norwitz et al., 2001).

Bisphenol A (BPA) is one of the highest-volume chemicals produced worldwide. Current estimates indicate that more than eight billion pounds of BPA is produced annually and that approximately 100 tons may be released into the atmosphere each year (Rubin, 2011; Vanderberg et al., 2010). BPA is used in the manufacture of plastics often used for food and beverage storage and is also a component of epoxy resins that are used to line food and beverage containers. Studies have shown that BPA can leach from these and other products in contact with food and drink and, as a result, be routinely ingested. BPA can also be used in the manufacture of some dental sealants and composites and of thermal receipt paper (Biedermann, Tschudin, & Grob, 2010). Thus, given the prevalence of BPA in our environment, almost all the population seems to be exposed. BPA has been detected in more than 90% of urine samples obtained from a representative sample of US residents (Calafat, Ye, Wong, Reidy, & Needham, 2008). Detectable concentrations of BPA have also been measured in human follicular fluid and amniotic fluid, suggesting that exposure may occur as early as the periconception period.

This chapter deals with the long-term effects of early postnatal exposure to low doses of BPA and focuses on the lasting consequences in female fertility and the endocrine pathways that regulate the preparation of the endometrium for embryo implantation.

2. UTERINE IMPLANTATION OF THE EMBRYO

Different molecular events are essential to the implantation process. Various tissue compartments within the uterus, including the luminal epithelium, glandular epithelium, and stroma, undergo sequential proliferation and differentiation as the embryo attaches to the luminal epithelium and invades the stroma. However, our current understanding of the molecular signaling pathways that link these tissue compartments to achieve a functional state of the uterus conducive to implantation is still limited (Das, 2010).

The cascade of signaling events that occur in both fetal and maternal tissues at the time of implantation establishes an appropriate milieu critical to the development and survival of the fetus. Defects in the formation of this network and the inability to sustain this cross talk are believed to result in various pregnancy-associated complications that may manifest throughout pregnancy.

Although numerous of the molecules involved in the implantation process have been identified, the understanding of this process is still far from complete. For example, many of the genes that are expressed in an implantation-specific manner and appear to be important for implantation cannot be studied in depth because deletion of these genes results in embryonic lethality. One additional difficulty in identifying the critical roles of signaling molecules within a gene family is the redundant or compensatory functions of the gene products within the family.

2.1. Implantation-associated gene expression

Hoxa10 is one of the implantation-associated genes. This gene is known to be upregulated by progesterone in the uterine stroma during preimplantation period and its levels are sustained during decidualization (Daikoku et al., 2004; Satokata, Benson, & Maas, 1995; Wang & Dey, 2006). These characteristics have made *Hoxa10* an obvious marker for experimentation in an attempt to elucidate the molecular mechanisms of implantation. The severe infertility phenotype observed in *Hoxa10*-deficient female mice is multifactorial, suggesting that *Hoxa10* has pleiotropic effects and regulates multiple pathways. *Hoxa10*-deficient mice exhibit female infertility, with the proximal region of the uterus showing partial homeosis into an oviduct-like structure. However, the cause of infertility in these females seems to be impaired stromal cell proliferation and decidualization (Lim, Ma, Ma, Maas, & Dey, 1999). Furthermore, embryo transfer experiments have conclusively shown that *Hoxa10* is required for both implantation and decidualization (Bagot, Troy, & Taylor, 2000, Benson et al., 1996). Stromal cell proliferation in *Hoxa10*$^{-/-}$ mice in response to ovarian progesterone and estrogen is severely compromised, while epithelial cell proliferation remains normal in response to estrogen (Yao et al., 2003). This impaired stromal cell responsiveness to progesterone suggests that *Hoxa10* induces genes that are vital for stromal cell proliferation and differentiation and behaves as a mediator of progesterone effects on implantation.

B3 integrin (*ITGB3*) and *empty spiracles homolog 2* (*EMX-2*) are *Hoxa10*-target genes, which are known to be operative downstream in endocrine hormone-regulated *Hox* gene pathways. *ITGB3* has been proposed to be a bridging molecule between the endometrium and the trophoblast, thereby constituting an early link between maternal and fetal tissues (Sueoka et al., 1997). Endometrial *ITGB3* expression coincides with a systemic peak of progesterone, and high endometrial *Hoxa10* levels occur in the midsecretory phase of the menstrual cycle, around the time of embryo implantation (Taylor, Arici, Olive, & Igarashi, 1998). *ITGB3* expression has been shown to be directly regulated by *Hoxa10* through a consensus Abd-B-type *HOX* binding site located 5′ of the *ITGB3* gene within its regulatory region (Daftary, Troy, Bagot, Young, & Taylor, 2002). *EMX-2*, on the other hand, is a homeobox gene located outside the *HOX* cluster, orthologous to the *Drosophila empty spiracles* gene (Kastury et al., 1994), which is negatively regulated by *Hoxa10* in reproductive tissue (Troy, Daftary, Bagot, & Taylor, 2003). In contrast, at the same time, *Hoxa10* directly binds a regulatory element in an enhancer region of the *EMX-2* gene and transcriptionally represses its expression (Troy et al., 2003). In baboons with experimental endometriosis, it has been found that *Hoxa10* expression is lower than that of disease-free animals and that this decreased expression is accompanied by abnormal expression of *EMX-2* and *ITGB3* (Kim et al., 2007).

Another important event associated with the preparation of the uterus for embryo implantation is mediated by the action of vascular endothelial growth factor (VEGF). VEGF constitutes the main factor responsible for the control of endothelial proliferation and vascular permeability. Immunoneutralization of VEGF inhibits pregnancy establishment in rhesus monkeys (Sengupta et al., 2007) and rats (Rabbani & Rogers, 2001; Rockwell, Pillai, Olson, & Koos, 2002). This protein is present in different uterine cellular compartments, and its differential expression is associated with ovarian steroid levels. Studies in three different rodent species have shown that the luminal epithelium shows increased VEGF expression in the uterus in response to estradiol (Karuri, Kumar, & Mukhopadhyay, 1998; Shweiki, Itin, Neufeld, Gitay-Goren, & Keshet, 1993; Yi et al., 1999). In addition, these studies have shown little or no VEGF expression in stromal tissue until after progesterone administration. Different results have shown that progesterone- and estradiol-induced uterine VEGF expression does not involve their nuclear receptor interactions with their classic consensus hormone response element (Kazi & Koos, 2007; Mueller et al., 2003). Thus, in the rat uterus, estradiol induces the recruitment of estrogen receptor α (ERα) to the proximal GC-rich region of the *VEGF* promoter, probably via interaction with specificity proteins (Kazi & Koos, 2007). Therefore, downstream VEGF regulation by ovarian hormones depends on the expression profiles and recruitment of different transcription factors to the *VEGF* promoter region.

2.2. Ovarian steroids and their nuclear receptors

One would be remiss to discuss the molecular mediators of implantation without first emphasizing the paramount roles of the ovarian steroids estradiol and progesterone. The nuclear ER and progesterone receptor (PR) are expressed in all compartments of the uterus, and embryo implantation has been shown to be critically dependent on their intricate balance and interaction (Rubel, Jeong, Tsai, Lydon, & Demayo, 2010; Tan, Paria, Dey, & Das, 1999; Tibbetts, Mendoza-Meneses, O'Malley, & Conneely, 1998).

The preimplantation period shows different changes in steroid levels and steroid hormone receptor expression in the uterus. In pregnant rodents, estradiol levels and ERα activity in the endometrium decrease temporarily on gestation day 2 and then increase near the moment of implantation. Transcription of targeted genes may be estrogen-sensitive and thus down-regulated during this time. By GD3, corpus luteum-synthesized progesterone initiates stromal cell proliferation and its increasing presence may cause indirect regulation of gene expression through direct *Hoxa10* regulation. It has been established that homeobox genes are pleiotropic transcriptional modulators and that *Hoxa10*, specifically, can act as a repressor and an activator of transcription (Dey et al., 2004).

Estradiol acts mainly through one of two ERs, ERα or ERβ, which are encoded by two separate genes. Progesterone acts through the PR, which consists of two isoforms, PR-A and PR-B. These two isoforms arise from differential transcription of the *PR* gene. Gene ablation studies have demonstrated that ERα and PR-A are primary regulators of the uterine function (Curtis Hewitt, Goulding, Eddy, & Korach, 2002). These studies have also shown that while ERα plays a permissive role in the regulation of uterine function, PR-A is critical for the uterus to support pregnancy (Tan et al., 1999; Tibbetts et al., 1998). These receptors do not act alone in the regulation of gene transcription but are aided by coregulator proteins. Activated steroid receptors recruit coactivators or corepressors to target gene promoters. Coactivators such as steroid receptor coactivator-3 (SRC-3) enhance the transcriptional activity of steroid hormone receptors via their intrinsic histone acetyltransferase activity by bridging nuclear receptors with the basal transcription machinery or by interacting with other histone acetyltransferases such as CBP/p300. On the other hand, corepressors, such as the silencing mediator for retinoic acid and thyroid hormone receptor (SMRT), are limiting factors that inhibit the transcriptional activity of steroid hormone receptors by recruiting histone deacetylases and disrupting receptor dimer interactions (Privalsky, 2004). Different coregulators regulate the transcriptional activity of a variety of nuclear receptors, including ERα, ERβ, and PR, and are expressed in several hormone-responsive tissues including the uterus (Jeong et al., 2007). Previous results have shown that these coregulators play a necessary role in coordinating steroid hormone regulation of normal reproductive uterine function.

2.3. Cell proliferation in the stroma and the endothelium

Stromal proliferation and endothelial proliferation are critical events associated with the preparation of the endometrium for embryo implantation.

Previous results have shown that an adequate proliferation rate of these compartments is a requisite for successful implantation because, as it has been shown in several mouse models, the failure of these processes affects the implantation rate. Progesterone, which is the essential stimulus needed for *in vivo* proliferation of stromal cells, acts as the switch for their specific decidual program (Huet-Hudson, Andrews, & Dey, 1989). In rats, progesterone switches proliferation from the epithelial to the stromal compartment on day 4 of pregnancy as a prerequisite for implantation and decidualization (reviewed in Carson et al., 2000). Although different genes have been associated with the control of stromal proliferation, *Hoxa10* is defined as a key molecule during the preimplantation period.

Endothelial proliferation is one of the most studied events associated with the uterine angiogenesis during the preimplantation period. Like stromal proliferation, endothelial proliferation is known to be influenced by estradiol and progesterone through the activation of their respective nuclear receptors. The sex steroid receptor complex exerts some biological effects indirectly via a variety of growth factors (Weitlauf, 1994). Among them, VEGF is likely the main factor responsible for the control of endothelial proliferation.

3. ENDOCRINE DISRUPTORS AND THE DEVELOPMENTAL PROGRAMMING HYPOTHESIS

The developmental programming hypothesis suggests that aberrant stimuli encountered during critical periods of development can permanently reprogram normal physiological responses and, thus, give rise to reproductive consequences later in life (Bartol, Wiley, & Bagnell, 2006). These acquired changes can persist transgenerationally and a possible explanation of such outcome is the epigenetic regulation of the genome. Exposure to environmental endocrine disruptors can affect the normal development of reproductive tissues and may contribute to declining conception rates and increased incidence of female reproductive disorders such as oocyte aneuploidy, polycystic ovarian syndrome, and altered cyclicity, as well as endometriosis, uterine fibroids, fetal growth retardation, and pregnancy loss (Crain et al., 2008).

As already mentioned, BPA is an estrogenic compound produced in large quantities and a study carried out by the Center for Disease Control and Prevention in the United States detected BPA in the urine of >90% of the Americans sampled (Calafat et al., 2008). However, few epidemiological studies have examined the effects of BPA in humans. For instance, toddlers exposed to high maternal levels of BPA during pregnancy have shown externalizing behaviors (Braun et al., 2009). Also, urinary BPA levels have been shown to be associated with increased cardiovascular disease and diabetes in adults (Lang et al., 2008) and sexual dysfunction in men (Li et al., 2010). Because the true impact of endocrine disruptors on human health is difficult to assess, it is important to test their effect under controlled exposure conditions in animal models (Maffini, Rubin, Sonnenschein, & Soto, 2006; Tharp et al., 2012). The model of the endocrine disruptor diethylstilbestrol (DES)-induced reproductive tract malformations and cancers serves as a novel paradigm to study the pathological consequences that arise in adults exposed early in life to hormonally active substances (Mericskay, Carta, & Sassoon, 2005). There is no clear sign that any gene has undergone a permanent mutation in response to DES exposure. Instead, a transient disruption of normal gene expression, which impacts all subsequent and normal development, occurs during a critical period. It has been shown that DES potently represses a number of developmental control genes, including several *Hox* and *Wnt* genes, during critical periods of reproductive tract patterning (Couse et al., 2001).

To evaluate the effects of endocrine-disrupting compounds with estrogenic activity such as BPA, endosulfan, and DES, we have used a rat model with a brief postnatal treatment on days 1, 3, 5, and 7 of life by subcutaneous injections in the nape of the neck (Bosquiazzo, Varayoud, Muñoz-de-Toro, Luque, & Ramos, 2010; Milesi, Varayoud, Bosquiazzo, Muñoz-de-Toro, & Luque, 2012; Monje, Varayoud, Luque, & Ramos, 2007; Monje, Varayoud, Muñoz-de-Toro, Luque, & Ramos, 2009, 2010; Rodriguez, Santambrosio, Santamaría, Muñoz-de-Toro, & Luque, 2010; Varayoud et al., 2011; Varayoud, Ramos, Bosquiazzo, Muñoz-de-Toro, & Luque, 2008). In the rat, the uterine development and differentiation is completed during the first postnatal week; thus, the early postnatal period is critical to evaluate the effects of endocrine disruptor exposure.

The route of BPA administration and the doses of BPA administered are important issues to determine BPA health risks in animal models (CERHR, 2007). In fetuses and neonates, the low expression of the enzyme that conjugates BPA (uridine diphosphate-glucuronosyl transferase) implies that oral and nonoral administration of BPA during neonatal life results in the same internal active dose (Taylor, Welshons, & vom Saal, 2008). Since the Society of the Plastics Industry and the US Environmental Protection Agency have recommended using the current accepted lowest-observed-adverse-effect level dose (50 mg/kg/day) of BPA to calculate a maximum acceptable or reference dose, thus, 0.05 mg/kg/day was chosen (U.S. Environmental Protection Agency, 1993). In our studies (Bosquiazzo et al., 2010; Varayoud et al., 2011, 2008), we examined the effects of two different doses of BPA: one identical to the reference dose (0.05 mg/kg/day; BPA.05) and the other 400-fold higher (20 mg/kg/day; BPA20), although 2.5-fold lower than the declared lowest-observed-adverse-effect level. The aim was to investigate whether a brief postnatal exposure to BPA disrupts transcriptional control of the development-related genes *Hoxa10* and *Hoxa11* in the uterus of rats on postnatal day 8. *Hoxa10* and its neighbor in the *Hoxa* gene cluster, *Hoxa11*, are abdominal B type homeobox genes, which normally regulate differentiation of the Müllerian duct (Taylor, 2000). Down-regulation of both *Hox* genes has been detected using mice as a model of postnatal exposure to DES (Couse et al., 2001). Methoxychlor, a pesticide that has adverse effects on the reproductive capability of mice, decreases *Hoxa10* mRNA levels in Ishikawa cells *in vitro* and decreases uterine *Hoxa10* expression in mice treated *in vivo* (Fei, Chung, & Taylor, 2005). Little is known about BPA effects on Hox gene expression. A study has shown a dose–response increase in *Hoxa10* levels in the uterus of 2- and 6-week-old mice exposed *in utero* to BPA (Smith & Taylor, 2007). We detected that the two studied doses of BPA during early postnatal days decrease *Hoxa10* and *Hoxa11* expression in the prepubertal rat uterus (Varayoud et al., 2008). Taken together, the previously mentioned results show that *Hox* genes are a common target of endocrine disruption (Fei et al., 2005) and suggest that exposure during different developmental periods could lead to a different characteristic effect.

3.1. BPA effects on reproductive performance

The BPA effects on reproductive performance can be evaluated using different models of exposure. In laboratory animals, the exposure to components leached from dental sealants containing BPA alters reproductive end points (Darmani & Al-Hiyasat, 2006). While no effects on the number of implantation sites have been observed, an increased number of embryo resorptions (postimplantation loss) have been reported (Darmani & Al-Hiyasat, 2006). Other authors have shown that BPA exposure during the sensitive period of blastocyst implantation disrupts pregnancy (Berger, Hancock, & deCatanzaro, 2007). In our experimental design, we used a brief postnatal exposure and evaluated the long-lasting effects on reproductive performance. After early postnatal exposure to both doses of BPA, we observed a trend to a decreased percentage of rats that became pregnant, although all females were sexually receptive. The number of corpora lutea (CL) in the ovaries from all BPA-treated pregnant rats was similar to that of controls (12–13 CL/rat). This result suggests that the ovulation rate and CL "activation" are not altered in most of the females after neonatal exposure to the xenoestrogen BPA. In contrast, the number of implantation sites was significantly lower in BPA-treated rats, suggesting an intrinsic uterine defect that preceded embryo arrival (Varayoud et al., 2011). Therefore, BPA effects on reproductive performance could be different depending on the animal model used, developmental stage at exposure, and/or the dose administered.

3.2. BPA alters endocrine signaling in the preimplantation uterus

The effects of BPA on reproductive performance can be associated with the disruption of different markers of uterine implantation mainly those regulated by ovarian steroid hormones. To evaluate whether the endocrine pathway is affected, we established the serum levels of sex steroids and uterine steroid hormone receptor expression (ERα and PR) on GD 5 (Varayoud et al., 2011). The uteri of control animals showed a high expression of ERα and PR in subepithelial stromal cells, whereas those of animals neonatally treated with BPA showed a lower expression of both receptors, without changes in serum levels of estradiol and progesterone. In addition, we found that neonatal exposure to BPA caused different effects on PR expression according with the BPA dose, suggesting that the uterine response to the hormonal milieu on GD 5 of pregnancy is differentially affected. The lower dose of BPA (BPA.05) diminished *PR* mRNA, but not PR protein, whereas the higher dose (BPA20) affected both mRNA and protein expression. In this context, we propose that BPA.05 could affect the ubiquitination of PR protein and consequent degradation. Other previous studies have shown that a reduced ubiquitination of PR contributes to its stabilization and is correlated with an increased response to progesterone (Lee, 2008). The estrogen influence on the ubiquitination system has been extensively shown (Ito et al., 2010). ERα is commonly associated with ubiquitin ligases (like Smurf) forming protein complexes that regulate the ubiquitination rate of many targets in an estrogen-dependent manner. In particular, PR is a substrate for the ubiquitin/proteasome pathway (Qiu & Lange, 2003). Ubiquitination of PR depends on S294 phosphorylation. This has been demonstrated using an S294A mutant, which does not undergo ubiquitination and degradation by the proteasome pathway after progesterone binding (Qiu & Lange, 2003). These (and other) results provide some empirical data to speculate about the possible influence of xenoestrogens on the control of the ubiquitination process.

3.3. BPA and the expression of implantation-associated genes

With the intention to evaluate whether the effects of BPA exposure on reproductive performance are associated with modifications of implantation-associated genes, we have also assessed the expression of *Hoxa10*, *ITGB3*, and *EMX-2* (Varayoud et al., 2011). *Hoxa10* is an ovarian steroid downstream target gene, with a key role during implantation. In our work, we detected that *Hoxa10* uterine expression decreased in BPA-treated animals on GD 5 and that this decrease was further evidenced in the absence of variation in circulating steroid hormone levels and appeared to be due to a decrease in PR and ERα expression in the subepithelial stroma (Varayoud et al., 2011). Another previous report demonstrated that both steroid hormone receptors are implicated in the regulation of *Hoxa10* expression, using *in vitro* and *in vivo* models (Daftary & Taylor, 2006). Estradiol regulation of *Hoxa10* is associated with the detection of ER binding of two putative estrogen response elements in the 5′ regulatory region of *Hoxa10* (Taylor et al., 1998). Progestational regulation of *Hoxa10* occurs via PR and is therefore blocked by RU486 (Ma, Benson, Lim, Dey, & Maas, 1998).

As already mentioned, *EMX-2* and *ITGB3* are two *Hoxa10* target genes that are known to be operative downstream in endocrine hormone-regulated *Hox* gene pathways. Alterations in both genes are associated with subfertility in different species (Daftary & Taylor, 2006). Our results have shown that BPA-exposed animals exhibiting a lower number of implantation sites and a disruption of *Hoxa10* additionally showed a lower expression of *ITGB3* and a higher expression of *EMX-2*. Alterations in the endocrine-regulated *Hoxa10* gene pathways (steroid receptors–*Hoxa10*–*ITGB3*/*EMX-2*) could explain, at least in part, the BPA effects on the implantation process. Further evidence demonstrating that *Hoxa10*, *ITBG3*, and *EMX-2* function in a common pathway has been found in diseases with implantation defects, such as endometriosis, where simultaneous misregulation of these three genes has been documented (Lessey et al., 1994; Taylor, Bagot, Kardana, Olive, & Arici, 1999). A schematic representation showing the steroid receptors–*Hoxa10*–*ITGB3*/*EMX-2* network during the preimplantation period and the effects of early postnatal BPA exposure on this network is shown in Fig. 10.1.

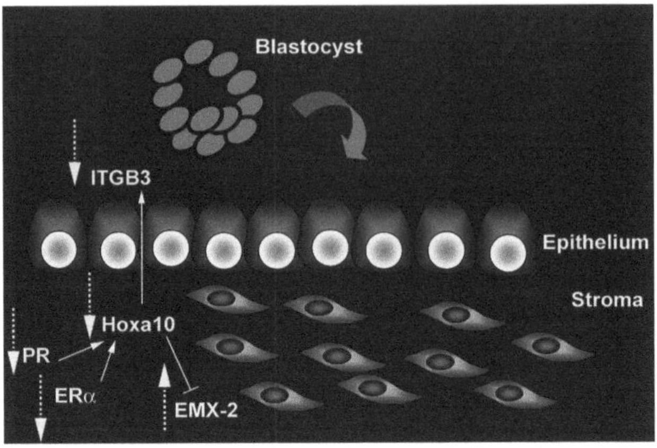

Figure 10.1 Schematic representation showing long-lasting effects of early postnatal bisphenol A (BPA) exposure on essential molecular events of the implantation process. In control conditions, the sex steroids estradiol and progesterone and their cognate receptors PR and ERα upregulate *Hoxa10* in the subepithelial uterine stroma, which in turn represses *EMX-2* expression. In addition, *Hoxa10* acting downstream of sex steroids upregulates *ITGB3* expression by endometrial epithelial cells, suggesting terminal differentiation in this cell type in preparation for embryo implantation. Dashed arrows indicate the neonatal BPA effects on implantation-associated gene expression evaluated in the rat uterine tissue on gestation day 5. Alterations in the endocrine-regulated *Hoxa10* gene pathways (steroid receptors-*Hoxa10*–*ITGB3*/*EMX-2*) could explain, at least in part, the BPA effects on the implantation process. ----▶ indicates induction and ⊣ indicates repression. PR (progesterone receptor), ERα (estrogen receptor alpha), *ITGB3* (*Beta 3 integrin*), and *EMX-2* (*empty spiracles homolog 2*). (See color plate.)

3.4. Early postnatal BPA exposure impairs the uterine response to ovarian steroids in the adult

The hormonal control of endometrial proliferation can be affected as a consequence of endocrine disruptor exposure. To evaluate whether a brief postnatal BPA exposure could adversely affect the uterine response to hormonal stimuli, we used a model of ovariectomized (OVX) adult rats with exogenous steroid hormone replacement with the intention to eliminate the variability in hormone levels characteristic of cycling animals (Varayoud et al., 2008). Progesterone pretreatment followed by a physiological dose of estradiol increased the number of synchronously proliferating subepithelial stromal cells (Rider, Thomson, & Seifert, 2003). In addition, mutant mice lacking normal *Hoxa10* expression showed defective progesterone-dependent uterine stromal proliferation (Yao et al., 2003). Figure 10.2A shows that rats neonatally exposed to BPA had an impaired response to normal ovarian steroid-mediated induction

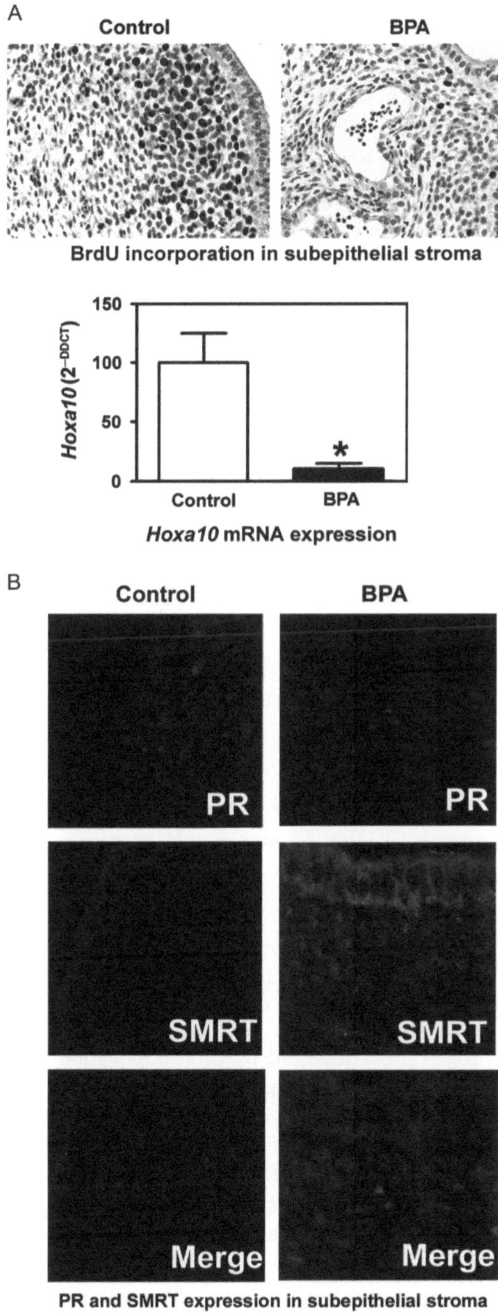

Figure 10.2 Long-term effects of postnatal exposure to BPA in the uterus of adult ovariectomized rats in response to steroid hormone replacement. (A) Subepithelial stromal *(Continued)*

of uterine stromal cell proliferation. In addition, steroid-mediated activation of *Hoxa10* failed in adult females postnatally exposed to BPA. It is notable that the increased cell number and endometrial tissue volume seen in controls may provide the necessary conditions for optimal embryo implantation. In support of this, increasing endometrial thickness correlates with higher implantation rates in humans (Zhang et al., 2005). Adult CD-1 mice exposed *in utero* to low doses of BPA show a decreased volume of the endometrial lamina propria (Markey, Wadia, Rubin, Sonnenschein, & Soto, 2005). Based on our results, we propose that alterations in the proliferative status of uterine stromal cells in response to steroid hormones could affect the synchrony between the endometrium and the embryo, likely leading to decreased fertility. These alterations have been demonstrated in mice in which the progesterone pathway is affected with clear consequences in fertility (Velarde, Geng, Eason, Simmen, & Simmen, 2005). Furthermore, several studies have supplied evidence about the possible relationship between this impaired proliferative response and the development of endocrine-related diseases such as endometriosis and endometrial tumors (Gargett & Chan, 2006).

Progesterone + estradiol treatment in OVX rats increases not only subepithelial proliferation but also endothelial proliferation. Previous works have shown that the uterine vascularization is another key process in the preparation of the endometrium for embryo implantation (Weitlauf, 1994). We found that the proliferative response of the uterine endothelial cells to ovarian steroids during adulthood is altered by neonatal exposure to BPA (Bosquiazzo et al., 2010). Moreover, BPA exposure downregulates *VEGF* expression in the subepithelial uterine stroma, another event closely related to the control of the vascular compartment (Fig. 10.3A). It is well known that VEGF is a secreted growth factor that operates by binding to specific receptors and that the VEGF/receptor signaling system is mainly

Figure 10.2—Cont'd proliferation detected by bromodeoxyuridine (BrdU) incorporation. Relative *Hoxa10* mRNA expression was measured via real-time quantitative PCR and fold expression from control values was calculated by the equation $2^{-\Delta\Delta CT}$. Control group was assigned to a reference level of 100 and values are given as mean ± SEM. Ribosomal protein L19 was used as internal control. *Asterisk* indicates $p < 0.05$. ($n = 8$/group). Note that BrdU incorporation and *Hoxa10* mRNA expression decrease in uterine tissue of rats postnatally exposed to BPA. Magnification: ×400. (B) Dual immunofluorescence staining for progesterone receptor (PR, red) and silencing mediator for retinoic acid and thyroid hormone receptor (SMRT, green). An increase in SMRT expression is observed in the subepithelial stroma of postnatally exposed BPA rats. The merge images show that SMRT colocalizes with PR in the subepithelial stroma. Magnification: ×1000. *For methodological details, see Varayoud et al. (2008).* (See color plate.)

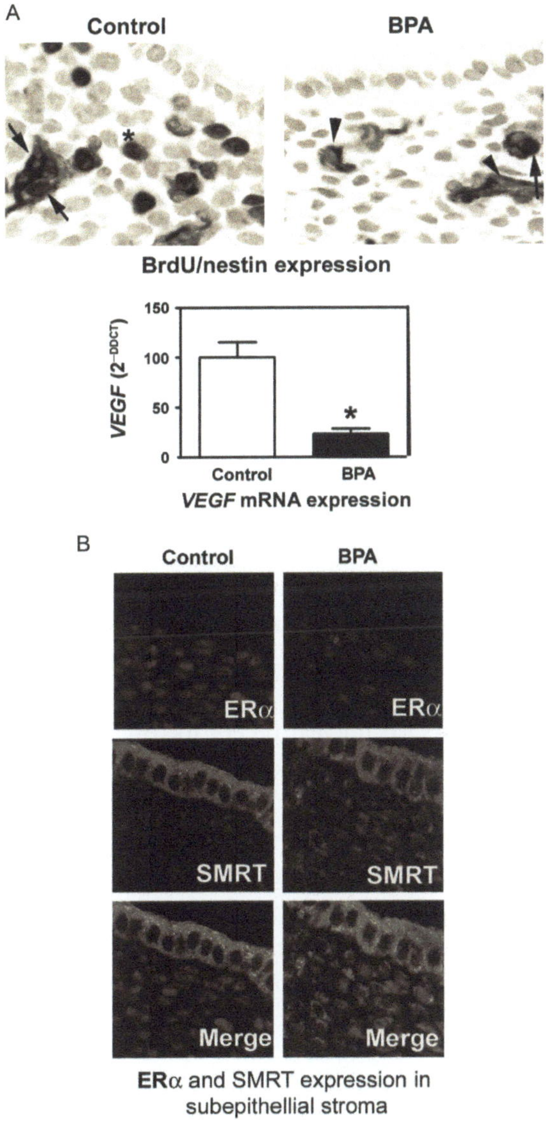

Figure 10.3 Effect of neonatal exposure to BPA on steroid regulation of vascular endothelial growth factor expression (*VEGF*) and endothelial cell proliferation. (A) Representative photomicrographs of uterine sections double-immunostained for BrdU (brown nuclei) and nestin (black cytoplasms) to evaluate endothelial proliferation. Arrows indicate double-positive cells (proliferating endothelial cells), and arrowheads indicate nonproliferating endothelial cells (positive for nestin in the cytoplasms with pink nuclei counterstained with nuclear fast red). Asterisk in the control photomicrograph indicates BrdU-positive fibroblastic stromal cell. Magnification: ×1000. Relative *VEGF* mRNA levels were measured by real-time quantitative PCR and fold expression from control values

(*Continued*)

involved in the regulation of endothelial cell proliferation (Ferrara, Gerber, & LeCouter, 2003). Therefore, our results suggest that the alteration in steroid-mediated activation of *VEGF* could be responsible for the impaired endothelial proliferative response found in BPA-exposed rats. The lack of changes in the processing of the *VEGF* mRNA splice variants suggests that xenoestrogens could modify *VEGF* mRNA expression by acting at the primary transcript level. Bredhult, Bäcklin, and Olovsson (2007) studied whether endocrine-disrupting chemicals affect the proliferation and viability of human endometrial endothelial cells *in vitro* and, in accordance with our results, observed that after treatment with 0.01, 1, or 100 μM BPA, endothelial proliferation was lower than in controls.

Taking into account that the steroid hormone responsiveness of the uterine stroma is affected in BPA-exposed animals, we determined stromal expression of PR and ERα in an OVX+progesterone+estradiol rat model and found no changes; however, we detected a decreased expression of both receptors in BPA-treated animals on GD 5. This indicates that results observed with regard to steroid hormone receptors are different between pregnant rats and the model of OVX rats with an exogenous ovarian steroid treatment that mimics the hormonal milieu during implantation. In addition, we determined the expression of coregulator proteins, because these proteins serve as partners for nuclear receptors, orchestrating the molecular events required for receptor-dependent transcriptional regulation (Hall & McDonnell, 2005). Therefore, the sensitivity to steroid hormones also depends on the availability of steroid receptor coregulators (Durrer, Maerkel, Schlumpf, & Lichtensteiger, 2005). The expression of the coactivator SRC-3 was similar in animals exposed to BPA and controls. However, our data demonstrate that neonatal exposure to BPA affects uterine stromal SMRT expression in response to progesterone+estradiol treatment, showing a clear upregulation of this corepressor in the subepithelial

Figure 10.3—Cont'd was calculated by the equation $2^{-\Delta\Delta CT}$. Control group was assigned to a reference level of 100 and values are given as mean ± SEM. Ribosomal protein L19 was used as internal control. *Asterisk* indicates $p < 0.05$. ($n = 8$/group). BrdU endothelial incorporation and *Vegf* mRNA expression decreased in rats neonatally exposed to BPA. (B) Dual immunofluorescence staining for estrogen receptor alpha (ERα, red) and silencing mediator for retinoic acid and thyroid hormone receptor (SMRT, green). An increase in SMRT expression is observed in the subepithelial stroma of BPA neonatally exposed rats. The merge images show that SMRT colocalizes with ERα in the subepithelial stroma. Magnification: ×1000. *For methodological details, see Bosquiazzo et al. (2010).* (See color plate.)

stroma (Figs. 10.2B and 10.3B). Moreover, immunofluorescence results showed the coexpression of SMRT/ERα and SMRT/PR in the uterine stromal cells (Figs. 10.2B and 10.3D). Nuclear receptor coregulators were revealed as targets for endocrine disruptors, as shown for SMRT in the prostate and SRC-1 in the uterus (Durrer et al., 2005, 2007). The increase in SMRT described here may have implications for gene expression on a broad scale because SMRT is recruited by many transcription factors, including steroid receptors (Hall & McDonnell, 2005), and is also a limiting factor inhibiting transcriptional activity of steroid hormone receptors (Privalsky, 2004). The fact that the abnormal overexpression of SMRT was found in the same subepithelial stromal cells where VEGF and Hoxa10 induction failed suggests that the high levels of SMRT could interfere with different steroid-dependent genes in BPA-exposed animals. Our results show that the exposure to xenoestrogen chemicals during critical periods of perinatal life changes the uterine hormonal response during adulthood by disrupting the assembly of the transcription machinery of PR- and ER-dependent genes. Future studies will address this issue by studying whether neonatal exposure to BPA affects the transcription factor assembly in the *Hoxa10* promoter region.

4. ENDOCRINE DISRUPTION AND FEMALE FERTILITY

The combination of data showing reduced conception rates in humans and the common occurrence of female reproductive disease raises concerns that environmental factors may be having a negative impact on female reproductive health. However, the effects of endocrine disruptors are difficult to determine, because the consequences are evident long after exposure has ended. In addition, it is becoming increasingly clear from epidemiological studies in humans (Christiansen et al., 2005), and from genetic studies in rodents (Wang & Dey, 2006), that failed pregnancies are largely due to faulty uterine function or miscommunication between the embryo and the mother before placentation. Our results corroborate this paradigm and should serve to alert on the fact that reproductive performance and altered uterine function due to neonatal exposure to BPA are probably related. Results obtained after DES or endosulfan exposure using the same animal model (Varayoud et al., 2011, 2012) show that different endocrine-disrupting compounds impair fertility by altering signaling pathways similar to those described for BPA.

5. CONCLUSIONS

BPA effects on reproduction and specifically on the uterus physiology have been the focus of numerous studies. Using a rat model of a brief early postnatal exposure, we detected that low doses of BPA affect the course of uterine development with lasting consequences. Subfertility was evidenced by a lower number of implantation sites and different alterations in the endocrine pathways that regulate the preparation of the endometrium for embryo implantation. According to our and other results, *Hoxa10* is a common target of endocrine disruptors in uterine tissue and is affected during the early postnatal period. BPA effects observed during the prepubertal period remained during adulthood, and some *Hoxa10*-downstream events were fully disrupted. We propose that an early alteration in *Hoxa10* gene expression affects functional differentiation of the uterus during pregnancy as part of an altered endocrine signal transduction pathway.

ACKNOWLEDGMENTS

This work was supported by Grants from the Universidad Nacional del Litoral (CAI+D program), the Argentine National Council for Science and Technology (CONICET), and the Argentine National Agency for the Promotion of Science and Technology (ANPCyT). J. V., J. G. R., and E. H. L. are career investigators of the CONICET.

REFERENCES

Bagot, C. N., Troy, P. J., & Taylor, H. S. (2000). Alteration of maternal *Hoxa10* expression by in vivo gene transfection affects implantation. *Gene Therapy*, 7, 1378–1384.

Bartol, F. F., Wiley, A. A., & Bagnell, C. A. (2006). Uterine development and endometrial programming. *Society of Reproduction and Fertility Supplement*, *62*, 113–130.

Benson, G. V., Lim, H., Paria, B. C., Satokata, I., Dey, S. K., & Maas, R. L. (1996). Mechanisms of reduced fertility in Hoxa-10 mutant mice: Uterine homeosis and loss of maternal Hoxa-10 expression. *Development*, *122*, 2687–2696.

Berger, R. G., Hancock, T., & deCatanzaro, D. (2007). Influence of oral and subcutaneous bisphenol-A on intrauterine implantation of fertilized ova in inseminated female mice. *Reproductive Toxicology*, *23*, 38–44.

Biedermann, S., Tschudin, P., & Grob, K. (2010). Transfer of bisphenol A from thermal printer paper to the skin. *Analytical and Bioanalytical Chemistry*, *398*, 571–576.

Bosquiazzo, V. L., Varayoud, J., Muñoz-de-Toro, M., Luque, E. H., & Ramos, J. G. (2010). Effects of neonatal exposure to bisphenol A on steroid regulation of vascular endothelial growth factor expression and endothelial cell proliferation in the adult rat uterus. *Biology of Reproduction*, *82*, 86–95.

Braun, J. M., Yolton, K., Dietrich, K. N., Hornung, R., Ye, X., & Calafat, A. M. (2009). Prenatal bisphenol A exposure and early childhood behavior. *Environmental Health Perspectives*, *117*, 1945–1952.

Bredhult, C., Bäcklin, B. M., & Olovsson, M. (2007). Effects of some endocrine disruptors on t he proliferation and viability of human endometrial endothelial cells in vitro. *Reproductive Toxicology*, *23*, 550–559.
Calafat, A. M., Ye, X., Wong, L. Y., Reidy, J. A., & Needham, L. L. (2008). Exposure of the U.S. population to bisphenol A and 4-tertiary-octylphenol: 2003–2004. *Environmental Health Perspectives*, *116*, 39–44.
Carson, D. D., Bagchi, I., Dey, S. K., Enders, A. C., Fazleabas, A. T., Lessey, B. A., et al. (2000). Embryo implantation. *Developmental Biology*, *223*, 217–237.
CERHR NTP-CERHR expert panel report on reproductive and developmental toxicity of bisphenol A. (2007). Center for the evaluation of risks to human reproduction (CERHR), U.S. National Toxicology Program (NTP). http://cerhr.niehs.nih.gov/chemicals/bisphenol/BPAFinalEPVF112607.pdf.
Christiansen, O. B., Nybo Andersen, A. M., Bosch, E., Daya, S., Delves, P. J., Hviid, T. V., et al. (2005). Evidence-based investigations and treatment of recurrent pregnancy loss. *Fertility and Sterility*, *83*, 821–839.
Couse, J. F., Dixon, D., Yates, M., Moore, A. B., Ma, L., Maas, R., et al. (2001). Estrogen receptor-a knockout mice exhibit resistance to the developmental effects of neonatal diethylstilbestrol exposure on the female reproductive tract. *Developmental Biology*, *238*, 224–238.
Crain, D. A., Janssen, S. J., Edwards, T. M., Heindel, J., Ho, S. M., Hunt, P., et al. (2008). Female reproductive disorders: The roles of endocrine-disrupting compounds and developmental timing. *Fertility and Sterility*, *90*, 911–940.
Curtis Hewitt, S., Goulding, E. H., Eddy, E. M., & Korach, K. S. (2002). Studies using the estrogen receptor alpha knockout uterus demonstrate that implantation but not decidualization-associated signaling is estrogen dependent. *Biology of Reproduction*, *67*, 1268–1277.
Daftary, G. S., & Taylor, H. S. (2006). Endocrine regulation of HOX genes. *Endocrine Reviews*, *27*, 331–355.
Daftary, G. S., Troy, P. J., Bagot, C. N., Young, S. L., & Taylor, H. S. (2002). Direct regulation of B3-integrin subunit gene expression by *HOXA10* in endometrial cells. *Molecular Endocrinology*, *16*, 571–579.
Daikoku, T., Song, H., Guo, Y., Riesewijk, A., Mosselman, S., Das, S. K., et al. (2004). Uterine Msx-1 and Wnt4 signaling becomes aberrant in mice with the loss of leukemia inhibitory factor or Hoxa-10: Evidence for a novel cytokine-homeobox-Wnt signaling in implantation. *Molecular Endocrinology*, *18*, 1238–1250.
Darmani, H., & Al-Hiyasat, A. S. (2006). The effects of BIS-GMA and TEGDMA on female mouse fertility. *Dental Materials*, *22*, 353–358.
Das, S. K. (2010). Regional development of uterine decidualization: Molecular signalling by Hoxa-10. *Molecular Reproduction and Development*, *77*, 387–396.
Dey, S. K., Lim, H., Das, S. K., Reese, J., Paria, B. C., Daikoku, T., et al. (2004). Molecular cues to implantation. *Endocrine Reviews*, *25*, 341–373.
Durrer, S., Ehnes, C., Fuetsch, M., Maerkel, K., Schlumpf, M., & Lichtensteiger, W. (2007). Estrogen sensitivity of target genes and expression of nuclear receptor coregulators in rat prostate after pre- and postnatal exposure to the ultraviolet filter 4-methylbenzylidene camphor. *Environmental Health Perspectives*, *115*, 42–50.
Durrer, S., Maerkel, K., Schlumpf, M., & Lichtensteiger, W. (2005). Estrogen target gene regulation and coactivator expression in rat uterus after developmental exposure to the ultraviolet filter 4-methylbenzylidene camphor. *Endocrinology*, *146*, 2130–2139.
Fei, X., Chung, H., & Taylor, H. S. (2005). Methoxychlor disrupts uterine *Hoxa10* gene expression. *Endocrinology*, *146*, 3445–3451.
Ferrara, N., Gerber, H. P., & LeCouter, J. (2003). The biology of VEGF and its receptors. *Nature Medicine*, *9*, 669–676.

Gargett, B. E., & Chan, R. W. (2006). Endometrial stem/progenitor cells and proliferative disorders of the endometrium. *Minerva Ginecologica, 58*, 511–526.

Hall, J. M., & McDonnell, D. P. (2005). Coregulators in nuclear estrogen receptor action: From concept to therapeutic targeting. *Molecular Interventions, 5*, 343–357.

Hayashi, Y., Saitou, M., & Yamanaka, S. (2012). Germline development from human pluripotent stem cells toward disease modeling of infertility. *Fertility and Sterility, 97*, 1250–1259.

Huet-Hudson, Y. M., Andrews, G. K., & Dey, S. K. (1989). Cell type-specific localization of c-myc protein in the uterus: Modulation by steroid hormones and analysis of the periimplantation period. *Endocrinology, 125*, 1683–1690.

Ito, I., Hanyu, A., Wayama, M., Goto, N., Katsuno, Y., Kawasaki, S., et al. (2010). Estrogen inhibits transforming growth factor beta signaling by promoting Smad2/3 degradation. *The Journal of Biological Chemistry, 285*, 14747–14755.

Jeong, J. W., Lee, K. Y., Han, S. J., Aronow, B. J., Lydon, J. P., O'Malley, B. W., et al. (2007). The p160 steroid receptor coactivator 2, SRC-2, regulates murine endometrial function and regulates progesterone-independent and dependent gene expression. *Endocrinology, 148*, 4238–4250.

Karuri, A. R., Kumar, A. M., & Mukhopadhyay, D. (1998). Differential expression and selective localization of vascular permeability factor/vascular endothelial growth factor in the rat uterus during the estrous cycle. *The Journal of Endocrinology, 159*, 489–499.

Kastury, K., Druck, T., Huebner, K., Barletta, C., Acampora, D., Simeone, A., et al. (1994). Chromosome locations of human EMX and OTX genes. *Genomics, 22*, 41–45.

Kazi, A. A., & Koos, R. D. (2007). Estrogen-induced activation of hypoxia-inducible factor-1alpha, vascular endothelial growth factor expression, and edema in the uterus are mediated by the phosphatidylinositol 3-kinase/Akt pathway. *Endocrinology, 148*, 2363–2374.

Kim, J. J., Taylor, H. S., Lu, Z., Ladhani, O., Hastings, J. M., Jackson, K. S., et al. (2007). Altered expression of *HOXA10* in endometriosis: Potential role in decidualization. *Human Reproduction, 13*, 323–332.

Lang, I. A., Galloway, T. S., Scarlett, A., Henley, W. E., Depledge, M., Wallace, R. B., et al. (2008). Association of urinary bisphenol A concentration with medical disorders and laboratory abnormalities in adults. *Journal of the American Medical Association, 300*, 1303–1310.

Lee, E. Y. (2008). Promotion of BRCA1-associated triple-negative breast cancer by ovarian hormones. *Current Opinion in Obstetrics & Gynecology, 20*, 68–73.

Lessey, B. A., Castelbaum, A. J., Sawin, S. W., Buck, C. A., Schinnar, R., Bilker, W., et al. (1994). Aberrant integrin expression in the endometrium of women with endometriosis. *The Journal of Clinical Endocrinology and Metabolism, 79*, 643–649.

Li, D. K., Zhou, Z., Miao, M., He, Y., Qing, D., Wu, T., et al. (2010). Relationship between urine bisphenol-A level and declining male sexual function. *Journal of Andrology, 31*, 500–506.

Lim, H., Ma, L., Ma, W. G., Maas, R. L., & Dey, S. K. (1999). Hoxa-10 regulates uterine stromal cell responsiveness to progesterone during implantation and decidualization in the mouse. *Molecular Endocrinology, 13*, 1005–1017.

Ma, L., Benson, G. V., Lim, H., Dey, S. K., & Maas, R. L. (1998). Abdominal B (AbdB) Hoxa genes: Regulation in adult uterus by estrogen and progesterone and repression in mullerian duct by the synthetic estrogen diethylstilbestrol (DES). *Developmental Biology, 197*, 141–154.

Macklon, N. S., Pieters, M. H., Hassan, M. A., Jeucken, P. H., Eijkemans, M. J., & Fauser, B. C. (2002). A prospective randomized comparison of sequential versus monoculture systems for in-vitro human blastocyst development. *Human Reproduction, 17*, 2700–2705.

Maffini, M. V., Rubin, B. S., Sonnenschein, C., & Soto, A. M. (2006). Endocrine disruptors and reproductive health: The case of bisphenol-A. *Molecular and Cellular Endocrinology, 255*, 179–186.

Markey, C. M., Wadia, P. R., Rubin, B. S., Sonnenschein, C., & Soto, A. M. (2005). Long-term effects of fetal exposure to low doses of the xenoestrogen bisphenol-A in the female mouse genital tract. *Biology of Reproduction, 72*, 1344–1351.

Mericskay, M., Carta, L., & Sassoon, D. (2005). Diethylstilbestrol exposure in utero: A paradigm for mechanisms leading to adult disease. *Birth Defects Research, Part A: Clinical and Molecular Teratology, 73*, 133–135.

Milesi, M. M., Varayoud, J., Bosquiazzo, V. L., Muñoz-de-Toro, M., & Luque, E. H. (2012). Neonatal exposure to low doses of endosulfan disrupts the expression of proteins regulating uterine development and differentiation. *Reproductive Toxicology, 33*, 85–93.

Monje, L., Varayoud, J., Luque, E. H., & Ramos, J. G. (2007). Neonatal exposure to bisphenol A modifies the abundance of estrogen receptor alpha transcripts with alternative 5′-untranslated regions in the female rat preoptic area. *The Journal of Endocrinology, 194*, 201–212.

Monje, L., Varayoud, J., Muñoz-de-Toro, M., Luque, E. H., & Ramos, J. G. (2009). Neonatal exposure to bisphenol A alters estrogen-dependent mechanisms governing sexual behavior in the adult female rat. *Reproductive Toxicology, 28*, 435–442.

Monje, L., Varayoud, J., Muñoz-de-Toro, M., Luque, E. H., & Ramos, J. G. (2010). Exposure of neonatal female rats to bisphenol A disrupts hypothalamic LHRH pre-mRNA processing and estrogen receptor alpha expression in nuclei controlling estrous cyclicity. *Reproductive Toxicology, 30*, 625–634.

Mueller, M. D., Vigne, J. L., Pritts, E. A., Chao, V., Dreher, E., & Taylor, R. N. (2003). Progestins activate vascular endothelial growth factor gene transcription in endometrial adenocarcinoma cells. *Fertility and Sterility, 79*, 386–392.

Norwitz, E. R., Schust, D. J., & Fisher, S. J. (2001). Implantation and the survival of early pregnancy. *The New England Journal of Medicine, 345*, 1400–1408.

Ola, B., & Li, T. C. (2006). Implantation failure following in-vitro fertilization. *Current Opinion in Obstetrics & Gynecology, 18*, 440–445.

Privalsky, M. L. (2004). The role of corepressors in transcriptional regulation by nuclear hormone receptors. *Annual Review of Physiology, 66*, 315–360.

Qiu, M., & Lange, C. A. (2003). MAP kinases couple multiple functions of human progesterone receptors: Degradation, transcriptional synergy, and nuclear association. *The Journal of Steroid Biochemistry and Molecular Biology, 85*, 147–157.

Rabbani, M. L., & Rogers, P. A. (2001). Role of vascular endothelial growth factor in endometrial vascular events before implantation in rats. *Reproduction, 122*, 85–90.

Rider, V., Thomson, E., & Seifert, C. (2003). Transit of rat uterine stromal cells through G1 phase of the cell cycle requires temporal and cell-specific hormone-dependent changes on cell cycle regulators. *Endocrinology, 144*, 5450–5458.

Rockwell, L. C., Pillai, S., Olson, C. E., & Koos, R. D. (2002). Inhibition of vascular endothelial growth factor/vascular permeability factor action blocks estrogen-induced uterine edema and implantation in rodents. *Biology of Reproduction, 67*, 1804–1810.

Rodriguez, H. A., Santambrosio, N., Santamaría, C. G., Muñoz-de-Toro, M., & Luque, E. H. (2010). Neonatal exposure to bisphenol A reduces the pool of primordial follicles in the rat ovary. *Reproductive Toxicology, 30*, 550–557.

Rubel, C. A., Jeong, J. W., Tsai, S. Y., Lydon, J. P., & Demayo, F. J. (2010). Epithelial-stromal interaction and progesterone receptors in the mouse uterus. *Seminars in Reproductive Medicine, 28*, 27–35.

Rubin, B. S. (2011). Bisphenol A: An endocrine disrupter with widespread exposure and multiple effects. *The Journal of Steroid Biochemistry and Molecular Biology, 127*, 27–34.

Satokata, I., Benson, G., & Maas, R. (1995). Sexually dimorphic sterility phenotypes in *Hoxa10*-deficient mice. *Nature, 374*, 460–463.

Sengupta, J., Lalitkumar, P. G., Najwa, A. R., Charnock-Jones, D. S., Evans, A. L., Sharkey, A. M., et al. (2007). Immunoneutralization of vascular endothelial growth factor inhibits pregnancy establishment in the rhesus monkey (Macaca mulatta). *Reproduction, 133*, 1199–1211.

Shweiki, D., Itin, A., Neufeld, G., Gitay-Goren, H., & Keshet, E. (1993). Patterns of expression of vascular endothelial growth factor (VEGF) and VEGF receptors in mice suggest a role in hormonally regulated angiogenesis. *The Journal of Clinical Investigation, 91*, 2235–2243.

Smith, C. C., & Taylor, H. S. (2007). Xenoestrogen exposure imprints expression of genes (*Hoxa10*) required for normal uterine development. *The FASEB Journal, 21*, 239–246.

Sueoka, K., Shiokawa, S., Miyazaki, T., Kuji, N., Tanaka, M., & Yoshimura, Y. (1997). Integrins and reproductive physiology: Expression and modulation in fertilization, embryogenesis, and implantation. *Fertility and Sterility, 67*, 799–811.

Tan, J., Paria, B. C., Dey, S. K., & Das, S. K. (1999). Differential uterine expression of estrogen and progesterone receptors correlated with uterine preparation for implantation and decidualization in the mouse. *Endocrinology, 140*, 5310–5321.

Taylor, H. S. (2000). The role of HOX genes in the development and function of the female reproductive tract. *Seminars in Reproductive Medicine, 18*, 81–89.

Taylor, H. S., Arici, A., Olive, D., & Igarashi, P. (1998). *HOXA10* is expressed in response to sex steroids at the time of implantation in the human endometrium. *The Journal of Clinical Investigation, 101*, 1379–1384.

Taylor, H. S., Bagot, C., Kardana, A., Olive, D., & Arici, A. (1999). HOX gene expression is altered in the endometrium of women with endometriosis. *Human Reproduction, 14*, 1328–1331.

Taylor, J. A., Welshons, W. V., & vom Saal, F. S. (2008). No effect of route of exposure (oral; subcutaneous injection) on plasma bisphenol A throughout 24 h after administration in neonatal female mice. *Reproductive Toxicology, 25*, 169–176.

Tharp, A. P., Maffini, M. V., Hunt, P. A., VandeVoort, C. A., Sonnenschein, C., & Soto, A. M. (2012). Bisphenol A alters the development of the rhesus monkey mammary gland. *Proceedings of the National Academy of Sciences of the United States of America, 109*, 8190–8195.

Tibbetts, T. A., Mendoza-Meneses, M., O'Malley, B. W., & Conneely, O. M. (1998). Mutual and intercompartmental regulation of estrogen receptor and progesterone receptor expression in the mouse uterus. *Biology of Reproduction, 59*, 1143–1152.

Troy, P. J., Daftary, G. S., Bagot, C. N., & Taylor, H. S. (2003). Transcriptional repression of peri-implantation EMX2 expression in mammalian reproduction by *HOXA10*. *Molecular and Cellular Biology, 23*, 1–13.

U.S. Environmental Protection Agency. (1993). Bisphenol A, CASRN 80-05-7, IRIS, Integrated Risk Information System. http://www.epa.gov/iris/subst/0356.htm.

Vanderberg, L. N., Chauhoud, J., Heindel, J. J., Padmanabhan, V., Paumgartten, F. J., & Schoenfelder, G. (2010). Urinary, circulating and tissue biomonitoring studies indicate widespread exposure to bisphenol A. *Environmental Health Perspectives, 118*, 1055–1070.

Varayoud, J., Milesi, M. M., Alarcón, R., Rivera, O. E., Muñoz-de-Toro, M., & Luque, E. H. (2012). Postnatal endosulfan exposure alters endocrine signalling and endometrial proliferation in the rat. *Biocell, 36*, 41–42.

Varayoud, J., Ramos, J. G., Bosquiazzo, V. L., Coger, M., Muñoz-de-Toro, M., & Luque, E. H. (2011). Neonatal exposure to bisphenol A alters rat uterine implantation-associated gene expression and reduces the number of implantation sites. *Endocrinology, 152*, 1101–1111.

Varayoud, J., Ramos, J. G., Bosquiazzo, V. L., Muñoz-de-Toro, M., & Luque, E. H. (2008). Developmental exposure to bisphenol A impairs the uterine response to ovarian steroids in the adult. *Endocrinology, 149*, 5848–5860.

Velarde, M. C., Geng, Y., Eason, R. R., Simmen, F. A., & Simmen, R. C. (2005). Null mutation of Kruppel-like factor9/basic transcription element binding protein-1 alters peri-implantation uterine development in mice. *Biology of Reproduction, 73*, 472–481.

Wang, H., & Dey, S. K. (2006). Roadmap to embryo implantation: Clues from mouse models. *Nature Reviews Genetics*, 7, 185–199.

Weitlauf, H. M. (1994). Biology of implantation. In E. Knobil & J. D. Neill (Eds.), *The physiology of reproduction* (pp. 391–440). New York: Raven Press.

Yao, M. W., Lim, H., Schust, D. J., Choe, S. E., Farago, A., Ding, Y., et al. (2003). Gene expression profiling reveals progesterone-mediated cell cycle and immunoregulatory roles of Hoxa-10 in the preimplantation uterus. *Molecular Endocrinology, 17*, 610–627.

Yi, X. J., Jiang, H. Y., Lee, K. K., O, W. S., Tang, P. L., & Chow, P. H. (1999). Expression of vascular endothelial growth factor (VEGF) and its receptors during embryonic implantation in the golden hamster (Mesocricetus auratus). *Cell and Tissue Research, 296*, 339–349.

Zhang, X., Chen, C. H., Confino, E., Barnes, R., Milad, M., & Kazer, R. R. (2005). Increased endometrial thickness is associated with improved treatment outcome for selected patients undergoing in vitro fertilization-embryo transfer. *Fertility and Sterility, 83*, 336–340.

CHAPTER ELEVEN

The Obesogen Tributyltin

Felix Grün[1]
The Center for Complex Biological Systems, University of California Irvine, Irvine, California, USA
[1]Corresponding author: e-mail address: fgrun@uci.edu

Contents

1. The Obesogen Hypothesis 277
2. Organotins Environmental Exposure 281
3. Mechanisms of Cellular Organotin Toxicity 285
4. Nuclear Hormone Receptors as Organotin Targets 291
5. TBT and Disrupted Adipose Biology 297
6. Epigenetic Perturbations in Adipogenesis and Metabolic Set Points 303
7. Conclusion and Perspective 308
Acknowledgments 311
References 312

Abstract

The obesogen hypothesis postulates the role of environmental chemical pollutants that disrupt homeostatic controls and adaptive mechanisms to promote adipose-dependent weight gain leading to obesity and metabolic syndrome complications. One of the most direct molecular mechanisms for coupling environmental chemical exposures to perturbed physiology invokes pollutants mimicking endogenous endocrine hormones or bioactive dietary signaling metabolites that serve as nuclear receptor ligands. The organotin pollutant tributyltin can exert toxicity through multiple mechanisms but most recently has been shown to bind, activate, and mediate RXR–PPARγ transcriptional regulation central to lipid metabolism and adipocyte biology. Data in support of long-term obesogenic effects on whole body adipose tissue are also reported. Organotins represent an important model test system for evaluating the impact and epidemiological significance of chemical insults as contributing factors for obesity and human metabolic health.

1. THE OBESOGEN HYPOTHESIS

Human metabolic physiology evolved during our paleolithic hunter-gatherer lifestyle to effectively buffer intermittent variations of excess or deficiency in caloric intake and balance the body's overall energy demands for growth, activity, and long-term energy reserves. The rapid and efficient

Vitamins and Hormones, Volume 94
ISSN 0083-6729
http://dx.doi.org/10.1016/B978-0-12-800095-3.00011-0

accumulation of fat reserves was a critical advantage prior to the development of more secure and predictable agrarian food sources. Today with the advent of modern food production and distribution practices, access to abundant, palatable, and nutritionally dense foods has become the norm for a large fraction of the world's population and our ancestral thrifty predisposition may be maladapted to such an environment (Neel, 1999; Stoger, 2008). Perhaps, it is not surprising that a perpetual state of caloric indulgence beyond the body's metabolic requirements has led to an explosion in obesity rates especially when adaptive mechanisms to restore balance—feedback inhibition of appetite, increased physical activity, and higher metabolic rates—are also under assault or have physiological limits. The mantra of "eat less, exercise more" is the appropriate response to this altered lifestyle but is difficult to implement in our modern societies.

But human societies have also changed in other important ways that are relevant to our physiology and health. We are no longer restricted in our exposure to a chemical environment based solely on dietary components and natural products synthesized by biological systems that have been tested and coevolved over eons. Our exposure to chemical space today is vastly expanded through industrial processes that generate novel functional groups, exotic combinations of elements, and metabolically stable chemicals that our biology is ill equipped to handle. Baillie-Hamilton (2002) postulated such a contributing role for chemical insults that damage many of the body's natural weight control mechanisms, arguing that inactivity and dietary changes were insufficient to fully account for the rapid ascendancy in obesity rates. The exponential rise in output of industrial chemicals was presented as a causal correlation to the parallel epidemiological rise in metabolic syndrome diseases. We may have been born in a "primeval soup," but today, we are swimming in a "synthetic soup" of toxins, carcinogens, and endocrine-disrupting chemicals (EDCs), all vying to confuse or derail our bodies' attempts to interpret nutritional and environmental cues. Thus, the obesogen hypothesis proposes chemical exposures that perturb mechanisms of lipid homeostasis and adipogenesis or change the body's energy balance by altering metabolic set points or misregulating appetite and satiety to promote fat accumulation and obesity (Grun & Blumberg, 2006, 2007). However, in addition to providing a sound biological rationale and molecular mechanism, the hypothesis of obesity driven by chemical insults at the population level must answer criticism of their environmental abundance and overall epidemiological relevance.

Despite these considerable evidentiary hurdles, solid data in support of obesogens as a contributing factor are mounting (Thayer, Heindel, Bucher, & Gallo, 2012). Two prominent examples serve to highlight these concepts. The best studied is the role of smoking as a significant modulator of body weight. Whereas smoking typically suppresses appetite, cessation can lead to a temporary increase in body weight as the body readjusts to withdrawal from addiction. Less publicly appreciated, however, are the observations of the dramatic consequences of maternal smoking during pregnancy on obesity risks (Thayer et al., 2012). Fetal exposure to noxious compounds from cigarette smoke during critical developmental windows leads to a long-term increased propensity to develop obesity and metabolic syndrome disorders. These observations strongly argue for a permanent maladjustment to environmental and nutritional cues.

A variety of mechanisms have been studied to account for these effects. Exposure to cigarette carbon monoxide (Carmines & Rajendran, 2008), heavy metals like cadmium (Menai et al., 2012), or other toxic smoke by-products has profound effects on placental function and neonatal cardiovascular development. Consequently, intrauterine fetal growth is restricted. Lowered birth weight and subsequent catch-up growth are a common hallmark of fetal metabolic stress associated with long-term complications and metabolic syndrome disease risks. Nicotine also exerts broad biological effects on multiple organ systems. It can disrupt adipose and pancreatic islet development consistent with a subsequent transition to increased adiposity (Gao et al., 2005; Somm et al., 2008). Furthermore, nicotine's neuropharmacological effects exert changes in gene expression and morphology of central nervous system neural circuits that impact reward-related behaviors leading to unhealthy eating habits (junk food addiction) (Chen, Saad, Sandow, & Bertrand, 2012; Haghighi et al., 2013). Irrespective of the exact molecular mechanisms, prenatal maternal smoking raises the adjusted odds ratio for obesity by 1.5–2.0 in this cohort of children and is one of the leading indicators for persistent overall poor metabolic health (Al Mamun et al., 2006; Oken, Levitan, & Gillman, 2008; Power, Atherton, & Thomas, 2010; Power & Jefferis, 2002; Toschke, Koletzko, Slikker, Hermann, & von Kries, 2002).

A second example of obesogenic action can be found among neuropharmaceuticals used to treat psychiatric disorders. A number of tricyclic antidepressants, selective serotonin reuptake inhibitors, atypical antipsychotics, and mood stabilizers lead to a dose-dependent obesity in patients as an unwanted side effect of chronic therapy (Newcomer,

2007). For example, therapeutic treatment with the atypical antipsychotic olanzapine drives weight gain by as much as 10 kg/year (Nemeroff, 1997). The weight-inducing mechanisms of antipsychotic drugs are principally through their cognate neurotransmitter receptor targets—particularly the histamine (H1), serotonin 2c (5HT2c), and dopamine D2 (DRD2) receptors—regulating neural circuits of appetite and satiety. However, peripheral actions of ADPs that alter insulin action, lipid metabolism, and adipogenesis may also play a role (Ferno et al., 2009; Vestri, Maianu, Moellering, & Garvey, 2007; Yang, Chen, Yu, & Chen, 2007). Both examples represent proof of concept for the central aspects of the obesogen hypothesis by illustrating chemical exposures in humans that clearly reach pharmacologically active levels and demographic populations that are nontrivial in size. Therefore, the question is not whether obesogens exist in theory, but rather how significant are the risks from exposure to a plethora of chemical pollutants present at low levels or through intermittent exposures commonly encountered in the environment.

The list of chemical pollutants with proven or suspected endocrine-disrupting potential is substantial (Vandenberg et al., 2012). A subset of these EDCs, covering a wide diversity of chemical classes, are reported to produce weight gains in toxicological studies. Some examples include plastic derivatives (bisphenol A, BPA) and plasticizers (phthalates), herbicides (e.g., atrazine), fungicides (e.g., triflumizole), organophosphate pesticides (e.g., chlorpyrifos, disulfoton, fenthion, tebupirimfos, and tribufos), polychlorinated and polybrominated pesticides and derivatives (flame retardants), synthetic estrogens (diethylstilbestrol), antibiotics, and antibacterial compounds (Brown, 2012; Hatch et al., 2008; Lassiter & Brimijoin, 2008; Lassiter et al., 2008; Lim et al., 2009; Newbold, Padilla-Banks, Jefferson, & Heindel, 2008; Patisaul et al., 2012; Rubin, Murray, Damassa, King, & Soto, 2001; Somm et al., 2009). Frequently, the difficulty in assessing the risk to human health from low-dose exposures to EDCs stems from their ability to interact via multiple points and mechanisms with the body's highly complex and dynamic physiology that evoke phenomena with nonmonotonic dose–response curves (Vandenberg et al., 2012). This certainly appears to hold true in the case of candidate obesogens, such as the organotin tributyltin (TBT), where the dose–response relationship to develop obesity is strongly dependent on additional factors: frequency and duration of exposure, critical developmental windows, gender, metabolism and bioaccumulation, nutritional environment, and potential behavioral changes in food intake.

Although the biological effects of organotins have been extensively studied for over 40 years, a focus on their potential to act as obesogens was only recently recognized (Grun & Blumberg, 2006). A complete exposition of their obesogenic properties is therefore not yet possible. There are many important gaps in the experimental record and new insights that future work needs to resolve. The data summarized and outlined in this chapter are therefore focused on highlighting knowledge about organotin exposures, their chemical properties in relation to their ability to perturb biological processes, selected molecular mechanisms, supporting data from cellular and animal studies, and promising areas for future research exploration.

2. ORGANOTINS ENVIRONMENTAL EXPOSURE

Organotins are tetravalent derivatives of tin(IV) with a general formula of $R_{(4-n)}SnX_n$, where R represents organic substituents and X can be a halide, anion, or an organic group linked covalently through a heteroatom (O, N, S, etc.). The most commonly encountered compounds usually consist of identical substituent groups that can be alkyl, aryl, or alicyclic in nature (Fig. 11.1). Mono-, di-, tri-, and tetraorganotin compounds have found many applications in industrial processes, including as catalysts, in glass coating processes and PVC plastic manufacturing, and as broad spectrum biocides. Several hundred different compounds are in routine use.

Triorganotin species generally raise the greatest concern for biological toxicity. Estimates of annual worldwide organotin production climbed from 5000 tons/year in 1955 to 30,000 tons/year by the mid-1980s and, since this time, have remained approximately constant (Blunden & Chapman, 1986). Currently, triorganotin compounds represent about 30% of total annual production. The dramatic rise in organotin use was driven by the expanded production in plastics manufacturing as well as their rapid adoption as effective biocidal agents. Tributyltin oxide (TBTO) was discovered to be a particularly potent algicide and molluscicide that became ubiquitous as the active component in marine antifouling ship paints (Bosselmann, 1996). Widespread environmental contamination of marine ecosystems with tributyltin began in the 1960s. By the mid-1970s, studies of population declines and abnormalities in bivalve and marine mollusks species were being associated with TBT contamination of harbors and shipping lanes along European and North American coastlines (Ruiz, Bachelet, Caumette, & Donard, 1996). A principal observation from these environmental studies, confirmed by laboratory and field experimentation, linked organotin exposure to the

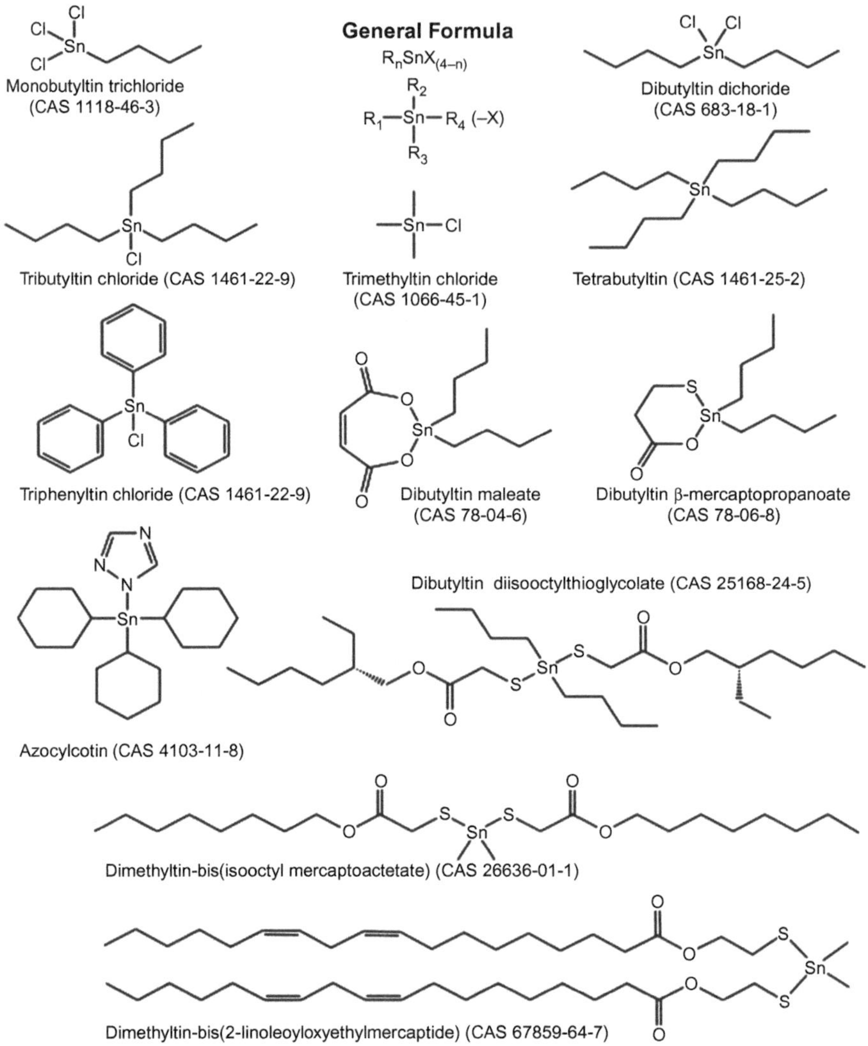

Figure 11.1 Common organotin derivatives.

dramatic rise in the incidence of imposex, sterility, and shell malformations (Blaber, 1970; Smith, 1981). Imposex is the pathological masculinization of hermaphroditic mollusks associated with a reduction in fecundity. TBT represents one of the best examples for a validated endocrine disruptor active on a broad scale and at realistic environmental exposure levels.

The specific phenotypes seen with organotin exposure suggested a role for perturbed sex hormone-dependent endocrine signaling as a likely molecular mechanism. Furthermore, the slow rate of environmental degradation and potential for bioaccumulation spread effects to upper trophic species in the food chain. Recorded levels of organotins in liver and fat depots of top marine predators such as tuna, pinnipeds, and cetaceans can exceed 1000 ng/g wet weight (Choi, Moon, An, Choi, & Choi, 2011; Kannan, Corsolini, Focardi, Tanabe, & Tatsukawa, 1996; Strand & Jacobsen, 2005). These tissue levels are in the range sufficient to compromise immune system function and elevate mortality rates (Nakayama et al., 2009; Strand, Larsen, & Lockyer, 2005). TBT's ability to induce imposex in marine invertebrates certainly underscores its potential to function as a potent endocrine disruptor, disrupt developmental tissue morphology, and do so at exceptionally low environmental levels. Naturally, this led to concerns for human health effects through consumption of contaminated seafood (Antizar-Ladislao, 2008; Guerin, Sirot, Volatier, & Leblanc, 2007). As a result of this broad-scale marine ecosystem impact and potential human health risk, member states to the International Maritime Organization enacted a global ban on the use of organotin-based antifouling paints from 2003 onward (Champ, 2003).

However, environmental contamination by triorganotins goes beyond aquatic ecosystems. TBTO and tributyltin naphthenate are in use as preservatives for industrial wood treatments. In agriculture, triorganotin derivatives such as triphenyltin hydroxide, tricyclohexyltin hydroxide, tricyclohexyltin triazole, and triphenyltin acetate have been employed as fungicides and acaricides on high-value food crops including potatoes, sugar beets, nut trees, and a variety of citrus, vegetable, and vine crops presenting another route for human dietary exposure (Hunter, 1976).

Although generally considered less biologically toxic, mono- and dialkyl tin species may still pose a significant risk on account of their greater environmental mobility and ubiquitous use in the manufacture of polyolefin (PVC) plastics that brings them into closer contact with drinking water and food supplies (Muncke, 2011). Organotin additives are employed as heat stabilizers for scavenging HCl released during PVC polymerization and assist lubrication during processing. Mono- or dialkyl derivatives based on octyl-, butyl-, or methyltin mercaptides, thioglycolic acid esters, reverse esters, and carboxylic acid compounds are most commonly used. A more limited set of organotin additives are approved in PVC plastics intended for food contact. Organotin additives are typically incorporated at fractions of 0.5–2% (w/w) of vinyl monomer with a maximum permissible cap of 3% (w/w) for PVC intended for food contact (US FDA, 2013; Muncke,

2011). In common household plastic products, the measured levels of extractable mono-, di-, and trialkyl tins range between 123 and 1380, 1770 and 13,200, and 6.6 and 139 mg/kg, respectively (Ohno, Suzuki, Nakashima, Aoyama, & Mitani, 2002). Leaching of organotins from PVC and CPVC water pipes raises concerns as a route for human exposure. Trialkyl species such as trimethyl and triethyltin are highly potent neurotoxins, so the presence of even small quantities in leachates has potential relevance to human health (Impellitteri, Evans, & Ravel, 2007; Philbert, Billingsley, & Reuhl, 2000; Shintani, Ogita, Hashimoto, & Baba, 2007). Even though the bulk of the leached organotin material is in the form of mono- and dialkyl species (Forsyth & Jay, 1997; Sadiki & Williams, 1999), compounds such as monomethyl-, dimethyl-, and dibutyltin have significant capacity to induce neurodevelopmental lesions and disrupt neurological functions as well (Ehman, Phillips, McDaniel, Barone, & Moser, 2007; Jenkins, Ehman, & Barone, 2004; Moser, Barone, Phillips, McDaniel, & Ehman, 2006).

A number of studies have attempted to address the prevalence and degree of human exposure to organotins in relation to health risk assessments. Regulatory scientific advisory panels recommend a group tolerable daily intake (TDI) for DBT, TBT, DOT, and TPhT of <100 ng Sn/kg bw/day (or equivalent to 270 ng TBT/kg bw/day) that are set 100-fold below the currently accepted NOAEL for oncogenicity and immunotoxicity determined from animal chronic feeding studies (Alexander et al., 2004; Boyer, 1989; RPA, 2005). Estimates from the 1990s indicated dietary and nonpoint source exposure at 2–5 μg/day for individual trialkyl components but possibly as high as 375 μg/day in some demographic groups such as coastal fishing communities (Sekizawa, 1998; Tsuda, Inoue, Kojima, & Aoki, 1995). As expected, levels continue to decline further below the recommended TDI values following introduction of stricter environmental guidelines, although organotins can still be found in seafood and vegetable market basket samples (Gueguen et al., 2011; Rantakokko, Kuningas, Saastamoinen, & Vartiainen, 2006; Santos et al., 2009). Another potential route of exposure comes from organotin-contaminated household dust (estimated average for total organotins of ~6 μg/g, range 0.3–28 μg/g) (Kannan, Takahashi, Fujiwara, Mizukawa, & Tanabe, 2010). In children, dust inhalation is calculated to account for about 15% of their TDI dose.

Several studies have reported on organotin concentrations in human liver biopsies and blood samples. Total organotins present in European livers during the 1990s were reported to be in the range of 1.1–33 ng Sn/g wet wt

(Kannan & Falandysz, 1997; Nielsen & Strand, 2002). Livers of Japanese averaged higher with values of 18, 66, and <2 ng Sn/g wet wt for MBT, DBT, and TBT, respectively (Takahashi et al., 1999). Three studies quantitated butyltins and phenyltins in blood samples from North America and Europe. The majority of individuals in the North American study had concentrations of MBT, DBT, and TBT above detectable levels (average 8.17 ± 8.56, 4.94 ± 3.83, and 8.18 ± 15.4 ng/mL, respectively); some individuals recorded substantially higher levels in the range of 39–85 ng/mL for TBT (Kannan, Senthilkumar, & Giesy, 1999). In contrast, an initial small European study found relatively few individuals with blood levels of TBT exceeding the detection limit of 0.02 ng Sn/mL; in contrast, TPhT was detectable in all samples tested (average 0.31 ± 0.16 ng Sn/mL; Lo et al., 2003). A later larger study of 300 individuals that focused on fishermen and their families found TPhT in 12% of samples (average 0.09 ng/mL) (Rantakokko et al., 2008). TPhT concentrations were positively correlated with fish consumption, age, and gender.

Although these historical studies are limited in size and demographic scope, the combined data highlight that human organotin exposure was quite variable but not uncommon. The nonuniform distribution reflected not only variability of dietary and nonpoint source exposure but also geographic regional differences in organotin use and regulation. Based on the studies' values, it is a reasonable expectation that nominal concentrations of TBT and TPhT in organs and blood reached sub to low nanomolar levels (0.3–10 nM) in a significant fraction of the population. Total organotin levels (that include mono- and diorganotin species) were likely higher in the range of 50–250 nM. Exposures today are anticipated to be considerably lower and to occur primarily as a result of the ubiquitous presence of organotins in PVC plastics. Hence, overall levels and the chemical nature of organotin exposures are shifting.

3. MECHANISMS OF CELLULAR ORGANOTIN TOXICITY

At the molecular level, organotins perturb biological systems via multiple mechanisms reflecting their distinct chemical and physical properties. Their biological activity is strongly dependent on the number and nature of the organic groups. In general, toxicity increases with the degree of organic substitution: inorganic Sn(IV) < mono < di = tetra < triorganic tin. Tetra-substituted organotins are chemically less reactive and generally considered to exhibit low toxicity. However, biotransformation gives rise to bioactive intermediate metabolites. In triorganotins, the anionic group at the fourth position is susceptible to exchange in aqueous environments and consequently has less influence toward toxicity. Overall, toxicity is high for alkyl chains up to six carbons but drops off quickly with further increases in length. These general trends are explained in part by the ability to associate with or traverse cellular membranes. Organotins, especially those with bulky alkyl or aryl groups, change the degree of hydration of lipid phosphate and carbonyl groups, alter lipid packing and fluidity, and disrupt protein organization within phospholipid membranes. Tributyltin appears the most effective at penetrating deep into the hydrophobic core (Bonarska-Kujawa, Kleszczynska, & Przestalski, 2012; Chicano, Ortiz, Teruel, & Aranda, 2001; Zylka et al., 2009).

Organotins also promote lipid peroxidation via a radical chain mechanism that is enhanced by formation of phospholipids complexes through dative Sn—O—P bonds (Petrosyan et al., 2003). Accumulation and release of the resulting lipid hydroperoxides damage cell membranes and stimulate lipid signaling pathways (Higdon, Diers, Oh, Landar, & Darley-Usmar, 2012). Nonspecific chemical peroxidation generates a wide variety of electrophilic reactive lipid species (RLS), for instance, 4-hydroxynonenal and cyclopentenone isoprostanes, that mediate inflammatory stress responses and upregulate cellular antioxidant defenses through activation of the antioxidant response element (ARE)-dependent Nrf2/Keap1 signaling pathway (Levonen et al., 2004). In contrast, cellular synthesis of closely related important bioactive lipid peroxide metabolites, for example, prostaglandins and leukotrienes, is tightly regulated through the combined actions of apolipase, cyclooxygenase, and lipoxygenase enzyme activities. In either case, these RLS share common properties with organotins in terms of a propensity for covalent bond formation with soft nucleophiles, including cellular small molecule antioxidants and protein thiols. Perhaps not coincidently, TBT along with a variety of lipid peroxide derivatives, including the cylcopentenone isoprostane 15-J2-isoP, its prostaglandin cousin 15-d-PGJ2, and even nitro fatty acids, shares the ability to covalently bind and activate peroxisome proliferator-activated receptor gamma (PPARγ), a member of the nuclear hormone receptor superfamily, via a ligand-binding pocket cysteine thiol (Grun et al., 2006; Musiek et al., 2005; Schopfer et al., 2010; Shiraki et al., 2005). Retinoid X receptor (RXR)–PPARγ transcriptional signaling is a master regulator of adipogenesis, and its inappropriate activation by organotins will be addressed in detail in later sections.

This same chemical reactivity also allows organotins to inhibit glutathione transferase activity and deplete reduced glutathione in a dose-dependent manner (Okada et al., 2000; Tahir, Guthenberg, & Mannervik, 1985; Tipping et al., 1979). Consequently, the combined action of lipid peroxidation and depletion of the cell's endogenous sulfhydryl antioxidants compromises the cell's antioxidative defense system leading to a rise in toxic reactive oxygen species that unchecked can trigger apoptosis (Milaeva, Petrosyan, Berberova, Pimenov, & Pellerito, 2004; Yoneyama et al., 2008). Significant evidence links the potent immuno- and neurotoxic effects observed with organotins to this damaging persistent chemical process (Ishihara, Kawami, Ishida, & Yamazaki, 2012; Yoneyama et al., 2008). Consistent with this explanation, reducing agents, in particular dithiol reagents, significantly protect against organotin toxicity in cellular and biochemical studies by boosting antioxidative capacity (Gray, Porvaznik, Lee, & Flemming, 1986; Nishikimi et al., 2001; Siebenlist & Taketa, 1983; Yoneyama et al., 2008).

Besides radical initiation, organotins can disrupt membrane functions in other ways as well. The solvolytic and hydrolytic equilibriums of trialkyltins in solution are conducive for the formation of weak bases and lipophilic cation species that act as electroneutral chloride/hydroxide (Cl^-/OH^-) anion exchangers and as proton carriers. These properties partially explain the ability of TBT to uncouple and disrupt electrochemical ion gradients of membrane organelles and mitochondria, thereby compromising their essential functions (Bragadin, Marton, Scutari, & Dell'Antone, 2000).

Furthermore, triorganotins have been shown to disrupt mitochondrial energy coupling and integrity by interacting directly with a number of mitochondrial membrane component proteins at submicromolar concentrations. For instance, the F_1F_0 ATP synthase is a target of TBT, TPhT, and DBT in both prokaryotic and eukaryotic species leading to an inhibition of proton flow and a significant reduction in intracellular ATP levels (Matsuno-Yagi & Hatefi, 1993; von Ballmoos, Brunner, & Dimroth, 2004). Structurally related F-ATPases (e.g., Mg-ATPase) and V-ATPases (vacuolar ATPases) can also be inhibited, disrupting the function of these proton and cation pumps in mitochondrial, lysosomal, endosomal, and Golgi membranes (Apps & Webster, 1996; Nesci et al., 2011). Indeed, organotin exposure leads to a rapid and substantial rise in cytosolic-free calcium levels through release from intracellular Ca^{2+} stores and an inhibition of calcium efflux (Chow, Kass, McCabe, & Orrenius, 1992). Other lines of evidence propose organotins interact with components of the mitochondrial transitional pore, such as the adenine nucleotide translocator (ANT), that regulates membrane permeability (Nishikimi et al., 2001). Together, the combination of these perturbations disrupts proton and ion gradients, blocks ATP synthesis, and induces mitochondrial swelling. As a result, the stress-induced release of mitochondrial cytochrome *c* and the aberrant rise of cytosolic Ca^{2+} levels provide another route for the induction of apoptosis that rationalizes the potent cytotoxic effects of triorganotins (Gogvadze, Stridh, Orrenius, & Cotgreave, 2002; Stridh, Gigliotti, Orrenius, & Cotgreave, 1999). Recent genetic and pharmacological antagonist data also argue for an alternate mechanism of apoptotic signaling at low doses in certain types of immune cell through a caspase-10- or caspase-3-dependent activation of the "death-inducing signaling complex" that normally mediates extrinsic apoptotic signaling (Katika, Hendriksen, de Ruijter, van Loveren, & Peijnenburg, 2012; Krug, 2012).

As previously indicated, the electrophilic nature of the Sn(IV) atom in organotin molecules permits several possible modes of covalent binding (Sn—O, Sn—N, and Sn—S) with nucleophilic groups in biomolecules (Saxena, 1987; Smith, Crowe, Das, & Duncan, 1979). Tin's large atom size and orbital arrangement are permissive for bond hybridization and formation of penta- or hexacoordinated complexes exhibiting trigonal bipyramidal or octahedral geometry. Some examples are shown in Fig. 11.2. In cases where organotins interact with one nucleophile, for example, cysteine, aspartic, or glutamic acid (Fig. 11.2A and B), the bonding geometry of the tin atom remains tetrahedral in nature. Studies probing functional sensitivity using chemical modifiers suggest organotins target F_0F_1-ATPases through formation of Sn—O bonds at critical conserved acidic amino acid residues (Guerrieri, Zanotti, Che, Scarfo, & Papa, 1987; Spruth, Reidlinger, & Müller, 1995). In other cases, studies propose organotins interact with two nucleophilic groups, for example, cysteine plus histidine or two histidines (Fig. 11.2D and E). ATPases and/or hemoglobins may have the appropriate 3D geometry of residues to support this type of complex formation (Aldridge & Rose, 1969; Emmanuel, Carver, Solaini, & Griffiths, 1984; Saxena, 1987; Siebenlist & Taketa, 1986).

Another mode of binding involves vicinal thiols that react to form stable chelate complexes with dialkyltins (or with trialkyltins via a dealkylation step) (Fig. 11.2C). This bonding mechanism is believed to be relevant to the interaction of organotins with the endogenous dithiol compound lipoic acid that serves as an essential cofactor of core metabolic enzymes, such as the pyruvate and α-keto-glutarate dehydrogenase complexes. Low-level

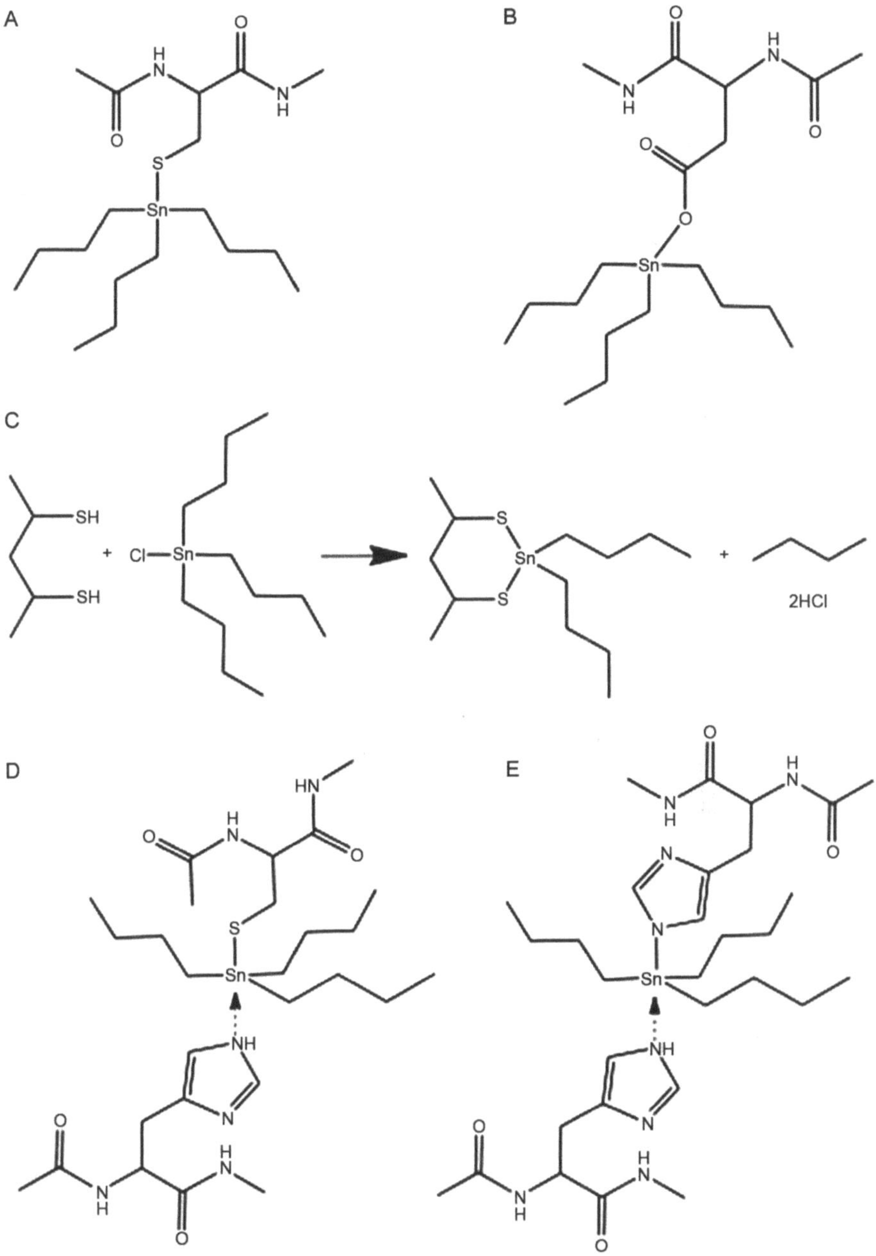

Figure 11.2 Modes of organotin covalent bonding. (A) Sn—S with cysteine, (B) Sn—O with aspartic/glutamic acid, (C) dealkylation of trialkyltins and binding to vicinal thiols, (D and E) penta-coordinate complex with cysteine and histidine or two histidine residues.

exposure to tri- and dialkyltins causes an accumulation of α-keto acids during oxidative metabolism of carbohydrate substrates consistent with a model of poisoning of enzymatic complexes in the tricarboxylic acid cycle (Penninks & Seinen, 1980). A further example is provided by the protein stannin (Snn) identified as a mediator of enhanced tissue-specific sensitivity toward trimethyltin (TMT) or triethyltin (TET) toxicity in subsets of neurons. Ectopic expression of stannin in fibroblasts can sensitize cells to TMT toxicity and apoptosis (Davidson, Reese, Billingsley, & Yun, 2004). Stannin is localized to the membranes of organelles, including mitochondria, and consists of a single transmembrane-spanning domain, a 14-3-3 protein binding domain with a proximal CXC motif at the membrane interface and a cytoplasmic helix (Fig. 11.3). TMT binds stannin at the CXC motif through dealkylation, and formation of a dithio-tin adduct induces a structural change in the 14-3-3ξ interaction domain contributing to aberrant TNF/inflammatory responses, inhibition of cell cycle progression, and induction of apoptosis (Billingsley et al., 2006; Buck et al., 2004; Buck-Koehntop et al., 2005).

The general characteristics described earlier outline how organotins interact with a wide variety of biological components to elicit multiple mechanisms of cellular toxicity, compromise cellular energy status, and exert

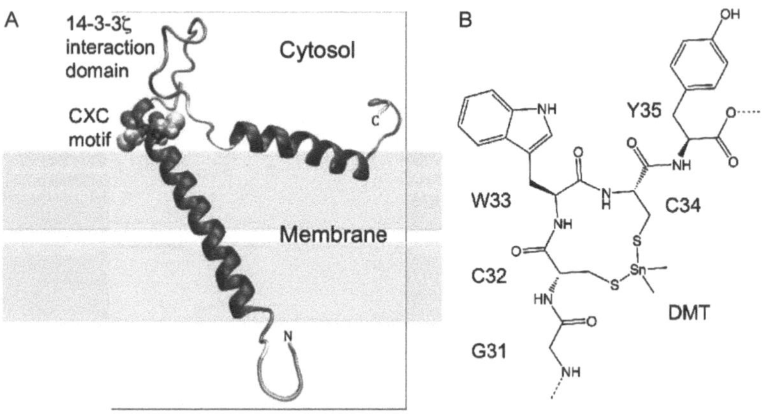

Figure 11.3 Stannin membrane topology and dimethyltin binding. (A) Solution NMR structure of stannin (Snn) indicates a transmembrane helix, CXC motif, 14-3-3 interaction domain, and helical cytoplasmic tail (Buck, Mascioni, Cramer, & Veglia, 2004; Buck-Koehntop, Mascioni, Buffy, & Veglia, 2005). (B) Dimethyltin (DMT) binding to vicinal cysteine residues (C32 and C34) induces a β-turn disrupting the adjacent 14-3-3ζ interaction domain. (See color plate.)

broad effects on numerous metabolic processes. However, direct mechanistic links for how organotins disrupt lipid metabolism and promote obesity arose from recent insights gained by identification of high-affinity targets of endocrine hormone signaling pathways relevant to adipogenesis and metabolic imbalances that favor increased fat storage. These are described next.

4. NUCLEAR HORMONE RECEPTORS AS ORGANOTIN TARGETS

Members of the nuclear hormone receptor family of transcription factors share a common architecture with conserved motifs defining their two principal functional domains: a DNA binding domain (DBD) with a zinc finger motif that recognizes sequence-specific promoter elements and a separate regulatory domain, referred to as the ligand binding domain (LBD), that in most cases binds a small lipophilic ligand required for the recruitment of coactivator proteins that help mediate transcriptional responses. Receptor ligands include a wide variety of small lipophilic hormone and signaling molecules including classical steroids such as estrogens, androgens, and glucocorticoids, nonsteroidal hormones and dietary vitamins, lipid metabolites, and xenobiotics such as EDCs. EDC pollutants can target NR signaling pathways by virtue of mimicking these endogenous ligands, and the resultant unregulated activation of NR gene networks leads to inappropriate nonphysiological responses.

The modular domain architecture of NRs lends itself to easy adaptation for *in vitro* and *in vivo* ligand-dependent assays and is a common tool employed for sensitive high-throughput chemical screening. Kanayama, Kobayashi, Mamiya, Nakanishi, and Nishikawa (2005) used an *in vitro* enzyme-linked coactivator recruitment assay to screen 16 nuclear receptors against 40 high-priority pollutants for endocrine disruptor potential. A number of EDCs were found capable of promoting coactivator recruitment with specific receptors, including TBT and TPhT acting on RXRs and the PPARγ.

Our group used a related strategy for a cell-based transcriptional assay using chimeric constructs of the yeast GAL4 DBD fused to various NR LBDs to drive a GAL4 UAS-dependent luciferase reporter gene. Dose-dependent and NR LBD-specific induction of reporter expression is strong evidence for direct ligand binding. We independently discovered that TBT and TPhT functioned as full agonists of RXRα, β, and γ (Grun et al., 2006). Activation was absent for monobutyltin, weak for dibutyltin, but exceptionally potent in the case of TBT with EC_{50}s for RXRs in the range of 3–8 nM (Fig. 11.4A). These values are on par with activation with the endogenous ligand 9-*cis* retinoic acid (9-*c* RA) and other potent rexinoids (synthetic RXR agonists). Competitive displacement-binding studies confirmed organotins are direct receptor ligands with K_Ds of equivalent magnitude. Besides RXR activation, we also observed significant activity with organotins on NR LBDs that serve as permissive heterodimeric partners of RXR, for example, PPARγ and NURR1, but not in those heterodimeric partners where RXR is typically a silent or subservient partner, for example, retinoic acid receptors. Activation of NURR1 was informative because its residual ligand-binding pocket is considered too small to accommodate a lipophilic ligand (Wang et al., 2003); the response in our cellular assays can be explained as activation and recruitment of the endogenous native RXRs by NURR1 LBD. However, in the case of PPARγ, activation was through direct ligand binding. Activation reached approximately 30% of maximal receptor activation at concentrations just below overt cellular toxicity; EC_{50} and K_D values are approximately 20 nM (Grun et al., 2006).

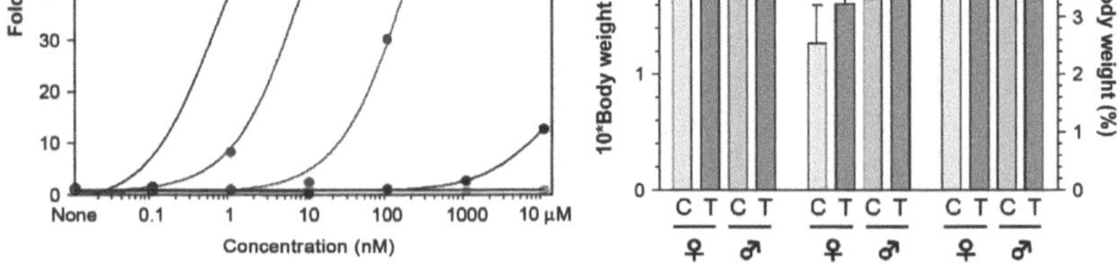

Figure 11.4 TBT activates RXRs and increases adiposity in mice. (A) Gal-RXR activation reporter assay with butyltins or the rexinoid LG268 control. TBT is a full agonist with $EC_{50} = 5$ nM. Data are redrawn from Grun et al., 2006 with permission. Copyright 2006, The Endocrine Society. (B–D) C58BL6 pregnant dams treated by oral gavage with 0.5 mg TBT/kg bw or vehicle control at E16.5, offspring maintained on normal chow diet and analyzed at 1 year for body weight (B), abdominal fat (C), and adiposity (ratio of abdominal fat/body weight, %). C, vehicle control; T, tributyltin. Data are plotted as means ± SEM, $n = 5$. One-tailed *t*-test with Welch's correction, *p-value <0.05. (See color plate.)

These data established organotins as potent *dual agonist ligands* of the RXR–PPARγ heterodimer. But the implications of aberrant NR signaling are much broader on account of the prevalent role RXR plays as the common partner in one-third of nuclear receptor dimer combinations. The dual agonist role for RXR–PPARγ activation is surprising since nuclear receptors, especially RXRs, typically exhibit exquisite discriminatory binding sites for their high-affinity cognate ligands based on size, overall geometry, and functional groups. Thus, features critical for the high-affinity binding of RXRs by 9-*c* RA include its hydrophobic core, composed of a β-ionone ring and isoprenoid tail that contribute to van der Waals interactions, and the ionic and H-bonding between the terminal carboxylic group and residues R316 and A327 and water molecule deep in the pocket. The geometric constraints prevent significant binding with all-*t* RA, while the 9-*cis* isomer configuration permits the correct fit to the pocket (Allenby et al., 1994). In contrast, TBT and TPhT are radically different from known endogenous or synthetic rexinoid ligands and their ability to serve as agonists was a surprise and not predictable *a priori*.

However, it seemed reasonable to presume that TBT would target NR LBD cysteine residues on the basis of organotin's propensity to form covalent adducts with sulfhydryl groups as previously indicated for other protein targets. Inspection of RXR structures focused attention on the conserved residues C432 and C269 as the most likely candidates. These residues project into the ligand pocket and are located in a position that straddle retinoic acid's β-ionone ring. A site-directed mutation in RXRα to glycine at position 432 (C432G) abolished organotin-dependent activation. Comparative reporter assays and MALDI-TOF mass spectrometric analyses of wild-type and mutant RXR LBDs provided evidence that C432 in helix 11 plays a critical role for TBT binding and receptor activation (Grun, 2010; Grün & Blumberg, 2006). le Maire et al. definitively confirmed this result in their crystal structure models of TBT and TPhT bound to the RXRα LBD and its coactivator peptide TIF2 (le Maire, Bourguet, & Balaguer, 2010; le Maire et al., 2009). Figure 11.5A and B shows the close similarity in overall structure between RXR LBD bound to 9-*c* RA and TBT, respectively. In either case, ligand binding allows for the appropriate rearrangement of helix 12 to form the surface groove necessary for recruitment of an LXXLL motif coactivator protein. As predicted, TBT formed a covalent thio–Sn bond with C432. Critical residues such as L436 are also orientated in a manner compatible with agonist activity. An agonist conformation of the LBD is further stabilized by van der Waals interactions between the organotin butyl

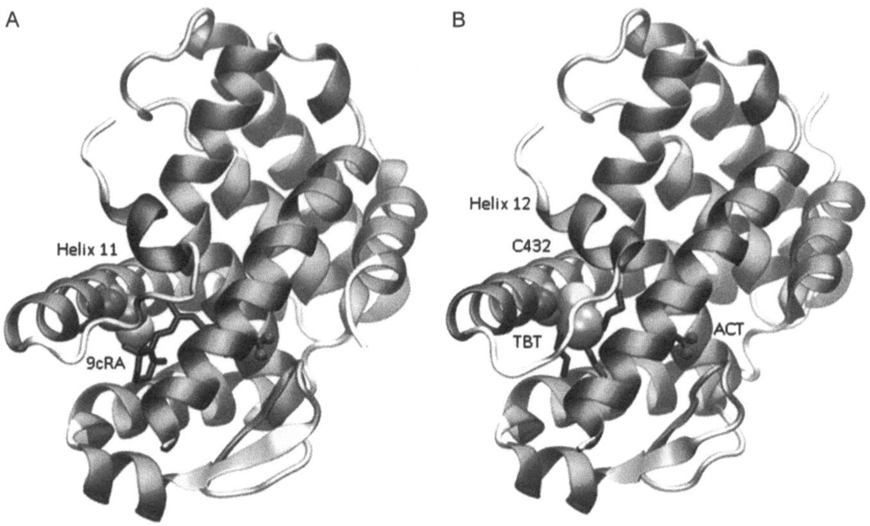

Figure 11.5 TBT is an agonist ligand of RXRs. (A) 3D crystal structure of RXRα ligand binding domain (LBD) bound to its agonist ligand 9-*cis* RA (blue). (B) 3D crystal structure of TBT bound to RXRα LBD via a thio–Sn bond with C432 in helix 11; an acetate molecule (ACT) is cocrystallized in the TBT–RXR structure. Helix 12 is positioned for coactivator peptide binding. TPHT binds and activates RXRα in a similar manner (le Maire et al., 2010, 2009). Color key: α-helix, purple; β-sheet, yellow; 9-*cis* RA ligand, blue stick; C432 residue, space filled with sulfur atom, yellow; 9-*cis* RA carboxylate group or acetate molecule, blue/red stick; TBT ligand, butyl carbon bonds, blue stick; Sn atom, space filled pink. Models derived from PDB: 1FBY and 3E94. (See color plate.)

(or phenyl groups of TPhT) and residue side chains in helices H3, H5, H7, and H11 lining the ligand pocket. A cocrystallized acetate molecule assumes the role of the terminal carboxylic acid group of rexinoid ligands. Together, these interactions account for the high-affinity binding and agonist properties of TBT and TPhT with RXR LBDs.

PPARγ lacks a cysteine residue at an equivalent location to C432 of RXRα. However, C313 of PPARγ2 (or C285 of PPARγ1) is comparable to RXR's C269, projects into the cavity, and is the prime candidate for covalent interaction. A conserved cysteine also occupies similar positions in PPARα and PPARδ. Mass spectrometric experiments with wild-type or mutant constructs of PPARγ2 at C313 and RXRα at C269 were consistent with the idea organotins can bind covalently at these residues (F. Grun, unpublished data; le Maire et al., 2009). There is precedent for covalent lipid interactions at this position modulating PPARγ activity. Endogenous oxidized eicosanoid and fatty acid derivatives that contain an alpha, beta-unsaturated ketone group are also compatible for covalent sulfide addition. Studies have demonstrated a number of metabolites, including prostaglandin-15-deoxy-$\Delta^{12,14}$–PGJ2, 4-oxodocasa-hexanenoic acid, and 6-oxooctadecatrienoic acid, as covalent agonists (Shiraki et al., 2005; Waku, Shiraki, Oyama, Fujimoto, et al., 2009; Waku, Shiraki, Oyama, & Morikawa, 2009). Furthermore, the synthetic partial agonist L-764406 and suicide inhibitor GW-9662 were reported to bind irreversibly to C313 of PPARγ2 (Elbrecht et al., 1999; Leesnitzer et al., 2002), although in the case of GW9662, the crystallographic data indicate the bond may not be covalent in nature (Chandra et al., 2008).

Additional evidence for organotins targeting nuclear receptors comes from a study by Gumy et al. (2008) that identified dibutyltin as an inhibitor of the glucocorticoid receptor (GR). DBT significantly inhibited stimulation by the synthetic agonist dexamethasone of GR activity in NR transactivation reporter assays and of endogenous GR target genes. In contrast, mildly synergistic effects with dexamethasone were noted with TBT and TPhT. Displacement binding assays determined the IC_{50} for DBT to be in the range of 50–150 nM. Although a crystal structure of GR with DBT has not been published, *in silico* docking studies identified two putative DBT binding sites: the canonical steroid binding site and an adjacent allosteric site where organotin binding would interfere with rearrangements of helices 3 and 5 during glucocorticoid binding, thereby affecting receptor activation. The issue of whether covalent bonding to cysteines may also be involved currently remains an unresolved issue although several residues (C736, C642, and C638) are situated in close proximity or contribute to the steroid-binding cavity. Beyond direct binding, organotins can impact GR signaling in an indirect manner as well. Local tissue activation and inactivation of glucocorticoid ligands are important features of glucocorticoid signaling in peripheral target tissues, including adipose tissue, and are mediated, respectively, by the activity of type I and type II 11β-hydroxysteroid dehydrogenases (11β-HSD). DBT, TBT, and TPhT inhibit the type II dehydrogenase, 11β-HSD2, that converts glucocorticoids to their inactive 11-ketoglucorticoids products (Atanasov, Nashev, Tam, Baker, & Odermatt, 2005). The involvement of cysteine residues in stabilizing substrate binding and catalysis was implicated based on protective effects by thiol reagents and kinetic studies of mutants. An inhibition of this enzymatic activity is expected to elevate local levels of active glucocorticoid ligands.

Similar indirect effects on other NR signaling pathways are expected due to additional points of interference in the metabolism of endogenous NR ligands by organotins. Indeed, the targeted disruption of steroidogenesis, steroid metabolism, or storage has been the primary mechanism frequently invoked to rationalize organotin endocrine disruption. Steroidogenic enzymes, including 17β-hydroxysteroid dehydrogenase and aromatase (CYP19), are sensitive to TBT and TPhT inhibition in invertebrates and mammals, including humans, albeit at μmolar levels (Cooke, 2002; Heidrich, Steckelbroeck, & Klingmuller, 2001; Le Curieux-Belfond, Moslemi, Mathieu, & Seralini, 2001; Ohno, Nakajima, & Nakajin, 2005). The decrease in aromatase activity, for instance, would alter the balance favoring androgen receptor (AR) over estrogen receptor (ER) signaling by skewing their respective ligand ratios and ostensibly give rise to the masculinized (imposex) phenotype in various sensitive species (McAllister & Kime, 2003; McGinnis & Crivello, 2011; Santos, ten Hallers-Tjabbes, Vieira, Boon, & Porte, 2002). Other studies reported aromatase transcriptional regulation is itself sensitive to RXR-NR (e.g., RXR–PPARγ). Mammalian aromatase expression can be either upregulated or repressed, dependent on the tissue-specific promoter context, by TBT, rexinoids, or PPARγ agonists (Nakanishi et al., 2002; Saitoh et al., 2001). Similarly, amphibian aromatase and fish aromatase are sensitive to RXR modulation and TBT-mediated intersex (Cheshenko, Pakdel, Segner, Kah, & Eggen, 2008; Grun et al., 2006; McAllister & Kime, 2003; Shi, Zhu, & Guo, 2012). Most impressively, activation of the RXR homolog by 9-*c* RA or other rexinoids has been demonstrated to be sufficient to phenocopy TBT-induced imposex in some marine mollusks, highlighting the conservation of a common mechanism over long evolutionary periods (Castro et al., 2007; Nishikawa et al., 2004; Stange, Sieratowicz, & Oehlmann, 2012). Any disruption in classical steroid receptor signaling pathways can be expected to contribute to altered differential sensitivity of adipose tissue responses, as well as gender-specific remodeling of adipose depots (Grove, Fried, Greenberg, Xiao, & Clegg, 2010; Joe, Yi, Even, Vogl, & Rossi, 2009; Lee, Wu, & Fried, 2010).

The conclusions that organotins act as high-affinity agonists for specific NRs (or antagonists in the case of DBT with GR) and disrupt NR ligand metabolism provide a crucial mechanistic insight directly linking low-level (nM) exposure to widespread perturbations of downstream target gene networks relevant to lipid homeostasis and adipose biology. This direct link to well-characterized nuclear receptor signaling pathways opens the possibility to predict and evaluate specific physiological outcomes based on comparisons to the numerous studies already available on endogenous endocrine hormones.

5. TBT AND DISRUPTED ADIPOSE BIOLOGY

Fat tissue can be divided into two principal distinct types, white adipose tissue (WAT) and brown adipose tissue (BAT), based on developmental lineage, morphology, and function (Fig. 11.6). Both lineages originate from multipotent mesenchymal stem cells (MSCs) capable of generating adipocytes, osteoblasts, chondrocytes, and myocytes. MSCs can give rise to committed preadipocytes that reside interspersed within the stromal vascular

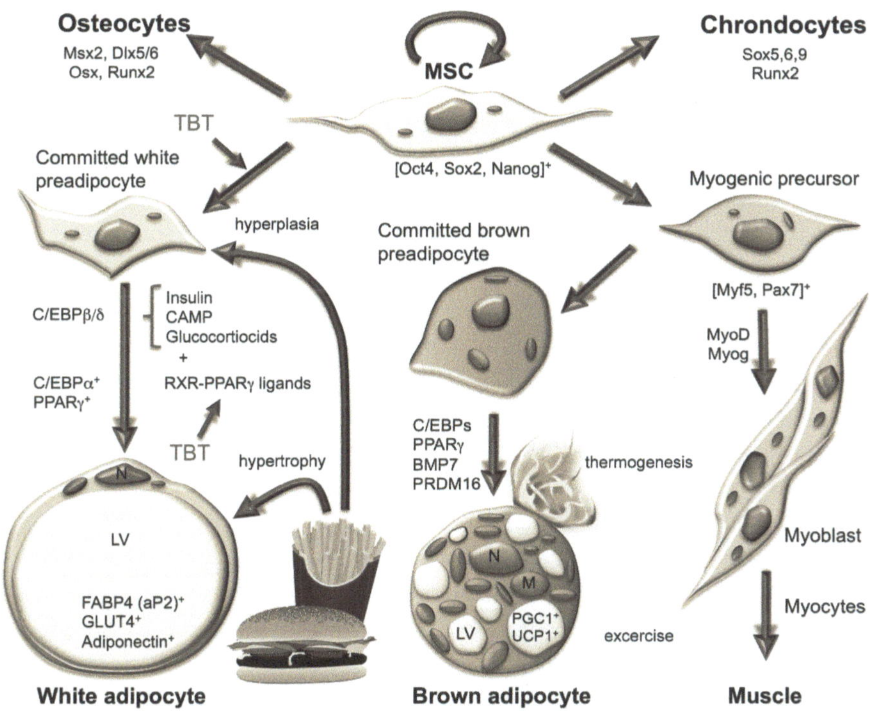

Figure 11.6 MSC lineages: Adipose mesenchymal stem cells (MSCs) give rise to osteocytes, chondrocytes, myocytes, and adipocyte lineages. Adipogenic signals act on committed white preadipocytes to induce a switch to C/EBPα and PPARy transcriptional regulation that causes terminal differentiation into mature white adipocytes. WAT secretes a variety of adipokine hormones and responds to metabolic cues to regulate the flow of lipid nutrients for storage or mobilization. Brown adipocytes are derived from a myogenic lineage precursor ($Myf5^{+}Pax7^{+}$), are rich in mitochondria (M) and multilocular lipid vesicles (LV), and express genes that control thermogenic responses. The obesogen tributyltin (TBT) promotes adipocyte differentiation by acting as a dual agonist ligand of RXR and PPARγ. In addition, TBT can skew cell fate decisions in favor of the adipogenic lineage at the expense of osteo-chondrogenesis. (See color plate.)

fraction of WAT. Upon adipogenic stimulation, preadipocytes differentiate into mature fat cells characterized by large unilocular lipid droplets. In contrast, the development of BAT differs and proceeds via an early MYF5-positive myogenic precursor that differentiates into adipose cells with numerous multilocular lipid droplets and an abundance of mitochondria (Cypess et al., 2009; Frontini & Cinti, 2010). These morphological differences help define their physiological functions: BAT is distributed as small discreet pockets active in thermogenesis, while WAT comprises the bulk of the body's fat storage system and participates as an endocrine organ in the regulation of insulin sensitivity, lipid metabolism, and satiety. WAT is also an active endocrine organ, secreting and responding to a variety of adipokine, endocrine, and proinflammatory signals (Galic, Oakhill, & Steinberg, 2010). Functional metabolic differences further define WAT depots (Ibrahim, 2010). Visceral fat in obesity is correlated with pathological inflammation and insulin resistance (Hamdy, Porramatikul, & Al-Ozairi, 2006), whereas excess accumulation in subcutaneous adipose depots is associated with improved glucose tolerance and provides some protective benefits against metabolic syndrome diseases (Tran, Yamamoto, Gesta, & Kahn, 2008).

How then do the molecular mechanisms and specific cellular targets outlined in the previous sections allow organotins to disrupt adipose tissue biology, specifically for WAT that is central to obesity and its pathological consequences? And how compelling is the evidence that their obesogenic potential does translate into a significant impact on weight gain and whole body fat mass relevant to human obesity? The best lines of evidence for tributyltin as an obesogen follow from the consequences of aberrant RXR–PPARγ activation in adipose lineage cells.

Formation of functional fat tissue requires the influence of numerous intrinsic and extrinsic signals in control of cell proliferation, commitment, and differentiation (Cristancho & Lazar, 2011). PPARγ is considered the master regulator of adipogenesis by controlling differentiation of committed preadipocytes into mature fat cells and maintaining the stable differentiated state (Tontonoz & Spiegelman, 2008). Preadipocytes respond to the combined action of adipogenic factors—including insulin, glucocorticoid, and cAMP signaling—by promoting a transient epigenomic transition that switches the *milieu* of transcription factors toward a competent state of cooperative CCAAT/enhancer-binding protein (C/EBP) and RXR–PPARγ transcriptional regulation of target genes (Steger et al., 2010). Appropriate lipid signaling via PPARγ agonists, either dietary fatty acids or endogenous metabolites, then permits effective differentiation and establishment of positive feedback loops that maintain C/EBP and PPARγ regulation (Tzameli et al., 2004; Wakabayashi et al., 2009). Genome-wide analyses have identified thousands of sites, enriched in genes for lipid and glucose metabolism, where such colocalized PPARγ and C/EBPβ binding is important for the adipocyte-specific pattern of gene expression (Lefterova et al., 2008; Nielsen et al., 2008). A broad influence by organotin exposure on adipocyte gene regulatory networks and differentiation is therefore predicted based on aberrant activation of RXR–PPARγ signaling.

Various studies using the murine 3T3-L1 preadipocyte cell line model confirm organotins as effective promoters of adipocyte differentiation at nanomolar concentrations, consistent with their role as RXR–PPARγ agonists, giving rise to mature adipocytes that acquire lipid droplets and expressing terminal differentiation markers such as fatty acid-binding protein 4 (FABP4 or aP2) (Grun et al., 2006; Inadera & Shimomura, 2005; Kanayama et al., 2005). Inhibitor competition studies verify that the principal effects by TBT are mediated through PPARγ signaling (Li, Ycaza, & Blumberg, 2011).

Interestingly, in contrast to pure PPARγ thiazolidinedione (TZD) agonists such as rosiglitazone, TBT differs by its ability to promote 3T3-L1 fibroblast differentiation, although to a reduced degree, even in the absence of the standard obligatory cocktail of insulin, glucocorticoid, and cAMP signals (Grun et al., 2006). This implies TBT exerts some of its proadipogenic properties at earlier stages, perhaps at the level of altered GR signaling or through the actions of other permissive RXR-NR dimmers, such as the NR4A family (Nurr77, Nurr1, and NOR1), liver X receptor, and PPARδ that are sensitive to organotin receptor activation (Grun et al., 2006; Yanik, Baker, Mann, & Schlezinger, 2011). There is precedent that some EDCs can potentiate GR signaling and support 3T3-L1 adipogenesis (Sargis, Johnson, Choudhury, & Brady, 2010). However, complicating this issue is that both pro- and antiadipogenic activities are to be expected for organotins. For instance, while not strictly obligatory for *in vitro* adipogenesis, NR4A family members nevertheless impact 3T3-L1 differentiation during early events of the clonal expansion stage (Zhao & Bruemmer, 2010). Transient increases in NR4A expression are reported to be proadipogenic, while chronic expression inhibits adipocyte differentiation (Chao, Bensinger, Villanueva, Wroblewski, & Tontonoz, 2008; Fumoto, Yamaguchi, Hirose, & Osumi, 2007). Furthermore, the expression levels of NR4A receptors themselves are sensitive to rapid induction through the cAMP response element-binding protein (CREB) pathway, while activity at target gene promoters is antagonized by direct interaction with GR (Carpentier, Sacchetti, Segard, Staels, & Lefebvre, 2008; Philips et al., 1997). Downstream transcriptional targets of NR4A receptors include FABP5, required for fatty acid-dependent adipogenesis mediated via PPARδ (Bastie, Luquet, Holst, Jehl-Pietri, & Grimaldi, 2000; Ma et al., 2010; Volakakis, Joodmardi, & Perlmann, 2009). Such complex network interactions, and many more, are potentially subject to organotin disruption: triorganotins cause rapid decreases in cyclic-AMP levels and alter PKA activity that diminishes CREB activity (Bariagaber & Whalen, 2003; Whalen & Loganathan, 2001), enhance GR activation either directly or by inhibition of inactivating glucocorticoid metabolic enzymes (Atanasov et al., 2005; Gumy et al., 2008), and serve as agonists of RXRs in certain RXR-NR heterodimers, including the NR4A member Nurr1 (Grun et al., 2006). The details and relative importance of concordant mechanisms will require further studies to resolve.

Irrespective of the additional specific pathways targeted, the preadipocyte cell line studies convincingly show TBT can drive adipogenesis through RXR–PPARγ signaling. The central issue is therefore whether such effects also translate *in vivo* into molecular and cellular changes that drive adipose tissue expansion and obesity. Data from a number of studies in different species indicate this to be the case. In our initial observations, we found that TBT exposure of adult male mice altered gene expression patterns of transcriptional regulators and metabolic genes in the liver, adipose, and testis, consistent with a perturbed profile of lipid regulation. Pups born following *in utero* exposure to 0.5 mg/kg bw TBT between E12 and 18 exhibited enhanced lipid accumulation in neonatal fat pads and liver steatosis (Grun et al., 2006). Although initial growth curves appeared normal up to 10 weeks of age, the epididymal fat pads of males were 20% larger. Subsequent exposure experiments found a progressive and sustained increase in adiposity, particularly in males, after 6 months of age, reaching 9% above controls by 1 year (F. Grün, unpublished data; Fig. 11.4B–D). Abdominal fat, such as the gonadal and retroperitoneal depots, was the largest contributor to the increased adipose mass and weight gain.

Corroborating evidence for this obesogenic phenotype has been reported in a chronic low-dose exposure study with peripubertal mice (Si et al., 2011). Mice receiving 50 μg/kg bw every 3 days from P24 to 45 had growth curves identical to controls during the dosing period but subsequently developed a consistent body weight gain of approximately 10%

during later stages (P45–84). Higher doses of TBT (0.5 mg/kg bw every 3 days) had no effect. Zuo et al. (2011) conducted a similar chronic 45-day feeding study and reported a maximal effect of 9% increased body weight at a lower dose of 5 μg/kg bw TBT. The index of fat weight/body weight for renal and epididymal adipose mass was elevated 1.37-fold compared to controls. Animals also exhibited significant liver steatosis in conjunction with increases in plasma levels of insulin, leptin, and resistin levels but a decrease in adiponectin. These data are compatible with a pattern of developing insulin resistance, hyperinsulinemia, and hyperleptinemia. Another study looked at high-dose effects on pubertal male rats after 30-day chronic dosing with TBT or TPhT (0.5–15 and 2–12 mg/kg bw, respectively). Animals receiving the lowest dose of TPhT (2 mg/kg bw) were statistically heavier. However, higher doses of TBT or TPhT led to a reduction in body weight or death, indicating the dosing regimen in this study reached overtly toxic levels (Grote et al., 2004).

Penza et al. (2011) had also investigated adipose and body weight changes in a 3-month controlled diet feeding study of peripubertal and sexually mature mice using environmentally relevant doses of TBT (range 0.05–500 μg/kg bw) finding both gender- and dose-dependent phenomena. Longitudinal EchoMRI analyses indicated young male mice responded rapidly to 0.5 μg TBT/kg chow by increasing total adipose mass without a change in overall body weight or growth profile. Hence, the elevated fat/body weight ratio indicates a significant increase in adiposity in response to low-dose TBT. Changes in adipose tissue architecture were also apparent and noticeable as greater variability in cell size, shape, and increased number of blood vessels. The increased adiposity was maintained throughout the feeding study; in contrast, females only showed a transient increase. At higher doses of TBT, the effects were diminished or reversed. Penza et al. ascribed this change in obesogenic response at higher doses and the gender differences to the activation of a secondary phenomenon whereby TBT stimulates estrogenic signaling that may function to counteract and suppress fat mass accumulation. They observed dose-dependent and tissue preferential action by TBT in male estrogen-responsive (ERE-tk-LUC) reporter mice at levels above 50 μg/kg but not at the adipogenic dose of 0.5 μg/kg. Acute exposures increased reporter activity in epididymal, renal, and brown fat, as well as the pancreas, while the testis and liver were equivalent or reduced compared to controls. Chronic exposure had effects primarily on reporter activity in the genital tract and abdominal region. The ability to target ER-dependent signaling was further confirmed in

3T3-L1 cell transcriptional reporter assays. TBT exhibited subtype-specific activation of ERs dependent on differentiation stage such that ERα was responsive in preadipocytes but ERβ was activated only in differentiated adipocytes.

Data supporting organotins as obesogens also come from the general conservation of molecular mechanism and phenotypes being described across a broad phylogenetic array of species. Marine snails acquire disturbances in lipid accumulation and lipid homeostasis (Janer, Navarro, & Porte, 2007; Lyssimachou, Navarro, Bachmann, & Porte, 2009). Mollusk RXR homologues are activated by TBT, and nonorganotin RXR ligands are shown to induce imposex (Nishikawa et al., 2004). In mammalian systems, transcriptional regulation of aromatase (CYP19) expression occurs via tissue-specific promoters, some of which are sensitive to RXR/PPARγ signaling and organotin modulation (Nakanishi et al., 2002, 2005; Saitoh et al., 2001). Amphibian RXRs are likewise responsive to organotins, and a consistent pattern in inhibition of aromatase expression is observed with TBT, rexinoids, or PPARγ ligands (Grun et al., 2006). In experiments with Xenopus tadpoles, chronic exposure to environmental levels of TBT or rexinoids/PPARγ agonists results in both ectopic adipocyte formation and gonadal abnormalities including intersex (Grun et al., 2006; Shi et al., 2012). A variety of fish species show similar types of responses to TBT with broad effects on steroidogenesis, the status of PPARs, and metabolism (Colliar, Sturm, & Leaver, 2011; Pavlikova, Kortner, & Arukwe, 2010). Ectopic lipid accumulation, adiposity, gonadal dysfunction, and sex reversal are documented (Shimasaki et al., 2003; Tingaud-Sequeira, Ouadah, & Babin, 2011; Zhang et al., 2009, 2013).

Meador, Sommers, Cooper, and Yanagida (2011) conducted a controlled 2-month feeding study in salmon and found a significant increase in body weight and specific growth rate (SGR) of 10% with TBT (range of 1.4–12 pmol TBT/g/fish/day) but depressed growth at the highest doses. Body weight continued to increase to 15–24% above controls during the two subsequent months that the authors attributed to slow metabolic turnover of TBT and persistence of residual organotins in tissues. Although total lipid plasma levels were substantially elevated (25–40%), the study noted a significant increase in the SGR of fish. Since food intake was tightly controlled and below satiety, the difference in SGR implied low-dose exposure to organotins enhanced food conversion efficiency and may represent a possible example of hormesis.

Combined, these exposure and feeding studies confirm that environmentally relevant levels of triorganotins do disturb lipid homeostasis, alter the flow of nutrient reserves between growth and storage, and can increase fat mass of specific adipose depots. Intriguingly, the studies hint at long-term effects on adipose tissue that are not reliant on continued exposure but that may follow from epigenomic changes in adipogenic lineage dynamics and/or metabolic set points.

6. EPIGENETIC PERTURBATIONS IN ADIPOGENESIS AND METABOLIC SET POINTS

Many models of the etiology of human metabolic syndrome diseases have focused on finding links between the nutritional environment, especially during fetal development, with changes in DNA and protein methylation status and subsequent health outcomes (Burdge & Lillycrop, 2010). Environmental influences on epigenetic DNA hyper- and hypomethylation of genes relevant to obesity have been described. For instance, DNA hypermethylation of the RXRα promoter has a positive association with childhood obesity (Godfrey et al., 2011), whereas fetal stress caused by gestational diabetes mellitus was associated with DNA demethylation of the imprinted mesoderm-specific transcript gene in children and was prevalent as an epigenomic mark in adults with morbid obesity (El Hajj et al., 2013).

Epigenetic modifications in response to organotin exposure could occur at a number of points that establish long-term patterns of maladapted responses leading to obesity: adipogenic lineage dynamics, adipocyte differentiation, and peripheral or central control over metabolic set points. Modifications at the level of the adipogenic progenitor pool are attractive because of the proximal relationship to adipose mass and cell number that directly couples to fat mass.

Lineage-tracing studies in animal models indicate the major development phase of adipogenic progenitors required for WAT depots occurs late during gestation with a postnatal surge in expansion based on nutrient availability (Tang et al., 2008). In humans, adipocyte numbers continue to increase through puberty but are generally considered stable in adult fat tissues. Maintaining constant adipose cell numbers is estimated to require a replacement rate of approximately 10% per year (Spalding et al., 2008). Mature adipose tissues do continue to respond dynamically to dietary caloric excess with an efficient hypertrophic increase of fat mass, while chronic excess also drives recruitment and adipocyte proliferation to increase cell number. Constraining this response is a proinflammatory environment that stimulates apoptosis of the large-sized adipocyte fraction, thereby limiting depot storage capacity (Faust, Johnson, Stern, & Hirsch, 1978; Klyde & Hirsch, 1979; Strissel et al., 2007). In contrast, it is less clear whether caloric deficiency causes a loss of adipose mass coupled to an overall decrease of adipose cell numbers over the near term (Jo et al., 2009, 2010; Miller, Faust, Goldberger, & Hirsch, 1983; Singh et al., 2012). Hence, this predisposition toward a net positive gain in adipose cell number upon stimulation would predispose an individual toward obesity and likely contributes to weight-cycling problems commonly encountered during dieting (Barbosa-da-Silva, Fraulob-Aquino, Lopes, Mandarim-de-Lacerda, & Aguila, 2012; Singh et al., 2012). Further complicating the issue are adipose depot and gender-specific differences in hyperplastic and hypertrophic responses (Joe et al., 2009; Tchoukalova et al., 2010). Whereas the acute effects on adipose tissue mass to chronic TBT exposure could be rationalized solely in terms of hypertrophy and preadipocyte terminal differentiation, a bias toward adipogenic progenitors or a heightened sensitivity to differentiation would be consistent with the data from the exposure studies that documented a persistent influence on adipogenesis even at times far removed from the point of TBT exposure.

Evidence for this hypothesis comes from previous studies with PPARγ agonists, for example, the class of TZD drugs, that modify adipose lineage dynamics and tissue remodeling (de Souza et al., 2001; Tang, Zeve, Seo, Jo, & Graff, 2011). *In vivo* TZDs drove proliferation and increased the flow of cells from the progenitor compartment to mature adipocytes twofold. But chronic exposure reduced adipogenesis by depleting the adipogenic capacity of the progenitor pool and generating descendants with an altered molecular signature (Tang et al., 2011). When treated with low doses of TBT (<7 nM), human bone marrow-derived stromal cell cultures respond with proliferation of granulocyte–macrophage progenitors and differentiation into adipocytes while decreasing critical chemokine and hematopoietic factors necessary for support of myeloid lineages (Carfi et al., 2008). Treatment of mouse bone marrow-derived MSCs with organotins (TBT, DBT, and TPhT) also induced adipocyte differentiation through a combination of PPARγ-dependent and PPARγ-independent mechanisms (Yanik et al., 2011). Kirchner, Kieu, Chow, Casey, and Blumberg (2010) tested the effect of TBT on both human and mouse multipotent adipose-derived stromal cells (ADSCs) with similar results. Moreover, prenatal exposure to TBT or the TZD rosiglitazone enhanced the adipogenic potential of bone marrow-derived MSC at the expense of osteogenic differentiation capacity when subsequently challenged with TBT or rosiglitazone. These results are consistent with a bias in the progenitor population. A comparative study by Biemann et al. (2012) investigated the ability of ECDs to influence adipogenic potential of MSCs at different stages of adipogenesis. BPA decreased subsequent adipocyte differentiation when exposure occurred during undifferentiated growth, while diethylhexylphthalate enhanced it when present during the hormonal induction period. TBT was active at all stages. The lack of a response on murine embryonic stem cells with any of these EDCs indicated an MSC identity was necessary for the effects. Overall, the results reported in these studies support a model of adipogenic potential and response that is sensitive to organotin disruption.

Adipocyte differentiation also requires extensive changes in genome-wide transcription factor binding profiles and histone modifications that exhibit susceptibility to epigenetic interference (Mikkelsen et al., 2010; Okamura, Inagaki, Tanaka, & Sakai, 2010). For instance, the epigenomic transition during hormonal induction of adipogenesis establishes histone H3/H4 acetylation and methylation marks at the PPARγ locus and target genes of PPARγ and C/EBPs (Mikkelsen et al., 2010; Steger et al., 2010; Wakabayashi et al., 2009). Some demethylases, such as jumonji-C domain-containing histone demethylase 2A, are linked to obesity although their normal function is protective (Tateishi, Okada, Kallin, & Zhang, 2009). A different histone methyltransferase, PR-Set7/Setd8, is required for activation of adipogenic target genes and subject to positive feedback regulation by RXR–PPARγ signaling at late stages of adipocyte differentiation (Wakabayashi et al., 2009). Misregulation of this player by aberrant TBT activation of RXR–PPARγ is a plausible scenario.

So far, only limited published data are available that directly address the potential for altered epigenetic modifications from organotin exposure. *In vitro* assays show several organotins, including TBT, increase histone acetyltransferase activity (Osada, Nishikawa, Nakanishi, Tanaka, & Nishihara, 2005). In their study, Kirchner et al. (2010) also reported DNA hypomethylation of the FABP4 promoter of undifferentiated ADSCs after prior exposure to TBT concluding target genes were already exhibiting an epigenetic bias toward adipogenesis. Consistent with such a possibility, a study by Wang looked at global DNA methylation status in fish livers following 48 h low-dose exposure (1–100 ng/L Sn) to TBT (Wang, Wang, Zhang, Chen, & Zuo, 2009). The global pattern of DNA hypomethylation observed correlated with a decrease in the methyl donor cosubstrate *S*-adenosylmethionine (SAM) used by DNA (cytosine-5) methyltransferase 1 and a concomitant rise in its reaction product *S*-adenosylhomocysteine

(SAH). The change in SAM/SAH ratio suggests TBT may impair recycling of the methyl donor and hence contribute to the demethylation of CpG islands at promoters leading to systemic changes in expression. Broad influences on methylation and acetylation reactions would be of greatest concern during early periods of life when metabolic programming is being established and most sensitive to disturbances.

Numerous studies have highlighted the role of the maternal and perinatal environment on programming of metabolic set points and obesity (Spencer, 2012). Of key importance are the development of the central neuroendocrine circuits of the hypothalamus–pituitary–adrenal (H–P–A) and hypothalamus–pituitary–thyroid (H–P–T) axes that regulate basal metabolic rate, growth, lipid metabolism, appetite, and satiety, as well as adaptive responses to subsequent metabolic stress. Again, maturation of these circuits occurs during the late stages of fetal and early postnatal life and can be permanently modified by many factors including the status of the insulin, leptin, and glucocorticoid signaling pathways (Bouret & Simerly, 2007; Dahlgren et al., 2001). Indeed, excess fetal glucocorticoid exposure has been invoked as a unifying mechanism to account for many of the deleterious effects of disparate stressors (nutrition, hormonal, social, and chemical) on metabolic health including obesity (Harris & Seckl, 2011; Koch, Sepa, & Ludvigsson, 2008).

In this respect, the placenta plays critical functions during fetal development as the gatekeeper of nutrient flow to the embryo and as a primary site of defense against maternal stress (Monk, Spicer, & Champagne, 2012). Maternal stress causes a systemic elevation of glucocorticoids that require inactivation by efficient placental 11β-HSD2 metabolism to buffer the embryo from excessive glucocorticoid signals deleterious to both peripheral embryonic tissues and proper development of central nervous circuits critical to energy homeostasis. Epigenetic modifications are central to these responses (Drake et al., 2012; Welberg, Seckl, & Holmes, 2000). Maternal adversity can derail glucocorticoid signaling through tissue-specific epigenetic modification of 11β-HSD2 and GR receptor expression. In the placenta, prenatal stress results in reduced 11β-HSD2 expression on account of increased DNA methyltransferase activity on its promoter (Jensen Pena, Monk, & Champagne, 2012). A failure to limit these glucocorticoid surges leaves the embryo vulnerable to inappropriate metabolic programming cues and results in gestational growth retardation that is a strong prognostic indicator of future metabolic syndrome health issues (Harris & Seckl, 2011). Atanasov et al. (2005) found that TBT directly inhibited 11β-HSD2 enzymatic activity, implicating organotins might compromise the placental fetomaternal barrier to glucocorticoid excess and entrain deleterious epigenetic changes.

The ability of organotins to target glucocorticoid signaling focuses attention on the H–P–A and H–P–T axes that have profound effects on the regulation of metabolism and growth. Either excess or deficiency of glucocorticoid signaling can alter the developmental trajectory of vulnerable brain structures, including neurons in the hippocampus and arcuate (ARC) nucleus and paraventricular nucleus (PVN) of the hypothalamus that are critical for integrating information about food intake and body energy stores. Stressors can influence both epigenetic changes in GR and MR expression (Shoener, Baig, & Page, 2006) and expression or secretion of proopiomelanocortin, neuropeptide Y (NPY), and agouti-related peptide (AGRP) that are all central to the control of food intake (Ikenasio-Thorpe, Breier, Vickers, & Fraser, 2007; Stevens et al., 2010). An important unaddressed question, therefore, is whether TBT exposure will impact the development and neuroendocrine physiology relevant to H–P–A and H–P–T functions that would increase the propensity for obesity.

At the anatomical level, organotins have long been known to elicit site-specific neurological pathologies. Potent neurotoxic organotins, such as TMT and TET, are used extensively in experimental models on account of their preferential selectivity in causing loss of pyramidal neurons of the hippocampus (and other limbic systems) (Philbert et al., 2000). Adrenalectomy can exacerbate this loss, while supplementation with glucocorticoids provides protection indicating an interconnection to glucocorticoid-sensitive signaling (Imai et al., 2001; Shuto et al., 2009). More recently, *in vivo* exposure of rats to TBT was shown to selectively induce the cell activation marker c-Fos in neurons of the arcuate nucleus, but not other nuclei regulating food intake (Bo, Viglietti-Panzica, & Panzica, 2011). Although speculative, it is plausible that the induction of site-specific lesions or cellular responses by organotins would contribute to maladaptations of neuroendocrine circuits regulating food intake or reward systems that become locked in with long-term consequences.

Some additional precedents for overlap with NR-mediated mechanisms in these pathways come from studies investigating the influence of poor maternal nutrition, either low-protein or high-fat (junk food) diets, on inappropriate fetal programming of food intake and dietary choices. In either case, offspring increase mesolimbic reward pathways that favor preferences for high-fat foods (Bellinger, Lilley, & Langley-Evans, 2004; Ong &

Muhlhausler, 2011). Furthermore, these epigenetic changes can be transmitted to subsequent generations (Dunn & Bale, 2011). In this context, studies with tissue-specific knockouts of PPARγ show its important role in the brain for controlling appetite and metabolism in response to high-fat diets (Lu et al., 2011; Myers & Burant, 2011; Ryan et al., 2011). Activation of brain PPARγ by TZDs caused an increase in feeding and body weight gain, while inhibition or loss-of-function experiments decreased food intake of high-fat but not normal diets. The potent activation of RXR–PPARγ by TBT should elicit a similar response.

Additional connections to disruptions of central metabolic regulation by obesogens are being made in the H–P–T axis (Decherf & Demeneix, 2011). Thyrotropin-releasing hormone (TRH) neurons in the PVN regulate basal metabolic rate, feeding, and lipid metabolism by acting as metabolic sensors sensitive to thyroid hormone (TH) and multiple neuronal inputs emanating from the ARC nucleus and discrete populations of α-MSH/CART and NPY/AGRP neurons within the PVN (Hollenberg, 2008). TBT treatment has been noted to lower serum thyroxine levels and induces hypothyroidism in progeny of treated dams (Adeeko et al., 2003; Cooke et al., 2004). TBT treatment also supported a T3-independent activation of the TRH promoter in the hypothalamus that was potentiated by overexpression of RXRα (Decherf, Seugnet, Fini, Clerget-Froidevaux, & Demeneix, 2010; Kouidhi et al., 2010). The ability to influence TH levels and feedback circuits suggests basal metabolic rate and energy partitioning could be affected by organotin exposure.

7. CONCLUSION AND PERSPECTIVE

So how and why does a broadly toxic and potent pollutant such as tributyltin promote adipose weight gain and obesity? The answer to this question is both complicated and still incomplete. A generalized answer to this paradoxical behavior is twofold and is summarized in Fig. 11.7. One part relates to the appropriate exposure dose, the other to timing that can discriminate between different molecular mechanisms. At sufficiently high intracellular levels (>1 μM), broad cytotoxic effects that overwhelm membrane integrity are anticipated to dominate. Although the rate of lipid radical initiation will be proportional to the organotin exposure dose, lipid peroxidation damage will be cumulative unless actively countered by effective antioxidant defenses. But these defenses are limited. Moreover, the "covalent advantage" of protein modification by deleterious lipid peroxide

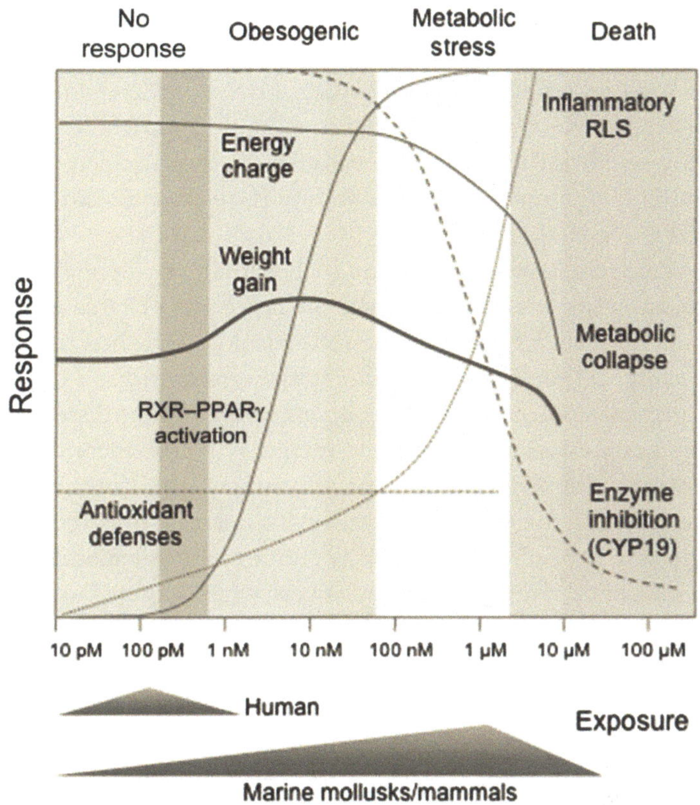

Figure 11.7 Conceptual overview of responses to TBT exposure. Low-dose obesogenic effects mediated by high-affinity targets, for example, RXR–PPARγ transcriptional regulation of adipogenic GRNs; $EC_{50} = 5$ nM (solid blue). Disruption of mitochondrial integrity (cell energy charge, solid red) and production of inflammatory reactive lipid species (RLS) by organotin-mediated peroxidation (dotted red) contribute to metabolic and chronic inflammatory signals. Beyond the threshold of cellular antioxidant capacity (dotted blue), TBT and RLS accumulation is cytotoxic, contributes to metabolic collapse, and triggers apoptosis and eventually death. Above micromolar levels, TBT directly inhibits biosynthetic enzymes of steroidogenesis and metabolism, for example, CYP19 and 11β-HSD2 (hashed red), but sensitivity to transcriptional misregulation may shift endocrine-disruptive responses 100-fold lower. Combinations of these factors likely contribute to the obesogenic response (increased adiposity and weight gain) at low environmental exposures that produces a nonmonotonic dose–response curve (inverted U-shape, solid green). Bioaccumulation by marine organisms can result in significant organotin exposures that disrupt endocrine systems (imposex) and are immunotoxic/cytotoxic and biocidal. Average human exposure is typically subnanomolar, although serum and tissues levels in the range of 10–100 nM are reported for some individuals. (See color plate.)

products is an explanation for their potency and efficacy (Dickinson, Darley-Usmar, & Landar, 2006), and the significant signaling by such bioactive lipid intermediaries may explain how even low-dose organotin exposure can be effective and harmful to adipose tissue homeostasis where chronic low-grade inflammation is a hallmark of disturbed adipogenesis and the comorbid pathologies seen with obesity (Calder et al., 2011; Rocha & Folco, 2011; Xu et al., 2003).

At intermediate levels or exposure (0.1–1 μM), universal effects on ion gradients, mitochondrial function, and the cell energy charge (ATP levels) are evident in cellular experiments (Agarwal, 2011; Nakatsu, Kotake, Hino, & Ohta, 2008). These metabolic stresses are sensed and can be countered by adaptations in metabolic flux unless severe. Strong disruptive effects on energy homeostasis and metabolic integrity will be incompatible with normal growth and weight gain. Not surprisingly, toxic metabolic stresses frequently manifest themselves as wasting or a decrease of body weight gain during growth. Indeed, animal toxicity studies with organotins, including TBT, demonstrate overt deleterious effects when exposed to high doses (>3 mg Sn/kg, equivalent to ~10 μM) or at lower doses during long-term chronic feeding studies where tissue bioaccumulation eventually reaches toxic levels (Adeeko et al., 2003; Cooke et al., 2004).

However, a different set of targets and phenomena may be more relevant at low subtoxic levels (1–100 nM) that show properties of adipogenic, progrowth, or altered nutrient flow. Differential tissue-specific sensitivity, for instance in thymocytes and neuronal subpopulations, to low nanomolar concentrations of organotins predicted some effects are mediated by high-affinity intracellular targets, for example, TMT toxicity in stannin-expressing neuronal cells (Toggas, Krady, & Billingsley, 1992). The finding that TBT, and other triorganotins, are potent nanomolar activators of both the RXRs and PPARγ is conclusive evidence for such tissue-specific targets and provides the clearest mechanistic link to enhanced adipogenesis and accumulation of excess fat over time. The pharmacological overlap and similar adipogenic consequences shared between NR-agonist organotins and unrelated PPARγ activators, such as the TZD drugs, demonstrate the basic mechanistic principals are sound.

In this context, perhaps, the responses elicited by low-dose organotin exposure are a combination of weaker interference at the level of mitochondrial function and proinflammatory signals and the ability for high-affinity interactions with metabolic sensors and endocrine signaling pathways that are misinterpreted to establish a state of increased food conversion efficiency and fat storage as a hedge against metabolic stress. Similar explanations have been invoked to account for the unanticipated actions of other toxic endocrine disruptors at low environmental levels that rely on the concept of hormesis or nonmonotonic dose responses (Kendig, Le, & Belcher, 2010; Mattson & Calabrese, 2009; Vandenberg et al., 2012).

Second, obesity is ultimately an accumulation of excess adipose tissue mass due to a change in the dynamics of adipocyte lipid accumulation (hypertrophy) and cell number (hyperplasia) over long periods of time. The correct dynamic balance of adipose tissue mass requires tight integration of nutrient, adipokine, neuroendocrine, and endocrine hormone signals between central and peripheral organs that regulate the flow of energy reserves into and out from fat tissues. Increased fat mass would therefore require a prolonged positive shift toward lipid storage, promote adipogenesis, or enhance adipocyte survival/longevity. In the case of organotins, the obesogen hypothesis would not seem to be a likely viable explanation if effects were solely dependent on substantial chronic environmental exposure over a person's lifetime. Environmental organotin exposure is characterized as low or at best intermittent—a pattern that may be insufficient by its own to drive this persistent response, especially in comparison to the regular large-scale fluctuations of nutrient intake and energy expenditures that are normally encountered. However, the fetal origins of health and disease paradigm postulate that long-term health outcomes are susceptible to early developmental events and environmental conditions that alter epigenetic programming (Seki, Williams, Vuguin, & Charron, 2012). Hence, an acute chemical insult that occurs during critical developmental windows can continue to shape the body's metabolic responses long after exposure ceases. The contributions of organotin exposures, and other candidate obesogens, to obesity at the population level are likely to be found in their influence over adipogenic developmental gene regulatory networks, neuroendocrine circuits, and programming of metabolic set points that occurs during this early life period.

Future work will no doubt focus on these unanswered questions and address the epidemiological relevance of environmental obesogens to the etiology and the magnitude of their contribution to current obesity trends.

ACKNOWLEDGMENTS

F. G. would like to thank S. Kawauchi for critical reading of the chapter. Funding support for cited experimental data from FG/BB was provided by grants from UC TSR&TP grant (UC-3757) and NIEHS (RO1 ES015849).

REFERENCES

Adeeko, A., Li, D., Forsyth, D. S., Casey, V., Cooke, G. M., Barthelemy, J., et al. (2003). Effects of in utero tributyltin chloride exposure in the rat on pregnancy outcome. *Toxicological Sciences*, *74*(2), 407–415.

Agarwal, B. (2011). A role for anions in ATP synthesis and its molecular mechanistic interpretation. *Journal of Bioenergetics and Biomembranes*, *43*(3), 299–310.

Aldridge, W. N., & Rose, M. S. (1969). The mechanism of oxidative phosphorylation A hypothesis derived from studies of trimethyltin and triethyltin compounds. *FEBS Letters*, *4*(2), 61–68.

Alexander, J. W., Autrup, H., Bard, D., Carere, A., Guido Costa, L., Cravedi, J.-P., et al. (2004). Opinion of the Scientific Panel on Contaminants in the Food Chain on a request from the Commission to assess the health risks to consumers associated with exposure to organotins in foodstuffs. *The EFSA Journal*, *102*, 1–119.

Allenby, G., Janocha, R., Kazmer, S., Speck, J., Grippo, J. F., & Levin, A. A. (1994). Binding of 9-cis-retinoic acid and all-trans-retinoic acid to retinoic acid receptors alpha, beta, and gamma. Retinoic acid receptor gamma binds all-trans-retinoic acid preferentially over 9-cis-retinoic acid. *The Journal of Biological Chemistry*, *269*(24), 16689–16695.

Al Mamun, A., Lawlor, D. A., Alati, R., O'Callaghan, M. J., Williams, G. M., & Najman, J. M. (2006). Does maternal smoking during pregnancy have a direct effect on future offspring obesity? Evidence from a prospective birth cohort study. *American Journal of Epidemiology*, *164*(4), 317–325.

Antizar-Ladislao, B. (2008). Environmental levels, toxicity and human exposure to tributyltin (TBT)-contaminated marine environment. a review. b_antizar@hotmail.com. *Environment International*, *34*(2), 292–308.

Apps, D. K., & Webster, L. C. (1996). Interaction of organotins with a vacuolar-type H(+)-ATPase. *Biochemical and Biophysical Research Communications*, *227*(3), 839–845.

Atanasov, A. G., Nashev, L. G., Tam, S., Baker, M. E., & Odermatt, A. (2005). Organotins disrupt the 11beta-hydroxysteroid dehydrogenase type 2-dependent local inactivation of glucocorticoids. *Environmental Health Perspectives*, *113*(11), 1600–1606.

Baillie-Hamilton, P. F. (2002). Chemical toxins: A hypothesis to explain the global obesity epidemic. *Journal of Alternative and Complementary Medicine*, *8*(2), 185–192.

Barbosa-da-Silva, S., Fraulob-Aquino, J. C., Lopes, J. R., Mandarim-de-Lacerda, C. A., & Aguila, M. B. (2012). Weight cycling enhances adipose tissue inflammatory responses in male mice. *PLoS One*, 7(7), e39837.

Bariagaber, A. K., & Whalen, M. M. (2003). Decreased adenylyl cyclase and cAMP-dependent protein kinase activities inhibit the cytotoxic function of human natural killer cells. *Human Immunology*, *64*(9), 866–873.

Bastie, C., Luquet, S., Holst, D., Jehl-Pietri, C., & Grimaldi, P. A. (2000). Alterations of peroxisome proliferator-activated receptor delta activity affect fatty acid-controlled adipose differentiation. *The Journal of Biological Chemistry*, *275*(49), 38768–38773.

Bellinger, L., Lilley, C., & Langley-Evans, S. C. (2004). Prenatal exposure to a maternal low-protein diet programmes a preference for high-fat foods in the young adult rat. *The British Journal of Nutrition*, *92*(3), 513–520.

Biemann, R., Navarrete Santos, A., Riemann, D., Knelangen, J., Bluher, M., Koch, H., et al. (2012). Endocrine disrupting chemicals affect the adipogenic differentiation of mesenchymal stem cells in distinct ontogenetic windows. *Biochemical and Biophysical Research Communications*, *417*(2), 747–752.

Billingsley, M. L., Yun, J., Reese, B. E., Davidson, C. E., Buck-Koehntop, B. A., & Veglia, G. (2006). Functional and structural properties of stannin: Roles in cellular growth, selective toxicity, and mitochondrial responses to injury. *Journal of Cellular Biochemistry*, *98*(2), 243–250.

Blaber, S. J. M. (1970). The occurrence of a penis-like outgrowth behind the right tentacle in spent females of Nucella lapillus. *Proceedings of the Malacological Society of London*, *39*, 231–233.

Blunden, S. J., & Chapman, A. (1986). Organotin compounds in the environment. In P. J. Craig (Ed.), *Organometallic compounds in the environment* (pp. 111–159). London: Longman Group Ltd.

Bo, E., Viglietti-Panzica, C., & Panzica, G. C. (2011). Acute exposure to tributyltin induces c-fos activation in the hypothalamic arcuate nucleus of adult male mice. *Neurotoxicology*, *32*(2), 277–280.

Bonarska-Kujawa, D., Kleszczynska, H., & Przestalski, S. (2012). The location of organotins within the erythrocyte membrane in relation to their toxicity. *Ecotoxicology and Environmental Safety*, *78*, 232–238.

Bosselmann, K. (1996). Environmental law and tributyltin in the environment. In S. de Mora (Ed.), *Tributyltin: Case Study of an Environmental Contaminant*. Cambridge: Cambridge University Press.

Bouret, S. G., & Simerly, R. B. (2007). Development of leptin-sensitive circuits. *Journal of Neuroendocrinology*, *19*(8), 575–582.

Boyer, I. J. (1989). Toxicity of dibutyltin, tributyltin and other organotin compounds to humans and to experimental animals. *Toxicology*, *55*(3), 253–298.

Bragadin, M., Marton, D., Scutari, G., & Dell'Antone, P. (2000). The interactions of trialkyltin compounds with lysosomes from rat liver. *Journal of Inorganic Biochemistry*, *78*(3), 205–207.

Brown, V. J. (2012). Potential obesogen identified: Fungicide triflumizole is associated with increased adipogenesis in mice. *Environmental Health Perspectives*, *120*(12), a474.

Buck, B. A., Mascioni, A., Cramer, C. J., & Veglia, G. (2004). Interactions of alkyltin salts with biological dithiols: Dealkylation and induction of a regular beta-turn structure in peptides. *Journal of the American Chemical Society*, *126*(44), 14400–14410.

Buck-Koehntop, B. A., Mascioni, A., Buffy, J. J., & Veglia, G. (2005). Structure, dynamics, and membrane topology of stannin: A mediator of neuronal cell apoptosis induced by trimethyltin chloride. *Journal of Molecular Biology*, *354*(3), 652–665.

Burdge, G. C., & Lillycrop, K. A. (2010). Nutrition, epigenetics, and developmental plasticity: Implications for understanding human disease. *Annual Review of Nutrition*, *30*, 315–339.

Calder, P. C., Ahluwalia, N., Brouns, F., Buetler, T., Clement, K., Cunningham, K., et al. (2011). Dietary factors and low-grade inflammation in relation to overweight and obesity. *The British Journal of Nutrition*, *106*(Suppl. 3), S5–S78.

Carfi, M., Croera, C., Ferrario, D., Campi, V., Bowe, G., Pieters, R., et al. (2008). TBTC induces adipocyte differentiation in human bone marrow long term culture. *Toxicology*, *249*(1), 11–18.

Carmines, E. L., & Rajendran, N. (2008). Evidence for carbon monoxide as the major factor contributing to lower fetal weights in rats exposed to cigarette smoke. *Toxicological Sciences*, *102*(2), 383–391.

Carpentier, R., Sacchetti, P., Segard, P., Staels, B., & Lefebvre, P. (2008). The glucocorticoid receptor is a co-regulator of the orphan nuclear receptor Nurr1. *Journal of Neurochemistry*, *104*(3), 777–789.

Castro, L. F., Lima, D., Machado, A., Melo, C., Hiromori, Y., Nishikawa, J., et al. (2007). Imposex induction is mediated through the Retinoid X Receptor signalling pathway in the neogastropod Nucella lapillus. *Aquatic Toxicology*, *85*(1), 57–66.

Champ, M. A. (2003). Economic and environmental impacts on ports and harbors from the convention to ban harmful marine anti-fouling systems. *Marine Pollution Bulletin*, *46*(8), 935–940.

Chandra, V., Huang, P., Hamuro, Y., Raghuram, S., Wang, Y., Burris, T. P., et al. (2008). Structure of the intact PPAR-gamma-RXR-alpha nuclear receptor complex on DNA. *Nature, 456*, 350–356.

Chao, L. C., Bensinger, S. J., Villanueva, C. J., Wroblewski, K., & Tontonoz, P. (2008). Inhibition of adipocyte differentiation by Nur77, Nurr1, and Nor1. *Molecular Endocrinology, 22*(12), 2596–2608.

Chen, H., Saad, S., Sandow, S. L., & Bertrand, P. P. (2012). Cigarette smoking and brain regulation of energy homeostasis. *Frontiers in Pharmacology, 3*, 147.

Cheshenko, K., Pakdel, F., Segner, H., Kah, O., & Eggen, R. I. (2008). Interference of endocrine disrupting chemicals with aromatase CYP19 expression or activity, and consequences for reproduction of teleost fish. *General and Comparative Endocrinology, 155*(1), 31–62.

Chicano, J. J., Ortiz, A., Teruel, J. A., & Aranda, F. J. (2001). Organotin compounds alter the physical organization of phosphatidylcholine membranes. *Biochimica et Biophysica Acta, 1510*(1–2), 330–341.

Choi, M., Moon, H. B., An, Y. R., Choi, S. G., & Choi, H. G. (2011). Accumulation of butyltin compounds in cetaceans from Korean coastal waters. *Marine Pollution Bulletin, 62*(5), 1120–1123.

Chow, S. C., Kass, G. E., McCabe, M. J., Jr., & Orrenius, S. (1992). Tributyltin increases cytosolic free Ca2+ concentration in thymocytes by mobilizing intracellular Ca2+, activating a Ca2+ entry pathway, and inhibiting Ca2+ efflux. *Archives of Biochemistry and Biophysics, 298*(1), 143–149.

Colliar, L., Sturm, A., & Leaver, M. J. (2011). Tributyltin is a potent inhibitor of piscine peroxisome proliferator-activated receptor alpha and beta. *Comparative Biochemistry and Physiology C, Toxicology and Pharmacology, 153*(1), 168–173.

Cooke, G. M. (2002). Effect of organotins on human aromatase activity in vitro. *Toxicology Letters, 126*(2), 121–130.

Cooke, G. M., Tryphonas, H., Pulido, O., Caldwell, D., Bondy, G. S., & Forsyth, D. (2004). Oral (gavage), in utero and postnatal exposure of Sprague-Dawley rats to low doses of tributyltin chloride. Part 1: Toxicology, histopathology and clinical chemistry. *Food and Chemical Toxicology, 42*(2), 211–220.

Cristancho, A. G., & Lazar, M. A. (2011). Forming functional fat: A growing understanding of adipocyte differentiation. *Nature Reviews. Molecular Cell Biology, 12*(11), 722–734.

Cypess, A. M., Lehman, S., Williams, G., Tal, I., Rodman, D., Goldfine, A. B., et al. (2009). Identification and importance of brown adipose tissue in adult humans. *The New England Journal of Medicine, 360*(15), 1509–1517.

Dahlgren, J., Nilsson, C., Jennische, E., Ho, H. P., Eriksson, E., Niklasson, A., et al. (2001). Prenatal cytokine exposure results in obesity and gender-specific programming. *American Journal of Physiology. Endocrinology and Metabolism, 281*(2), E326–E334.

Davidson, C. E., Reese, B. E., Billingsley, M. L., & Yun, J. K. (2004). Stannin, a protein that localizes to the mitochondria and sensitizes NIH-3T3 cells to trimethyltin and dimethyltin toxicity. *Molecular Pharmacology, 66*(4), 855–863.

Decherf, S., & Demeneix, B. A. (2011). The obesogen hypothesis: A shift of focus from the periphery to the hypothalamus. *Journal of Toxicology and Environmental Health. Part B, Critical Reviews, 14*(5–7), 423–448.

Decherf, S., Seugnet, I., Fini, J. B., Clerget-Froidevaux, M. S., & Demeneix, B. A. (2010). Disruption of thyroid hormone-dependent hypothalamic set-points by environmental contaminants. *Molecular and Cellular Endocrinology, 323*(2), 172–182.

de Souza, C. J., Eckhardt, M., Gagen, K., Dong, M., Chen, W., Laurent, D., et al. (2001). Effects of pioglitazone on adipose tissue remodeling within the setting of obesity and insulin resistance. *Diabetes, 50*(8), 1863–1871.

Dickinson, D. A., Darley-Usmar, V. M., & Landar, A. (2006). The covalent advantage: A new paradigm for cell signaling by thiol reactive lipid oxidation products. In I. Dalle-Donne,

A. Scalone, & D. A. Buttefield (Eds.), *Redox proteomics: from protein modifications to cellular dysfunction and diseases* (pp. 345–367). Indianapolis: John Wiley & Sons.

Drake, A. J., McPherson, R. C., Godfrey, K. M., Cooper, C., Lillycrop, K. A., Hanson, M. A., et al. (2012). An unbalanced maternal diet in pregnancy associates with offspring epigenetic changes in genes controlling glucocorticoid action and foetal growth. *Clinical Endocrinology*, 77(6), 808–815.

Dunn, G. A., & Bale, T. L. (2011). Maternal high-fat diet effects on third-generation female body size via the paternal lineage. *Endocrinology*, *152*(6), 2228–2236.

Ehman, K. D., Phillips, P. M., McDaniel, K. L., Barone, S., Jr., & Moser, V. C. (2007). Evaluation of developmental neurotoxicity of organotins via drinking water in rats: Dimethyl tin. *Neurotoxicology and Teratology*, *29*(6), 622–633.

Elbrecht, A., Chen, Y., Adams, A., Berger, J., Griffin, P., Klatt, T., et al. (1999). L-764406 is a partial agonist of human peroxisome proliferator-activated receptor gamma. The role of Cys313 in ligand binding. *The Journal of Biological Chemistry*, *274*(12), 7913–7922.

El Hajj, N., Pliushch, G., Schneider, E., Dittrich, M., Muller, T., Korenkov, M., et al. (2013). Metabolic programming of MEST DNA methylation by intrauterine exposure to gestational diabetes mellitus. *Diabetes*, *62*(4), 1320–1328.

Emmanuel, E. L., Carver, M. A., Solaini, G. C., & Griffiths, D. E. (1984). Differential inhibition of F0F1-ATPase catalysed reactions in bovine-heart submitochondrial particles by organotin compounds. *Biochimica et Biophysica Acta*, *766*, 209–214.

Faust, I. M., Johnson, P. R., Stern, J. S., & Hirsch, J. (1978). Diet-induced adipocyte number increase in adult rats: A new model of obesity. *The American Journal of Physiology*, *235*(3), E279–E286.

Ferno, J., Vik-Mo, A. O., Jassim, G., Havik, B., Berge, K., Skrede, S., et al. (2009). Acute clozapine exposure in vivo induces lipid accumulation and marked sequential changes in the expression of SREBP, PPAR, and LXR target genes in rat liver. *Psychopharmacology*, *203*(1), 73–84.

Forsyth, D. S., & Jay, B. (1997). Organotin leachates in drinking water from chlorinated poly(vinyl)chloride (CPVC) pipe. *Applied Organometallic Chemistry*, *11*(7), 551–558.

Frontini, A., & Cinti, S. (2010). Distribution and development of brown adipocytes in the murine and human adipose organ. *Cell Metabolism*, *11*(4), 253–256.

Fumoto, T., Yamaguchi, T., Hirose, F., & Osumi, T. (2007). Orphan nuclear receptor Nur77 accelerates the initial phase of adipocyte differentiation in 3T3-L1 cells by promoting mitotic clonal expansion. *Journal of Biochemistry*, *141*(2), 181–192.

Galic, S., Oakhill, J. S., & Steinberg, G. R. (2010). Adipose tissue as an endocrine organ. *Molecular and Cellular Endocrinology*, *316*(2), 129–139.

Gao, Y. J., Holloway, A. C., Zeng, Z. H., Lim, G. E., Petrik, J. J., Foster, W. G., et al. (2005). Prenatal exposure to nicotine causes postnatal obesity and altered perivascular adipose tissue function. *Obesity Research*, *13*(4), 687–692.

Godfrey, K. M., Sheppard, A., Gluckman, P. D., Lillycrop, K. A., Burdge, G. C., McLean, C., et al. (2011). Epigenetic gene promoter methylation at birth is associated with child's later adiposity. *Diabetes*, *60*(5), 1528–1534.

Gogvadze, V., Stridh, H., Orrenius, S., & Cotgreave, I. (2002). Tributyltin causes cytochrome C release from isolated mitochondria by two discrete mechanisms. *Biochemical and Biophysical Research Communications*, *292*(4), 904–908.

Gray, B. H., Porvaznik, M., Lee, L. H., & Flemming, C. (1986). Inhibition of tributyltin mediated hemolysis by mercapto compounds. *Journal of Applied Toxicology*, *6*(5), 363–370.

Grote, K., Stahlschmidt, B., Talsness, C. E., Gericke, C., Appel, K. E., & Chahoud, I. (2004). Effects of organotin compounds on pubertal male rats. *Toxicology*, *202*(3), 145–158.

Grove, K. L., Fried, S. K., Greenberg, A. S., Xiao, X. Q., & Clegg, D. J. (2010). A microarray analysis of sexual dimorphism of adipose tissues in high-fat-diet-induced obese mice. *International Journal of Obesity*, *34*(6), 989–1000.

Grun, F. (2010). Covalent interactions of oganotins with nuclear receptors. In A. Pagliarani, V. Ventrella, & A. Trombetti (Eds.), *Biochemical and biological effects of organotins* (pp. 74–95). Sharjah: Bentham Science Publishers Ltd.

Grun, F., & Blumberg, B. (2006). Environmental obesogens: Organotins and endocrine disruption via nuclear receptor signaling. *Endocrinology, 147*(6 Suppl.), S50–S55.

Grün, F., & Blumberg, B. (2006). Environmental obesogens: Organotins and endocrine disruption of RXR:PPARγ signaling in adipogenesis. In *Paper presented at the FASEB summer research conference: Retinoids, Indian Wells, CA*.

Grun, F., & Blumberg, B. (2007). Perturbed nuclear receptor signaling by environmental obesogens as emerging factors in the obesity crisis. *Reviews in Endocrine & Metabolic Disorders, 8*(2), 161–171.

Grun, F., Watanabe, H., Zamanian, Z., Maeda, L., Arima, K., Cubacha, R., et al. (2006). Endocrine-disrupting organotin compounds are potent inducers of adipogenesis in vertebrates. *Molecular Endocrinology, 20*(9), 2141–2155.

Gueguen, M., Amiard, J. C., Arnich, N., Badot, P. M., Claisse, D., Guerin, T., et al. (2011). Shellfish and residual chemical contaminants: Hazards, monitoring, and health risk assessment along French coasts. *Reviews of Environmental Contamination and Toxicology, 213*, 55–111.

Guerin, T., Sirot, V., Volatier, J. L., & Leblanc, J. C. (2007). Organotin levels in seafood and its implications for health risk in high-seafood consumers. *The Science of the Total Environment, 388*(1–3), 66–77.

Guerrieri, F., Zanotti, F., Che, Y. W., Scarfo, R., & Papa, S. (1987). Inactivation of the mitochondrial ATPase inhibitor protein by chemical modification with diethylpyrocarbonate. *Biochimica et Biophysica Acta, 892*(3), 284–293.

Gumy, C., Chandsawangbhuwana, C., Dzyakanchuk, A. A., Kratschmar, D. V., Baker, M. E., & Odermatt, A. (2008). Dibutyltin disrupts glucocorticoid receptor function and impairs glucocorticoid-induced suppression of cytokine production. *PLoS One, 3*(10), e3545.

Haghighi, A., Schwartz, D. H., Abrahamowicz, M., Leonard, G. T., Perron, M., Richer, L., et al. (2013). Prenatal exposure to maternal cigarette smoking, amygdala volume, and fat intake in adolescence. *JAMA Psychiatry, 70*(1), 98–105.

Hamdy, O., Porramatikul, S., & Al-Ozairi, E. (2006). Metabolic obesity: The paradox between visceral and subcutaneous fat. *Current Diabetes Reviews, 2*(4), 367–373.

Harris, A., & Seckl, J. (2011). Glucocorticoids, prenatal stress and the programming of disease. *Hormones and Behavior, 59*(3), 279–289.

Hatch, E. E., Nelson, J. W., Qureshi, M. M., Weinberg, J., Moore, L. L., Singer, M., et al. (2008). Association of urinary phthalate metabolite concentrations with body mass index and waist circumference: A cross-sectional study of NHANES data, 1999-2002. *Environmental Health, 7*, 27.

Heidrich, D. D., Steckelbroeck, S., & Klingmuller, D. (2001). Inhibition of human cytochrome P450 aromatase activity by butyltins. *Steroids, 66*(10), 763–769.

Higdon, A., Diers, A. R., Oh, J. Y., Landar, A., & Darley-Usmar, V. M. (2012). Cell signalling by reactive lipid species: New concepts and molecular mechanisms. *The Biochemical Journal, 442*(3), 453–464.

Hollenberg, A. N. (2008). The role of the thyrotropin-releasing hormone (TRH) neuron as a metabolic sensor. *Thyroid, 18*(2), 131–139.

Hunter, R. C. (1976). Organotin compounds and their use for insect and mite control. *Environmental Health Perspectives, 14*, 47–50.

Ibrahim, M. M. (2010). Subcutaneous and visceral adipose tissue: Structural and functional differences. *Obesity Reviews, 11*(1), 11–18.

Ikenasio-Thorpe, B. A., Breier, B. H., Vickers, M. H., & Fraser, M. (2007). Prenatal influences on susceptibility to diet-induced obesity are mediated by altered neuroendocrine gene expression. *The Journal of Endocrinology, 193*(1), 31–37.

Imai, H., Nishimura, T., Sadamatsu, M., Liu, Y., Kabuto, M., & Kato, N. (2001). Type II glucocorticoid receptors are involved in neuronal death and astrocyte activation induced by trimethyltin in the rat hippocampus. *Experimental Neurology, 171*(1), 22–28.

Impellitteri, C. A., Evans, O., & Ravel, B. (2007). Speciation of organotins in polyvinyl chloride pipe via X-ray absorption spectroscopy and in leachates using GC-PFPD after derivatisation. *Journal of Environmental Monitoring, 9*(4), 358–365.

Inadera, H., & Shimomura, A. (2005). Environmental chemical tributyltin augments adipocyte differentiation. *Toxicology Letters, 159*(3), 226–234.

Ishihara, Y., Kawami, T., Ishida, A., & Yamazaki, T. (2012). Tributyltin induces oxidative stress and neuronal injury by inhibiting glutathione S-transferase in rat organotypic hippocampal slice cultures. *Neurochemistry International, 60*(8), 782–790.

Janer, G., Navarro, J. C., & Porte, C. (2007). Exposure to TBT increases accumulation of lipids and alters fatty acid homeostasis in the ramshorn snail Marisa cornuarietis. *Comparative Biochemistry and Physiology C, Toxicology and Pharmacology, 146*(3), 368–374.

Jenkins, S. M., Ehman, K., & Barone, S., Jr. (2004). Structure-activity comparison of organotin species: Dibutyltin is a developmental neurotoxicant in vitro and in vivo. *Brain Research. Developmental Brain Research, 151*(1–2), 1–12.

Jensen Pena, C., Monk, C., & Champagne, F. A. (2012). Epigenetic effects of prenatal stress on 11beta-hydroxysteroid dehydrogenase-2 in the placenta and fetal brain. *PLoS One, 7*(6), e39791.

Jo, J., Gavrilova, O., Pack, S., Jou, W., Mullen, S., Sumner, A. E., et al. (2009). Hypertrophy and/or hyperplasia: Dynamics of adipose tissue growth. *PLoS Computational Biology, 5*(3), e1000324.

Jo, J., Guo, J., Liu, T., Mullen, S., Hall, K. D., Cushman, S. W., et al. (2010). Hypertrophy-driven adipocyte death overwhelms recruitment under prolonged weight gain. *Biophysical Journal, 99*(11), 3535–3544.

Joe, A. W., Yi, L., Even, Y., Vogl, A. W., & Rossi, F. M. (2009). Depot-specific differences in adipogenic progenitor abundance and proliferative response to high-fat diet. *Stem Cells, 27*(10), 2563–2570.

Kanayama, T., Kobayashi, N., Mamiya, S., Nakanishi, T., & Nishikawa, J. (2005). Organotin compounds promote adipocyte differentiation as agonists of the peroxisome proliferator-activated receptor gamma/retinoid X receptor pathway. *Molecular Pharmacology, 67*(3), 766–774.

Kannan, K., Corsolini, S., Focardi, S., Tanabe, S., & Tatsukawa, R. (1996). Accumulation pattern of butyltin compounds in dolphin, tuna, and shark collected from Italian coastal waters. *Archives of Environmental Contamination and Toxicology, 31*(1), 19–23.

Kannan, A., & Falandysz, Z. (1997). Butyltin residues in sediment, fish, fish eating birds, harbour porpoise and human tissues from the Polish coast of the Baltic Sea. *Marine Pollution Bulletin, 34*(3), 203–207.

Kannan, K., Senthilkumar, K., & Giesy, J. (1999). Occurrence of butyltin compounds in human blood. *Environmental Science and Technology, 33*(10), 1776–1779.

Kannan, K., Takahashi, S., Fujiwara, N., Mizukawa, H., & Tanabe, S. (2010). Organotin compounds, including butyltins and octyltins, in house dust from Albany, New York, USA. *Archives of Environmental Contamination and Toxicology, 58*(4), 901–907.

Katika, M. R., Hendriksen, P. J., de Ruijter, N. C., van Loveren, H., & Peijnenburg, A. (2012). Immunocytological and biochemical analysis of the mode of action of bis (tri-n-butyltin) tri-oxide (TBTO) in Jurkat cells. *Toxicology Letters, 212*(2), 126–136.

Kendig, E. L., Le, H. H., & Belcher, S. M. (2010). Defining hormesis: Evaluation of a complex concentration response phenomenon. *International Journal of Toxicology, 29*(3), 235–246.

Kirchner, S., Kieu, T., Chow, C., Casey, S., & Blumberg, B. (2010). Prenatal exposure to the environmental obesogen tributyltin predisposes multipotent stem cells to become adipocytes. *Molecular Endocrinology, 24*(3), 526–539.

Klyde, B. J., & Hirsch, J. (1979). Increased cellular proliferation in adipose tissue of adult rats fed a high-fat diet. *Journal of Lipid Research, 20*(6), 705–715.

Koch, F. S., Sepa, A., & Ludvigsson, J. (2008). Psychological stress and obesity. *The Journal of Pediatrics, 153*(6), 839–844.

Kouidhi, S., Seugnet, I., Decherf, S., Guissouma, H., Elgaaied, A. B., Demeneix, B., et al. (2010). Peroxisome proliferator-activated receptor-gamma (PPARgamma) modulates hypothalamic Trh regulation in vivo. *Molecular and Cellular Endocrinology, 317*(1–2), 44–52.

Krug, H. F. (2012). Caspase-10 is the key initiator caspase involved in tributyltin-mediated apoptosis in human immune cells. *Journal of Toxicology, 2012*, 395482.

Lassiter, T. L., & Brimijoin, S. (2008). Rats gain excess weight after developmental exposure to the organophosphorothionate pesticide, chlorpyrifos. *Neurotoxicology and Teratology, 30*(2), 125–130.

Lassiter, T. L., Ryde, I. T., Mackillop, E. A., Brown, K. K., Levin, E. D., Seidler, F. J., et al. (2008). Exposure of neonatal rats to parathion elicits sex-selective reprogramming of metabolism and alters the response to a high-fat diet in adulthood. *Environmental Health Perspectives, 116*(11), 1456–1462.

Le Curieux-Belfond, O., Moslemi, S., Mathieu, M., & Seralini, G. E. (2001). Androgen metabolism in oyster Crassostrea gigas: Evidence for 17beta-HSD activities and characterization of an aromatase-like activity inhibited by pharmacological compounds and a marine pollutant. *The Journal of Steroid Biochemistry and Molecular Biology, 78*(4), 359–366.

Lee, M. J., Wu, Y., & Fried, S. K. (2010). Adipose tissue remodeling in pathophysiology of obesity. *Current Opinion in Clinical Nutrition and Metabolic Care, 13*(4), 371–376.

Leesnitzer, L. M., Parks, D. J., Bledsoe, R. K., Cobb, J. E., Collins, J. L., Consler, T. G., et al. (2002). Functional consequences of cysteine modification in the ligand binding sites of peroxisome proliferator activated receptors by GW9662. *Biochemistry, 41*(21), 6640–6650.

Lefterova, M. I., Zhang, Y., Steger, D. J., Schupp, M., Schug, J., Cristancho, A., et al. (2008). PPARgamma and C/EBP factors orchestrate adipocyte biology via adjacent binding on a genome-wide scale. *Genes & Development, 22*(21), 2941–2952.

le Maire, A., Bourguet, W., & Balaguer, P. (2010). A structural view of nuclear hormone receptor: Endocrine disruptor interactions. *Cellular and Molecular Life Sciences, 67*(8), 1219–1237.

le Maire, A., Grimaldi, M., Roecklin, D., Dagnino, S., Vivat-Hannah, V., Balaguer, P., et al. (2009). Activation of RXR-PPAR heterodimers by organotin environmental endocrine disruptors. *EMBO Reports, 10*(4), 367–373.

Levonen, A. L., Landar, A., Ramachandran, A., Ceaser, E. K., Dickinson, D. A., Zanoni, G., et al. (2004). Cellular mechanisms of redox cell signalling: Role of cysteine modification in controlling antioxidant defences in response to electrophilic lipid oxidation products. *The Biochemical Journal, 378*(Pt 2), 373–382.

Li, X., Ycaza, J., & Blumberg, B. (2011). The environmental obesogen tributyltin chloride acts via peroxisome proliferator activated receptor gamma to induce adipogenesis in murine 3T3-L1 preadipocytes. *The Journal of Steroid Biochemistry and Molecular Biology, 127*(1–2), 9–15.

Lim, S., Ahn, S. Y., Song, I. C., Chung, M. H., Jang, H. C., Park, K. S., et al. (2009). Chronic exposure to the herbicide, atrazine, causes mitochondrial dysfunction and insulin resistance. *PLoS One, 4*(4), e5186.

Lo, S., Allera, A., Albers, P., Heimbrecht, J., Jantzen, E., Klingmuller, D., et al. (2003). Dithioerythritol (DTE) prevents inhibitory effects of triphenyltin (TPT) on the key

enzymes of the human sex steroid hormone metabolism. *The Journal of Steroid Biochemistry and Molecular Biology, 84*(5), 569–576.
Lu, M., Sarruf, D. A., Talukdar, S., Sharma, S., Li, P., Bandyopadhyay, G., et al. (2011). Brain PPAR-gamma promotes obesity and is required for the insulin-sensitizing effect of thiazolidinediones. *Nature Medicine, 17*(5), 618–622.
Lyssimachou, A., Navarro, J. C., Bachmann, J., & Porte, C. (2009). Triphenyltin alters lipid homeostasis in females of the ramshorn snail Marisa cornuarietis. *Environmental Pollution, 157*(5), 1714–1720.
Ma, X., Ren, X., Han, P., Hu, S., Wang, J., & Yin, J. (2010). SiRNA against Fabp5 induces 3T3-L1 cells apoptosis during adipocytic induction. *Molecular Biology Reports, 37*(8), 4003–4011.
Matsuno-Yagi, A., & Hatefi, Y. (1993). Studies on the mechanism of oxidative phosphorylation. ATP synthesis by submitochondrial particles inhibited at F0 by venturicidin and organotin compounds. *The Journal of Biological Chemistry, 268*(9), 6168–6173.
Mattson, M., & Calabrese, E. (2009). *Hormesis: A revolution in biology, toxicology and medicine.* New York: Humana Press.
McAllister, B. G., & Kime, D. E. (2003). Early life exposure to environmental levels of the aromatase inhibitor tributyltin causes masculinisation and irreversible sperm damage in zebrafish (Danio rerio). *Aquatic Toxicology, 65*(3), 309–316.
McGinnis, C. L., & Crivello, J. F. (2011). Elucidating the mechanism of action of tributyltin (TBT) in zebrafish. *Aquatic Toxicology, 103*(1–2), 25–31.
Meador, J. P., Sommers, F. C., Cooper, K. A., & Yanagida, G. (2011). Tributyltin and the obesogen metabolic syndrome in a salmonid. *Environmental Research, 111*(1), 50–56.
Menai, M., Heude, B., Slama, R., Forhan, A., Sahuquillo, J., Charles, M. A., et al. (2012). Association between maternal blood cadmium during pregnancy and birth weight and the risk of fetal growth restriction: The EDEN mother-child cohort study. *Reproductive Toxicology, 34*(4), 622–627.
Mikkelsen, T. S., Xu, Z., Zhang, X., Wang, L., Gimble, J. M., Lander, E. S., et al. (2010). Comparative epigenomic analysis of murine and human adipogenesis. *Cell, 143*(1), 156–169.
Milaeva, E., Petrosyan, V., Berberova, N., Pimenov, Y., & Pellerito, L. (2004). Organic derivatives of mercury and tin as promoters of membrane lipid peroxidation. *Bioinorganic Chemistry and Applications, 2*(1–2), 69–91.
Miller, W. H., Jr., Faust, I. M., Goldberger, A. C., & Hirsch, J. (1983). Effects of severe long-term food deprivation and refeeding on adipose tissue cells in the rat. *The American Journal of Physiology, 245*(1), E74–E80.
Monk, C., Spicer, J., & Champagne, F. A. (2012). Linking prenatal maternal adversity to developmental outcomes in infants: The role of epigenetic pathways. *Development and Psychopathology, 24*(4), 1361–1376.
Moser, V. C., Barone, S., Jr., Phillips, P. M., McDaniel, K. L., & Ehman, K. D. (2006). Evaluation of developmental neurotoxicity of organotins via drinking water in rats: Monomethyltin. *Neurotoxicology, 27*(3), 409–420.
Muncke, J. (2011). Endocrine disrupting chemicals and other substances of concern in food contact materials: An updated review of exposure, effect and risk assessment. *The Journal of Steroid Biochemistry and Molecular Biology, 127*(1–2), 118–127.
Musiek, E. S., Gao, L., Milne, G. L., Han, W., Everhart, M. B., Wang, D., et al. (2005). Cyclopentenone isoprostanes inhibit the inflammatory response in macrophages. *The Journal of Biological Chemistry, 280*(42), 35562–35570.
Myers, M. G., Jr., & Burant, C. F. (2011). PPAR-gamma action: It's all in your head. *Nature Medicine, 17*(5), 544–545.
Nakanishi, T., Kohroki, J., Suzuki, S., Ishizaki, J., Hiromori, Y., Takasuga, S., et al. (2002). Trialkyltin compounds enhance human CG secretion and aromatase activity in human

placental choriocarcinoma cells. *The Journal of Clinical Endocrinology and Metabolism, 87*(6), 2830–2837.

Nakanishi, T., Nishikawa, J. I., Hiromori, Y., Yokoyama, H., Koyanagi, M., Takasuga, S., et al. (2005). Trialkyltin compounds bind retinoid X receptor to alter human placental endocrine functions. *Molecular Endocrinology, 19*(10), 2502–2516.

Nakatsu, Y., Kotake, Y., Hino, A., & Ohta, S. (2008). Activation of AMP-activated protein kinase by tributyltin induces neuronal cell death. *Toxicology and Applied Pharmacology, 230*(3), 358–363.

Nakayama, K., Matsudaira, C., Tajima, Y., Yamada, T. K., Yoshioka, M., Isobe, T., et al. (2009). Temporal and spatial trends of organotin contamination in the livers of finless porpoises (Neophocaena phocaenoides) and their association with parasitic infection status. *The Science of the Total Environment, 407*(24), 6173–6178.

Neel, J. V. (1999). The "thrifty genotype" in 1998. *Nutrition Reviews, 57*(5 Pt 2), S2–S9.

Nemeroff, C. B. (1997). Dosing the antipsychotic medication olanzapine. *The Journal of Clinical Psychiatry, 58*(Suppl. 10), 45–49.

Nesci, S., Ventrella, V., Trombetti, F., Pirini, M., Borgatti, A. R., & Pagliarani, A. (2011). Tributyltin (TBT) and dibutyltin (DBT) differently inhibit the mitochondrial Mg-ATPase activity in mussel digestive gland. *Toxicology In Vitro, 25*(1), 117–124.

Newbold, R. R., Padilla-Banks, E., Jefferson, W. N., & Heindel, J. J. (2008). Effects of endocrine disruptors on obesity. *International Journal of Andrology, 31*(2), 201–208.

Newcomer, J. W. (2007). Antipsychotic medications: Metabolic and cardiovascular risk. *The Journal of Clinical Psychiatry, 68*(Suppl. 4), 8–13.

Nielsen, R., Pedersen, T. A., Hagenbeek, D., Moulos, P., Siersbaek, R., Megens, E., et al. (2008). Genome-wide profiling of PPARgamma:RXR and RNA polymerase II occupancy reveals temporal activation of distinct metabolic pathways and changes in RXR dimer composition during adipogenesis. *Genes & Development, 22*(21), 2953–2967.

Nielsen, J. B., & Strand, J. (2002). Butyltin compounds in human liver. *Environmental Research, 88*(2), 129–133.

Nishikawa, J., Mamiya, S., Kanayama, T., Nishikawa, T., Shiraishi, F., & Horiguchi, T. (2004). Involvement of the retinoid X receptor in the development of imposex caused by organotins in gastropods. *Environmental Science & Technology, 38*(23), 6271–6276.

Nishikimi, A., Kira, Y., Kasahara, E., Sato, E. F., Kanno, T., Utsumi, K., et al. (2001). Tributyltin interacts with mitochondria and induces cytochrome c release. *The Biochemical Journal, 356*(Pt 2), 621–626.

Ohno, S., Nakajima, Y., & Nakajin, S. (2005). Triphenyltin and Tributyltin inhibit pig testicular 17beta-hydroxysteroid dehydrogenase activity and suppress testicular testosterone biosynthesis. *Steroids, 70*(9), 645–651.

Ohno, H., Suzuki, M., Nakashima, S., Aoyama, T., & Mitani, K. (2002). Determination of organotin compounds in plastic products by GC/MS after ethyl derivatization with sodium tetraethylborate. *Shokuhin Eiseigaku Zasshi, 43*(4), 208–214.

Okada, Y., Oyama, Y., Chikahisa, L., Satoh, M., Kanemaru, K., Sakai, H., et al. (2000). Tri-n-butyltin-induced change in cellular level of glutathione in rat thymocytes: A flow cytometric study. *Toxicology Letters, 117*(3), 123–128.

Okamura, M., Inagaki, T., Tanaka, T., & Sakai, J. (2010). Role of histone methylation and demethylation in adipogenesis and obesity. *Organogenesis, 6*(1), 24–32.

Oken, E., Levitan, E. B., & Gillman, M. W. (2008). Maternal smoking during pregnancy and child overweight: Systematic review and meta-analysis. *International Journal of Obesity, 32*(2), 201–210.

Ong, Z. Y., & Muhlhausler, B. S. (2011). Maternal "junk-food" feeding of rat dams alters food choices and development of the mesolimbic reward pathway in the offspring. *The FASEB Journal, 25*(7), 2167–2179.

Osada, S., Nishikawa, J., Nakanishi, T., Tanaka, K., & Nishihara, T. (2005). Some organotin compounds enhance histone acetyltransferase activity. *Toxicology Letters, 155*(2), 329–335.

Patisaul, H. B., Roberts, S. C., Mabrey, N., McCaffrey, K. A., Gear, R. B., Braun, J., et al. (2012). Accumulation and endocrine disrupting effects of the flame retardant mixture firemaster((R)) 550 in rats: An exploratory assessment. *Journal of Biochemical and Molecular Toxicology, 27*(2), 124–136.

Pavlikova, N., Kortner, T. M., & Arukwe, A. (2010). Modulation of acute steroidogenesis, peroxisome proliferator-activated receptors and CYP3A/PXR in salmon interrenal tissues by tributyltin and the second messenger activator, forskolin. *Chemico-Biological Interactions, 185*(2), 119–127.

Penninks, A. H., & Seinen, W. (1980). Toxicity of organotin compounds. IV. Impairment of energy metabolism of rat thymocytes by various dialkyltin compounds. *Toxicology and Applied Pharmacology, 56*(2), 221–231.

Penza, M., Jeremic, M., Marrazzo, E., Maggi, A., Ciana, P., Rando, G., et al. (2011). The environmental chemical tributyltin chloride (TBT) shows both estrogenic and adipogenic activities in mice which might depend on the exposure dose. *Toxicology and Applied Pharmacology, 255*(1), 65–75.

Petrosyan, V. S., Gracheva, Y. A., Tyurin, V. Y., Grigor'ev, E. V., Millaeva, E. R., & Pellerito, L. (2003). Effect of organotin compounds and their complexes with phosphatidylcholine on peroxide oxidation of lipid structural elements. *Journal of Organic Chemistry, 39*(3), 353–356.

Philbert, M. A., Billingsley, M. L., & Reuhl, K. R. (2000). Mechanisms of injury in the central nervous system. *Toxicologic Pathology, 28*(1), 43–53.

Philips, A., Maira, M., Mullick, A., Chamberland, M., Lesage, S., Hugo, P., et al. (1997). Antagonism between Nur77 and glucocorticoid receptor for control of transcription. *Molecular and Cellular Biology, 17*(10), 5952–5959.

Power, C., Atherton, K., & Thomas, C. (2010). Maternal smoking in pregnancy, adult adiposity and other risk factors for cardiovascular disease. *Atherosclerosis, 211*(2), 643–648.

Power, C., & Jefferis, B. J. (2002). Fetal environment and subsequent obesity: A study of maternal smoking. *International Journal of Epidemiology, 31*(2), 413–419.

Rantakokko, P., Kuningas, T., Saastamoinen, K., & Vartiainen, T. (2006). Dietary intake of organotin compounds in Finland: A market-basket study. *Food Additives and Contaminants, 23*(8), 749–756.

Rantakokko, P., Turunen, A., Verkasalo, P. K., Kiviranta, H., Mannisto, S., & Vartiainen, T. (2008). Blood levels of organotin compounds and their relation to fish consumption in Finland. *The Science of the Total Environment, 399*(1–3), 90–95.

Rocha, V. Z., & Folco, E. J. (2011). Inflammatory concepts of obesity. *International Journal of Inflammation, 2011*, 529061.

RPA. (2005). *Risk assessment of targeted consumer applications of certain organotin compounds. A report of the European Commission.* Risk and Policy Analysts Limited.

Rubin, B. S., Murray, M. K., Damassa, D. A., King, J. C., & Soto, A. M. (2001). Perinatal exposure to low doses of bisphenol A affects body weight, patterns of estrous cyclicity, and plasma LH levels. *Environmental Health Perspectives, 109*(7), 675–680.

Ruiz, J. M., Bachelet, G., Caumette, P., & Donard, O. F. (1996). Three decades of tributyltin in the coastal environment with emphasis on Arcachon Bay, France. *Environmental Pollution, 93*(2), 195–203.

Ryan, K. K., Li, B., Grayson, B. E., Matter, E. K., Woods, S. C., & Seeley, R. J. (2011). A role for central nervous system PPAR-gamma in the regulation of energy balance. *Nature Medicine, 17*(5), 623–626.

Sadiki, A. I., & Williams, D. T. (1999). A study on organotin levels in Canadian drinking water distributed through PVC pipes. *Chemosphere, 38*(7), 1541–1548.

Saitoh, M., Yanase, T., Morinaga, H., Tanabe, M., Mu, Y. M., Nishi, Y., et al. (2001). Tributyltin or triphenyltin inhibits aromatase activity in the human granulosa-like tumor cell line KGN. *Biochemical and Biophysical Research Communications*, *289*(1), 198–204.

Santos, M. M., Enes, P., Reis-Henriques, M. A., Kuballa, J., Castro, L. F., & Vieira, M. N. (2009). Organotin levels in seafood from Portuguese markets and the risk for consumers. *Chemosphere*, *75*(5), 661–666.

Santos, M. M., ten Hallers-Tjabbes, C. C., Vieira, N., Boon, J. P., & Porte, C. (2002). Cytochrome P450 differences in normal and imposex-affected female whelk Buccinum undatum from the open North Sea. *Marine Environmental Research*, *54*(3–5), 661–665.

Sargis, R. M., Johnson, D. N., Choudhury, R. A., & Brady, M. J. (2010). Environmental endocrine disruptors promote adipogenesis in the 3T3-L1 cell line through glucocorticoid receptor activation. *Obesity (Silver Spring)*, *18*(7), 1283–1288.

Saxena, A. K. (1987). Organotin compounds: Toxicology and biomedicinal applications. *Applied Organometallic Chemistry*, *1*, 39–56.

Schopfer, F. J., Cole, M. P., Groeger, A. L., Chen, C. S., Khoo, N. K., Woodcock, S. R., et al. (2010). Covalent peroxisome proliferator-activated receptor gamma adduction by nitro-fatty acids: Selective ligand activity and anti-diabetic signaling actions. *The Journal of Biological Chemistry*, *285*(16), 12321–12333.

Seki, Y., Williams, L., Vuguin, P. M., & Charron, M. J. (2012). Minireview: Epigenetic programming of diabetes and obesity: Animal models. *Endocrinology*, *153*(3), 1031–1038.

Sekizawa, J. (1998). Health and environmental risk assessment of organotin pollution in Japan. *Kokuritsu Iyakuhin Shokuhin Eisei Kenkyūjo Hōkoku*, *116*, 126–131.

Shi, H., Zhu, P., & Guo, S. (2012). Effects of tributyltin on metamorphosis and gonadal differentiation of Xenopus laevis at environmentally relevant concentrations. *Toxicology and Industrial Health*. http://dx.doi.org/10.1177/0748233712457440.

Shimasaki, Y., Kitano, T., Oshima, Y., Inoue, S., Imada, N., & Honjo, T. (2003). Tributyltin causes masculinization in fish. *Environmental Toxicology and Chemistry*, *22*(1), 141–144.

Shintani, N., Ogita, K., Hashimoto, H., & Baba, A. (2007). Recent studies on the trimethyltin actions in central nervous systems. *Yakugaku Zasshi*, *127*(3), 451–461.

Shiraki, T., Kamiya, N., Shiki, S., Kodama, T. S., Kakizuka, A., & Jingami, H. (2005). Alpha, beta-unsaturated ketone is a core moiety of natural ligands for covalent binding to peroxisome proliferator-activated receptor gamma. *The Journal of Biological Chemistry*, *280*(14), 14145–14153.

Shoener, J. A., Baig, R., & Page, K. C. (2006). Prenatal exposure to dexamethasone alters hippocampal drive on hypothalamic-pituitary-adrenal axis activity in adult male rats. *American Journal of Physiology. Regulatory, Integrative and Comparative Physiology*, *290*(5), R1366–R1373.

Shuto, M., Higuchi, K., Sugiyama, C., Yoneyama, M., Kuramoto, N., Nagashima, R., et al. (2009). Endogenous and exogenous glucocorticoids prevent trimethyltin from causing neuronal degeneration of the mouse brain in vivo: Involvement of oxidative stress pathways. *Journal of Pharmacological Sciences*, *110*(4), 424–436.

Si, J., Wu, X., Wan, C., Zeng, T., Zhang, M., Xie, K., et al. (2011). Peripubertal exposure to low doses of tributyltin chloride affects the homeostasis of serum T, E2, LH, and body weight of male mice. *Environmental Toxicology*, *26*(3), 307–314.

Siebenlist, K. R., & Taketa, F. (1983). Inactivation of yeast hexokinase B by triethyltin bromide and reactivation by dithiothreitol and glucose. *Biochemistry*, *22*(20), 4642–4646.

Siebenlist, K. R., & Taketa, F. (1986). Organotin-protein interactions. Binding of triethyltin bromide to cat haemoglobin. *The Biochemical Journal*, *233*(2), 471–477.

Singh, P., Somers, V. K., Romero-Corral, A., Sert-Kuniyoshi, F. H., Pusalavidyasagar, S., Davison, D. E., et al. (2012). Effects of weight gain and weight loss on regional fat distribution. *The American Journal of Clinical Nutrition*, *96*(2), 229–233.

Smith, B. S. (1981). Male characteristics on female mud snails caused by antifouling bottom paints. *Journal of Applied Toxicology, 1*(1), 22–25.

Smith, P. J., Crowe, A. J., Das, V. K., & Duncan, J. (1979). Structure-activity relationship for some organotin molluscicides. *Pesticide Science, 10*(5), 419–422.

Somm, E., Schwitzgebel, V. M., Toulotte, A., Cederroth, C. R., Combescure, C., Nef, S., et al. (2009). Perinatal exposure to bisphenol a alters early adipogenesis in the rat. *Environmental Health Perspectives, 117*(10), 1549–1555.

Somm, E., Schwitzgebel, V. M., Vauthay, D. M., Camm, E. J., Chen, C. Y., Giacobino, J. P., et al. (2008). Prenatal nicotine exposure alters early pancreatic islet and adipose tissue development with consequences on the control of body weight and glucose metabolism later in life. *Endocrinology, 149*(12), 6289–6299.

Spalding, K. L., Arner, E., Westermark, P. O., Bernard, S., Buchholz, B. A., Bergmann, O., et al. (2008). Dynamics of fat cell turnover in humans. *Nature, 453*(7196), 783–787.

Spencer, S. J. (2012). Early life programming of obesity: The impact of the perinatal environment on the development of obesity and metabolic dysfunction in the offspring. *Current Diabetes Reviews, 8*(1), 55–68.

Spruth, M., Reidlinger, J., & Müller, V. (1995). Sodium ion dependence of inhibition of the Na+-translocating F1F0-ATPase from Acetobacterium woodii. Probing the site(s) involved in ion transport. *Biochimica et Biophysica Acta, 1229*, 96–102.

Stange, D., Sieratowicz, A., & Oehlmann, J. (2012). Imposex development in Nucella lapillus—Evidence for the involvement of retinoid X receptor and androgen signalling pathways in vivo. *Aquatic Toxicology, 106–107*, 20–24.

Steger, D. J., Grant, G. R., Schupp, M., Tomaru, T., Lefterova, M. I., Schug, J., et al. (2010). Propagation of adipogenic signals through an epigenomic transition state. *Genes & Development, 24*(10), 1035–1044.

Stevens, A., Begum, G., Cook, A., Connor, K., Rumball, C., Oliver, M., et al. (2010). Epigenetic changes in the hypothalamic proopiomelanocortin and glucocorticoid receptor genes in the ovine fetus after periconceptional undernutrition. *Endocrinology, 151*(8), 3652–3664.

Stoger, R. (2008). The thrifty epigenotype: An acquired and heritable predisposition for obesity and diabetes? *Bioessays, 30*(2), 156–166.

Strand, J., & Jacobsen, J. A. (2005). Accumulation and trophic transfer of organotins in a marine food web from the Danish coastal waters. *The Science of the Total Environment, 350*(1–3), 72–85.

Strand, J., Larsen, M. M., & Lockyer, C. (2005). Accumulation of organotin compounds and mercury in harbour porpoises (Phocoena phocoena) from the Danish waters and West Greenland. *The Science of the Total Environment, 350*(1–3), 59–71.

Stridh, H., Gigliotti, D., Orrenius, S., & Cotgreave, I. (1999). The role of calcium in pre- and postmitochondrial events in tributyltin-induced T-cell apoptosis. *Biochemical and Biophysical Research Communications, 266*(2), 460–465.

Strissel, K. J., Stancheva, Z., Miyoshi, H., Perfield, J. W., 2nd., DeFuria, J., Jick, Z., et al. (2007). Adipocyte death, adipose tissue remodeling, and obesity complications. *Diabetes, 56*(12), 2910–2918.

Tahir, M. K., Guthenberg, C., & Mannervik, B. (1985). Inhibitors for distinction of three types of human glutathione transferase. *FEBS Letters, 181*(2), 249–252.

Takahashi, S., Mukai, H., Tanabe, S., Sakayama, K., Miyazaki, T., & Masuno, H. (1999). Butyltin residues in livers of humans and wild terrestrial mammals and in plastic products. *Environmental Pollution, 106*(2), 213–218.

Tang, W., Zeve, D., Seo, J., Jo, A. Y., & Graff, J. M. (2011). Thiazolidinediones regulate adipose lineage dynamics. *Cell Metabolism, 14*(1), 116–122.

Tang, W., Zeve, D., Suh, J. M., Bosnakovski, D., Kyba, M., Hammer, R. E., et al. (2008). White fat progenitor cells reside in the adipose vasculature. *Science, 322*(5901), 583–586.

Tateishi, K., Okada, Y., Kallin, E. M., & Zhang, Y. (2009). Role of Jhdm2a in regulating metabolic gene expression and obesity resistance. *Nature, 458*(7239), 757–761.

Tchoukalova, Y. D., Votruba, S. B., Tchkonia, T., Giorgadze, N., Kirkland, J. L., & Jensen, M. D. (2010). Regional differences in cellular mechanisms of adipose tissue gain with overfeeding. *Proceedings of the National Academy of Sciences of the United States of America, 107*(42), 18226–18231.

Thayer, K. A., Heindel, J. J., Bucher, J. R., & Gallo, M. A. (2012). Role of environmental chemicals in diabetes and obesity: A National Toxicology Program workshop review. *Environmental Health Perspectives, 120*(6), 779–789.

Tingaud-Sequeira, A., Ouadah, N., & Babin, P. J. (2011). Zebrafish obesogenic test: A tool for screening molecules that target adiposity. *Journal of Lipid Research, 52*(9), 1765–1772.

Tipping, E., Ketterer, B., Christodoulides, L., Elliott, B. M., Aldridge, W. N., & Bridges, J. W. (1979). The interactions of triethyltin with rat glutathione-S-transferases A, B and C. Enzyme-inhibition and equilibrium-dialysis studies. *Chemico-Biological Interaction, 24*(3), 317–327.

Toggas, S. M., Krady, J. K., & Billingsley, M. L. (1992). Molecular neurotoxicology of trimethyltin: Identification of stannin, a novel protein expressed in trimethyltin-sensitive cells. *Molecular Pharmacology, 42*(1), 44–56.

Tontonoz, P., & Spiegelman, B. M. (2008). Fat and beyond: The diverse biology of PPARgamma. *Annual Review of Biochemistry*, 77, 289–312.

Toschke, A. M., Koletzko, B., Slikker, W., Jr., Hermann, M., & von Kries, R. (2002). Childhood obesity is associated with maternal smoking in pregnancy. *European Journal of Pediatrics, 161*(8), 445–448.

Tran, T. T., Yamamoto, Y., Gesta, S., & Kahn, C. R. (2008). Beneficial effects of subcutaneous fat transplantation on metabolism. *Cell Metabolism*, 7(5), 410–420.

Tsuda, T., Inoue, T., Kojima, M., & Aoki, S. (1995). Daily intakes of tributyltin and triphenyltin compounds from meals. *Journal of AOAC International, 78*(4), 941–943.

Tzameli, I., Fang, H., Ollero, M., Shi, H., Hamm, J. K., Kievit, P., et al. (2004). Regulated production of a peroxisome proliferator-activated receptor-gamma ligand during an early phase of adipocyte differentiation in 3T3-L1 adipocytes. *The Journal of Biological Chemistry, 279*(34), 36093–36102.

US FDA. (2013). *Code of federal regulations (21CFR178.2650): Organotin stabilizers in vinyl chloride plastics.* Silver Spring, MD: US Food and Drug Administration.

Vandenberg, L. N., Colborn, T., Hayes, T. B., Heindel, J. J., Jacobs, D. R., Jr., Lee, D. H., et al. (2012). Hormones and endocrine-disrupting chemicals: Low-dose effects and nonmonotonic dose responses. *Endocrine Reviews, 33*(3), 378–455.

Vestri, H. S., Maianu, L., Moellering, D. R., & Garvey, W. T. (2007). Atypical antipsychotic drugs directly impair insulin action in adipocytes: Effects on glucose transport, lipogenesis, and antilipolysis. *Neuropsychopharmacology, 32*(4), 765–772.

Volakakis, N., Joodmardi, E., & Perlmann, T. (2009). NR4A orphan nuclear receptors influence retinoic acid and docosahexaenoic acid signaling via up-regulation of fatty acid binding protein 5. *Biochemical and Biophysical Research Communications, 390*(4), 1186–1191.

von Ballmoos, C., Brunner, J., & Dimroth, P. (2004). The ion channel of F-ATP synthase is the target of toxic organotin compounds. *Proceedings of the National Academy of Sciences of the United States of America, 101*(31), 11239–11244.

Wakabayashi, K., Okamura, M., Tsutsumi, S., Nishikawa, N. S., Tanaka, T., Sakakibara, I., et al. (2009). The peroxisome proliferator-activated receptor gamma/retinoid X receptor alpha heterodimer targets the histone modification enzyme PR-Set7/Setd8 gene and regulates adipogenesis through a positive feedback loop. *Molecular and Cellular Biology, 29*(13), 3544–3555.

Waku, T., Shiraki, T., Oyama, T., Fujimoto, Y., Maebara, K., Kamiya, N., et al. (2009). Structural insight into PPARgamma activation through covalent modification with endogenous fatty acids. *Journal of Molecular Biology*, *385*(1), 188–199.

Waku, T., Shiraki, T., Oyama, T., & Morikawa, K. (2009). Atomic structure of mutant PPARgamma LBD complexed with 15d-PGJ2: Novel modulation mechanism of PPARgamma/RXRalpha function by covalently bound ligands. *FEBS Letters*, *583*(2), 320–324.

Wang, Z., Benoit, G., Liu, J., Prasad, S., Aarnisalo, P., Liu, X., et al. (2003). Structure and function of Nurr1 identifies a class of ligand-independent nuclear receptors. *Nature*, *423*(6939), 555–560.

Wang, Y., Wang, C., Zhang, J., Chen, Y., & Zuo, Z. (2009). DNA hypomethylation induced by tributyltin, triphenyltin, and a mixture of these in Sebastiscus marmoratus liver. *Aquatic Toxicology*, *95*(2), 93–98.

Welberg, L. A., Seckl, J. R., & Holmes, M. C. (2000). Inhibition of 11beta-hydroxysteroid dehydrogenase, the foeto-placental barrier to maternal glucocorticoids, permanently programs amygdala GR mRNA expression and anxiety-like behaviour in the offspring. *The European Journal of Neuroscience*, *12*(3), 1047–1054.

Whalen, M. M., & Loganathan, B. G. (2001). Butyltin exposure causes a rapid decrease in cyclic AMP levels in human lymphocytes. *Toxicology and Applied Pharmacology*, *171*(3), 141–148.

Xu, H., Barnes, G. T., Yang, Q., Tan, G., Yang, D., Chou, C. J., et al. (2003). Chronic inflammation in fat plays a crucial role in the development of obesity-related insulin resistance. *The Journal of Clinical Investigation*, *112*(12), 1821–1830.

Yang, L. H., Chen, T. M., Yu, S. T., & Chen, Y. H. (2007). Olanzapine induces SREBP-1-related adipogenesis in 3T3-L1 cells. *Pharmacological Research*, *56*(3), 202–208.

Yanik, S. C., Baker, A. H., Mann, K. K., & Schlezinger, J. J. (2011). Organotins are potent activators of PPARgamma and adipocyte differentiation in bone marrow multipotent mesenchymal stromal cells. *Toxicological Sciences*, *122*(2), 476–488.

Yoneyama, M., Nishiyama, N., Shuto, M., Sugiyama, C., Kawada, K., Seko, K., et al. (2008). In vivo depletion of endogenous glutathione facilitates trimethyltin-induced neuronal damage in the dentate gyrus of mice by enhancing oxidative stress. *Neurochemistry International*, *52*(4–5), 761–769.

Zhang, J., Zuo, Z., He, C., Cai, J., Wang, Y., Chen, Y., et al. (2009). Effect of tributyltin on testicular development in Sebastiscus marmoratus and the mechanism involved. *Environmental Toxicology and Chemistry*, *28*(7), 1528–1535.

Zhang, J., Zuo, Z., Xiong, J., Sun, P., Chen, Y., & Wang, C. (2013). Tributyltin exposure causes lipotoxicity responses in the ovaries of rockfish, Sebastiscus marmoratus. *Chemosphere*, *90*(3), 1294–1299.

Zhao, Y., & Bruemmer, D. (2010). NR4A orphan nuclear receptors: Transcriptional regulators of gene expression in metabolism and vascular biology. *Arteriosclerosis, Thrombosis, and Vascular Biology*, *30*(8), 1535–1541.

Zuo, Z., Chen, S., Wu, T., Zhang, J., Su, Y., Chen, Y., et al. (2011). Tributyltin causes obesity and hepatic steatosis in male mice. *Environmental Toxicology*, *26*(1), 79–85.

Zylka, R., Kleszczynska, H., Kupiec, J., Bonarska-Kujawa, D., Hladyszowski, J., & Przestalski, S. (2009). Modifications of erythrocyte membrane hydration induced by organic tin compounds. *Cell Biology International*, *33*(7), 801–806.

CHAPTER TWELVE

Human Testicular Insulin-Like Factor 3 and Endocrine Disrupters

Katrine Bay[*,1], **Ravinder Anand-Ivell**[†]
[*]University Department of Growth and Reproduction, Rigshospitalet, Copenhagen, Denmark
[†]Division of Animal Science, School of Biosciences, University of Nottingham, UK
[1]Corresponding author: e-mail address: katrine.bay@regionh.dk

Contents

1. Introduction 328
2. INSL3: Expression and Regulation 328
   2.1 Expression of INSL3 and its receptor RXFP2 328
   2.2 INSL3 production in fetal, neonatal, and adult Leydig cells 329
   2.3 INSL3 regulation in adult Leydig cells 330
3. Functions of INSL3 331
   3.1 Testicular descent and hormonal control 331
   3.2 Species differences in timing of testicular descent 332
   3.3 Evidence from human studies 334
   3.4 Testicular functions of INSL3 334
   3.5 INSL3 and bone formation 336
4. INSL3 and Endocrine Disrupters 336
   4.1 Cryptorchidism in humans 336
   4.2 INSL3 and antiandrogenic effects 336
   4.3 INSL3 and estrogenic compounds 339
5. Conclusions and Future Directions 341
References 341

Abstract

The hormone insulin-like factor 3 (INSL3) is produced by testicular Leydig cells. Production of INSL3 is dependent on the state of Leydig cell differentiation and is stimulated by the long-term trophic effects of luteinizing hormone. INSL3 is, along with the other major Leydig cell hormone testosterone, essential for testicular descent, which in humans should be completed before birth. The incidence of cryptorchidism (incomplete descent of the testis) may have increased in some developed countries during recent decades. Experimental studies have shown that maternal exposure to endocrine-disrupting chemicals (EDCs), such as phthalates, can result in cryptorchidism among male offspring and that INSL3 production, like steroidogenesis, is susceptible to phthalate exposure. Inhibition of these hormones may occur via a general phthalate-induced impairment of Leydig cell development and maturation. Recent studies have also addressed the sensitivity of human Leydig cells to EDCs, though with varied conclusions.

Vitamins and Hormones, Volume 94
ISSN 0083-6729
http://dx.doi.org/10.1016/B978-0-12-800095-3.00012-2

1. INTRODUCTION

Insulin-like factor 3 (INSL3) plays a crucial role in the process of testicular descent specifically in the first phase of abdominal testis translocation (Nef & Parada, 1999; Zimmermann et al., 1999). Like testosterone, INSL3 is produced by testicular Leydig cells, both in pre- and in postnatal life (Ivell et al., 1997). Whereas the production of INSL3 *in utero* is coupled to its role in testis descent, the function of the substantial amounts produced and secreted by adult Leydig cells is less characterized. Suggestions have, however, been put forward for a role of INSL3 in germ cell survival (Kawamura et al., 2004) and in bone metabolism (Ferlin, Pepe, et al., 2008).

Cryptorchidism (incomplete descent of the testis) is a common urogenital malformation in newborn boys, with reported prevalences between 2% and 9%, depending on the geographic area investigated and whether the mildest form of cryptorchidism is included or not (Bay, Main, Toppari, & Skakkebaek, 2011). In some countries, an increasing incidence of cryptorchidism has been observed over the last decades (Acerini, Miles, Dunger, Ong, & Hughes, 2009; Boisen et al., 2004). The reason for this is unknown, though indirect evidence suggests some kind of environmental interference. One category of environmental influence under suspicion is exposure of the pregnant mother, and thus of the unborn child, to endocrine-disrupting chemicals (EDCs). Experimental studies have shown that this can provoke cryptorchidism and other abnormalities of the male reproductive organs (Virtanen & Adamsson, 2012). Whereas the impact of EDCs on fetal testosterone production, which is also fundamental for testicular descent, has been studied for a number of years, the hypothesis that INSL3 may also be susceptible to some of these chemicals is relatively new. This chapter describes our current knowledge of INSL3, including its potential vulnerability to EDC exposure.

2. INSL3: EXPRESSION AND REGULATION

2.1. Expression of INSL3 and its receptor RXFP2

As appears from the name, INSL3 is structurally related to insulin and belongs to the insulin superfamily of peptide hormones. Within this superfamily, INSL3 belongs to the relaxin subfamily, comprising five other peptides in addition to INSL3 and relaxin. In an evolutionary context, both relaxin and INSL3 have evolved relatively recently and can therefore be referred to as neohormones (Ivell & Bathgate, 2006; Park et al., 2008).

INSL3 is produced, along with testosterone, by the testicular Leydig cells in a wide range of species, including humans (Adham, Burkhardt, Benahmed, & Engel, 1993; Burkhardt et al., 1994; Ivell et al., 1997; Spiess et al., 1999; Zimmermann, Schottler, Engel, & Adham, 1997). In humans, the Leydig cell populations follow a triphasic expression pattern, with a fetal, a perinatal, and an adult cell population (Codesal, Regadera, Nistal, Regadera-Sejas, & Paniagua, 1990; Prince, 2001). Both testosterone and INSL3 are produced in all three population types.

The receptor for INSL3, relaxin-family peptide receptor 2 (RXFP2), is a 7-transmembrane G-protein-coupled receptor, which is expressed in a number of human tissues. Within the urogenital system, the receptor can be found on the Leydig cells themselves, on meiotic and postmeiotic germ cells, in the epididymis, vas deferens, seminal vesicles, and the gubernaculum. Beyond the urogenital system, RXFP2 expression has been localized to the brain, kidney, thyroid, peripheral blood cells, bone marrow, osteoblasts, and muscle (Anand-Ivell, Relan, et al., 2006; Ferlin, Pepe, et al., 2008; Filonzi et al., 2007). Though less studied in women, there is low expression of INSL3 in the follicular theca cells of the ovary and possibly in the corpus luteum. The receptor, RXFP2, has been identified also in different parts of the female reproductive system (Hsu et al., 2002; Li et al., 2011). While a clear-cut function for INSL3 has only been characterized in a few of these male and female tissues, the widespread expression of the receptor implies a range of autocrine, paracrine, and endocrine functions of the hormone.

2.2. INSL3 production in fetal, neonatal, and adult Leydig cells

INSL3 produced by the fetal Leydig cells is responsible for one of the primary functions of the hormone, namely, mediation of transabdominal testis translocation (see later). In humans, *INSL3* mRNA is expressed at least from gestational week (gw) 12 (O'Shaughnessy et al., 2007). Most likely, however, the human fetal testis expresses the hormone even earlier, since transabdominal testis translocation begins already around gw 8–10, and in rodents, *Insl3* expression coincides with or even precedes this process (McKinnell et al., 2005; Zimmermann et al., 1997). For comparison, testosterone production begins around gw 6–7 in male human fetuses (Tapanainen, Kellokumpu-Lehtinen, Pelliniemi, & Huhtaniemi, 1981).

Studies assessing INSL3 peptide in human amniotic fluid indicate expression already in gw 12 (earlier samples were not available), with highest levels being detected around gw 14–18. Hereafter, INSL3 levels decreased and became undetectable after gw 22 (Anand-Ivell, Ivell, Driscoll, & Manson, 2008; Bay et al., 2008). A decline in INSL3 levels at this time point coincides with the observed decline in the numbers of differentiated fetal Leydig cells (Codesal et al., 1990). However, clearly detectable levels have also been measured in cord blood samples from male boys born at term (Bay et al., 2007), suggesting that INSL3 continues to be produced by the fetus in late pregnancy. The failure to detect INSL3 in third trimester amniotic fluid could perhaps be due in part to dilution in the increasing volume of amniotic fluid at that time, to the limits of our assay systems, or to the decreasing permeability of the fetal cardiovascular system, which increasingly restricts the loss of fetal peptides and proteins.

After birth, INSL3 can be measured in male serum during the transient activation of the hypothalamus–pituitary–gonadal axis, also called the minipuberty, which occurs around 3 months after birth. After this transient production, INSL3 appears to be below the limits of detection during childhood (Bay et al., 2007) and then starts to increase at puberty, coinciding with adult-type Leydig cell differentiation (Ferlin et al., 2006; Wikstrom, Bay, Hero, Andersson, & Dunkel, 2006). A young adult man on average has about 1 ng/ml of this hormone in his peripheral circulation (Bay et al., 2005; Foresta et al., 2004). Serum levels then decline gradually with aging (Anand-Ivell, Wohlgemuth, et al., 2006), losing about 10% per decade between the years of 40 and 80. For an overview, please see the review by Bay and Andersson (2011).

2.3. INSL3 regulation in adult Leydig cells

In adult-type Leydig cells, INSL3 appears to be an excellent marker of cell number and/or differentiation status, in that production of the hormone depends on the maturation of the Leydig cells, which again is mediated via the long-term trophic effects of luteinizing hormone (LH) (Balvers et al., 1998; Bay et al., 2005; Ivell et al., 1997; Zimmermann et al., 1997). In line with this, INSL3 concentrations in puberty coincide with circulating LH and steroid levels (Ferlin et al., 2006; Wikstrom et al., 2006). Further, we have shown that male patients with hypogonadotropic hypogonadism on testosterone replacement therapy have very low INSL3 serum levels, whereas those receiving long-term stimulatory therapy in the form of human chorionic gonadotropin (hCG) have much higher INSL3 levels (Bay et al., 2005). Histologically, human biopsies of Leydig cell neoplasia or hyperplasia, where cells appears to be less differentiated, stain only weakly for INSL3, whereas normally differentiated adult Leydig cells have a strong INSL3 expression (Klonisch et al., 1999).

As such, the INSL3 expression pattern is very similar to that of the other main Leydig cell hormone, testosterone. However, unlike testosterone, INSL3 is not sensitive to the acute stimulatory action of LH. In adult men with fully differentiated Leydig cells, additional LH/hCG can acutely cause synthesis and secretion of testosterone, whereas INSL3 serum levels remain stable (Bay, Matthiesson, McLachlan, & Andersson, 2006). Also, some *in vitro* studies have concluded that factors like hCG/LH, testosterone, and estradiol are not capable of affecting *Insl3* transcription in the short term (Balvers et al., 1998; McKinnell et al., 2005; Sadeghian, Anand-Ivell, Balvers, Relan, & Ivell, 2005). However, other studies report that testosterone and estradiol can cause a mild modulation of *Insl3* transcription by androgen receptor (AR) or estrogen receptor α-dependent mechanisms (Lague & Tremblay, 2008, 2009; Zhou et al., 2011). It may be noted here though, that in the latter studies, the Leydig cells used were either immature or not fully differentiated adult types. Thus, human INSL3 serum levels appear to reflect a constitutive expression of the hormone in fully differentiated adult Leydig cells.

3. FUNCTIONS OF INSL3

3.1. Testicular descent and hormonal control

The fetal testis is initially located in a perirenal position and attached to the inguinal canal via the cylindrical gubernacular ligament. The first phase of testis descent (the transabdominal phase) ensures the repositioning of the testis to a position near the internal inguinal ring and is mediated via an extensive remodeling of the gubernaculum (Barteczko & Jacob, 2000). Studies conducted on transgenic *Insl3*$^{-/-}$ mice revealed that, at least in rodents, Insl3 is essential for this first phase of testicular descent (Nef & Parada, 1999; Zimmermann et al., 1999). Such Insl3 knockout mice are born with testes located in a perirenal position, due to the lack of any gubernacular development. Also, mice with a mutated *Rxfp2* had a similar phenotype (Kumagai et al., 2002; Overbeek et al., 2001). Conversely, transgenic female mice falsely expressing Insl3 during pregnancy showed descent of the ovaries (Adham et al., 2002; Koskimies et al., 2003). Apparently, testosterone is not needed for abdominal translocation, as evidenced by clinical data on male patients with complete or partial androgen insensitivity syndrome (AIS) who often have testes positioned around the inner inguinal ring (Ahmed et al., 2000; Hannema et al., 2006; Quigley et al., 1995). Also, rodent data suggest that this process occurs independently of androgens (Adham et al., 2002; Kaftanovskaya et al., 2012).

The subsequent transinguinal and inguinoscrotal phases (traditionally regarded as a single inguinoscrotal phase) ensure the passage of the testis through the inguinal canal and further down to its final position at the bottom of the scrotum. For these phases, a prior dilation of the inguinal ring is required in addition to eversion of the gubernacular ligament, which gives rise to the processus vaginalis, and formation of the cremasteric sac (Barteczko & Jacob, 2000). Testosterone is essential for these processes, as again suggested by the position of the testes in patients with complete or partial AIS (Ahmed et al., 2000; Hannema et al., 2006; Quigley et al., 1995). Moreover, a recent study investigating the phenotype of mice with an ablated AR in the gubernacular ligament shows that androgens acting on this structure are essential to formation of the processus vaginalis (Kaftanovskaya et al., 2012). Experimental data suggest that INSL3, along with testosterone, is also important for these processes, suggesting that the two Leydig cell hormones interact closely to ensure these last phases of testis descent (Adham et al., 2002; Kaftanovskaya et al., 2011; Tomiyama, Hutson, Truong, & Agoulnik, 2003) (Fig. 12.1). At least in mice, it appears that the Insl3 receptor, Rxfp2, is expressed in an androgen-dependent fashion (Yuan et al., 2010), which may explain the evident synergy between these two factors.

3.2. Species differences in timing of testicular descent

The timing of testicular descent varies considerably between species (Fig. 12.2). In humans, the complete process of relocation including transit into the scrotum should be completed before birth. The first transabdominal phase is initiated very early, at around gw 8–10 (Amann & Veeramachaneni, 2007; Hughes & Acerini, 2008; Hutson & Hasthorpe, 2005), and is completed already at week 15, according to some (Hutson & Hasthorpe, 2005; Hutson, Williams, Fallat, & Attah, 1990), or later, according to others (Costa, Sampaio, Favorito, & Cardoso, 2002; Klonisch, Fowler, & Hombach-Klonisch, 2004). A time interval then separates the first transabdominal phase from the following transinguinal and inguinoscrotal phases, which in humans occur in late pregnancy (Barteczko & Jacob, 2000;

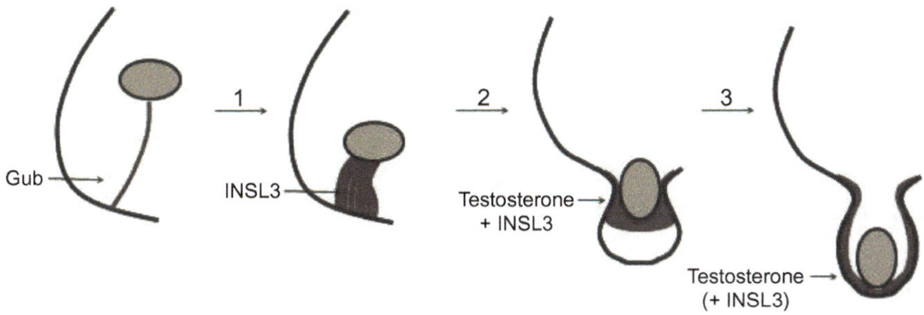

Figure 12.1 Hormonal regulation of testicular descent. INSL3 is essential for the initial abdominal testis translocation (1) via outgrowth of gubernaculum (gub). Important steps in the transinguinal passage (2) involve both INSL3 and testosterone. The final, inguinoscrotal testis descent (3) is mediated primarily by androgens, though INSL3 may also be involved. *Modified from Bay and Andersson (2011).* (See color plate.)

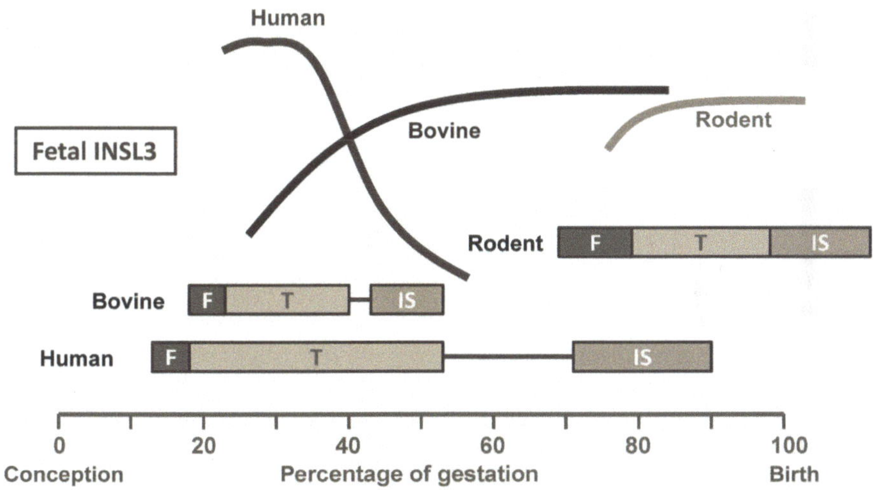

Figure 12.2 Scheme to indicate the relative timing of testis formation (F), the trans-abdominal (TA), and inguinoscrotal (IS) phases of testicular descent in humans, cows, and rodents (Amann & Veeramachaneni, 2007; Hughes & Acerini, 2008). Full-term gestation is indicated as 100%. Above this scheme are indicated the approximate levels of fetal INSL3 in male embryos based on amniotic fluid samples (Anand-Ivell et al., 2008; Bay et al., 2008) or fetal and/or maternal blood concentrations (R. Anand-Ivell and R. Ivell, unpublished data). (See color plate.)

Rotondi et al., 2001; Sampaio & Favorito, 1998). In rodents, in contrast, the entire process is more continuous and begins only in the second half of gestation, with the inguinoscrotal phase taking place after birth (Hughes & Acerini, 2008). In ruminants, the process is initiated early, as in humans, but is also completed rather early, usually by midgestation (Amann & Veeramachaneni, 2007). An overview is illustrated in Fig. 12.2, which also shows when during gestation INSL3 is expressed by the male fetus for the various species. These species differences are important to take into account, when investigating the effects of prenatal exposure to EDCs on the process of testicular descent and for the selection of appropriate animal models.

3.3. Evidence from human studies

The involvement of INSL3 in testicular descent, as described earlier, relies almost completely on experimental data. An involvement of INSL3 in testicular descent in humans is still not conclusively proven, though it is assumed to play a role similar to what has been shown in other mammals. Numerous human studies focusing on mutations or SNP analyses in *INSL3* and *RXFP2* have been conducted (Bogatcheva et al., 2007; Feng et al., 2004; Ferlin et al., 2009; Koskimies et al., 2000; Lim, Rajpert-De Meyts, Skakkebæk, Hawkins, & Hughes, 2001; Roh et al., 2003). Though data vary with geographic region, it seems that mutations in INSL3 are rarely (1.8%) associated with the cryptorchid phenotype, whereas the cumulative frequency of RXFP2 mutations in cryptorchid cases is higher (2.8%) but still modest (Ferlin, Zuccarello, et al., 2008). Of the mutations observed in the RXFP2 gene, *T222P* is the most frequent one and has been associated with cryptorchidism in Italian men (Ferlin et al., 2003; Gorlov et al., 2002). This one is also of particular interest, since *in vitro* data show that this mutation hinders the expression of RXFP2 on the cell surface (Bogatcheva et al., 2007). Overall, the described phenotypes of cryptorchid men with a mutation in the INSL3 and RXFP2 genes vary considerably, including both mild cases of unilateral cryptorchidism where the testis descends spontaneously in early infancy and severe cases of consistent bilateral cryptorchidism (Ferlin et al., 2003; Foresta, Zuccarello, Garolla, & Ferlin, 2008). The variation may very well be due to the fact that all mutations reported in humans are heterozygous, making the situation different from that seen in homozygous knockout mice.

3.4. Testicular functions of INSL3

Elucidation of potential autocrine and paracrine functions of INSL3 within the testis has been complicated by the cryptorchid phenotype of the *Insl3*$^{-/-}$

mouse model, since cryptorchidism per se, and consequent exposure of testes to abdominal temperature, exerts a crucial impact on the overall function of the testes and thereby disguises possible roles for intratesticular INSL3. One study has, however, reported that treatment of isolated rat seminiferous tubules with Insl3 protects the meiotic germ cells from undergoing apoptosis (Kawamura et al., 2004). This is in accordance with RXFP2 being expressed on pre- and postmeiotic germ cells (Anand-Ivell, Relan, et al., 2006; Feng et al., 2007) and the observation that INSL3 is able to cross the blood–testis barrier and enter the seminiferous compartment (Anand-Ivell, Heng, Hafen, Setchell, & Ivell, 2009). In addition, the 20% testis weight reduction observed in mice treated with an Insl3-antagonist was suggested to be caused by an inhibition of Insl3-induced germ cell survival (Del Borgo et al., 2006). On the other hand, orchiopexy performed in mice lacking Insl3 or Rxfp2 can at least partially restore male fertility, pointing to a functional, but not essential, role for INSL3 in spermatogenesis (Nguyen et al., 2002; Overbeek et al., 2001; Zimmermann et al., 1999). Recently, a conditional knockout mouse model in which *Rxfp2* gene ablation was specifically restricted only to the male germ cells, and which consequently did not exhibit cryptorchidism, failed to indicate gross aberration of spermatogenesis, at least in sexually mature adult male mice (Huang, Rivas, & Agoulnik, 2012).

In agreement with expression of Rxfp2 on Leydig cells, it has also recently been reported that Insl3 can stimulate testosterone secretion from mouse Leydig cells via a cAMP-dependent mechanism, thus suggesting a possible autocrine role for the hormone (Pathirana et al., 2012). This study made use of highly diluted cell cultures, such that endogenously produced Insl3 could be ignored. This could explain why earlier studies, using cell cultures at high density, were unable to detect such stimulation (Anand-Ivell, Relan, et al., 2006) and why adult *Insl3* knockout mice appear with normal serum testosterone levels (Nef & Parada, 1999). The dynamics of puberty in these animals have not been looked at.

Also in females, where small amounts of INSL3 are produced by adult ovarian theca cells, INSL3 has been reported to initiate meiotic progression of the arrested oocytes (Kawamura et al., 2004). This is in accordance with a prolonged estrous cycle and impaired fertility in female mice lacking Insl3 (Nef & Parada, 1999). Because of the low serum INSL3 levels observed in adult women (Foresta et al., 2004; own unpublished data), it seems likely that in females, INSL3 action is paracrine only.

3.5. INSL3 and bone formation

The high serum levels of INSL3 in adult men suggest that the hormone may also serve some kind of endocrine role, such as in bone metabolism. One study has linked *RXFP2* gene mutations with osteoporosis and osteopenia in mice and men (Ferlin, Pepe, et al., 2008). A follow-up study has characterized further the involved signaling pathways and coupled the mechanisms to effects of INSL3 on both osteoblast maturation and osteoclast differentiation (Ferlin, Perilli, Gianesello, Taglialavoro, & Foresta, 2011).

4. INSL3 AND ENDOCRINE DISRUPTERS

4.1. Cryptorchidism in humans

The vast majority of cryptorchidism cases cannot be explained by genetic factors. This, of course, stimulates the search for alternative explanations. Substantial evidence suggests that the intrauterine milieu is important for the development of cryptorchidism. For example, growth restriction and being born small for gestational age are important risk factors for cryptorchidism (Akre, Lipworth, Cnattingius, Sparen, & Ekbom, 1999; Berkowitz et al., 1993; Biggs, Baer, & Critchlow, 2002; Boisen et al., 2004; Ghirri et al., 2002; Jensen et al., 2012). Maternal smoking is a known risk factor for intrauterine growth restriction, and accordingly, a number of studies have shown that maternal smoking is also a risk factor for cryptorchidism (Akre et al., 1999; Biggs et al., 2002; Jensen, Toft, Thulstrup, Bonde, & Olsen, 2007; McBride, Van den Steen, Lamb, & Gallagher, 1991). Maternal exposure to EDCs is also suspected to contribute to the relatively high incidence of cryptorchidism observed in some developed countries. A large number of epidemiological studies have therefore also looked at possible associations between maternal exposure to various EDCs and the presence of cryptorchidism in their newborn sons. Some find positive associations suggestive of a role for such exposure (Brucker-Davis et al., 2008; Damgaard et al., 2006; Weidner, Moller, Jensen, & Skakkebaek, 1998), whereas others find no associations (McGlynn et al., 2009; Zhu, Hjollund, Andersen, & Olsen, 2006). For details, see the recent review by Virtanen and Adamsson (2012).

4.2. INSL3 and antiandrogenic effects

Animal experiments unequivocally show that some EDCs can induce cryptorchidism in rats and mice. Primarily, chemicals with antiandrogenic potential have been investigated. Classical antiandrogens (some of which are true AR antagonists) like the pesticides vinclozolin, procymidone, linuron, and prochloraz are indeed capable of inducing cryptorchidism but apparently do this primarily by interfering with the action of testosterone, whereas they appear to have no effect on Insl3 expression (Laier et al., 2006; Wilson, Blystone, Hotchkiss, Rider, & Gray, 2008; Wilson et al., 2004). Furthermore, the mild analgesic paracetamol appears to inhibit testosterone production specifically, leaving Insl3 levels unaffected (Kristensen et al., 2012). However, for one group of chemicals, namely, the phthalates, the mode of action seems to be somewhat different and to involve also INSL3. Even though phthalates are well known for their antiandrogenic properties, a comparison of the effects in rats of prenatal exposure to the phthalate di(*n*-butyl)phthalate (DBP) and the well-characterized AR antagonist flutamide revealed significant differences. Especially, whereas the inguinoscrotal part of testicular descent was blocked by flutamide, exposure to DBP affected primarily the androgen-independent, but INSL3-dependent, earlier process of transabdominal testis descent (Mylchreest, Sar, Cattley, & Foster, 1999). This is in accordance with studies showing that phthalates, like di-*n*-ethylhexyl phthalate (DEHP), DBP, and benzyl butyl phthalate, can indeed inhibit Insl3 production and thereby impair the outgrowth of the gubernaculum required for transabdominal descent (Borch, Metzdorff, Vinggaard, Brokken, & Dalgaard, 2006; Howdeshell et al., 2007; McKinnell et al., 2005; Shono, Shima, Kondo, & Suita, 2005; Wilson et al., 2004). Phthalates act as antiandrogens by inhibiting steroidogenesis, for example, by targeting the enzyme CYP17, which converts 17 alpha-hydroxyprogesterone to androstenedione, and StAR, which mediates the transfer of cholesterol into the mitochondria (Chauvigne et al., 2011; Hannas et al., 2011). However, they are not true AR antagonists. The mechanism by which they inhibit Insl3 production is not clearly understood. A proposed mode of action is via a general inhibition of the fetal Leydig cell maturation, which secondarily causes reduced Insl3 and testosterone levels (Mahood et al., 2005; Wilson et al., 2004). This model may also be true for adult-type Leydig cells, since new data indicate a changed Leydig cell maturation trajectory in adult rats acutely exposed to phthalates, where Leydig cells regenerating following ablation being the specific alkylating agent ethane-dimethanesulfonate (EDS) (Heng, Anand-Ivell, Teerds, & Ivell, 2012). Another study shows comparable effects of maternal phthalate exposure on natural Leydig cell differentiation during puberty, again in rats (Ivell, Heng, Nicholson, & Anand-Ivell, 2013) (Fig. 12.3). It is also possible

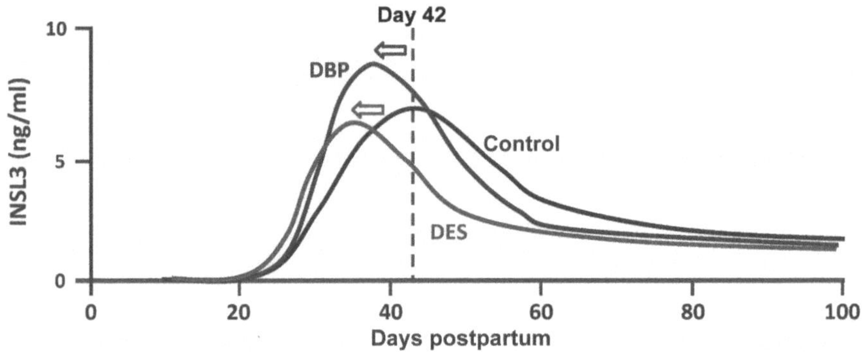

Figure 12.3 Effect on subsequent pubertal development of brief maternal exposure to dibutyl phthalate (DBP) or diethylstilbestrol (DES) in late pregnancy and the commencement of lactation in developing male rats. Early exposure of adult-type Leydig stem cells to these endocrine disruptors leads to a shift in the dynamics of later Leydig cell differentiation during puberty, as assessed by circulating INSL3 concentrations. Whereas in control rats there is a peak in INSL3 concentration on day 42, concomitant with the first appearance of sperm in the epididymis, DES and DBP advance this time, without, however, influencing later mature levels of INSL3 (Ivell et al., 2013). Very similar results were obtained also using the EDS model of adult-type Leydig cell regeneration (Heng et al., 2012). (See color plate.)

that such EDC molecules serve to inhibit key transcription factors, such as SF-1, which are important both for *Insl3* transcription and steroidogenesis (Borch et al., 2006).

Whereas all the previously mentioned details deal with rodent models, only few and recent studies have addressed directly the effect of phthalates on *human* testis development and function. However, the few studies that have looked at the human species suggest that effects of phthalates on INSL3, and partly also on testosterone, in human testis tissue may be quite attenuated, compared to those observed in rodents. For example, a single study has investigated the effect of phthalate exposure on organocultured *adult* human testis tissue. Here, testosterone production was clearly impaired by DEHP exposure. In contrast, INSL3 levels remained unaffected, suggesting that inhibition was specific for steroidogenesis (Desdoits-Lethimonier et al., 2012). For *fetal* tissues, DBP exposure of fetal human testis xenografts, grafted on castrated male nude mice, did not affect steroidogenesis. In contrast, corresponding experiments made with xenografts of rodent origin showed a phthalate-induced inhibition of testosterone production (Mitchell et al., 2012). Unfortunately, this study did not look at INSL3 production. INSL3 was, however, included in a similar experiment, comparing

DPB-exposed mice, rat, and human fetal testis. Here, INSL3 and testosterone were impaired in rodent fetal testis, whereas neither testosterone nor INSL3 was affected in the human fetal xenografts (Heger et al., 2012). According to these experimental studies, therefore, human fetal testis may not be as sensitive to phthalate exposure, as is the rodent fetal testis. Results from epidemiological studies, looking at associations between prenatal phthalate exposure and cryptorchidism in newborn sons, are somewhat inconclusive. A Danish cohort study found no association between phthalates in breast milk samples and congenital cryptorchidism, though hormone levels might have been affected (Main et al., 2006). A French study found borderline significantly higher levels of phthalates in colostrum from boys with cryptorchidism as compared to controls. Similar trends could, however, not be found for cord serum phthalate levels (Brucker-Davis et al., 2008). A newer Danish register study found no association between possible maternal occupational phthalate exposure and cryptorchidism in the sons (Morales-Suarez-Varela et al., 2011), whereas a recent French case–control study found a positive association between maternal self-reported occupational phthalate exposure and cryptorchidism in the sons (Wagner-Mahler et al., 2011).

4.3. INSL3 and estrogenic compounds

Not only antiandrogens but also the xenoestrogen diethylstilbestrol (DES) has been shown capable of inducing cryptorchidism in mice models (McLachlan, 1977). DES was widely used for decades to prevent abortions and pregnancy complications, until it was banned in the early 1970s. Later studies have found an increased incidence of cryptorchidism in sons of mothers using DES during pregnancy (Gill, Schumacher, Bibbo, Straus, & Schoenberg, 1979; Martin et al., 2008). After the recognition that INSL3 is essential for gubernacular development and early testicular descent, studies have investigated the effects of DES on INSL3 production. Indeed, fetal exposure to DES and to the natural estrogens 17α- and β-estradiol inhibits *Insl3* in rodent models (Emmen et al., 2000; Nef, Shipman, & Parada, 2000). Again, as for phthalates, the effect may occur via a general inhibition of Leydig cell maturation (Sharpe, Rivas, Walker, McKinnell, & Fisher, 2003), as also suggested by the changed Leydig cell maturation trajectory in EDS-treated adult rats acutely exposed to DES (Heng et al., 2012), and comparable effects on natural Leydig cell differentiation during puberty after *in utero* exposure to DES in rats (Ivell et al., 2013)

(Fig. 12.3). *In vitro* studies also suggest a more direct molecular effect of estradiol, via repression of *Insl3* expression and promoter activity (Lague & Tremblay, 2009). Again, however, the situation may be somewhat different in humans. A very recent study comparing the effect of DES exposure on human and rodent fetal organ culture systems suggests that in comparison to the rodent fetal testis, the corresponding human tissue may not be as sensitive to DES exposure (N'tumba-Byn et al., 2012). Interestingly, the same study also investigated the effect of another endocrine-disrupting compound, namely, bisphenol A (BPA), which has been defined as a weak xenoestrogen. Indeed, here, the conclusion was opposite in that the human fetal testis was much more sensitive to BPA exposure as compared to both mice and rat fetal testis tissue (Fig. 12.4). Thus, very low concentrations of BPA inhibited INSL3 and testosterone production in the human fetal testis, whereas higher doses were needed to provide similar results in the tested rodent species (N'tumba-Byn et al., 2012). The authors suggest that the effect of BPA may not be mediated via the estrogen receptor α (as the effects of DES are known to be), but rather via the membrane estrogen receptor GPR 30 or the estrogen-related receptor gamma. The latter has previously shown to have higher affinity for BPA than for DES (Takayanagi et al., 2006).

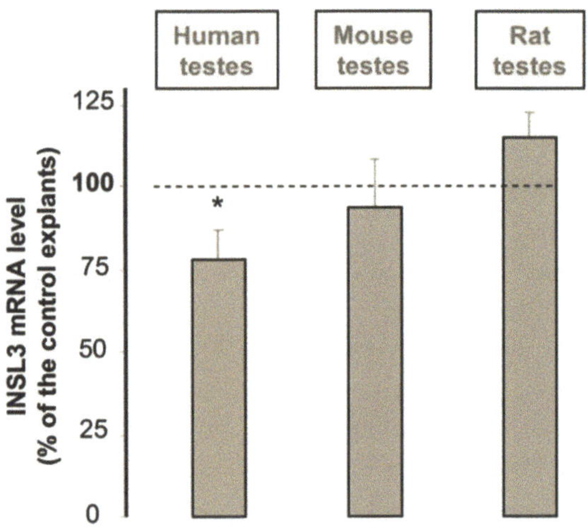

Figure 12.4 Effect of 10^{-8} M bisphenol A on *INSL3* mRNA levels in human, mouse, and rat fetal testes explants. Values are the mean ± SEM of *INSL3* mRNA levels normalized to β-actin one and expressed as percentage of control values from seven (human), five (mouse), and six (rat) independent experiments. $^{*}p < 0.05$ in the statistical comparison between BPA-treated and control testes (Wilcoxon's nonparametric paired test). *The figure is originally from N'tumba-Byn et al. (2012). For details of the experimental setup, please see this chapter.* (See color plate.)

5. CONCLUSIONS AND FUTURE DIRECTIONS

It appears from the present overview that data on INSL3 in response to EDC exposure are indeed limited. Animal studies suggest that the hormone is sensitive to phthalates, whereas its effect on human fetal testis, including fetal INSL3 production, is questionable. The important issue of species differences has only really been addressed in recent years. If initial findings are confirmed in future studies, this has important implications for human risk assessment. Especially, the suggestions of a higher sensitivity towards BPA, a high-volume industrial chemical, in humans as compared to rodents should stimulate further studies, both in experimental and in epidemiological settings.

The basic biology of INSL3 is still incompletely characterized, largely due to the relatively recent characterization of the hormone and its receptor RXFP2. There are still large gaps in our knowledge of this interesting hormone–receptor system including its postnatal functions, both within and beyond the testis, and the relationship between INSL3 and testosterone.

REFERENCES

Acerini, C. L., Miles, H. L., Dunger, D. B., Ong, K. K., & Hughes, I. A. (2009). The descriptive epidemiology of congenital and acquired cryptorchidism in a UK infant cohort. *Archives of Disease in Childhood*, *94*, 868–872.

Adham, I. M., Burkhardt, E., Benahmed, M., & Engel, W. (1993). Cloning of a cDNA for a novel insulin-like peptide of the testicular Leydig cells. *Journal of Biological Chemistry*, *268*, 26668–26672.

Adham, I. M., Steding, G., Thamm, T., Bullesbach, E. E., Schwabe, C., Paprotta, I., et al. (2002). The overexpression of the insl3 in female mice causes descent of the ovaries. *Molecular Endocrinology*, *16*, 244–252.

Ahmed, S. F., Cheng, A., Dovey, L., Hawkins, J. R., Martin, H., Rowland, J., et al. (2000). Phenotypic features, androgen receptor binding, and mutational analysis in 278 clinical cases reported as androgen insensitivity syndrome. *Journal of Clinical Endocrinology and Metabolism*, *85*, 658–665.

Akre, O., Lipworth, L., Cnattingius, S., Sparen, P., & Ekbom, A. (1999). Risk factor patterns for cryptorchidism and hypospadias. *Epidemiology*, *10*, 364–369.

Amann, R. P., & Veeramachaneni, D. N. (2007). Cryptorchidism in common eutherian mammals. *Reproduction*, *133*, 541–561.

Anand-Ivell, R., Heng, K., Hafen, B., Setchell, B., & Ivell, R. (2009). Dynamics of INSL3 peptide expression in the rodent testis. *Biology of Reproduction*, *81*, 480–487.

Anand-Ivell, R., Ivell, R., Driscoll, D., & Manson, J. (2008). Insulin-like factor 3 levels in amniotic fluid of human male fetuses. *Human Reproduction*, *23*, 1180–1186.

Anand-Ivell, R. J., Relan, V., Balvers, M., Coiffec-Dorval, I., Fritsch, M., Bathgate, R. A., et al. (2006). Expression of the insulin-like peptide 3 (INSL3) hormone-receptor (LGR8) system in the testis. *Biology of Reproduction*, *74*, 945–953.

Anand-Ivell, R., Wohlgemuth, J., Haren, M. T., Hope, P. J., Hatzinikolas, G., Wittert, G., et al. (2006). Peripheral INSL3 concentrations decline with age in a large population of Australian men. *International Journal of Andrology, 29*, 618–626.

Balvers, M., Spiess, A. N., Domagalski, R., Hunt, N., Kilic, E., Mukhopadhyay, A. K., et al. (1998). Relaxin-like factor expression as a marker of differentiation in the mouse testis and ovary. *Endocrinology, 139*, 2960–2970.

Barteczko, K. J., & Jacob, M. I. (2000). The testicular descent in human. Origin, development and fate of the gubernaculum Hunteri, processus vaginalis peritonei, and gonadal ligaments. *Advances in Anatomy, Embryology, and Cell Biology, 156*(III–X), 1–98.

Bay, K., & Andersson, A. M. (2011). Human testicular insulin-like factor 3: In relation to development, reproductive hormones and andrological disorders. *International Journal of Andrology, 34*, 97–109.

Bay, K., Cohen, A. S., Jorgensen, F. S., Jorgensen, C., Lind, A. M., Skakkebaek, N. E., et al. (2008). Insulin-like factor 3 levels in second-trimester amniotic fluid. *Journal of Clinical Endocrinology and Metabolism, 93*, 4048–4051.

Bay, K., Hartung, S., Ivell, R., Schumacher, M., Jurgensen, D., Jorgensen, N., et al. (2005). Insulin-like factor 3 (INSL3) serum levels in 135 normal men and 85 men with testicular disorders: Relationship to the LH-Testosterone axis. *Journal of Clinical Endocrinology and Metabolism, 90*, 3410–3418.

Bay, K., Main, K. M., Toppari, J., & Skakkebaek, N. E. (2011). Testicular descent: INSL3, testosterone, genes and the intrauterine milieu. *Nature Reviews. Urology, 8*, 187–196.

Bay, K., Matthiesson, K. L., McLachlan, R. I., & Andersson, A. M. (2006). The effects of gonadotropin suppression and selective replacement on insulin-like factor 3 secretion in normal adult men. *Journal of Clinical Endocrinology and Metabolism, 91*, 1108–1111.

Bay, K., Virtanen, H. E., Hartung, S., Ivell, R., Main, K. M., Skakkebaek, N. E., et al. (2007). Insulin-like factor 3 levels in cord blood and serum from children: Effects of age, postnatal hypothalamic-pituitary-gonadal axis activation, and cryptorchidism. *Journal of Clinical Endocrinology and Metabolism, 92*, 4020–4027.

Berkowitz, G. S., Lapinski, R. H., Dolgin, S. E., Gazella, J. G., Bodian, C. A., & Holzman, I. R. (1993). Prevalence and natural history of cryptorchidism. *Pediatrics, 92*, 44–49.

Biggs, M. L., Baer, A., & Critchlow, C. W. (2002). Maternal, delivery, and perinatal characteristics associated with cryptorchidism: A population-based case-control study among births in Washington State. *Epidemiology, 13*, 197–204.

Bogatcheva, N. V., Ferlin, A., Feng, S., Truong, A., Gianesello, L., Foresta, C., et al. (2007). T222P mutation of the insulin-like 3 hormone receptor LGR8 is associated with testicular maldescent and hinders receptor expression on the cell surface membrane. *American Journal of Physiology. Endocrinology and Metabolism, 292*, E138–E144.

Boisen, K. A., Kaleva, M., Main, K. M., Virtanen, H. E., Haavisto, A. M., Schmidt, I. M., et al. (2004). Difference in prevalence of congenital cryptorchidism in infants between two Nordic countries. *Lancet, 363*, 1264–1269.

Borch, J., Metzdorff, S. B., Vinggaard, A. M., Brokken, L., & Dalgaard, M. (2006). Mechanisms underlying the anti-androgenic effects of diethylhexyl phthalate in fetal rat testis. *Toxicology, 223*, 144–155.

Brucker-Davis, F., Wagner-Mahler, K., Delattre, I., Ducot, B., Ferrari, P., Bongain, A., et al. (2008). Cryptorchidism at birth in Nice area (France) is associated with higher prenatal exposure to PCBs and DDE, as assessed by colostrum concentrations. *Human Reproduction, 23*, 1708–1718.

Burkhardt, E., Adham, I. M., Hobohm, U., Murphy, D., Sander, C., & Engel, W. (1994). A human cDNA coding for the Leydig insulin-like peptide (Ley I-L). *Human Genetics, 94*, 91–94.

Chauvigne, F., Plummer, S., Lesne, L., Cravedi, J. P., Dejucq-Rainsford, N., Fostier, A., et al. (2011). Mono-(2-ethylhexyl) phthalate directly alters the expression of Leydig cell genes and CYP17 lyase activity in cultured rat fetal testis. *PLoS One*, *6*, e27172.

Codesal, J., Regadera, J., Nistal, M., Regadera-Sejas, J., & Paniagua, R. (1990). Involution of human fetal Leydig cells. An immunohistochemical, ultrastructural and quantitative study. *Journal of Anatomy*, *172*, 103–114.

Costa, W. S., Sampaio, F. J., Favorito, L. A., & Cardoso, L. E. (2002). Testicular migration: Remodeling of connective tissue and muscle cells in human gubernaculum testis. *Journal of Urology*, *167*, 2171–2176.

Damgaard, I. N., Skakkebaek, N. E., Toppari, J., Virtanen, H. E., Shen, H., Schramm, K. W., et al. (2006). Persistent pesticides in human breast milk and cryptorchidism. *Environmental Health Perspectives*, *114*, 1133–1138.

Del Borgo, M. P., Hughes, R. A., Bathgate, R. A., Lin, F., Kawamura, K., & Wade, J. D. (2006). Analogs of insulin-like peptide 3 (INSL3) B-chain are LGR8 antagonists in vitro and in vivo. *Journal of Biological Chemistry*, *281*, 13068–13074.

Desdoits-Lethimonier, C., Albert, O., Le Bizec, B., Perdu, E., Zalko, D., Courant, F., et al. (2012). Human testis steroidogenesis is inhibited by phthalates. *Human Reproduction*, *27*, 1451–1459.

Emmen, J. M., McLuskey, A., Adham, I. M., Engel, W., Verhoef-Post, M., Themmen, A. P., et al. (2000). Involvement of insulin-like factor 3 (Insl3) in diethylstilbestrol-induced cryptorchidism. *Endocrinology*, *141*, 846–849.

Feng, S., Bogatcheva, N. V., Truong, A., Korchin, B., Bishop, C. E., Klonisch, T., et al. (2007). Developmental expression and gene regulation of insulin-like 3 receptor RXFP2 in mouse male reproductive organs. *Biology of Reproduction*, 77, 671–680.

Feng, S., Cortessis, V. K., Hwang, A., Hardy, B., Koh, C. J., Bogatcheva, N. V., et al. (2004). Mutation analysis of INSL3 and GREAT/LGR8 genes in familial cryptorchidism. *Urology*, *64*, 1032–1036.

Ferlin, A., Garolla, A., Rigon, F., Rasi, C. L., Lenzi, A., & Foresta, C. (2006). Changes in serum insulin-like factor 3 during normal male puberty. *Journal of Clinical Endocrinology and Metabolism*, *91*, 3426–3431.

Ferlin, A., Pepe, A., Gianesello, L., Garolla, A., Feng, S., Giannini, S., et al. (2008). Mutations in the insulin-like factor 3 receptor are associated with osteoporosis. *Journal of Bone and Mineral Research*, *23*, 683–693.

Ferlin, A., Perilli, L., Gianesello, L., Taglialavoro, G., & Foresta, C. (2011). Profiling insulin like factor 3 (INSL3) signaling in human osteoblasts. *PLoS One*, *6*, e29733.

Ferlin, A., Simonato, M., Bartoloni, L., Rizzo, G., Bettella, A., Dottorini, T., et al. (2003). The INSL3-LGR8/GREAT ligand-receptor pair in human cryptorchidism. *Journal of Clinical Endocrinology and Metabolism*, *88*, 4273–4279.

Ferlin, A., Zuccarello, D., Garolla, A., Selice, R., Vinanzi, C., Ganz, F., et al. (2009). Mutations in INSL3 and RXFP2 genes in cryptorchid boys. *Annals of the New York Academy of Sciences*, *1160*, 213–214.

Ferlin, A., Zuccarello, D., Zuccarello, B., Chirico, M. R., Zanon, G. F., & Foresta, C. (2008). Genetic alterations associated with cryptorchidism. *JAMA*, *300*, 2271–2276.

Filonzi, M., Cardoso, L. C., Pimenta, M. T., Queiroz, D. B., Avellar, M. C., Porto, C. S., et al. (2007). Relaxin family peptide receptors Rxfp1 and Rxfp2: Mapping of the mRNA and protein distribution in the reproductive tract of the male rat. *Reproductive Biology and Endocrinology*, *5*, 29.

Foresta, C., Bettella, A., Vinanzi, C., Dabrilli, P., Meriggiola, M. C., Garolla, A., et al. (2004). A novel circulating hormone of testis origin in humans. *Journal of Clinical Endocrinology and Metabolism*, *89*, 5952–5958.

Foresta, C., Zuccarello, D., Garolla, A., & Ferlin, A. (2008). Role of hormones, genes, and environment in human cryptorchidism. *Endocrine Reviews*, *29*, 560–580.

Ghirri, P., Ciulli, C., Vuerich, M., Cuttano, A., Faraoni, M., Guerrini, L., et al. (2002). Incidence at birth and natural history of cryptorchidism: A study of 10,730 consecutive male infants. *Journal of Endocrinological Investigation*, *25*, 709–715.

Gill, W. B., Schumacher, G. F., Bibbo, M., Straus, F. H., & Schoenberg, H. W. (1979). Association of diethylstilbestrol exposure in utero with cryptorchidism, testicular hypoplasia and semen abnormalities. *Journal of Urology*, *122*, 36–39.

Gorlov, I. P., Kamat, A., Bogatcheva, N. V., Jones, E., Lamb, D. J., Truong, A., et al. (2002). Mutations of the GREAT gene cause cryptorchidism. *Human Molecular Genetics*, *11*, 2309–2318.

Hannas, B. R., Lambright, C. S., Furr, J., Howdeshell, K. L., Wilson, V. S., & Gray, L. E., Jr. (2011). Dose-response assessment of fetal testosterone production and gene expression levels in rat testes following in utero exposure to diethylhexyl phthalate, diisobutyl phthalate, diisoheptyl phthalate, and diisononyl phthalate. *Toxicological Sciences*, *123*, 206–216.

Hannema, S. E., Scott, I. S., Rajpert-De Meyts, E., Skakkebaek, N. E., Coleman, N., & Hughes, I. A. (2006). Testicular development in the complete androgen insensitivity syndrome. *Journal of Pathology*, *208*, 518–527.

Heger, N. E., Hall, S. J., Sandrof, M. A., McDonnell, E. V., Hensley, J. B., McDowell, E. N., et al. (2012). Human fetal testis xenografts are resistant to phthalate-induced endocrine disruption. *Environmental Health Perspectives*, *120*, 1137–1143.

Heng, K., Anand-Ivell, R., Teerds, K., & Ivell, R. (2012). The endocrine disruptors dibutyl phthalate (DBP) and diethylstilbestrol (DES) influence Leydig cell regeneration following ethane dimethane sulphonate treatment of adult male rats. *International Journal of Andrology*, *35*, 353–363.

Howdeshell, K. L., Furr, J., Lambright, C. R., Rider, C. V., Wilson, V. S., & Gray, L. E., Jr. (2007). Cumulative effects of dibutyl phthalate and diethylhexyl phthalate on male rat reproductive tract development: Altered fetal steroid hormones and genes. *Toxicological Sciences*, *99*, 190–202.

Hsu, S. Y., Nakabayashi, K., Nishi, S., Kumagai, J., Kudo, M., Sherwood, O. D., et al. (2002). Activation of orphan receptors by the hormone relaxin. *Science*, *295*, 671–674.

Huang, Z., Rivas, B., & Agoulnik, A. I. (2012). Insulin-like 3 signaling is important for testicular descent but dispensable for spermatogenesis and germ cell survival in adult mice. *Biology of Reproduction*, *87*, 143.

Hughes, I. A., & Acerini, C. L. (2008). Factors controlling testis descent. *European Journal of Endocrinology*, *159*(Suppl. 1), S75–82.

Hutson, J. M., & Hasthorpe, S. (2005). Abnormalities of testicular descent. *Cell and Tissue Research*, *322*, 155–158.

Hutson, J. M., Williams, M. P., Fallat, M. E., & Attah, A. (1990). Testicular descent: New insights into its hormonal control. *Oxford Reviews of Reproductive Biology*, *12*, 1–56.

Ivell, R., Balvers, M., Domagalski, R., Ungefroren, H., Hunt, N., & Schulze, W. (1997). Relaxin-like factor: A highly specific and constitutive new marker for Leydig cells in the human testis. *Molecular Human Reproduction*, *3*, 459–466.

Ivell, R., & Bathgate, R. (2006). Neohormone systems as exciting targets for drug development. *Trends in Endocrinology and Metabolism*, *17*, 123.

Ivell, R., Heng, K., Nicholson, H., & Anand-Ivell, R. (2013). Brief maternal exposure of rats to the xenobiotics dibutyl phthalate or diethylstilbestrol alters adult-type Leydig cell development in male offspring. *Asian Journal of Andrology*, *15*(2), 261–268.

Jensen, M. S., Toft, G., Thulstrup, A. M., Bonde, J. P., & Olsen, J. (2007). Cryptorchidism according to maternal gestational smoking. *Epidemiology*, *18*, 220–225.

Jensen, M. S., Wilcox, A. J., Olsen, J., Bonde, J. P., Thulstrup, A. M., Ramlau-Hansen, C. H., et al. (2012). Cryptorchidism and hypospadias in a cohort of 934,538 Danish boys: The role of birth weight, gestational age, body dimensions, and fetal growth. *American Journal of Epidemiology, 175*, 917–925.

Kaftanovskaya, E. M., Feng, S., Huang, Z., Tan, Y., Barbara, A. M., Kaur, S., et al. (2011). Suppression of Insulin-like3 receptor reveals the role of beta-catenin and Notch signaling in gubernaculum development. *Molecular Endocrinology, 25*, 170–183.

Kaftanovskaya, E. M., Huang, Z., Barbara, A. M., De Gendt, K., Verhoeven, G., Gorlov, I. P., et al. (2012). Cryptorchidism in mice with an androgen receptor ablation in gubernaculum testis. *Molecular Endocrinology, 26*, 598–607.

Kawamura, K., Kumagai, J., Sudo, S., Chun, S. Y., Pisarska, M., Morita, H., et al. (2004). Paracrine regulation of mammalian oocyte maturation and male germ cell survival. *Proceedings of the National Academy of Sciences of the United States of America, 101*, 7323–7328.

Klonisch, T., Fowler, P. A., & Hombach-Klonisch, S. (2004). Molecular and genetic regulation of testis descent and external genitalia development. *Developmental Biology, 270*, 1–18.

Klonisch, T., Ivell, R., Balvers, M., Kliesch, S., Fischer, B., Bergmann, M., et al. (1999). Expression of relaxin-like factor is down-regulated in human testicular Leydig cell neoplasia. *Molecular Human Reproduction, 5*, 104–108.

Koskimies, P., Suvanto, M., Nokkala, E., Huhtaniemi, I. T., McLuskey, A., Themmen, A. P., et al. (2003). Female mice carrying a ubiquitin promoter-Insl3 transgene have descended ovaries and inguinal hernias but normal fertility. *Molecular and Cellular Endocrinology, 206*, 159–166.

Koskimies, P., Virtanen, H., Lindstrom, M., Kaleva, M., Poutanen, M., Huhtaniemi, I., et al. (2000). A common polymorphism in the human relaxin-like factor (RLF) gene: No relationship with cryptorchidism. *Pediatric Research, 47*, 538–541.

Kristensen, D. M., Lesne, L., Le Fol, V., Desdoits-Lethimonier, C., Dejucq-Rainsford, N., Leffers, H., et al. (2012). Paracetamol (acetaminophen), aspirin (acetylsalicylic acid) and indomethacin are anti-androgenic in the rat foetal testis. *International Journal of Andrology, 35*, 377–384.

Kumagai, J., Hsu, S. Y., Matsumi, H., Roh, J. S., Fu, P., Wade, J. D., et al. (2002). INSL3/ Leydig insulin-like peptide activates the LGR8 receptor important in testis descent. *Journal of Biological Chemistry, 277*, 31283–31286.

Lague, E., & Tremblay, J. J. (2008). Antagonistic effects of testosterone and the endocrine disruptor mono-(2-ethylhexyl) phthalate on INSL3 transcription in Leydig cells. *Endocrinology, 149*, 4688–4694.

Lague, E., & Tremblay, J. J. (2009). Estradiol represses Insulin-like 3 expression and promoter activity in MA-10 Leydig cells. *Toxicology, 258*, 101–105.

Laier, P., Metzdorff, S. B., Borch, J., Hagen, M. L., Hass, U., Christiansen, S., et al. (2006). Mechanisms of action underlying the antiandrogenic effects of the fungicide prochloraz. *Toxicology and Applied Pharmacology, 213*, 160–171.

Li, Z., Feng, S., Lopez, V., Elhammady, G., Anderson, M. L., Kaftanovskaya, E. M., et al. (2011). Uterine cysts in female mice deficient for caveolin-1 and insulin-like 3 receptor RXFP2. *Endocrinology, 152*, 2474–2482.

Lim, H. N., Rajpert-De Meyts, E., Skakkebæk, N. E., Hawkins, J. R., & Hughes, I. A. (2001). Genetic analysis of the INSL3 gene in patients with maldescent of the testis. *European Journal of Endocrinology, 144*, 129–137.

Mahood, I. K., Hallmark, N., McKinnell, C., Walker, M., Fisher, J. S., & Sharpe, R. M. (2005). Abnormal Leydig cell aggregation in the fetal testis of rats exposed to di (n-butyl) phthalate and its possible role in testicular dysgenesis. *Endocrinology, 146*, 613–623.

Main, K. M., Mortensen, G. K., Kaleva, M. M., Boisen, K. A., Damgaard, I. N., Chellakooty, M., et al. (2006). Human breast milk contamination with phthalates and alterations of endogenous reproductive hormones in infants three months of age. *Environmental Health Perspectives, 114*, 270–276.

Martin, O. V., Shialis, T., Lester, J. N., Scrimshaw, M. D., Boobis, A. R., & Voulvoulis, N. (2008). Testicular dysgenesis syndrome and the estrogen hypothesis: A quantitative meta-analysis. *Environmental Health Perspectives, 116*, 149–157.

McBride, M. L., Van den Steen, N., Lamb, C. W., & Gallagher, R. P. (1991). Maternal and gestational factors in cryptorchidism. *International Journal of Epidemiology, 20*, 964–970.

McGlynn, K. A., Guo, X., Graubard, B. I., Brock, J. W., Klebanoff, M. A., & Longnecker, M. P. (2009). Maternal pregnancy levels of polychlorinated biphenyls and risk of hypospadias and cryptorchidism in male offspring. *Environmental Health Perspectives, 117*, 1472–1476.

McKinnell, C., Sharpe, R. M., Mahood, K., Hallmark, N., Scott, H., Ivell, R., et al. (2005). Expression of insulin-like factor 3 protein in the rat testis during fetal and postnatal development and in relation to cryptorchidism induced by in utero exposure to di (n-butyl) phthalate. *Endocrinology, 146*, 4536–4544.

McLachlan, J. A. (1977). Prenatal exposure to diethylstilbestrol in mice: Toxicological studies. *Journal of Toxicology and Environmental Health, 2*, 527–537.

Mitchell, R. T., Childs, A. J., Anderson, R. A., van den Driesche, S., Saunders, P. T., McKinnell, C., et al. (2012). Do phthalates affect steroidogenesis by the human fetal testis? Exposure of human fetal testis xenografts to di-n-butyl phthalate. *Journal of Clinical Endocrinology and Metabolism, 97*, E341–E348.

Morales-Suarez-Varela, M. M., Toft, G. V., Jensen, M. S., Ramlau-Hansen, C., Kaerlev, L., Thulstrup, A. M., et al. (2011). Parental occupational exposure to endocrine disrupting chemicals and male genital malformations: A study in the Danish National Birth Cohort study. *Environmental Health, 10*, 3–10.

Mylchreest, E., Sar, M., Cattley, R. C., & Foster, P. M. (1999). Disruption of androgen-regulated male reproductive development by di(n-butyl) phthalate during late gestation in rats is different from flutamide. *Toxicology and Applied Pharmacology, 156*, 81–95.

Nef, S., & Parada, L. F. (1999). Cryptorchidism in mice mutant for Insl3. *Nature Genetics, 22*, 295–299.

Nef, S., Shipman, T., & Parada, L. F. (2000). A molecular basis for estrogen-induced cryptorchidism. *Developmental Biology, 224*, 354–361.

Nguyen, M. T., Showalter, P. R., Timmons, C. F., Nef, S., Parada, L. F., & Baker, L. A. (2002). Effects of orchiopexy on congenitally cryptorchid insulin-3 knockout mice. *Journal of Urology, 168*, 1779–1783.

N'tumba-Byn, T., Moison, D., Lacroix, M., Lecureuil, C., Lesage, L., Prud'homme, S. M., et al. (2012). Differential effects of bisphenol a and diethylstilbestrol on human, rat and mouse fetal Leydig cell function. *PLoS One, 7*, e51579.

O'Shaughnessy, P. J., Baker, P. J., Monteiro, A., Cassie, S., Bhattacharya, S., & Fowler, P. A. (2007). Developmental changes in human fetal testicular cell numbers and messenger ribonucleic acid levels during the second trimester. *Journal of Clinical Endocrinology and Metabolism, 92*, 4792–4801.

Overbeek, P. A., Gorlov, I. P., Sutherland, R. W., Houston, J. B., Harrison, W. R., Boettger-Tong, H. L., et al. (2001). A transgenic insertion causing cryptorchidism in mice. *Genesis, 30*, 26–35.

Park, J. I., Semyonov, J., Chang, C. L., Yi, W., Warren, W., & Hsu, S. Y. (2008). Origin of INSL3-mediated testicular descent in therian mammals. *Genome Research, 18*, 974–985.

Pathirana, I. N., Kawate, N., Bullesbach, E. E., Takahashi, M., Hatoya, S., Inaba, T., et al. (2012). Insulin-like peptide 3 stimulates testosterone secretion in mouse Leydig cells via cAMP pathway. *Regulatory Peptides, 178*, 102–106.

Prince, F. P. (2001). The triphasic nature of Leydig cell development in humans, and comments on nomenclature. *Journal of Endocrinology, 168*, 213–216.

Quigley, C. A., De Bellis, A., Marschke, K. B., el-Awady, M. K., Wilson, E. M., & French, F. S. (1995). Androgen receptor defects: Historical, clinical, and molecular perspectives. *Endocrine Reviews*, *16*, 271–321.

Roh, J., Virtanen, H., Kumagai, J., Sudo, S., Kaleva, M., Toppari, J., et al. (2003). Lack of LGR8 gene mutation in Finnish patients with a family history of cryptorchidism. *Reproductive Biomedicine Online*, 7, 400–406.

Rotondi, M., Valenzano, F., Bilancioni, E., Spano, G., Rotondi, M., & Giorlandino, C. (2001). Prenatal measurement of testicular diameter by ultrasonography: Development of fetal male gender and evaluation of testicular descent. *Prenatal Diagnosis*, *21*, 112–115.

Sadeghian, H., Anand-Ivell, R., Balvers, M., Relan, V., & Ivell, R. (2005). Constitutive regulation of the Insl3 gene in rat Leydig cells. *Molecular and Cellular Endocrinology*, *241*, 10–20.

Sampaio, F. J., & Favorito, L. A. (1998). Analysis of testicular migration during the fetal period in humans. *Journal of Urology*, *159*, 540–542.

Sharpe, R. M., Rivas, A., Walker, M., McKinnell, C., & Fisher, J. S. (2003). Effect of neonatal treatment of rats with potent or weak (environmental) oestrogens, or with a GnRH antagonist, on Leydig cell development and function through puberty into adulthood. *International Journal of Andrology*, *26*, 26–36.

Shono, T., Shima, Y., Kondo, T., & Suita, S. (2005). In utero exposure to mono-n-butyl phthalate impairs insulin-like factor 3 gene expression and the transabdominal phase of testicular descent in fetal rats. *Journal of Pediatric Surgery*, *40*, 1861–1864.

Spiess, A. N., Balvers, M., Tena-Sempere, M., Huhtaniemi, I., Parry, L., & Ivell, R. (1999). Structure and expression of the rat relaxin-like factor (RLF) gene. *Molecular Reproduction and Development*, *54*, 319–325.

Takayanagi, S., Tokunaga, T., Liu, X., Okada, H., Matsushima, A., & Shimohigashi, Y. (2006). Endocrine disruptor bisphenol A strongly binds to human estrogen-related receptor gamma (ERRgamma) with high constitutive activity. *Toxicology Letters*, *167*, 95–105.

Tapanainen, J., Kellokumpu-Lehtinen, P., Pelliniemi, L., & Huhtaniemi, I. (1981). Age-related changes in endogenous steroids of human fetal testis during early and midpregnancy. *Journal of Clinical Endocrinology and Metabolism*, *52*, 98–102.

Tomiyama, H., Hutson, J. M., Truong, A., & Agoulnik, A. I. (2003). Transabdominal testicular descent is disrupted in mice with deletion of insulinlike factor 3 receptor. *Journal of Pediatric Surgery*, *38*, 1793–1798.

Virtanen, H. E., & Adamsson, A. (2012). Cryptorchidism and endocrine disrupting chemicals. *Molecular and Cellular Endocrinology*, *355*, 208–220.

Wagner-Mahler, K., Kurzenne, J. Y., Delattre, I., Berard, E., Mas, J. C., Bornebush, L., et al. (2011). Prospective study on the prevalence and associated risk factors of cryptorchidism in 6246 newborn boys from Nice area. *International Journal of Andrology*, *34*, e499–e510.

Weidner, I. S., Moller, H., Jensen, T. K., & Skakkebaek, N. E. (1998). Cryptorchidism and hypospadias in sons of gardeners and farmers. *Environmental Health Perspectives*, *106*, 793–796.

Wikstrom, A. M., Bay, K., Hero, M., Andersson, A. M., & Dunkel, L. (2006). Serum insulin-like factor 3 levels during puberty in healthy boys and boys with Klinefelter syndrome. *Journal of Clinical Endocrinology and Metabolism*, *91*, 4705–4708.

Wilson, V. S., Blystone, C. R., Hotchkiss, A. K., Rider, C. V., & Gray, L. E., Jr. (2008). Diverse mechanisms of anti-androgen action: Impact on male rat reproductive tract development. *International Journal of Andrology*, *31*, 178–187.

Wilson, V. S., Lambright, C., Furr, J., Ostby, J., Wood, C., Held, G., et al. (2004). Phthalate ester-induced gubernacular lesions are associated with reduced insl3 gene expression in the fetal rat testis. *Toxicology Letters*, *146*, 207–215.

Yuan, F. P., Li, X., Lin, J., Schwabe, C., Bullesbach, E. E., Rao, C. V., et al. (2010). The role of RXFP2 in mediating androgen-induced inguinoscrotal testis descent in LH receptor knockout mice. *Reproduction, 139*, 759–769.

Zhou, W., Bolden-Tiller, O. U., Shao, S. H., Weng, C. C., Shetty, G., AbuElhija, M., et al. (2011). Estrogen-regulated genes in rat testes and their relationship to recovery of spermatogenesis after irradiation. *Biology of Reproduction, 85*, 823–833.

Zhu, J. L., Hjollund, N. H., Andersen, A. M., & Olsen, J. (2006). Occupational exposure to pesticides and pregnancy outcomes in gardeners and farmers: A study within the Danish National Birth Cohort. *Journal of Occupational and Environmental Medicine, 48*, 347–352.

Zimmermann, S., Schottler, P., Engel, W., & Adham, I. M. (1997). Mouse Leydig insulin-like (Ley I-L) gene: Structure and expression during testis and ovary development. *Molecular Reproduction and Development, 47*, 30–38.

Zimmermann, S., Steding, G., Emmen, J. M., Brinkmann, A. O., Nayernia, K., Holstein, A. F., et al. (1999). Targeted disruption of the Insl3 gene causes bilateral cryptorchidism. *Molecular Endocrinology, 13*, 681–691.

CHAPTER THIRTEEN

Environmental Pollutants and Hydroxysteroid Dehydrogenases

Leping Ye, Jingjing Guo, Ren-Shan Ge[1]
The 2nd Affiliated Hospital and Research Academy of Reproductive Biomedicine of Wenzhou Medical University, Wenzhou, Zhejiang, PR China
[1]Corresponding author: e-mail address: r_ge@yahoo.com

Contents

1. Introduction 350
2. 3β-Hydroxysteroid Dehydrogenase/Isomerase 352
   2.1 3β-HSD2 353
3. 11β-Hydroxysteroid Dehydrogenase 358
   3.1 11β-HSD1 358
   3.2 11β-HSD2 364
4. 17β-Hydroxysteroid Dehydrogenase 370
   4.1 17β-HSD1 370
   4.2 17β-HSD3 372
5. 20α-Hydroxysteroid Dehydrogenase 375
   5.1 20α-HSD (AKR1C1) 375
6. Summary and Conclusion 377
Acknowledgments 377
References 378

Abstract

Hydroxysteroid dehydrogenases (HSD) are a group of steroidogenic enzymes that are involved in the steroid biosynthesis and metabolism. Four classes of HSDs, namely, 3β-, 11β-, 17β-, and 20α-HSDs, are discussed. 3β-HSDs catalyze the conversion of pregnenolone, 17α-hydroxypregnenolone, and dehydroepiandrosterone to progesterone, 17α-hydroxyprogesterone, and androstenedione, respectively. 11β-HSDs catalyze the interconversion between active cortisol and inactive cortisone. 17β-HSDs catalyze the interconversion between 17β-hydroxyl steroids and 17-ketoandrogens and estrogens. 20α-HSDs catalyze the conversion of progesterone into 20α-hydroxyprogesterone. Many environmental pollutants directly inhibit one or more enzymes of these HSDs, thus interfering with endogenous active steroid hormone levels. These chemicals include industrial materials (perfluoroalkyl compounds, phthalates, bisphenol A, and benzophenone), pesticides/biocides (methoxychlor, organotins, 1,2-dibromo-3-chloropropane, and prochloraz), and plant constituents (genistein, gossypol, and licorice). This chapter reviews these inhibitors targeting on HSDs.

Vitamins and Hormones, Volume 94
ISSN 0083-6729
http://dx.doi.org/10.1016/B978-0-12-800095-3.00013-4

1. INTRODUCTION

The active endogenous progestogen, androgen, estrogen, glucocorticoid, and mineralocorticoid are progesterone, testosterone, estradiol, cortisol, and aldosterone. They are steroid hormones. These hormones bind to their respective nuclear receptors to exert their biological roles. Many steroidogenic enzymes are involved in steroid biosynthesis and metabolism. One group of steroidogenic enzymes is the hydroxysteroid dehydrogenases (HSDs). HSDs belong to short-chain alcohol oxidoreductase family in which members act upon an alcohol functional group or a keto functional group.

HSD catalyzes the interconversion between the hydroxysteroid and the ketosteroid. There are four types of HSDs, classified by carbon number acted upon (Table 13.1). These HSDs include 3β-hydroxysteroid dehydrogenase/isomerase (3β-HSD), 11β-hydroxysteroid dehydrogenases (11β-HSD), 17β-hydroxysteroid dehydrogenases (17β-HSD), and 20α-hydroxysteroid dehydrogenase (20α-HSD). Each group of these HSDs contains different isoforms, which have different tissue localization and functions.

Environmental pollutants that interfere with these HSDs could affect the biosynthesis and metabolism of progestogens, androgens, estrogens, glucocorticoids, and mineralocorticoids. Many environmental pollutants are considered to be endocrine disruptors. These environmental pollutants include plasticizers (phthalates and bisphenol A), surfactants (perfluoroalkyl substances), insecticides (methoxychlor and dichlorodiphenyltrichloroethane), and plant constituents (genistein, gossypol, and licorice). In the present book chapter, we focus on environmental pollutants that directly inhibit HSDs (Table 13.2). Many data are from human HSDs. Therefore, we mainly discuss the effects of environmental pollutants on human HSDs. The inhibitory

Table 13.1 Classification of hydroxysteroid dehydrogenases based on carbon number

Carbon	Substrate	Product
3	Pregnenolone (17-hydroxypregnenolone, dehydroepiandrosterone)	Progesterone (17-hydroxyprogesterone, androstenedione)
11	Cortisol	Cortisone
17	Androstenedione	Testosterone
20	Progesterone	20α-Hydroxyprogesterone

Table 13.2 Inhibitors of enzymes for human hydroxysteroid dehydrogenases

Enzyme	Environmental pollutants	Use	Mode of inhibition
3β-HSD2	Bisphenol A	Plasticizer	Competitive
	Methoxychlor and HPTE	Insecticide	Noncompetitive
	Triphenyltin	Biocide	Unknown
	Tributyltin	Biocide	Unknown
	Genistein	Plant constituent	Competitive
	Gossypol	Plant constituent	Competitive
	Phthalates	Plasticizers	Competitive
11β-HSD1	Perfluorooctane sulfonate	Surfactant	Competitive
	Perfluorooctane acid	Surfactant	Competitive
	Bisphenol A	Plasticizer	Competitive
	Methoxychlor and HPTE	Insecticide	Competitive
	(+)Gossypol	Plant constituent	Competitive
	Glycyrrhetinic acid	Plant constituent	Competitive
11β-HSD2	Perfluorooctane sulfonate	Surfactant	Competitive
	Perfluorooctane acid	Surfactant	Competitive
	Perfluorohexyl sulfonate	Surfactant	Competitive
	HPTE	Insecticide	Competitive
	(+) and (−) Gossypol	Plant constituent	Unknown
	Organotins	Biocide	Unknown
	Glycyrrhetinic acid	Plant constituent	Competitive
	Phthalates	Plasticizers	Competitive
	Alkylphenols	Surfactants	Unknown
	Thiram	Fungicide	Unknown
17β-HSD1	Diethylstilbestrol	Drug	Unknown
	Gossypol	Plant constituent	Competitive
	Benzophenone 1	UV protector	Unknown
	Genistein	Plant constituent	Unknown
	Genkwanin and diosmetin	Plant constituent	Unknown

Continued

Table 13.2 Inhibitors of enzymes for human hydroxysteroid dehydrogenases—cont'd

Enzyme	Environmental pollutants	Use	Mode of inhibition
17β-HSD3	Perfluorooctane sulfonate	Surfactant	Noncompetitive
	Perfluorooctane acid	Surfactant	Noncompetitive
	HPTE	Insecticide	Competitive
	Triphenyltin	Biocide	Unknown
	Tributyltin	Biocide	Unknown
	(+) and (−) Gossypol	Plant constituent	Competitive
	Bisphenol A	Plasticizer	Competitive
	Benzophenones	UV blocker	Unknown
	Methoxychlor and HPTE	Insecticide	Noncompetitive
	Gossypol	Plant constituent	Competitive
	Benzyl octyl phthalate	Plasticizer	Competitive
	Dicyclohexyl phthalate	Plasticizer	Competitive
	Benzophenone 1	UV blocker	Unknown
20α-HSD	Phenolphthalein	Drug	Unknown
	Coumestrol	Plant constituent	Unknown
	Glycyrrhetinic acid	Plant constituent	Unknown
	Quercitrin	Plant constituent	Unknown
	Benzbromarone	Drug	Unknown

HPTE, 2,2-bis(*p*-hydroxyphenyl)-1,1,1-trichloroethane.

potencies of environmental pollutants on human enzymes will also be compared to those of rodent (rat and mouse) enzymes.

2. 3β-HYDROXYSTEROID DEHYDROGENASE/ ISOMERASE

3β-HSD is a group of HSDs that are responsible for the oxidation and isomerization of Δ5-3β-hydroxysteroids, pregnenolone, 17α-hydroxypregnenolone, and dehydroepiandrosterone to Δ4-ketosteroids, progesterone, 17α-hydroxyprogesterone, and androstenedione, respectively (Mason et al., 1997; Simard et al., 1996). 3β-HSDs are membrane-bound enzymes and are located in both mitochondrial and microsomal membranes. Two isoforms have been identified in the human (human 3β-HSD1 and 3β-HSD2). The tissue localization of human 3β-HSD isoforms and their affinities to steroid substrates are different. In normal tissues, human 3β-HSD1 is primarily localized in human placenta (Thomas, Myers, & Strickler, 1989), while 3β-HSD2 is predominantly present in gonadal tissues and adrenal glands (Tang, Tsai-Morris, & Dufau, 1998). Human 3β-HSD1 has higher K_m value than 3β-HSD2 isoform (Thomas, Mason, Brandt, Spencer, & Norris, 2002). Many environmental pollutants have been tested to inhibit 3β-HSD2 activity, while the reports of the inhibition on 3β-HSD1 were few. Therefore, in the present chapter, we discuss the inhibitors on human 3β-HSD2.

2.1. 3β-HSD2

2.1.1 Enzyme reaction

The enzymatic reaction of 3β-HSD2 is the critical step for the formation of many active steroids. These steroids include progesterone, testosterone, cortisol, aldosterone, or estradiol, which is derived from testosterone. 3β-HSD2 catalyzes two sequential reactions: (1) the first step of dehydrogenation of the 3β-equatorial hydroxysteroid that requires the cofactor NAD+ to produce a Δ5-3-ketosteroid intermediate and reduced NADH and (2) NADH that then activates the isomerization of the Δ5-3-ketosteroid into the Δ4-3-ketosteroid. A single protein catalyzes the two steps without the release of the intermediate steroid or coenzyme (Thomas et al., 2003). Human 3β-HSD2 primarily uses NAD+ as cofactor, but the enzyme also weakly binds NADP+ (Clarke, Rao, Fallest, & Shupnik, 1993). 3β-HSD2 acts on the CH–OH group of donor with NAD+ as acceptor as follows: Δ5-3-ketosteroid + NAD + → Δ5-3-ketosteroid + NADH + H+ and Δ5-3-ketosteroid → Δ4-3-ketosteroid (Fig. 13.1).

2.1.2 Gene

Each human 3β-HSD isoform is the product of a distinct gene. The human 3β-HSD2 is encoded by the *HSD3B2* gene. Human *HSD3B2* gene is located on chromosome 1p13.1 (Bain, Meisler, Taylor, & Payne, 1993; Simard et al., 1996). The human *HSD3B2* gene is about 7.8 kb in length (Simard et al., 1996). *HSD3B2* cDNA was first cloned from a human adrenal cDNA library in 1991, and the gene has 4 exons (Rheaume et al., 1991). Human 3β-HSD2 protein shares 93.5% sequence homology with human 3β-HSD1 (Rheaume et al., 1991). Human *HSD3B1* and *HSD3B2* cDNAs have 93.6% sequence

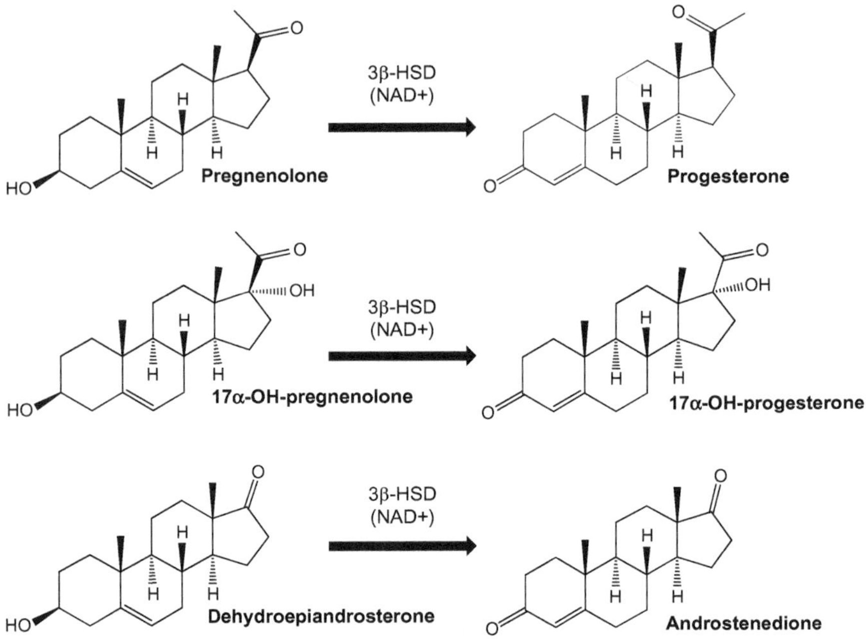

Figure 13.1 The reaction catalyzed by 3β-hydroxysteroid dehydrogenase (3β-HSD).

identity, including the 5′ and 3′ untranslated regions (Doi et al., 2010). Mutation of *HSD3B2* causes a male pseudohermaphrodite with salt-wasting classic 3β-HSD deficiency congenital adrenal hyperplasia (Chang et al., 1993), suggesting that 3β-HSD2 is a critical enzyme for reproductive tract development and adrenal functions.

2.1.3 Protein structure

3β-HSD2 has 371 amino acids (Rheaume et al., 1991). The human 3β-HSD2 catalyzes two-step reactions and requires different protein-active sites. The dehydrogenase activity of the human 3β-HSD2 requires Y156-X-K158 domain and Y156 in the catalytic domain (Thomas et al., 2002). Tyr156 resides in the α-helical subunit of the enzyme. This residue does not interact directly with bound substrate but apparently influences subunit interactions that modify the topography of the active site (Thomas, Boswell, Scaccia, Pletnev, & Umland, 2005). The amino-terminal sequence contains the cofactor-binding site (Thomas et al., 2003). The amino acid Asp36 in the human 3β-HSD2 is responsible for NAD+ binding (Thomas et al., 2003).

2.1.4 Tissue localization and possible function

Human 3β-HSD2 is primarily localized in gonadal tissues and adrenal glands (Tang et al., 1998). This enzyme catalyzes the critical step for the formation of many active steroids, including progesterone, testosterone, cortisol, aldosterone, and estradiol, which is derived from testosterone. Therefore, 3β-HSD2 inhibition can cause the defects in the reproductive system and adrenal function. The environmental pollutants that inhibit 3β-HSD2 activity can interfere with these normal physiological processes.

2.1.5 Environmental pollutants that inhibit 3β-HSD2

2.1.5.1 Perfluoroalkyl substance

Perfluoroalkyl substance is widely used for industrial and consumer products (Zhao, Chu, Hardy, Li, & Ge, 2010). These chemicals are used as surfactants, adhesives, and insecticides (Abdellatif, Preat, Vamecq, Nilsson, & Roberfroid, 1990; Jensen & Leffers, 2008; Johnson, Gibson, & Ober, 1984). These chemicals are persistent in the environment and accumulated in wildlife and humans due to their very long elimination half-lives (Jensen & Leffers, 2008; Olsen et al., 2007). Perfluoroalkyl substance has been shown to be associated with lower serum testosterone concentrations (Gilliland & Mandel, 1993; Olsen et al., 1998). Rats exposed to perfluoroalkyl substance had reduced serum testosterone concentrations (Biegel, Liu, Hurtt, & Cook, 1995; Shi, Zhang, Liu, Xu, & Dai, 2007). The effects of perfluoroalkyl substance on gonadal 3β-HSD have been tested. Perfluoroalkyl substance directly inhibited rat Leydig cell 3β-HSD activity (Zhao, Chu, Hardy, et al., 2010). Structure–activity response analysis showed that the inhibitory potency of perfluoroalkyl substance depended on the length of carbon and sulfur chain. Perfluorooctane sulfonate (8 carbons and 1 sulfur) and perfluorooctanoic acid (8 carbons) had inhibitory action on rat 3β-HSD with IC_{50} values of 1.3 and 53.2 μM, respectively, while perfluorohexanesulfonate (6 carbons and 1 sulfur) and perfluorobutanesulfonate (4 carbons and 1 sulfur) had no inhibition even at concentration of 250 μM (Zhao, Hu, Chu, et al., 2010). This indicates that 8-carbon length is required for perfluoroalkyl substance to inhibit this enzyme. Perfluorooctane sulfonate and perfluorooctanoic acid are competitive inhibitors of rat 3β-HSD (Zhao, Hu, Chu, et al., 2010). Surprisingly, perfluoroalkyl substances had almost no inhibitory effects on human gonadal 3β-HSD2 activity (Zhao, Hu, Chu, et al., 2010).

2.1.5.2 Bisphenol A

Bisphenol A is used primarily in the manufacture of polycarbonate plastic and epoxy resins. Human exposure to bisphenol A includes indoor air, dust ingestion, and contamination of foods (Loganathan & Kannan, 2011). Human urine samples had 95% detection of bisphenol A, indicating that bisphenol A exposure is widely spread (Calafat et al., 2005, Calafat, Ye, Wong, Reidy, & Needham, 2008; Ouchi & Watanabe, 2002). Bisphenol A has antiandrogenic effects. Both *in vivo* and *in vitro* exposures to bisphenol A in rodents significantly decreased testosterone production (Akingbemi, Sottas, Koulova, Klinefelter, & Hardy, 2004; Murono, Derk, & de Leon, 2001). Apparently, bisphenol A inhibited human testicular 3β-HSD2 and rat 3β-HSD with IC_{50} values of 7.9 and 26.5 μM (Ye et al., 2011), respectively. Bisphenol A is a competitive inhibitor of human 3β-HSD2 and rat testis 3β-HSD against substrate pregnenolone (Ye et al., 2011).

2.1.5.3 Methoxychlor

Methoxychlor is an organochlorine pesticide and is developed as a replacement for the banned pesticide 2, 2-bis (*p*-chlorophenyl)-1,1,1-trichloroethane. *In vitro* exposure to methoxychlor caused the decrease of luteinizing hormone-stimulated testosterone production in rat Leydig cells (Akingbemi, Ge, Klinefelter, Gunsalus, & Hardy, 2000; Gray et al., 1989; Murono & Derk, 2005). Some effects of methoxychlor is also mediated by its bioactive metabolite 2,2-bis(*p*-hydroxyphenyl)-1,1,1-trichloroethane (HPTE) (Akingbemi et al., 2000). Methoxychlor inhibited human 3β-HSD2 and rat testicular 3β-HSD activities, with IC_{50} values of 53.2 and 46.15 μM, respectively. HPTE is more potent than methoxychlor with IC_{50} values of 8.2 and 13.8 μM, respectively. Methoxychlor and HPTE are noncompetitive inhibitors of human 3β-HSD2 against pregnenolone (Hu et al., 2011).

2.1.5.4 Organotins

Organotins are the organometallic compounds and have been widely used as antifouling biocides for ships and fishing nets, agricultural fungicides, and rodent repellents (Bhosle et al., 2004). Increasing amounts of organotins have been accumulated in the environment. Organotins have antiandrogenic effects. Tributyltin exposure caused defects in testicular development *in vivo* (Zhang et al., 2009). Tributyltin is a primarily competitive inhibitor of rat testicular 3β-HSD activity with Ki of 2.4 μM

(McVey & Cooke, 2003). Triphenyltin inhibited human 3β-HSD2 activity (Lo et al., 2003) with IC_{50} value of 4.0 μM (Lo et al., 2003).

2.1.5.5 Genistein

Genistein is a soy isoflavone. The highest amount of flavonoids has been found in soybeans and soy food (Reinli & Block, 1996). Genistein inhibited rat Leydig cell function by decreasing testosterone production (Svechnikov et al., 2005). Genistein competitively inhibited human 3β-HSD2 with IC_{50} of 90 nM (Hu et al., 2010). It inhibited rat testicular 3β-HSD activity with the IC_{50} of 640 nM (Hu et al., 2010). Another isoflavone equol inhibited human testicular 3β-HSD2 by 42% at 100 μM, but it is less potent than genistein (Hu et al., 2010).

2.1.5.6 Gossypol

Gossypol is a yellowish compound isolated from cottonseeds (Yu & Chan, 1998). The exposure to gossypol could be from ingestion of cottonseed oils and materials. Food and animal agricultural industries must manage cotton-derivative product levels to avoid gossypol toxicity. Gossypol inhibited ovary 3β-HSD activities (Gu, Lin, & Rikihisa, 1990). Gossypol potently inhibited human 3β-HSD2 activity with IC_{50} of 3–5 μM and inhibited rat 3β-HSD with the IC_{50} value of 200 nM (Hu et al., 2009).

2.1.5.7 Phthalates

Phthalates are widely used as plasticizers in polyvinyl chloride consumer products (Kohn et al., 2000). Phthalates are not chemically linked to polyvinyl chloride, and they readily leach out to the environment (Binder, Baumgartner, Zavala, Deg, & Grossman, 1984). Phthalates are made about one billion pounds per year (Boxmeer et al., 2007). Structurally, phthalates differ in the length of carbon chain in the alcohol moiety. The most abundantly used are the diethylhexyl phthalate and di-*n*-butyl phthalate (Ge, Chen, Tanrikut, & Hardy, 2007). When entering human body, phthalate diesters are rapidly converted into monoester metabolites (Albro, Corbett, Schroeder, Jordan, & Matthews, 1982). Some phthalates have antiandrogenic effects. These phthalates act not via blocking the androgen receptor but via other mechanisms (Ge et al., 2007). *In vivo* exposure to some phthalates including diethylhexyl phthalate and di-*n*-butyl phthalate caused androgen deficiency of male rodent pups (Creasy, Beech, Gray, & Butler, 1987; Gray & Beamand, 1984; Gray & Butterworth, 1980; Gray & Gangolli, 1986; Howdeshell et al., 2007; Sjoberg, Bondesson, Gray, &

Ploen, 1986). Epidemiological studies also showed the association of phthalates with abnormal reproductive development due to androgen deficiency (Akingbemi & Hardy, 2001; Sharpe, 2001; Zhang et al., 2009). Some phthalates inhibited both human and rat gonadal 3β-HSD. The IC_{50} values of dipropyl, dibutyl, dipentyl, bis (2-butoxyethyl), and dicyclohexyl phthalate were 123.0, 24.1, 25.5, 50.3, and 25.5 μM for human 3β-HSD2 and 62.7, 30.3, 33.8, 82.6, and 24.7 μM for rat testis 3β-HSD, respectively (Yuan et al., 2012). Structure–activity response analysis showed that phthalates with 1–2 or 7–8 carbon atoms in ethanol moieties had no effects on both human 3β-HSD2 activities at concentrations up to 1 mM (Yuan et al., 2012). Dipropyl, dibutyl, dipentyl, bis (2-butoxyethyl), and dicyclohexyl phthalate are competitive inhibitors of human 3β-HSD2 (Yuan et al., 2012).

3. 11β-HYDROXYSTEROID DEHYDROGENASE

11β-HSD is a group of HSDs that catalyze the interconversion between inert 11 ketosteroid (cortisone) and active 11β-hydroxyl steroid (cortisol) (Zhou, Hu, Lian, Morris, & Ge, 2012). 11β-HSDs are membrane-bound enzymes and located in microsomal membranes. Two isoforms have been identified in the human (human 11β-HSD1 and 11β-HSD2). The tissue localization of human 11β-HSD isoforms and their affinities to steroids are different. In normal tissues, human 11β-HSD1 is primarily localized in many glucocorticoid target tissues including the liver, fat, testis, and brain (Monder, 1991), while 11β-HSD2 is primarily present in mineralocorticoid target tissues including the kidney, colon, epididymis, and interstitial cells in the testis (Ge et al., 2005a; Krozowski, MaGuire, et al., 1995; Whorwood, Mason, Ricketts, Howie, & Stewart, 1995). Human 11β-HSD1 has higher K_m value than 11β-HSD2 isoform (Thomas et al., 2002). Many environmental pollutants have been tested to inhibit both 11β-HSD1 and 11β-HSD2 activities. Therefore, in the present chapter, we discuss the inhibitors of both 11β-HSD1 and 11β-HSD2.

3.1. 11β-HSD1

3.1.1 Enzyme reaction

Human 11β-HSD1 is low-affinity (K_m ~2 μM for cortisol) enzyme (Monder & White, 1993). Human 11β-HSD1 primarily uses NADP+ or NADPH as cofactors (Monder & White, 1993). 11β-HSD1 is a bidirectional enzyme and acts on the CH–OH group of donor with NADP+ as

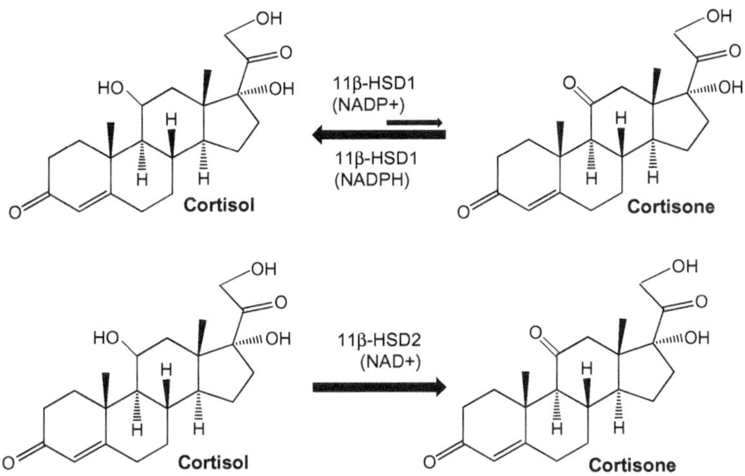

Figure 13.2 The reaction catalyzed by 11β-hydroxysteroid dehydrogenases. The top panel shows the catalysis by type I isoform (11β-HSD1) and the bottom panel shows the catalysis by type II isoform (11β-HSD2).

acceptor or C=O group of donor with NADPH as acceptor as follows: 11β-hydroxysteroid + NADP+ ↔ 11-oxosteroid + NADPH + H+ (Fig. 13.2). Purified 11β-HSD1 from rat liver showed bidirectional reaction too (Monder & Lakshmi, 1989). The oxidative activity was much higher than the reductive activity in the purified enzyme, and this suggests that the reductive activity of the enzyme is unstable *in vitro* (Monder & Lakshmi, 1989). When rat 11β-HSD1 (*Hsd11b1*) cDNA was expressed in CHO cells, the encoded enzyme catalyzed bidirectional reaction (Agarwal, Monder, Eckstein, & White, 1989). However, when *Hsd11b1* cDNA was transfected to toad bladder cells and COS7 cells, the encoded enzyme showed an exclusive reductive activity in intact cells (Duperrex et al., 1993; Low et al., 1994). Furthermore, when transfected with *Hsd11b1* cDNA, 11β-HSD1 in CHOP cells behaved a predominant oxidase, while the encoded enzyme in COS1 cells behaved primarily as reductase (Ge & Hardy, 2000). These results indicate that the cellular metabolic milieu is a key determinant of the behavior of the enzyme. It has been demonstrated that the oxidative and reductive activities of 11β-HSD1 rely on concentrations of pyridine nucleotide cofactor NADP+/NADPH redox potential in the microsomal lumen. The subpool of NADP+/NADPH was influenced by another smooth endoplasmic reticulum enzyme, hexose-6-phosphate dehydrogenase (H6PDH), thus rendering the directionality of 11β-HSD1 (Atanasov, Nashev, Schweizer, Frick, & Odermatt, 2004; Bujalska et al.,

2005; Draper et al., 2003; Piccirella et al., 2006). 11β-HSD1 is bound to microsomal membrane and has its cofactor-binding site and catalytic active site in the lumen. H6PDH is homogenously soluble in the lumen (Atanasov et al., 2004; Banhegyi, Benedetti, Fulceri, & Senesi, 2004). H6PDH uses NADP+ and glucose-6-phosphate (Atanasov et al., 2008). Glucose-6-phosphate is used by H6PDH to generate NADPH, which alters the sub-pool NADP+/NADPH ratio to drive 11β-HSD1 toward a reductive activity (Banhegyi et al., 2004; Frick, Atanasov, Arnold, Ozols, & Odermatt, 2004). The determination of H6PDH on 11β-HSD1 directionality in the liver has been proven in H6PDH knockout mice in which the 11β-HSD1 of liver cells switched from reductive activity to oxidative activity (Lavery et al., 2006). In this regard, the default direction of 11β-HSD1 is an oxidase by nature (Lavery et al., 2006). Therefore, the direction of 11β-HSD1 largely relies on the abundance of H6PDH.

3.1.2 Gene

Each 11β-HSD human isoform is the product of a distinct gene. The human 11β-HSD1 is encoded by the *HSD11B1* gene. Human *HSD11B1* gene is located on chromosome 1q32–q41 (Schutte et al., 2000). The human *HSD11B1* gene is about 9 kb in length (Tannin, Agarwal, Monder, New, & White, 1991). *HSD11B1* cDNA was first cloned from a human testis cDNA library in 1991, and the gene has 6 exons (Tannin, Agarwal, Monder, New, & White, 1991). Mutation of *HSD11B1* causes corticosterone reductase deficiency (Draper et al., 2003).

3.1.3 Protein structure

11β-HSD1 has 292 amino acids (Tannin et al., 1991). 11β-HSD1 has an N-terminal nucleotide cofactor-binding domain and a catalytic active site in the central region (Oppermann, Persson, & Jornvall, 1997). The nucleotide cofactor-binding region of the family contains GASKGIG motif that binds specifically to NADP+ and NADPH (Oppermann et al., 1997). The catalytic active site of the enzyme contains tyrosine (Tyr) and lysine (Lys) residues that bind to a ligand (Oppermann et al., 1997). The 11β-HSD1 peptide contains a single hydrophobic N-terminal extension, which possibly anchors in the smooth endoplasmic reticulum. The majority of 11β-HSD1 peptide resides in the luminal space of the smooth endoplasmic reticulum with only five amino acids on the cytosolic side and the catalytic domain-containing C terminus protrudes into the lumen (Odermatt, Arnold, Stauffer, Frey, & Frey, 1999). The amino acid Lys5 but not Lys6 of 11β-HSD1 peptide is critical for the topology of 11β-HSD1. Glu25 and Glu26 in 11β-HSD1 are also responsible for determining its luminal orientation (Frick et al., 2004). N-terminally truncated form of rat 11β-HSD1 loses its catalytic activity (Mercer, Obeyesekere, Smith, & Krozowski, 1993; Obeid & White, 1992). 11β-HSD1 can form important disulfide bonds within the 11β-HSD1 second peptide structure and the luminal milieu promotes the formation of disulfide bonds (Ozols, 1995).

Purified rat 11β-HSD1 is a glycosylated protein (Lakshmi & Monder, 1988). Partial inhibition of glycosylation of recombinant protein decreased its oxidase activity by 50% without affecting reductive activity (Agarwal, Tusie-Luna, Monder, & White, 1990). Two potential N-linked glycosylation sites, Asn158-X-Ser160 and Asn203-X-Ser205, were identified in the translated peptide (Agarwal et al., 1990). Mutation of Asn203-X-Ser205 of rat 11β-HSD1 almost completely abolished both activities (Agarwal, Mune, Monder, & White, 1995), indicating that Asn203 glycosylation plays a major role and Asn158 a minor role in catalysis. Human 11β-HSD1 contains three potential glycosylation sites, Asn123-X-Ser125, Asn162-X-Ser164, and Asn207-X-Ser209. When human 11β-HSD1 cDNA (*HSD11B1*) is expressed in *Escherichia coli*, in which glycosylation does not occur, the enzyme lost its activity completely in one study (Blum, Martin, & Maser, 2000b) or maintained its activities in another study (Walker, Clark, Hewison, Ride, & Stewart, 2001). Mutagenesis of these three potential glycosylation sites revealed that all of these mutants lost their functions in yeast cells (Blum, Martin, & Maser, 2000a). Surprisingly, when the sugar residues were removed, the purified human 11β-HSD1 still retained complete enzyme activities (Blum et al., 2000a), indicating that glycosylation is not required for human 11β-HSD1 activity.

3.1.4 Tissue localization and possible function

11β-HSD1 is localized in glucocorticoid target tissues, including the lung, liver, testis, and brain. In the developing lung, 11β-HSD1 is a predominant reductase, because of the higher level of H6PDH (Gomez-Sanchez et al., 2009). Fetal lungs have significant higher enzyme activity of 11β-HSD1 toward the end of gestation (Suzuki et al., 2003). Importantly, 11β-HSD1 activity was significantly higher than 11β-HSD2 throughout gestation and after birth, since 11β-HSD2 does the opposite reaction (Suzuki et al., 2003). 11β-HSD1 has been found to be critical for lung development, since the null mutation of *Hsd11b1* gene or inhibition of the enzyme in mice delayed the lung maturity (Hundertmark et al., 2002). This suggests that lung 11β-HSD1 increases lung glucocorticoid availability by converting the receptor-inactive glucocorticoid to its active forms. Glucocorticoid plays a critical role in the modulation of phosphatidylcholine and surfactant protein synthesis in alveolar type II cells of fetal lung at the late gestation (Rooney, Young, & Mendelson, 1994). Phosphatidylcholine reduces surface tension of the alveolar wall and prevents atelectasis and may play an important role in maintaining normal alveolar structure. Surfactant proteins are known to be essential in the host defense system after birth (Mendelson et al., 1998).

11β-HSD1 is also abundantly present in human and rat livers (Agarwal, Rogerson, Mune, & White, 1995a; Ge, Gao, Nacharaju, Gunsalus, & Hardy, 1997) and acts as a reductase to generate active glucocorticoid locally due to higher expression of H6PDH (Agarwal, Rogerson, Mune, et al., 1995a; Ge et al., 1997). The glucocorticoid has been found to profoundly regulate the glucose metabolism in the liver (Yabaluri & Bashyam, 2010).

11β-HSD1 is abundantly present in Leydig cells of the testis (Ge et al., 1997; Phillips, Lakshmi, & Monder, 1989). In contrast to the lung and liver, Leydig cell 11β-HSD1 behaves as a primary oxidase (Ge et al., 1997). Leydig cell 11β-HSD1 oxidase directionality is possibly caused by its coupling to 17β-hydroxysteroid dehydrogenase 3 (17β-HSD3) (Latif et al., 2011). Leydig cell 17β-HSD3 uses NADPH as cofactor and generates NADP+, which derives 11β-HSD1 as a primary oxidase (Latif et al., 2011). The oxidase activity of 11β-HSD1 is very critical for Leydig cells to prevent from the inhibitory effects of endogenous glucocorticoids by inactivating them (Monder, Hardy, Blanchard, & Blanchard, 1994). Therefore, environmental pollutants that inhibit 11β-HSD1 can produce different effects on reproduction and development.

3.1.5 Environmental pollutants that inhibit 11β-HSD1

3.1.5.1 Perfluoroalkyl substance

The effects of perfluoroalkyl substance on 11β-HSD1 have been tested. Perfluorooctane sulfonate and perfluorooctanoic acid inhibited neonatal rat lung 11β-HSD1 activity with IC_{50} values of 3.4 and 45.3 μM and inhibited human liver 11β-HSD1 activity with IC_{50} values of 7.5 and 37.6 μM, respectively. However, the 4- and 6-carbon perfluoroalkyl substances did not inhibit the enzyme activity even at 250 μM. Both perfluorooctane sulfonate and perfluorooctanoic acid are competitive inhibitors against steroid substrates (Ye et al., 2012).

3.1.5.2 Bisphenol A

Bisphenol A inhibited human and rat 11β-HSD1 activities with IC_{50} values of 14.8 ± 0.1 μM for the human liver and 19.4 ± 0.1 μM for rat testis enzyme, respectively. Bisphenol A also inhibited rat 11β-HSD1 activity in intact rat Leydig cells. Bisphenol A is a competitive inhibitor for both human and rat 11β-HSD1 against 11ketoglucocorticoids (Guo et al., 2012).

3.1.5.3 Methoxychlor

Methoxychlor inhibited human 11β-HSD1 more potently than its metabolite HPTE, with IC_{50} values of 1.9 ± 0.1 and 8.9 ± 0.1 μM, respectively (Ge R.S., personal communication). However, methoxychlor and HPTE showed the opposite potency on rat enzyme. HPTE inhibited rat 11β-HSD1 with IC_{50} values of 9.2 ± 0.1 μM, and methoxychlor had no effect on rat enzyme at all. The modes of action of methoxychlor and HPTE on human 11β-HSD1 activities were competitive against steroid substrate.

3.1.5.4 Organotins

Although organotins potently inhibited 11β-HSD2 activity (Atanasov, Nashev, Tam, Baker, & Odermatt, 2005), they did not inhibit 11β-HSD1 at all (Atanasov et al., 2005).

3.1.5.5 Gossypol

Gossypol showed some inhibition on 11β-HSD1 activity. The inhibitory potency of gossypol depends on its enantiomer structure. (+) Gossypol inhibited both human and rat 11β-HSD1 reductase with IC_{50} values of 80.6 and 15.1 μM, respectively. However, (−) gossypol did not inhibit both human and rat 11β-HSD1 activities (Chen et al., 2009). Racemic gossypol inhibited NADP+-dependent 11β-HSD1 activity, with IC_{50} being 147 μM when 0.06 mM cortisol was used in the human kidney (Song, Lorenzo, & Reidenberg, 1992). Gossypol also inhibited guinea pig 11β-HSD1. Racemic gossypol was found to be a competitive inhibitor of guinea pig 11β-HSD1 with a Ki of 67 ± 5 μM, with the (+) enantiomer a little more potent than the (−) enantiomer of the gossypol (Sang, Lorenzo, & Reidenberg, 1991).

3.1.5.6 Licorice components

Licorice is the root of *Glycyrrhiza glabra*, from which a sweet flavor can be extracted and added to candies and soft drinks. Licorice is also widely used in Chinese traditional herbs as a flavor. Excessive consumption of licorice is known to be toxic, producing hypertension and edema (Atanasov et al., 2005). The licorice-caused apparent mineralocorticoid-like syndrome was first observed in 1953 (Borst, Ten Holt, De Vries, & Molhuysen, 1953).

There was an addictive effect of licorice and cortisone in the treatment of adrenal insufficiency (Borst et al., 1953). In 1989, licorice was demonstrated to inhibit rat liver 11β-HSD1 (Monder et al., 1989). The active component of licorice was found to be mainly glycyrrhetinic acid, which potently inhibited rat liver 11β-HSD1 (Marandici & Monder, 1993). The similar potency was found for the synthetic analog of glycyrrhetinic acid, carbenoxolone (Chen et al., 2009; Ge et al., 1997). Although carbenoxolone can produce apparent mineralocorticoid-like syndrome, the exact mechanism was not understood until the cloning of 11β-HSD2 in 1995. We found that carbenoxolone and glycyrrhetinic acid inhibited human 11β-HSD1 with IC_{50} values of 1.8 and 1.5 μM, respectively (Chen et al., 2009). Both carbenoxolone and glycyrrhetinic acid are competitive inhibitors of 11β-HSD1.

3.2. 11β-HSD2

3.2.1 Enzyme reaction

Human 11β-HSD2 is a high-affinity (K_m~25 nM for cortisol) enzyme (Albiston, Obeyesekere, Smith, & Krozowski, 1994). Human 11β-HSD2 primarily uses NAD+ as a cofactor (Albiston et al., 1994). 11β-HSD2 is a unidirectional enzyme and acts on the CH–OH group of donor with NAD+ as acceptor as follows: 11β-hydroxysteroid + NAD+ → 11-oxosteroid + NADH + H+ (Fig. 13.2). The function of 11β-HSD2 is the inactivation of active glucocorticoid cortisol in local tissues.

3.2.2 Gene

The human 11β-HSD2 is encoded by the *HSD11B2* gene. Human *HSD11B2* gene is located on chromosome 16q22 (Agarwal, Rogerson, Mune, & White, 1995b). The human *HSD11B2* gene is about 6.2 kb in length (Agarwal, Rogerson, Mune, et al., 1995b). Mutation of *HSD11B2* caused an apparent mineralocorticoid excess with manifestation of hypokalemia, hypertension, and lower or normal aldosterone concentrations (White, Mune, & Agarwal, 1997), suggesting that 11β-HSD2 is a critical enzyme for the regulation of water and salt balance.

3.2.3 Protein structure

11β-HSD2 has 405 amino acids (Agarwal, Rogerson, Mune, et al., 1995b). 11β-HSD2 also has an N-terminal nucleotide cofactor-binding domain and a catalytic active site in the central region like 11β-HSD1 (Oppermann et al., 1997). Using Boltzmann-weighted randomized modeling procedure and the X-ray crystal structure of 11β-HSD1 as a template, 11β-HSD2 homology was modeled and the model showed a significant 3D similarity to 11β-HSD1 (Yamaguchi et al., 2011). The secondary structure of human 11β-HSD2 had a central 6-stranded all-parallel β-sheet sandwich-like structure, flanked on both sides by 3-helices (Yamaguchi et al., 2011). The model revealed that Asp91, Phe94, Tyr232, and Thr267 residues could be important for interaction between NAD+ and 11β-HSD2 (Yamaguchi et al., 2012). Asp91 and Glu115 amino residues render the selectivity of human 11β-HSD2 of the cofactor NAD+ rather than NADP+ (Arnold et al., 2003). A mutation in the cofactor-binding domain Glu115 of 11β-HSD2 is associated with apparent mineralocorticoid excess (Odermatt et al., 2001). The mutation study showed that Tyr338His may maintain thermodynamic stability and folding of 11β-HSD2 (Atanasov et al., 2007).

3.2.4 Tissue localization and possible function

11β-HSD2 is located in the kidney, placenta, testis, epididymis, and vascular epithelium. The kidney cells contain mineralocorticoid receptor (Cole, 1995; Kyossev, Walker, & Reeves, 1996). In the kidney, 11β-HSD2 is located in the renal collecting ducts in the cortex, most of the medulla, the connecting tubule, and the distal convoluted tubule (Krozowski, MaGuire, et al., 1995; Whorwood et al., 1995). The endogenous ligand for mineralocorticoid receptor is aldosterone. Aldosterone binds to mineralocorticoid receptor to induce gene transcription of target genes to increase sodium and water retention and increase blood pressure. The native mineralocorticoid receptor binds to mineralocorticoid aldosterone and glucocorticoid cortisol with similar affinities (Arriza et al., 1987). 11β-HSD2 in these cells inactivates cortisol, thus letting aldosterone binding to its receptor. The mutation of 11β-HSD2 (*HSD11B2*) gene caused apparent mineralocorticoid excess, in which patients have hypertension and hypokalemia, because mutant 11β-HSD2 is unable to metabolize cortisol that is built up in the mineralocorticoid target tissues (Edwards et al., 1988; White, Mune, Rogerson, Kayes, & Agarwal, 1997b). Apparent mineralocorticoid excess can be caused not only by mutational inactivation of the *HSD11B2* but also by the enzyme inhibitors (Funder, Pearce, Smith, & Smith, 1988; Stewart et al., 1987; White, Mune, Rogerson, Kayes, & Agarwal, 1997a). The phenotype of apparent mineralocorticoid excess was mimicked by *Hsd11b2* knockout in the mice (Kotelevtsev et al., 1999).

In the placenta, 11β-HSD2 is localized in glucocorticoid target tissue syncytiotrophoblast, where maternal–fetal exchange takes place (Krozowski,

Albiston, Obeyesekere, Andrews, & Smith, 1995). The placental 11β-HSD2 is responsible for pregnancy maintenance and fetal maturation. Placental 11β-HSD2 protects the fetus from overexposure to maternal cortisol, which may check fetal development and cause cardiovascular, metabolic, and neuropsychiatric disorders, by inactivating it (Doyle, Faber, Callanan, & Morley, 2003; Seckl, 2004; Seckl & Holmes, 2007). In the *Hsd11b2* knockout mouse, body weight of fetus and placental weight were significantly reduced, indicating that fetal intrauterine restriction takes place (Waddell, Hisheh, Krozowski, & Burton, 2003; Wyrwoll, Seckl, & Holmes, 2009).

11β-HSD2 is also present in Leydig cells and is critical for lowering intracellular glucocorticoid level (Ge et al., 2005b; Haeussler & Claus, 2007). The expression of 11β-HSD2 was localized to Leydig cells and blood capillaries (Claus et al., 2007). 11β-HSD2 is also present in other organs of the male reproductive tract including the epididymis (Moore, Hoong, & Cole, 2000; Waddell et al., 2003). The clear cells but not the principal cells of epididymal epithelium contain 11β-HSD2 (Waddell et al., 2003). The presence of 11β-HSD2 in the epididymal epithelium has been suggested to render mineralocorticoid receptor selectivity (Waddell et al., 2003) since the organ has mineralocorticoid receptor (Pearce, Lipkevicius, & Funder, 1986).

11β-HSD2 is present in endothelial cells of arterioles and veins in both human (Jang et al., 2007; Smith, Little, Maguire, Stein-Oakley, & Krozowski, 1996) and rodents (Christy et al., 2003). Mineralocorticoid receptor is colocalized with 11β-HSD2 in endothelial cells (Krug et al., 2007). Inhibition of 11β-HSD2 lets glucocorticoid cortisol to activate mineralocorticoid receptor in aortic endothelial cells (Caprio et al., 2008). Vascular specific mutation of *Hsd11b2* led to atherogenesis associated with activation of mineralocorticoid receptor (Deuchar et al., 2011).

3.2.5 Environmental pollutants that inhibit 11β-HSD2

3.2.5.1 Perfluoroalkyl substance

Many perfluoroalkyl substances are potent inhibitors of human and rat 11β-HSD2 activities. Perfluorooctyl sulfonate, perfluorooctanoic acid, and perfluorohexyl sulfonate inhibited human 11β-HSD2 with IC_{50} values of 48 nM, 24.4 μM, and 19.0 μM, respectively. They also inhibited rat 11β-HSD2 with IC_{50} values of 293 nM, 3.8 μM, and 62.9 μM, respectively (Zhao et al., 2011). However, perfluorobutyl sulfonate had no effects even at concentration of 250 μM (Zhao et al., 2011). Apparently, rats and mice exposed to perfluorooctyl sulfonate have elevated levels of circulating glucocorticoid corticosterone (Austin et al., 2003; Zheng, Dong, Jin, & He, 2009), indicating the *in vivo* inhibition of glucocorticoid metabolism.

3.2.5.2 Bisphenol A

Bisphenol A weakly inhibited both human and rat 11β-HSD2 activities. At 100 μM, BPA inhibited human and rat enzymes by 51.16% and 41.61%, respectively. Therefore, bisphenol A is a more selective inhibitor for 11β-HSD1 (Guo et al., 2012).

3.2.5.3 Methoxychlor

Methoxychlor metabolite HPTE also inhibited human and rat 11β-HSD2 with IC_{50} values of 55.57 ± 0.08 and 12.95 ± 0.11 μM, respectively (Ge, personal communication). Therefore, HPTE is more selective against 11β-HSD1. However, methoxychlor had no effects at 250 μM. HPTE is a competitive inhibitor of human and rat 11β-HSD2 against steroid substrate.

3.2.5.4 Organotins

Organotins potently inhibited human 11β-HSD2 activity. Tributyltin, dibutyltin, triphenyltin, and diphenyltin inhibited human 11β-HSD2 with IC_{50} values of 1.90 ± 0.66, 1.95 ± 0.27, 3.19 ± 0.73, and 1.42 ± 0.17 μM, respectively. The inhibition of human 11β-HSD2 activity by triphenyltin and tributyltin was also confirmed in human kidney microsomes, although the IC_{50} was slightly higher with 16.5 μM for tributyltin (Ohshima, Ohno, & Nakajin, 2005). Mutational analysis indicates that cysteines (Cys90, Cys228, and Cys264) in 11β-HSD2 are essential for enzymatic stability and catalytic activity (Atanasov et al., 2005). Organotins possibly disrupt the interaction by binding to cysteines of the enzyme (Atanasov et al., 2005).

3.2.5.5 Gossypol

Of enantiomers, (+)-gossypol inhibited human and rat 11β-HSD2 twofold more potent than (−)-gossypol. The IC_{50} values of (+)-gossypol for human and rat 11β-HSD2 activity are 1.05 and 0.61 μM compared to those of (−)-gossypol, which are 1.95 and 1.33 μM, respectively (Chen et al., 2009). Apparently, racemic gossypol selectively inhibited 11β-HSD2 because the IC_{50}values for 11β-HSD1 from human, rat, and guinea pig kidney were over 50 μM (Chen et al., 2009; Sang et al., 1991; Song et al., 1992).

3.2.5.6 Licorice and its components

It is longer ago that licorice was found to be associated with apparent mineralocorticoid-like syndrome (Borst et al., 1953). We compared the inhibitory potency of carbenoxolone on human 11β-HSD1 and 2 and found that carbenoxolone is a more specific 11β-HSD2 inhibitor, which has IC_{50}s of 20 and 50 nM for human and rat 11β-HSD2, respectively (Chen et al., 2009). Glycyrrhetinic acid is also a more specific inhibitor for human 11β-HSD2 with IC_{50} of 11 nM (Brown et al., 1996). Structure–activity relationship study of the glycyrrhetinic acid derivatives revealed that 3-hydroxyl and/or the carboxyl is required specific inhibition of 11β-HSD2 (Kratschmar et al., 2011).

3.2.5.7 Phthalates

Mono(2-ethylhexyl) phthalate significantly inhibited human 11β-HSD2 with IC_{50} of 110.8 μM (Zhao, Chu, Huang, et al., 2010), rat one with IC_{50} of 121.8 μM (Zhao, Chu, Huang, et al., 2010), and mouse enzyme with IC_{50} of 327.9 μM (Hong et al., 2009), even though its parent compound di(2-ethylhexyl) phthalate did not. Mono(2-ethylhexyl) phthalate was a competitive inhibitor of human and rat 11β-HSD2 when substrate glucocorticoids were used (Zhao, Chu, Huang, et al., 2010). 12 phthalate diesters and four monoesters for the inhibition of human and rat kidney 11β-HSD2 activities were examined (Zhao, Chu, Huang, et al., 2010). Of the phthalate diesters, dipropyl phthalate and di-*n*-butyl phthalate significantly inhibited both human and rat 11β-HSD2 activities with IC_{50} values of 85.6 μM for dipropyl phthalate and 13.7 μM for di-*n*-butyl phthalate in the inhibition of rat 11β-HSD2 activity. Compared to dipropyl phthalate and di-*n*-butyl phthalate, noninhibitory phthalates have either fewer carbons (1 or 2 carbons) or more carbons (5–10 carbons) in the alcohol moiety of phthalates. However, a phthalate could become an inhibitor of 11β-HSD2 activity with six carbons in the alcohol moiety if the carbon is cyclized as in dicyclohexyl phthalate, which inhibited rat 11β-HSD2 activity with an IC_{50} of 32.64 μM (Zhao, Chu, Huang, et al., 2010) or human 11β-HSD2 activity with an IC_{50} of 46.5 μM (Ohshima et al., 2005). Thus, whether a phthalate is an inhibitor may reflect the size and shape of the compound (Zhao, Chu, Huang, et al., 2010). Indeed, prepubertal male rats exposed to di-*n*-butyl phthalate for 30 days had significant increase of serum glucocorticoid concentration (Xiao-feng, Nai-qiang, Jing, Zi, & Yang, 2009), which was possibly contributed from the inhibition of kidney 11β-HSD2, since the inhibition of

11β-HSD2 by glycyrrhetinic acid has been reported to increase serum glucocorticoid level (Hu et al., 2008). Increased glucocorticoids may have many impacts on fetal development (Benediktsson, Calder, Edwards, & Seckl, 1997; Benediktsson, Lindsay, Noble, Seckl, & Edwards, 1993; Hahn et al., 1999; Seckl, 1997). A nested case–control study of Chinese newborns showed that low body weight of babies was correlated with higher di(2-ethylhexyl) phthalate and di-*n*-butyl phthalate levels in mother's blood (Zhang et al., 2009), suggesting that phthalates may negatively disrupt placental function.

3.2.5.8 Alkylphenols

Alkylphenols are used to make alkylphenol ethoxylates, which are widely used as industrial surfactants. They are used as emulsifiers for polymerization, as detergents and pesticides, and in the processing of wool and metals. Many alkylphenols including 4-*t*-octylphenol, 4-nonylphenol, 4-*n*-octylphenol, and 4-*n*-nonylphenol have been classified endocrine disruptors due to their weak estrogen-like activities (Soaresam, Guieysseb, Jeffersona, Cartmella, & Lestera, 2008). Many alkylphenols have been shown to directly inhibit human kidney 11β-HSD2 activity with IC_{50}s of 8.9 μM for 4-*t*-octylphenol, 20.3 μM for 4-nonylphenol, 23.5 μM for 4-*n*-octylphenol, and 26.2 μM for 4-*n*-nonylphenol (Ohshima et al., 2005). The exact mode of inhibition of these chemicals is unclear.

3.2.5.9 Dithiocarbamates

Dithiocarbamates are important therapeutic and industrial chemicals and they are leached out into the environment in a large amount. One of dithiocarbamates, thiram, is used as a fungicide both in the field and as a seed protectant. It has been applied on fruits and been applied postharvest on a number of seed crops. Thiram (50 μM) completely inhibited human 11β-HSD2 activity. The inhibition was irreversible (Atanasov, Tam, Rocken, Baker, & Odermatt, 2003). The sulfhydryl-protecting reagent dithiothreitol reversed thiram-mediated inhibition and NAD+ partially protected 11β-HSD2 activity, indicating that thiram acts at the cofactor-binding site. Cys90 amino acid in the NAD+-binding site is a likely target of thiram (Atanasov et al., 2003). Through the inhibition of 11β-HSD2, thiram regulates glucocorticoid-mediated responses in the human lung epithelial cells (Garbrecht, Krozowski, Snyder, & Schmidt, 2006).

4. 17β-HYDROXYSTEROID DEHYDROGENASE

17β-HSD is a subfamily of HSDs that catalyze the interconversion between 17-ketosteroids, dehydroepiandrosterone, androstenedione estrone, and 17β-hydroxyl steroids, androstenediol, testosterone, and estradiol (Labrie et al., 1997). A total 15 isoforms in the human (human 17β-HSD1–17β-HSD15) have been identified. Many environmental pollutants have been tested to inhibit 17β-HSD1 and 17β-HSD3 activities. Therefore, the present chapter discusses the inhibitors on only 17β-HSD1 and 17β-HSD3 activities.

4.1. 17β-HSD1

17β-HSD1 was the first of the 17HSD/ketosteroid reductases to be cloned and characterized. 17β-HSD1 was first purified from human placenta. It was cloned originally from a human placental library and subsequently found to be expressed in the ovary and the mammary gland.

4.1.1 Enzyme reaction

Human 17β-HSD1 primarily catalyzes the 17-ketoreduction for estrogens. This preferably uses NADPH cofactor and catalyzes conversion of estrone to estradiol to increase estrogenic action (Penning, 1997). 17β-HSD1 acts on the C=O group of donor with NADPH as acceptor as follows: estrone + NADPH → estradiol + NADP+ (Fig. 13.3). Human 17β-HSD1

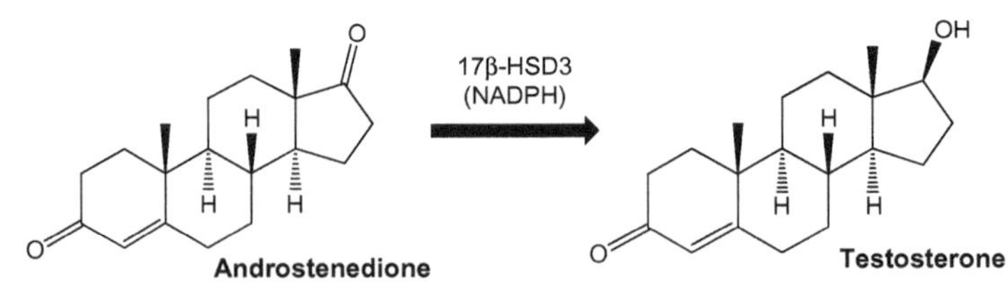

Figure 13.3 The reaction catalyzed by 17β-hydroxysteroid dehydrogenases. The top panel shows the catalysis by type I isoform (17β-HSD1) and the bottom panel shows the catalysis by type III isoform (17β-HSD3).

has much higher affinity for C18 steroids than C19 steroids. However, mouse and rat 17β-HSD1 also efficiently catalyzes C19 steroid androstenedione to testosterone (Puranen, Poutanen, Ghosh, Vihko, & Vihko, 1997b).

4.1.2 Gene

Each 17β-HSD human isoform is the product of a distinct gene. Human 17β-HSD1 is encoded by the human gene *HSD17B1*. The gene is located in chromosome 17q11–q21 (Luu-The et al., 1989). The human *HSD17B1* gene is about 13 kb in length (Luu-The et al., 1990).

4.1.3 Protein structure

17β-HSD1 has 327 amino acids and a molecular mass of 34.9 kDa (Luu-The et al., 1990). 17β-HSD1 is a member of the short-chain alcohol dehydrogenase reductase superfamily. 17β-HSD1 is present as a homodimer, which consists of noncovalently bound subunits (Ghosh et al., 1995). There are two dimerization helices in each monomer forming a four-helix bundle (Ghosh et al., 1995). The disruption of the helices in the enzyme causes improper protein folding and aggregation (Puranen, Poutanen, Ghosh, Vihko, & Vihko, 1997a). 17β-HSD1 contains three α-helices and a helix–turn–helix motif. The inserted helices are located at one end of the substrate-binding cleft away from the catalytic triad, restricting access to the active site of substrate (Duax, Ghosh, & Pletnev, 2000; Ghosh et al., 1995). The histidine on the helical insert of residues 209–229 forms a hydrogen bond to oxygen at position 3 of the steroid A-ring and creates specific binding of steroids (Duax et al., 2000; Ghosh et al., 1995). His-221 is essential for catalytic activity (Puranen, Poutanen, Peltoketo, Vihko, & Vihko, 1994).

4.1.4 Tissue localization and possible function

17β-HSD1 is abundantly expressed in the granulosa cells of developing follicles of placenta in the human (Green, Speirs, Landolt, Foy, & Atkin, 1999). 17β-HSD1 does not exist in rat placenta. 17β-HSD1 is mainly located in the syncytiotrophoblast of human placenta and in granulosa cells of human ovary (Green et al., 1999).

4.1.5 Environmental pollutants that inhibit 17β-HSD1

Diethylstilbestrol is a nonsteroidal estrogen. It is an endocrine disruptor. Humans are exposed to diethylstilbestrol via various sources such as dietary ingestion from supplemented cattle feed and medical treatment.

Diethylstilbestrol has been shown to cause a rare vaginal tumor in girls and young women who had been exposed to this drug *in utero* (Herbst, Ulfelder, & Poskanzer, 1971). These girls may also have an increased risk of moderate to severe cervical squamous cell dysplasia and an increased risk of breast cancer (Troisi et al., 2007). Diethylstilbestrol has been shown to cause malformations in daughters and sons who were exposed *in utero* (Hoover et al., 2011). Diethylstilbestrol has been demonstrated to inhibit human 17β-HSD1 with Ki of 3.3 μM (Poirier, 2003).

Many flavonoids have been tested to have inhibitory effects on human 17β-HSD1 activity. Soy isoflavone genistein inhibited human 17β-HSD1 with IC_{50} value of 50 μM (Brooks & Thompson, 2005). Cottonseed flavonoid gossypol competitively inhibited human 17β-HSD1 with Ki as low as 2 μM (Brown et al., 2003). Genkwanin and diosmetin are o-methylated flavones, isolated from the seeds of *Alnus glutinosa* and plants of Caucasian vetch, respectively. Scutellarein is a flavone found in *Scutellaria lateriflora.* Chrysoeriol is a flavonoid found in several tropical medicinal plants. Fisetin is a flavonol and found in many plants to serve as a coloring agent. All these flavonoids showed about 80% inhibition on human 17β-HSD1 at 6 μM (Brozic et al., 2009).

Benzophenones are the synthesized chemicals that block UV and are widely used in inks, imaging, and clear coatings in the printing industry. Benzophenones are exposed because they migrate into food from packing (Rodriguez-Bernaldo de Quiros et al., 2009). Many benzophenones may have endocrine-disrupting activities. Of nine benzophenones (1–8 and 12) tested, benzophenone 1 is a potent inhibitor of human 17β-HSD1 with IC_{50} about 20 μM (Nashev et al., 2010).

4.2. 17β-HSD3

4.2.1 Enzyme reaction

There are over 15 17β-HSD isoforms (Penning, 1997). Only 17β-HSD3 is located in Leydig cells for the final conversion of androstenedione into testosterone (Ge & Hardy, 1998). 17β-HSD3 requires NADPH as its cofactor. 17β-HSD3 acts on the C=O group of donor with NADPH as acceptor as follows: androstenedione + NADPH → testosterone + NADP+ (Fig. 13.3). The mutation of *HSD17B3* causes various phenotypes including pseudohermaphroditism with very low circulating testosterone concentrations in males (Andersson et al., 1996; Rosler, Silverstein, & Abeliovich, 1996).

4.2.2 Gene

The human 17β-HSD3 is encoded by the *HSD17B3* gene. Human *HSD17B3* gene is located on chromosome 9q22. The human *HSD17B3* gene is about 60 kb in length and contains 11 exons. Mutation of *HSD17B3* caused male pseudohermaphrodites (Geissler et al., 1994), suggesting that 17β-HSD3 is a critical enzyme for the regulation of reproduction.

4.2.3 Protein structure

17β-HSD3 has 310 amino acids and the protein has a molecular mass of 34.5 kDa (Geissler et al., 1994). Site-directed mutational analysis showed that Tyr80 was critical for cofactor binding and that substitution with different amino acid caused switching from NADPH to NADH (McKeever et al., 2002).

4.2.4 Tissue localization and possible function

17β-HSD3 is primarily localized in the testes (Ge & Hardy, 1998). The protein exclusively resides in immature and adult Leydig cells but not progenitor and stem Leydig cells in the adult Leydig cell population (Ge et al., 2006; Ge & Hardy, 1998). When *Hsd17b3* mRNA expression was examined in the developing mouse testis, it was found that *Hsd17b3* was also expressed in seminiferous tubules until postnatal day 10 (O'Shaughnessy, Baker, Heikkila, Vainio, & McMahon, 2000). Between postnatal days 10 and 20, there was no expression of *Hsd17b3* in the mouse testis and there was an increased expression in the immature Leydig cells of interstitial tissues (O'Shaughnessy et al., 2000). 17β-HSD3 enzyme activity paralleled the distribution of *Hsd17b3* mRNA.

4.2.5 Environmental pollutants that inhibit 17β-HSD3

4.2.5.1 Perfluoroalkyl substance

Perfluorooctane sulfonate is a very potent human 17β-HSD3 inhibitor. There is clear structure–activity response difference, with the potencies of perfluorooctane sulfonate ($IC_{50}=6.0\ \mu M$) > perfluorooctanoic acid ($IC_{50}=127.6\ \mu M$) > perfluorohexyl sulfonate (no inhibition at 250 μM) = perfluorobutyl sulfonate (no inhibition at 250 μM) (Zhao, Hu, Chu, et al., 2010). Perfluorooctane sulfonate is a noncompetitive inhibitor of human 17β-HSD3 (Zhao, Hu, Chu, et al., 2010). Of perfluoroalkyl substances, only perfluorooctanoic acid potently inhibited rat Leydig cell 17β-HSD3 with IC_{50} of 17 μM (Zhao, Hu, Chu, et al., 2010). The inhibition of

17β-HSD3 activities in Leydig cells clearly led to the decrease of testosterone production (Zhao, Hu, Chu, et al., 2010).

4.2.5.2 Bisphenol A

BPA is also a weak human and rat 17β-HSD3 activity inhibitor with IC_{50} values about 100 μM (Adu-Kumi et al., 2012).

4.2.5.3 Methoxychlor

At the concentration as high as 100 μM, methoxychlor does not have inhibitory effects on human and rat 17β-HSD3 activities, while its metabolite HPTE significantly inhibited human and rat 17β-HSD3 activities with IC_{50} values of 12.1 μM (human) and 32.0 μM (rat), suggesting that methoxychlor is metabolically activated into HPTE to inhibit 17β-HSD3 activity (Hu et al., 2011).

4.2.5.4 Organotins

Triphenyltin and tributyltin inhibited 17β-HSD3 activities from pig Leydig cells with IC_{50}s of 48 and 148 nM, respectively (Ohno, Nakajima, & Nakajin, 2005). Triphenyltin was investigated to test its *in vitro* effects on human testosterone biosynthetic enzyme 17β-HSD3 activity (Lo et al., 2003). The IC_{50} of triphenyltin inhibiting 17β-HSD3 was 4.2 μM (Lo et al., 2003).

4.2.5.5 Gossypol

Gossypol potently inhibited human and rat 17β-HSD3 with clear enantiomer-specific differences. (−)-Gossypol inhibited human and rat 17β-HSD3 activities with IC_{50} values of 0.36 and 3.43 μM, respectively, while the (+)-gossypol is slightly less potent and inhibited human and rat 17β-HSD3 activities with IC_{50} of 1.13 and 10.93 μM, respectively (Hu et al., 2009).

4.2.5.6 Phthalates

We also demonstrated that dipropyl phthalate, di-*n*-butyl phthalate, dipentyl phthalate, dicyclohexyl phthalate, benzyl octyl phthalate, and butyl benzyl phthalate significantly inhibited both human and rat testicular 17β-HSD3 activities at concentrations of 100 μM. Only benzyl octyl phthalate and dicyclohexyl phthalate potently inhibited human (IC_{50} values, 23.3 and 8.2 μM) and rat (IC_{50} values, 30.24 and 9. 1 μM) 17β-HSD3 activities potently. The mode of action of dicyclohexyl phthalate on 17β-HSD3 activity was competitive with the substrate androstenedione but non-competitive with the cofactor NADPH (Yuan et al., 2012).

4.2.5.7 Benzophenone

Of nine benzophenones (1–8 and 12) tested, benzophenone 1 is the most potent inhibitor of human 17β-HSD3 activities with IC_{50} of 1 μM, while others have IC_{50}s around 47–111 μM (Nashev et al., 2010). Apparently, the inhibition of benzophenone 1 on human 17β-HSD3 activity is selective, since it inhibits 17β-HSD1 and 17β-HSD2 activities with IC_{50} values over 20 μM and has no inhibition on 17β-HSD5 activity (Nashev et al., 2010). Rodent models also show that benzophenone 1 significantly inhibited testosterone production in mouse and rat testes (Nashev et al., 2010).

5. 20α-HYDROXYSTEROID DEHYDROGENASE

20α-HSD is an enzyme that catalyzes the conversion of progesterone into 20α-hydroxyprogesterone. 20α-HSD is involved in the metabolism of progesterone in the ovary, uterus, and cervix. Although human 20α-HSD is encoded by the *AKR1C1* gene, which belongs to the *AKR1C* subfamily, including four human enzymes 20α-HSD (AKR1C1), AKR1C2, AKR1C3, and AKR1C4, only AKR1C1 acts primarily as 20α-HSD. Only several environmental pollutants have been tested to inhibit 20α-HSD. Therefore, the present chapter will discuss 20α-HSD (AKR1C1).

5.1. 20α-HSD (AKR1C1)

5.1.1 Enzyme reaction

20α-HSD catalyzes the conversion of progesterone to 20α-hydroxyprogesterone. This enzyme belongs to the family of oxidoreductases. Human 20α-HSD primarily uses NADPH as a cofactor. 20α-HSD acts on the C=O group of donor with NADPH as acceptor as follows: progesterone + NADPH → 20α-hydroxyprogesterone + NADP+ (Fig. 13.4). The function of 20α-HSD is the inactivation of active progesterone in local tissues.

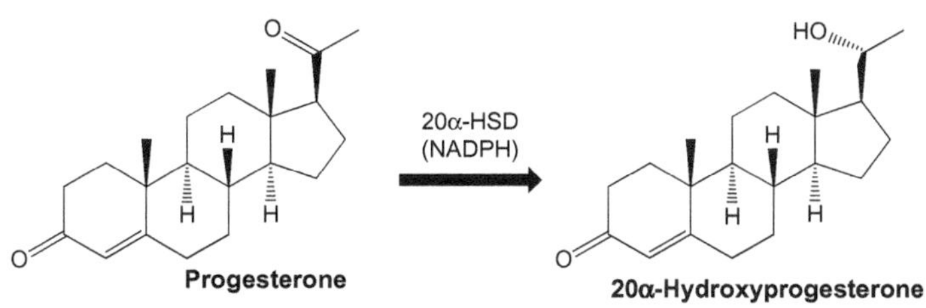

Figure 13.4 The reaction catalyzed by 20α-hydroxysteroid dehydrogenase (AKR1C1).

5.1.2 Gene

The human 20α-HSD is encoded by the *AKR1C1* gene. It belongs to the *AKR1C* subfamily, which includes four human enzymes AKR1C1, AKR1C2, AKR1C3, and AKR1C4. These enzymes share high percentages of amino acid homology (84–98%). However, they have a completely different enzymatic catalysis for steroids. For example, AKR1C1 and AKR1C2 differ in only seven amino acid residues, but AKR1C1 is 20α-HSD, and AKR1C2 is 3α-HSD (Usami et al., 2002). Each *AKR1C* gene is located on chromosome 10p15–p14.

5.1.3 Protein structure

20α-HSD is a cytosolic soluble protein with 37 kDa. 20α-HSD has (α/β8)-barrel and a catalytic tetrad of Tyr55, Asp50, Lys84, and His117 (Jez, Bennett, Schlegel, Lewis, & Penning, 1997). Although 20α-HSD can oxidize hydroxysteroids *in vitro*, however, it acts primarily as a ketosteroid reductase *in vivo*. For 20α-HSD catalysis, 20-ketosteroid substrate must bind backward relative to progesterone for 20α-hydroxysteroid to form.

5.1.4 Tissue localization and possible function

20α-HSD (AKR1C1) has been detected in myometrium (Lee et al., 2008; Nakajima et al., 2003). The increased 20α-HSD activity may be responsible for the increased 20α-hydroxyprogesterone concentration that is associated with spontaneous labor (Lee et al., 2008; Nakajima et al., 2003). 20α-HSD (AKR1C1) is also expressed in the human cervix (Andersson, Minjarez, Yost, & Word, 2008). In human cervical fibroblasts, interleukin-1β significantly induced 20α-HSD (AKR1C1) expression, thus accelerating progesterone metabolism to 20α-hydroxyprogesterone in cervical fibroblasts (Andersson et al., 2008). The increased 20α-HSD may have impact on cervical structure to increase the chance of a preterm birth (Roberson, Hyatt, Kenkel, Hanson, & Myers, 2011).

5.1.5 Environmental pollutants that inhibit 20α-HSD

Phenolphthalein is used in toys as a component of disappearing inks and has been commonly used as a laxative. Phenolphthalein is synthesized by condensation of phthalic anhydride with phenols. It was reported to cause multiple types of cancers on animal models (Dunnick & Hailey, 1996). Phenolphthalein inhibited human 20α-HSD with IC_{50} of 330 nM (Higaki et al., 2003). Phenolphthalein derivatives 3′,3″,5′,5″-tetrabromophenolphthalein and 3′,3″,5′,5″-tetraiodophenolphthalein are more potent with IC_{50} values of 33 and 120 nM, respectively (Higaki et al., 2003).

Coumestrol is a natural organic compound and is abundant in some foods such as soybeans. Coumestrol is classified as a phytoestrogen, which mimics the physiological actions of estradiol (Blomquist, Lima, & Hotchkiss, 2005). This compound is reported to inhibit 3α-HSD and aromatase activities (Blomquist et al., 2005). Coumestrol also inhibited human 20α-HSD with IC_{50} of 200 nM (Poirier, 2003). Therefore, it could interfere with progesterone metabolism.

Licorice component glycyrrhetinic acid has been reported to inhibit many HSDs including 3β-HSD2, 11β-HSD1, 11β-HSD2, and 17β-HSD3 (Ma, Lian, Dong, & Ge, 2011; Monder et al., 1989; Ye, Su, & Ge, 2011). Glycyrrhetinic acid also inhibited human 20α-HSD with IC_{50} of 2.2 μM (Higaki et al., 2003).

Quercitrin is a glycoside formed from the flavonoid quercetin and the deoxy sugar rhamnose. It is used as a constituent of the dye quercitron. It inhibited mouse liver 20α-HSD by 85% when 20 μM quercitrin is used (Shimada, Ohtaguro, Miura, & Imamura, 2007).

Benzbromarone is a uricosuric agent used in the treatment of gout and it also potently inhibited human 20α-HSD, with IC_{50} of 48 nM (Higaki et al., 2003).

6. SUMMARY AND CONCLUSION

HSDs are responsible for the biosynthesis and metabolism of many steroid hormones, which are critical for developmental and reproductive and adrenal function. Four types of HSDs are reported. Disruption of HSDs by environmental pollutants can interfere with steroid biosynthesis and metabolism, leading to sexual dysfunction, infertility, and adrenal dysfunction. Many environmental pollutants inhibit one or more types of HSDs. Because there are many isoforms of each type of HSDs, increased efforts are required to identify the inhibitory effects of environmental pollutants on different isoforms of these types of HSDs.

ACKNOWLEDGMENTS

Supported in part by NSFC 81102150 to L. Y. and NSFC 30871434 and 31171425 and Health Bureau of Zhejiang Province 11-CX29 to R. S. G.

REFERENCES

Abdellatif, A. G., Preat, V., Vamecq, J., Nilsson, R., & Roberfroid, M. (1990). Peroxisome proliferation and modulation of rat liver carcinogenesis by 2,4-dichlorophenoxyacetic acid, 2,4,5-trichlorophenoxyacetic acid, perfluorooctanoic acid and nafenopin. *Carcinogenesis, 11*, 1899–1902.

Adu-Kumi, S., Kares, R., Literak, J., Boruvkova, J., Yeboah, P. O., Carboo, D., et al. (2012). Levels and seasonal variations of organochlorine pesticides in urban and rural background air of southern Ghana. *Environmental Science and Pollution Research International, 19*, 1963–1970.

Agarwal, A. K., Monder, C., Eckstein, B., & White, P. C. (1989). Cloning and expression of rat cDNA encoding corticosteroid 11β-dehydrogenase. *The Journal of Biological Chemistry, 264*, 18939–18943.

Agarwal, A. K., Mune, T., Monder, C., & White, P. C. (1995). Mutations in putative glycosylation sites of rat 11 beta-hydroxysteroid dehydrogenase affect enzymatic activity. *Biochimica et Biophysica Acta, 1248*, 70–74.

Agarwal, A. K., Rogerson, F. M., Mune, T., & White, P. C. (1995a). Analysis of the human gene encoding the kidney isozyme of 11 beta-hydroxysteroid dehydrogenase. *Journal of Steroid Biochemistry and Molecular Biology, 55*, 473–479.

Agarwal, A. K., Rogerson, F. M., Mune, T., & White, P. C. (1995b). Gene structure and chromosomal localization of the human HSD11K gene encoding the kidney (type 2) isozyme of 11 beta-hydroxysteroid dehydrogenase. *Genomics, 29*, 195–199.

Agarwal, A. K., Tusie-Luna, M. T., Monder, C., & White, P. C. (1990). Expression of 11 beta-hydroxysteroid dehydrogenase using recombinant vaccinia virus. *Molecular Endocrinology, 4*, 1827–1832.

Akingbemi, B. T., Ge, R. S., Klinefelter, G. R., Gunsalus, G. L., & Hardy, M. P. (2000). A metabolite of methoxychlor, 2,2-bis(p-hydroxyphenyl)-1,1, 1-trichloroethane, reduces testosterone biosynthesis in rat leydig cells through suppression of steady-state messenger ribonucleic acid levels of the cholesterol side-chain cleavage enzyme. *Biology of Reproduction, 62*, 571–578.

Akingbemi, B. T., & Hardy, M. P. (2001). Oestrogenic and antiandrogenic chemicals in the environment: Effects on male reproductive health. *Annals of Medicine, 33*, 391–403.

Akingbemi, B. T., Sottas, C. M., Koulova, A. I., Klinefelter, G. R., & Hardy, M. P. (2004). Inhibition of testicular steroidogenesis by the xenoestrogen bisphenol A is associated with reduced pituitary luteinizing hormone secretion and decreased steroidogenic enzyme gene expression in rat Leydig cells. *Endocrinology, 145*, 592–603.

Albiston, A. L., Obeyesekere, V. R., Smith, R. E., & Krozowski, Z. S. (1994). Cloning and tissue distribution of the human 11 beta-hydroxysteroid dehydrogenase type 2 enzyme. *Molecular and Cellular Endocrinology, 105*, R11–R17.

Albro, P. W., Corbett, J. T., Schroeder, J. L., Jordan, S., & Matthews, H. B. (1982). Pharmacokinetics, interactions with macromolecules and species differences in metabolism of DEHP. *Environmental Health Perspectives, 45*, 19–25.

Andersson, S., Geissler, W. M., Wu, L., Davis, D. L., Grumbach, M. M., New, M. I., et al. (1996). Molecular genetics and pathophysiology of 17 beta-hydroxysteroid dehydrogenase 3 deficiency. *Journal of Clinical Endocrinology and Metabolism, 81*, 130–136.

Andersson, S., Minjarez, D., Yost, N. P., & Word, R. A. (2008). Estrogen and progesterone metabolism in the cervix during pregnancy and parturition. *Journal of Clinical Endocrinology and Metabolism, 93*, 2366–2374.

Arnold, P., Tam, S., Yan, L., Baker, M. E., Frey, F. J., & Odermatt, A. (2003). Glutamate-115 renders specificity of human 11beta-hydroxysteroid dehydrogenase type 2 for the cofactor NAD+. *Molecular and Cellular Endocrinology, 201*, 177–187.

Arriza, J. L., Weinberger, C., Cerelli, G., Glaser, T. M., Handelin, B. L., Housman, D. E., et al. (1987). Cloning of human mineralocorticoid receptor complementary

DNA: Structural and functional kinship with the glucocorticoid receptor. *Science*, *237*, 268–275.

Atanasov, A. G., Ignatova, I. D., Nashev, L. G., Dick, B., Ferrari, P., Frey, F. J., et al. (2007). Impaired protein stability of 11beta-hydroxysteroid dehydrogenase type 2: A novel mechanism of apparent mineralocorticoid excess. *Journal of the American Society of Nephrology*, *18*, 1262–1270.

Atanasov, A. G., Nashev, L. G., Gelman, L., Legeza, B., Sack, R., Portmann, R., et al. (2008). Direct protein-protein interaction of 11beta-hydroxysteroid dehydrogenase type 1 and hexose-6-phosphate dehydrogenase in the endoplasmic reticulum lumen. *Biochimica et Biophysica Acta*, *1783*, 1536–1543.

Atanasov, A. G., Nashev, L. G., Schweizer, R. A., Frick, C., & Odermatt, A. (2004). Hexose-6-phosphate dehydrogenase determines the reaction direction of 11β-hydroxysteroid dehydrogenase type 1 as an oxoreductase. *FEBS Letters*, *571*, 129–133.

Atanasov, A. G., Nashev, L. G., Tam, S., Baker, M. E., & Odermatt, A. (2005). Organotins disrupt the 11beta-hydroxysteroid dehydrogenase type 2-dependent local inactivation of glucocorticoids. *Environmental Health Perspectives*, *113*, 1600–1606.

Atanasov, A. G., Tam, S., Rocken, J. M., Baker, M. E., & Odermatt, A. (2003). Inhibition of 11 beta-hydroxysteroid dehydrogenase type 2 by dithiocarbamates. *Biochemical and Biophysical Research Communications*, *308*, 257–262.

Austin, M. E., Kasturi, B. S., Barber, M., Kannan, K., MohanKumar, P. S., & MohanKumar, S. M. (2003). Neuroendocrine effects of perfluorooctane sulfonate in rats. *Environmental Health Perspectives*, *111*, 1485–1489.

Bain, P. A., Meisler, M. H., Taylor, B. A., & Payne, A. H. (1993). The genes encoding gonadal and nongonadal forms of 3 beta-hydroxysteroid dehydrogenase/delta 5-delta 4 isomerase are closely linked on mouse chromosome 3. *Genomics*, *16*, 219–223.

Banhegyi, G., Benedetti, A., Fulceri, R., & Senesi, S. (2004). Cooperativity between 11beta-hydroxysteroid dehydrogenase type 1 and hexose-6-phosphate dehydrogenase in the lumen of the endoplasmic reticulum. *The Journal of Biological Chemistry*, *279*, 27017–27021.

Benediktsson, R., Calder, A. A., Edwards, C. R., & Seckl, J. R. (1997). Placental 11 beta-hydroxysteroid dehydrogenase: A key regulator of fetal glucocorticoid exposure. *Clinical Endocrinology*, *46*, 161–166.

Benediktsson, R., Lindsay, R. S., Noble, J., Seckl, J. R., & Edwards, C. R. (1993). Glucocorticoid exposure *in utero*: New model for adult hypertension. *Lancet*, *341*, 339–341.

Bhosle, N. B., Garg, A., Jadhav, S., Harjee, R., Sawant, S. S., Venkat, K., et al. (2004). Butyltins in water, biofilm, animals and sediments of the west coast of India. *Chemosphere*, *57*, 897–907.

Biegel, L. B., Liu, R. C., Hurtt, M. E., & Cook, J. C. (1995). Effects of ammonium perfluorooctanoate on Leydig cell function: *In vitro*, *in vivo*, and *ex vivo* studies. *Toxicology and Applied Pharmacology*, *134*, 18–25.

Binder, P. S., Baumgartner, S. D., Zavala, E. Y., Deg, J. K., & Grossman, K. R. (1984). Refractive keratoplasty: Myopic keratomileusis in baboons. *Current Eye Research*, *3*, 1187–1197.

Blomquist, C. H., Lima, P. H., & Hotchkiss, J. R. (2005). Inhibition of 3alpha-hydroxysteroid dehydrogenase (3alpha-HSD) activity of human lung microsomes by genistein, daidzein, coumestrol and C(18)-, C(19)- and C(21)-hydroxysteroids and ketosteroids. *Steroids*, *70*, 507–514.

Blum, A., Martin, H. J., & Maser, E. (2000a). Human 11beta-hydroxysteroid dehydrogenase 1/carbonyl reductase: Recombinant expression in the yeast *Pichia pastoris* and *Escherichia coli*. *Toxicology*, *144*, 113–120.

Blum, A., Martin, H. J., & Maser, E. (2000b). Human 11beta-hydroxysteroid dehydrogenase type 1 is enzymatically active in its nonglycosylated form. *Biochemical and Biophysical Research Communications, 276*, 428–434.

Borst, J. G., Ten Holt, S. P., De Vries, L. A., & Molhuysen, J. A. (1953). Synergistic action of liquorice and cortisone in Addison's and Simmonds's disease. *Lancet, 1*, 657–663.

Boxmeer, J. C., Smit, M., Weber, R. F., Lindemans, J., Romijn, J. C., Eijkemans, M. J., et al. (2007). Seminal plasma cobalamin significantly correlates with sperm concentration in men undergoing IVF or ICSI procedures. *Journal of Andrology, 28*, 521–527.

Brooks, J. D., & Thompson, L. U. (2005). Mammalian lignans and genistein decrease the activities of aromatase and 17beta-hydroxysteroid dehydrogenase in MCF-7 cells. *Journal of Steroid Biochemistry and Molecular Biology, 94*, 461–467.

Brown, R. W., Chapman, K. E., Kotelevtsev, Y., Yau, J. L., Lindsay, R. S., Brett, L., et al. (1996). Cloning and production of antisera to human placental 11 beta-hydroxysteroid dehydrogenase type 2. *The Biochemical Journal, 313*(Pt 3), 1007–1017.

Brown, W. M., Metzger, L. E., Barlow, J. P., Hunsaker, L. A., Deck, L. M., Royer, R. E., et al. (2003). 17-beta-Hydroxysteroid dehydrogenase type 1: Computational design of active site inhibitors targeted to the Rossmann fold. *Chemico-Biological Interactions, 143–144*, 481–491.

Brozic, P., Kocbek, P., Sova, M., Kristl, J., Martens, S., Adamski, J., et al. (2009). Flavonoids and cinnamic acid derivatives as inhibitors of 17beta-hydroxysteroid dehydrogenase type 1. *Molecular and Cellular Endocrinology, 301*, 229–234.

Bujalska, I. J., Draper, N., Michailidou, Z., Tomlinson, J. W., White, P. C., Chapman, K. E., et al. (2005). Hexose-6-phosphate dehydrogenase confers oxo-reductase activity upon 11 beta-hydroxysteroid dehydrogenase type 1. *Journal of Molecular Endocrinology, 34*, 675–684.

Calafat, A. M., Kuklenyik, Z., Reidy, J. A., Caudill, S. P., Ekong, J., & Needham, L. L. (2005). Urinary concentrations of bisphenol A and 4-nonylphenol in a human reference population. *Environmental Health Perspectives, 113*, 391–395.

Calafat, A. M., Ye, X., Wong, L. Y., Reidy, J. A., & Needham, L. L. (2008). Exposure of the U.S. population to bisphenol A and 4-tertiary-octylphenol: 2003–2004. *Environmental Health Perspectives, 116*, 39–44.

Caprio, M., Newfell, B. G., la Sala, A., Baur, W., Fabbri, A., Rosano, G., et al. (2008). Functional mineralocorticoid receptors in human vascular endothelial cells regulate intercellular adhesion molecule-1 expression and promote leukocyte adhesion. *Circulation Research, 102*, 1359–1367.

Chang, Y. T., Kappy, M. S., Iwamoto, K., Wang, J., Yang, X., & Pang, S. (1993). Mutations in the type II 3 beta-hydroxysteroid dehydrogenase gene in a patient with classic salt-wasting 3 beta-hydroxysteroid dehydrogenase deficiency congenital adrenal hyperplasia. *Pediatric Research, 34*, 698–700.

Chen, B. B., Lin, H., Hu, G. X., Su, Y., Zhou, H. Y., Lian, Q. Q., et al. (2009). The (+)- and (-)-gossypols potently inhibit human and rat 11beta-hydroxysteroid dehydrogenase type 2. *Journal of Steroid Biochemistry and Molecular Biology, 113*, 177–181.

Christy, C., Hadoke, P. W., Paterson, J. M., Mullins, J. J., Seckl, J. R., & Walker, B. R. (2003). 11beta-hydroxysteroid dehydrogenase type 2 in mouse aorta: Localization and influence on response to glucocorticoids. *Hypertension, 42*, 580–587.

Clarke, I. J., Rao, A., Fallest, P. C., & Shupnik, M. A. (1993). Transcription rate of the follicle stimulating hormone (FSH) beta subunit gene is reduced by inhibin in sheep but this does not fully explain the decrease in mRNA. *Molecular and Cellular Endocrinology, 91*, 211–216.

Claus, R., Lacorn, M., Welter, H., Lekhkota, O., Messe, N., Wagner, A., et al. (2007). Expression of 11beta-hydroxysteroid-dehydrogenase 2 in Sertoli cells of boar testes. *Molecular and Cellular Endocrinology, 272*, 86–92.

Cole, T. J. (1995). Cloning of the mouse 11 beta-hydroxysteroid dehydrogenase type 2 gene: Tissue specific expression and localization in distal convoluted tubules and collecting ducts of the kidney. *Endocrinology*, *136*, 4693–4696.

Creasy, D. M., Beech, L. M., Gray, T. J., & Butler, W. H. (1987). The ultrastructural effects of di-n-pentyl phthalate on the testis of the mature rat. *Experimental and Molecular Pathology*, *46*, 357–371.

Deuchar, G. A., McLean, D., Hadoke, P. W., Brownstein, D. G., Webb, D. J., Mullins, J. J., et al. (2011). 11beta-Hydroxysteroid dehydrogenase type 2 deficiency accelerates atherogenesis and causes proinflammatory changes in the endothelium in apoe −/− mice. *Endocrinology*, *152*, 236–246.

Doi, M., Takahashi, Y., Komatsu, R., Yamazaki, F., Yamada, H., Haraguchi, S., et al. (2010). Salt-sensitive hypertension in circadian clock-deficient Cry-null mice involves dysregulated adrenal Hsd3b6. *Nature Medicine*, *16*, 67–74.

Doyle, L. W., Faber, B., Callanan, C., & Morley, R. (2003). Blood pressure in late adolescence and very low birth weight. *Pediatrics*, *111*, 252–257.

Draper, N., Walker, E. A., Bujalska, I. J., Tomlinson, J. W., Chalder, S. M., Arlt, W., et al. (2003). Mutations in the genes encoding 11β-hydroxysteroid dehydrogenase type 1 and hexose-6-phosphate dehydrogenase interact to cause cortisone reductase deficiency. *Nature Genetics*, *34*, 434–439.

Duax, W. L., Ghosh, D., & Pletnev, V. (2000). Steroid dehydrogenase structures, mechanism of action, and disease. *Vitamins and Hormones*, *58*, 121–148.

Dunnick, J. K., & Hailey, J. R. (1996). Phenolphthalein exposure causes multiple carcinogenic effects in experimental model systems. *Cancer Research*, *56*, 4922–4926.

Duperrex, H., Kenouch, S., Gaeggeler, H. P., Seckl, J. R., Edwards, C. R., Farman, N., et al. (1993). Rat liver 11 beta-hydroxysteroid dehydrogenase complementary deoxyribonucleic acid encodes oxoreductase activity in a mineralocorticoid-responsive toad bladder cell line. *Endocrinology*, *132*, 612–619.

Edwards, C. R., Stewart, P. M., Burt, D., Brett, L., McIntyre, M. A., Sutanto, W. S., et al. (1988). Localisation of 11 beta-hydroxysteroid dehydrogenase—Tissue specific protector of the mineralocorticoid receptor. *Lancet*, *2*, 986–989.

Frick, C., Atanasov, A. G., Arnold, P., Ozols, J., & Odermatt, A. (2004). Appropriate function of 11beta-hydroxysteroid dehydrogenase type 1 in the endoplasmic reticulum lumen is dependent on its N-terminal region sharing similar topological determinants with 50-kDa esterase. *The Journal of Biological Chemistry*, *279*, 31131–31138.

Funder, J. W., Pearce, P. T., Smith, R., & Smith, A. I. (1988). Mineralocorticoid action: Target tissue specificity is enzyme, not receptor, mediated. *Science*, *242*, 583–585.

Garbrecht, M. R., Krozowski, Z. S., Snyder, J. M., & Schmidt, T. J. (2006). Reduction of glucocorticoid receptor ligand binding by the 11-beta hydroxysteroid dehydrogenase type 2 inhibitor, Thiram. *Steroids*, *71*, 895–901.

Ge, R. S., Chen, G. R., Tanrikut, C., & Hardy, M. P. (2007). Phthalate ester toxicity in Leydig cells: Developmental timing and dosage considerations. *Reproductive Toxicology*, *23*, 366–373.

Ge, R.-S., Dong, Q., Niu, E.-m., Sottas, C. M., Hardy, D. O., Catterall, J. F., et al. (2005a). 11β-Hydroxysteroid dehydrogenase 2 in rat Leydig cells: Its role in blunting glucocorticoid action at physiological levels of substrate. *Endocrinology*, *146*, 2657–2664.

Ge, R. S., Dong, Q., Niu, E. M., Sottas, C. M., Hardy, D. O., Catterall, J. F., et al. (2005b). 11{beta}-Hydroxysteroid dehydrogenase 2 in rat leydig cells: Its role in blunting glucocorticoid action at physiological levels of substrate. *Endocrinology*, *146*, 2657–2664.

Ge, R. S., Dong, Q., Sottas, C. M., Papadopoulos, V., Zirkin, B. R., & Hardy, M. P. (2006). In search of rat stem Leydig cells: Identification, isolation, and lineage-specific development. *Proceedings of the National Academy of Sciences of the United States of America*, *103*, 2719–2724.

Ge, R. S., Gao, H. B., Nacharaju, V. L., Gunsalus, G. L., & Hardy, M. P. (1997). Identification of a kinetically distinct activity of 11beta-hydroxysteroid dehydrogenase in rat Leydig cells. *Endocrinology, 138*, 2435–2442.

Ge, R. S., & Hardy, M. P. (1998). Variation in the end products of androgen biosynthesis and metabolism during postnatal differentiation of rat Leydig cells. *Endocrinology, 139*, 3787–3795.

Ge, R. S., & Hardy, M. P. (2000). Initial predominance of the oxidative activity of type I 11beta-hydroxysteroid dehydrogenase in primary rat Leydig cells and transfected cell lines. *Journal of Andrology, 21*, 303–310.

Geissler, W. M., Davis, D. L., Wu, L., Bradshaw, K. D., Patel, S., Mendonca, B. B., et al. (1994). Male pseudohermaphroditism caused by mutations of testicular 17 beta-hydroxysteroid dehydrogenase 3. *Nature Genetics*, 7, 34–39.

Ghosh, D., Pletnev, V. Z., Zhu, D. W., Wawrzak, Z., Duax, W. L., Pangborn, W., et al. (1995). Structure of human estrogenic 17 beta-hydroxysteroid dehydrogenase at 2.20 A resolution. *Structure, 3*, 503–513.

Gilliland, F. D., & Mandel, J. S. (1993). Mortality among employees of a perfluorooctanoic acid production plant. *Journal of Occupational Medicine, 35*, 950–954.

Gomez-Sanchez, E. P., Gomez-Sanchez, M. T., de Rodriguez, A. F., Romero, D. G., Warden, M. P., Plonczynski, M. W., et al. (2009). Immunohistochemical demonstration of the mineralocorticoid receptor, 11{beta}-hydroxysteroid dehydrogenase 1 and 2, and hexose-6-phosphate dehydrogenase in rat ovary. *Journal of Histochemistry and Cytochemistry, 57*, 633–641.

Gray, T. J., & Beamand, J. A. (1984). Effect of some phthalate esters and other testicular toxins on primary cultures of testicular cells. *Food and Chemical Toxicology, 22*, 123–131.

Gray, T. J., & Butterworth, K. R. (1980). Testicular atrophy produced by phthalate esters. *Archives of Toxicology Supplement, 4*, 452–455.

Gray, T. J., & Gangolli, S. D. (1986). Aspects of the testicular toxicity of phthalate esters. *Environmental Health Perspectives, 65*, 229–235.

Gray, L. E., Jr., Ostby, J., Ferrell, J., Sigmon, R., Cooper, R., Linder, R., et al. (1989). Correlation of sperm and endocrine measures with reproductive success in rodents. *Progress in Clinical and Biological Research, 302*, 193–206, Discussion 206–209.

Green, V. L., Speirs, V., Landolt, A. M., Foy, P. M., & Atkin, S. L. (1999). 17Beta-hydroxysteroid dehydrogenase type 1, 2, 3, and 4 expression and enzyme activity in human anterior pituitary adenomas. *Journal of Clinical Endocrinology and Metabolism, 84*, 1340–1345.

Gu, Y., Lin, Y. C., & Rikihisa, Y. (1990). Inhibitory effect of gossypol on steroidogenic pathways in cultured bovine luteal cells. *Biochemical and Biophysical Research Communications, 169*, 455–461.

Guo, J., Yuan, X., Qiu, L., Zhu, W., Wang, C., Hu, G., et al. (2012). Inhibition of human and rat 11beta-hydroxysteroid dehydrogenases activities by bisphenol A. *Toxicology Letters, 215*, 126–130.

Haeussler, S., & Claus, R. (2007). Expression of the glucocorticoid receptor and 11 beta-hydroxysteroid dehydrogenase 2 in pig testes cells along fetal development. *Reproduction, Fertility, and Development, 19*, 664–669.

Hahn, T., Barth, S., Graf, R., Engelmann, M., Beslagic, D., Reul, J. M., et al. (1999). Placental glucose transporter expression is regulated by glucocorticoids. *Journal of Clinical Endocrinology and Metabolism, 84*, 1445–1452.

Herbst, A. L., Ulfelder, H., & Poskanzer, D. C. (1971). Adenocarcinoma of the vagina. Association of maternal stilbestrol therapy with tumor appearance in young women. *The New England Journal of Medicine, 284*, 878–881.

Higaki, Y., Usami, N., Shintani, S., Ishikura, S., El-Kabbani, O., & Hara, A. (2003). Selective and potent inhibitors of human 20alpha-hydroxysteroid dehydrogenase (AKR1C1) that metabolizes neurosteroids derived from progesterone. *Chemico-Biological Interactions, 143–144*, 503–513.

Hong, D., Li, X. W., Lian, Q. Q., Lamba, P., Bernard, D. J., Hardy, D. O., et al. (2009). Mono-(2-ethylhexyl) phthalate (MEHP) regulates glucocorticoid metabolism through 11beta-hydroxysteroid dehydrogenase 2 in murine gonadotrope cells. *Biochemical and Biophysical Research Communications, 389*, 305–309.

Hoover, R. N., Hyer, M., Pfeiffer, R. M., Adam, E., Bond, B., Cheville, A. L., et al. (2011). Adverse health outcomes in women exposed *in utero* to diethylstilbestrol. *The New England Journal of Medicine, 365*, 1304–1314.

Howdeshell, K. L., Furr, J., Lambright, C. R., Rider, C. V., Wilson, V. S., & Gray, L. E., Jr. (2007). Cumulative effects of dibutyl phthalate and diethylhexyl phthalate on male rat reproductive tract development: Altered fetal steroid hormones and genes. *Toxicological Sciences, 99*, 190–202.

Hu, G. X., Lin, H., Sottas, C. M., Morris, D. J., Hardy, M. P., & Ge, R. S. (2008). Inhibition of 11beta-hydroxysteroid dehydrogenase enzymatic activities by glycyrrhetinic acid *in vivo* supports direct glucocorticoid-mediated suppression of steroidogenesis in Leydig cells. *Journal of Andrology, 29*, 345–351.

Hu, G. X., Zhao, B., Chu, Y., Li, X. H., Akingbemi, B. T., Zheng, Z. Q., et al. (2011). Effects of methoxychlor and 2,2-bis(p-hydroxyphenyl)-1,1,1-trichloroethane on 3beta-hydroxysteroid dehydrogenase and 17beta-hydroxysteroid dehydrogenase-3 activities in human and rat testes. *International Journal of Andrology, 34*, 138–144.

Hu, G. X., Zhao, B. H., Chu, Y. H., Zhou, H. Y., Akingbemi, B. T., Zheng, Z. Q., et al. (2010). Effects of genistein and equol on human and rat testicular 3beta-hydroxysteroid dehydrogenase and 17beta-hydroxysteroid dehydrogenase 3 activities. *Asian Journal of Andrology, 12*, 519–526.

Hu, G. X., Zhou, H. Y., Li, X. W., Chen, B. B., Xiao, Y. C., Lian, Q. Q., et al. (2009). The (+)- and (-)-gossypols potently inhibit both 3beta-hydroxysteroid dehydrogenase and 17beta-hydroxysteroid dehydrogenase 3 in human and rat testes. *Journal of Steroid Biochemistry and Molecular Biology, 115*, 14–19.

Hundertmark, S., Dill, A., Ebert, A., Zimmermann, B., Kotelevtsev, Y. V., Mullins, J. J., et al. (2002). Foetal lung maturation in 11beta-hydroxysteroid dehydrogenase type 1 knockout mice. *Hormone and Metabolic Research, 34*, 545–549.

Jang, C., Obeyesekere, V. R., Dilley, R. J., Krozowski, Z., Inder, W. J., & Alford, F. P. (2007). Altered activity of 11beta-hydroxysteroid dehydrogenase types 1 and 2 in skeletal muscle confers metabolic protection in subjects with type 2 diabetes. *Journal of Clinical Endocrinology and Metabolism, 92*, 3314–3320.

Jensen, A. A., & Leffers, H. (2008). Emerging endocrine disrupters: Perfluoroalkylated substances. *International Journal of Andrology, 31*, 161–169.

Jez, J. M., Bennett, M. J., Schlegel, B. P., Lewis, M., & Penning, T. M. (1997). Comparative anatomy of the aldo-keto reductase superfamily. *The Biochemical Journal, 326*(Pt 3), 625–636.

Johnson, J. D., Gibson, S. J., & Ober, R. E. (1984). Cholestyramine-enhanced fecal elimination of carbon-14 in rats after administration of ammonium [14C]perfluorooctanoate or potassium [14C]perfluorooctanesulfonate. *Fundamental and Applied Toxicology, 4*, 972–976.

Kohn, M. C., Parham, F., Masten, S. A., Portier, C. J., Shelby, M. D., Brock, J. W., et al. (2000). Human exposure estimates for phthalates. *Environmental Health Perspectives, 108*, A440–A442.

Kotelevtsev, Y., Brown, R. W., Fleming, S., Kenyon, C., Edwards, C. R., Seckl, J. R., et al. (1999). Hypertension in mice lacking 11beta-hydroxysteroid dehydrogenase type 2. *The Journal of Clinical Investigation, 103*, 683–689.

Kratschmar, D. V., Vuorinen, A., Da Cunha, T., Wolber, G., Classen-Houben, D., Doblhoff, O., et al. (2011). Characterization of activity and binding mode of glycyrrhetinic acid derivatives inhibiting 11beta-hydroxysteroid dehydrogenase type 2. *Journal of Steroid Biochemistry and Molecular Biology, 125*, 129–142.

Krozowski, Z., Albiston, A. L., Obeyesekere, V. R., Andrews, R. K., & Smith, R. E. (1995). The human 11 beta-hydroxysteroid dehydrogenase type II enzyme: Comparisons with other species and localization to the distal nephron. *Journal of Steroid Biochemistry and Molecular Biology, 55*, 457–464.

Krozowski, Z., MaGuire, J. A., Stein-Oakley, A. N., Dowling, J., Smith, R. E., & Andrews, R. K. (1995). Immunohistochemical localization of the 11 beta-hydroxysteroid dehydrogenase type II enzyme in human kidney and placenta. *Journal of Clinical Endocrinology and Metabolism, 80*, 2203–2209.

Krug, A. W., Kopprasch, S., Ziegler, C. G., Dippong, S., Catar, R. A., Bornstein, S. R., et al. (2007). Aldosterone rapidly induces leukocyte adhesion to endothelial cells: A new link between aldosterone and arteriosclerosis? *Hypertension, 50*, e156–e157.

Kyossev, Z., Walker, P. D., & Reeves, W. B. (1996). Immunolocalization of NAD-dependent 11 beta-hydroxysteroid dehydrogenase in human kidney and colon. *Kidney International, 49*, 271–281.

Labrie, F., Luu-The, V., Lin, S. X., Labrie, C., Simard, J., Breton, R., et al. (1997). The key role of 17 beta-hydroxysteroid dehydrogenases in sex steroid biology. *Steroids, 62*, 148–158.

Lakshmi, V., & Monder, C. (1988). Purification and characterization of the corticosteroid 11 beta-dehydrogenase component of the rat liver 11 beta-hydroxysteroid dehydrogenase complex. *Endocrinology, 123*, 2390–2398.

Latif, S. A., Shen, M., Ge, R. S., Sottas, C. M., Hardy, M. P., & Morris, D. J. (2011). Role of 11beta-OH-C(19) and C(21) steroids in the coupling of 11beta-HSD1 and 17beta-HSD3 in regulation of testosterone biosynthesis in rat Leydig cells. *Steroids, 76*, 682–689.

Lavery, G. G., Walker, E. A., Draper, N., Jeyasuria, P., Marcos, J., Shackleton, C. H., et al. (2006). Hexose-6-phosphate dehydrogenase knock-out mice lack 11 beta-hydroxysteroid dehydrogenase type 1-mediated glucocorticoid generation. *The Journal of Biological Chemistry, 281*, 6546–6551.

Lee, R. H., Stanczyk, F. Z., Stolz, A., Ji, Q., Yang, G., & Goodwin, T. M. (2008). AKR1C1 and SRD5A1 messenger RNA expression at term in the human myometrium and chorioamniotic membranes. *American Journal of Perinatology, 25*, 577–582.

Lo, S., Allera, A., Albers, P., Heimbrecht, J., Jantzen, E., Klingmuller, D., et al. (2003). Dithioerythritol (DTE) prevents inhibitory effects of triphenyltin (TPT) on the key enzymes of the human sex steroid hormone metabolism. *Journal of Steroid Biochemistry and Molecular Biology, 84*, 569–576.

Loganathan, S. N., & Kannan, K. (2011). Occurrence of bisphenol a in indoor dust from two locations in the eastern United States and implications for human exposures. *Archives of Environmental Contamination and Toxicology, 61*, 68–73.

Low, S. C., Chapman, K. E., Edwards, C. R., Wells, T., Robinson, I. C., & Seckl, J. R. (1994). Sexual dimorphism of hepatic 11 beta-hydroxysteroid dehydrogenase in the rat: The role of growth hormone patterns. *The Journal of Endocrinology, 143*, 541–548.

Luu-The, V., Labrie, C., Zhao, H. F., Couet, J., Lachance, Y., Simard, J., et al. (1989). Characterization of cDNAs for human estradiol 17 beta-dehydrogenase and assignment of the gene to chromosome 17: Evidence of two mRNA species with distinct 5'-termini in human placenta. *Molecular Endocrinology, 3*, 1301–1309.

Luu-The, V., Labrie, C., Simard, J., Lachance, Y., Zhao, H. F., Couet, J., et al. (1990). Structure of two in tandem human 17 beta-hydroxysteroid dehydrogenase genes. *Molecular Endocrinology, 4*, 268–275.

Ma, X., Lian, Q. Q., Dong, Q., & Ge, R. S. (2011). Environmental inhibitors of 11beta-hydroxysteroid dehydrogenase type 2. *Toxicology, 285*, 83–89.

Marandici, A., & Monder, C. (1993). Inhibition by glycyrrhetinic acid of rat tissue 11 beta-hydroxysteroid dehydrogenase *in vivo*. *Steroids, 58*, 153–156.

Mason, J. I., Keeney, D. S., Bird, I. M., Rainey, W. E., Morohashi, K., Leers-Sucheta, S., et al. (1997). The regulation of 3 beta-hydroxysteroid dehydrogenase expression. *Steroids, 62*, 164–168.

McKeever, B. M., Hawkins, B. K., Geissler, W. M., Wu, L., Sheridan, R. P., Mosley, R. T., et al. (2002). Amino acid substitution of arginine 80 in 17beta-hydroxysteroid dehydrogenase type 3 and its effect on NADPH cofactor binding and oxidation/reduction kinetics. *Biochimica et Biophysica Acta, 1601*, 29–37.

McVey, M. J., & Cooke, G. M. (2003). Inhibition of rat testis microsomal 3beta-hydroxysteroid dehydrogenase activity by tributyltin. *Journal of Steroid Biochemistry and Molecular Biology, 86*, 99–105.

Mendelson, C. R., Gao, E., Li, J., Young, P. P., Michael, L. F., & Alcorn, J. L. (1998). Regulation of expression of surfactant protein-A. *Biochimica et Biophysica Acta, 1408*, 132–149.

Mercer, W., Obeyesekere, V., Smith, R., & Krozowski, Z. (1993). Characterization of 11 beta-HSD1B gene expression and enzymatic activity. *Molecular and Cellular Endocrinology, 92*, 247–251.

Monder, C. (1991). Corticosteroids, receptors, and the organ-specific functions of 11 beta-hydroxysteroid dehydrogenase. *The FASEB Journal, 5*, 3047–3054.

Monder, C., Hardy, M. P., Blanchard, R. J., & Blanchard, D. C. (1994). Comparative aspects of 11 beta-hydroxysteroid dehydrogenase. Testicular 11 beta-hydroxysteroid dehydrogenase: Development of a model for the mediation of Leydig cell function by corticosteroids. *Steroids, 59*, 69–73.

Monder, C., & Lakshmi, V. (1989). Evidence for kinetically distinct forms of corticosteroid 11 β-dehydrogenase in rat liver microsomes. *Journal of Steroid Biochemistry, 32*, 77–83.

Monder, C., Stewart, P. M., Lakshmi, V., Valentino, R., Burt, D., & Edwards, C. R. (1989). Licorice inhibits corticosteroid 11β-dehydrogenase of rat kidney and liver: *In vivo* and *in vitro* studies. *Endocrinology, 125*, 1046–1053.

Monder, C., & White, P. C. (1993). 11 beta-hydroxysteroid dehydrogenase. *Vitamins and Hormones, 47*, 187–271.

Moore, X. L., Hoong, I., & Cole, T. J. (2000). Expression of the 11β-hydroxysteroid dehydrogenase 2 gene in the mouse. *Kidney International, 57*, 1307–1312.

Murono, E. P., & Derk, R. C. (2005). The reported active metabolite of methoxychlor, 2,2-bis(*p*-hydroxyphenyl)-1,1,1-trichloroethane, inhibits testosterone formation by cultured Leydig cells from neonatal rats. *Reproductive Toxicology, 20*, 503–513.

Murono, E. P., Derk, R. C., & de Leon, J. H. (2001). Differential effects of octylphenol, 17beta-estradiol, endosulfan, or bisphenol A on the steroidogenic competence of cultured adult rat Leydig cells. *Reproductive Toxicology, 15*, 551–560.

Nakajima, T., Yasuda, K., Nishizawa, M., Okada, H., Yoshimura, T., Ito, S., et al. (2003). Expression of 20alpha-hydroxysteroid dehydrogenase mRNA in human endometrium and decidua. *Endocrine Journal, 50*, 105–111.

Nashev, L. G., Schuster, D., Laggner, C., Sodha, S., Langer, T., Wolber, G., et al. (2010). The UV-filter benzophenone-1 inhibits 17beta-hydroxysteroid dehydrogenase type 3: Virtual screening as a strategy to identify potential endocrine disrupting chemicals. *Biochemical Pharmacology, 79*, 1189–1199.

Obeid, J., & White, P. C. (1992). Tyr-179 and Lys-183 are essential for enzymatic activity of 11 beta-hydroxysteroid dehydrogenase. *Biochemical and Biophysical Research Communications, 188*, 222–227.

Odermatt, A., Arnold, P., Stauffer, A., Frey, B. M., & Frey, F. J. (1999). The N-terminal anchor sequences of 11beta-hydroxysteroid dehydrogenases determine their orientation in the endoplasmic reticulum membrane. *The Journal of Biological Chemistry, 274*, 28762–28770.

Odermatt, A., Dick, B., Arnold, P., Zaehner, T., Plueschke, V., Deregibus, M. N., et al. (2001). A mutation in the cofactor-binding domain of 11beta-hydroxysteroid dehydrogenase type 2 associated with mineralocorticoid hypertension. *Journal of Clinical Endocrinology and Metabolism, 86*, 1247–1252.

Ohno, S., Nakajima, Y., & Nakajin, S. (2005). Triphenyltin and Tributyltin inhibit pig testicular 17beta-hydroxysteroid dehydrogenase activity and suppress testicular testosterone biosynthesis. *Steroids, 70*, 645–651.

Ohshima, M., Ohno, S., & Nakajin, S. (2005). Inhibitory effects of some possible endocrine-disrupting chemicals on the isozymes of human 11beta-hydroxysteroid dehydrogenase and expression of their mRNA in gonads and adrenal glands. *Environmental Sciences, 12*, 219–230.

Olsen, G. W., Burris, J. M., Ehresman, D. J., Froehlich, J. W., Seacat, A. M., Butenhoff, J. L., et al. (2007). Half-life of serum elimination of perfluorooctanesulfonate, perfluorohexanesulfonate, and perfluorooctanoate in retired fluorochemical production workers. *Environmental Health Perspectives, 115*, 1298–1305.

Olsen, G. W., Gilliland, F. D., Burlew, M. M., Burris, J. M., Mandel, J. S., & Mandel, J. H. (1998). An epidemiologic investigation of reproductive hormones in men with occupational exposure to perfluorooctanoic acid. *Journal of Occupational and Environmental Medicine, 40*, 614–622.

Oppermann, U. C., Persson, B., & Jornvall, H. (1997). Function, gene organization and protein structures of 11β-hydroxysteroid dehydrogenase isoforms. *European Journal of Biochemistry, 249*, 355–360.

O'Shaughnessy, P. J., Baker, P. J., Heikkila, M., Vainio, S., & McMahon, A. P. (2000). Localization of 17beta-hydroxysteroid dehydrogenase/17-ketosteroid reductase isoform expression in the developing mouse testis—Androstenedione is the major androgen secreted by fetal/neonatal leydig cells. *Endocrinology, 141*, 2631–2637.

Ouchi, K., & Watanabe, S. (2002). Measurement of bisphenol A in human urine using liquid chromatography with multi-channel coulometric electrochemical detection. *Journal of Chromatography B, Analytical Technologies in the Biomedical and Life Sciences, 780*, 365–370.

Ozols, J. (1995). Lumenal orientation and post-translational modifications of the liver microsomal 11 beta-hydroxysteroid dehydrogenase. *The Journal of Biological Chemistry, 270*, 2305–2312, [Published erratum appears in (1995 Apr 28) *The Journal of Biological Chemistry, 270*(17), 10360].

Pearce, P. T., Lipkevicius, O. R., & Funder, J. W. (1986). High affinity (type 1) aldosterone-binding sites in rat epididymis. *Endocrinology, 118*, 2072–2075.

Penning, T. M. (1997). Molecular endocrinology of hydroxysteroid dehydrogenases. *Endocrine Reviews, 18*, 281–305.

Phillips, D. M., Lakshmi, V., & Monder, C. (1989). Corticosteroid 11β-dehydrogenase in rat testis. *Endocrinology, 125*, 209–216.

Piccirella, S., Czegle, I., Lizak, B., Margittai, E., Senesi, S., Papp, E., et al. (2006). Uncoupled redox systems in the lumen of the endoplasmic reticulum. Pyridine nucleotides stay reduced in an oxidative environment. *The Journal of Biological Chemistry, 281*, 4671–4677.

Poirier, D. (2003). Inhibitors of 17 beta-hydroxysteroid dehydrogenases. *Current Medicinal Chemistry, 10*, 453–477.

Puranen, T., Poutanen, M., Ghosh, D., Vihko, P., & Vihko, R. (1997a). Characterization of structural and functional properties of human 17 beta-hydroxysteroid dehydrogenase type 1 using recombinant enzymes and site-directed mutagenesis. *Molecular Endocrinology, 11*, 77–86.

Puranen, T., Poutanen, M., Ghosh, D., Vihko, R., & Vihko, P. (1997b). Origin of substrate specificity of human and rat 17beta-hydroxysteroid dehydrogenase type 1, using chimeric enzymes and site-directed substitutions. *Endocrinology, 138*, 3532–3539.

Puranen, T. J., Poutanen, M. H., Peltoketo, H. E., Vihko, P. T., & Vihko, R. K. (1994). Site-directed mutagenesis of the putative active site of human 17 beta-hydroxysteroid dehydrogenase type 1. *The Biochemical Journal*, *304*(Pt 1), 289–293.

Reinli, K., & Block, G. (1996). Phytoestrogen content of foods—A compendium of literature values. *Nutrition and Cancer*, *26*, 123–148.

Rheaume, E., Lachance, Y., Zhao, H. F., Breton, N., Dumont, M., de Launoit, Y., et al. (1991). Structure and expression of a new complementary DNA encoding the almost exclusive 3 beta-hydroxysteroid dehydrogenase/delta 5-delta 4-isomerase in human adrenals and gonads. *Molecular Endocrinology*, *5*, 1147–1157.

Roberson, A. E., Hyatt, K., Kenkel, C., Hanson, K., & Myers, D. A. (2011). Interleukin 1beta regulates progesterone metabolism in human cervical fibroblasts. *Reproductive Sciences*, *19*, 271–281.

Rodriguez-Bernaldo de Quiros, A., Paseiro-Cerrato, R., Pastorelli, S., Koivikko, R., Simoneau, C., & Paseiro-Losada, P. (2009). Migration of photoinitiators by gas phase into dry foods. *Journal of Agricultural and Food Chemistry*, *57*, 10211–10215.

Rooney, S. A., Young, S. L., & Mendelson, C. R. (1994). Molecular and cellular processing of lung surfactant. *The FASEB Journal*, *8*, 957–967.

Rosler, A., Silverstein, S., & Abeliovich, D. (1996). A (R80Q) mutation in 17 beta-hydroxysteroid dehydrogenase type 3 gene among Arabs of Israel is associated with pseudohermaphroditism in males and normal asymptomatic females. *Journal of Clinical Endocrinology and Metabolism*, *81*, 1827–1831.

Sang, G. W., Lorenzo, B., & Reidenberg, M. M. (1991). Inhibitory effects of gossypol on corticosteroid 11-beta-hydroxysteroid dehydrogenase from guinea pig kidney: A possible mechanism for causing hypokalemia. *Journal of Steroid Biochemistry and Molecular Biology*, *39*, 169–176.

Schutte, B. C., Bjork, B. C., Coppage, K. B., Malik, M. I., Gregory, S. G., Scott, D. J., et al. (2000). A preliminary gene map for the Van der Woude syndrome critical region derived from 900 kb of genomic sequence at 1q32–q41. *Genome Research*, *10*, 81–94.

Seckl, J. R. (1997). Glucocorticoids, feto-placental 11 beta-hydroxysteroid dehydrogenase type 2, and the early life origins of adult disease. *Steroids*, *62*, 89–94.

Seckl, J. R. (2004). Prenatal glucocorticoids and long-term programming. *European Journal of Endocrinology*, *151*(Suppl. 3), U49–U62.

Seckl, J. R., & Holmes, M. C. (2007). Mechanisms of disease: Glucocorticoids, their placental metabolism and fetal 'programming' of adult pathophysiology. *Nature Clinical Practice Endocrinology & Metabolism*, *3*, 479–488.

Sharpe, R. M. (2001). Hormones and testis development and the possible adverse effects of environmental chemicals. *Toxicology Letters*, *120*, 221–232.

Shi, Z., Zhang, H., Liu, Y., Xu, M., & Dai, J. (2007). Alterations in gene expression and testosterone synthesis in the testes of male rats exposed to perfluorododecanoic acid. *Toxicological Sciences*, *98*, 206–215.

Shimada, H., Ohtaguro, M., Miura, K., & Imamura, Y. (2007). Inhibitory effects of diesel exhaust components and flavonoids on 20alpha-hydroxysteroid dehydrogenase activity in mouse tissues. *Journal of Enzyme Inhibition and Medicinal Chemistry*, *22*, 445–449.

Simard, J., Durocher, F., Mebarki, F., Turgeon, C., Sanchez, R., Labrie, Y., et al. (1996). Molecular biology and genetics of the 3 beta-hydroxysteroid dehydrogenase/delta5-delta4 isomerase gene family. *The Journal of Endocrinology*, *150*(Suppl.), S189–S207.

Sjoberg, P., Bondesson, U., Gray, T. J., & Ploen, L. (1986). Effects of di-(2-ethylhexyl) phthalate and five of its metabolites on rat testis *in vivo* and in *in vitro*. *Acta Pharmacologica et Toxicologica*, *58*, 225–233.

Smith, R. E., Little, P. J., Maguire, J. A., Stein-Oakley, A. N., & Krozowski, Z. S. (1996). Vascular localization of the 11 beta-hydroxysteroid dehydrogenase type II enzyme. *Clinical and Experimental Pharmacology & Physiology*, *23*, 549–551.

Soaresam, A., Guieysseb, B., Jeffersona, B., Cartmella, E., & Lestera, J. N. (2008). Nonylphenol in the environment: A critical review on occurrence, fate, toxicity and treatment in wastewaters. *Environment International, 34*, 1033–1049.

Song, D., Lorenzo, B., & Reidenberg, M. M. (1992). Inhibition of 11 beta-hydroxysteroid dehydrogenase by gossypol and bioflavonoids. *The Journal of Laboratory and Clinical Medicine, 120*, 792–797.

Stewart, P. M., Wallace, A. M., Valentino, R., Burt, D., Shackleton, C. H., & Edwards, C. R. (1987). Mineralocorticoid activity of liquorice: 11-Beta-hydroxysteroid dehydrogenase deficiency comes of age. *Lancet, 2*, 821–824.

Suzuki, S., Tsubochi, H., Darnel, A., Suzuki, T., Sasano, H., Krozowski, Z. S., et al. (2003). Expression of 11 beta-hydroxysteroid dehydrogenase type 1 in alveolar epithelial cells in rats. *Endocrine Journal, 50*, 445–451.

Svechnikov, K., Supornsilchai, V., Strand, M. L., Wahlgren, A., Seidlova-Wuttke, D., Wuttke, W., et al. (2005). Influence of long-term dietary administration of procymidone, a fungicide with anti-androgenic effects, or the phytoestrogen genistein to rats on the pituitary–gonadal axis and Leydig cell steroidogenesis. *The Journal of Endocrinology, 187*, 117–124.

Tang, P. Z., Tsai-Morris, C. H., & Dufau, M. L. (1998). Regulation of 3beta-hydroxysteroid dehydrogenase in gonadotropin-induced steroidogenic desensitization of Leydig cells. *Endocrinology, 139*, 4496–4505.

Tannin, G. M., Agarwal, A. K., Monder, C., New, M. I., & White, P. C. (1991). The human gene for 11 beta-hydroxysteroid dehydrogenase. Structure, tissue distribution, and chromosomal localization. *The Journal of Biological Chemistry, 266*, 16653–16658.

Thomas, J. L., Boswell, E. L., Scaccia, L. A., Pletnev, V., & Umland, T. C. (2005). Identification of key amino acids responsible for the substantially higher affinities of human type 1 3beta-hydroxysteroid dehydrogenase/isomerase (3beta-HSD1) for substrates, coenzymes, and inhibitors relative to human 3beta-HSD2. *The Journal of Biological Chemistry, 280*, 21321–21328.

Thomas, J. L., Duax, W. L., Addlagatta, A., Brandt, S., Fuller, R. R., & Norris, W. (2003). Structure/function relationships responsible for coenzyme specificity and the isomerase activity of human type 1 3 beta-hydroxysteroid dehydrogenase/isomerase. *The Journal of Biological Chemistry, 278*, 35483–35490.

Thomas, J. L., Mason, J. I., Brandt, S., Spencer, B. R., Jr., & Norris, W. (2002). Structure/function relationships responsible for the kinetic differences between human type 1 and type 2 3beta-hydroxysteroid dehydrogenase and for the catalysis of the type 1 activity. *The Journal of Biological Chemistry, 277*, 42795–42801.

Thomas, J. L., Myers, R. P., & Strickler, R. C. (1989). Human placental 3 beta-hydroxy-5-ene-steroid dehydrogenase and steroid 5–4-ene-isomerase: Purification from mitochondria and kinetic profiles, biophysical characterization of the purified mitochondrial and microsomal enzymes. *Journal of Steroid Biochemistry, 33*, 209–217.

Troisi, R., Hatch, E. E., Titus-Ernstoff, L., Hyer, M., Palmer, J. R., Robboy, S. J., et al. (2007). Cancer risk in women prenatally exposed to diethylstilbestrol. *International Journal of Cancer, 121*, 356–360.

Usami, N., Yamamoto, T., Shintani, S., Ishikura, S., Higaki, Y., Katagiri, Y., et al. (2002). Substrate specificity of human 3(20)alpha-hydroxysteroid dehydrogenase for neurosteroids and its inhibition by benzodiazepines. *Biological and Pharmaceutical Bulletin, 25*, 441–445.

Waddell, B. J., Hisheh, S., Krozowski, Z. S., & Burton, P. J. (2003). Localization of 11β-hydroxysteroid dehydrogenase types 1 and 2 in the male reproductive tract. *Endocrinology, 144*, 3101–3106.

Walker, E. A., Clark, A. M., Hewison, M., Ride, J. P., & Stewart, P. M. (2001). Functional expression, characterization, and purification of the catalytic domain of human

11-beta -hydroxysteroid dehydrogenase type 1. *The Journal of Biological Chemistry*, *276*, 21343–21350.

White, P. C., Mune, T., & Agarwal, A. K. (1997). 11 beta-Hydroxysteroid dehydrogenase and the syndrome of apparent mineralocorticoid excess. *Endocrine Reviews*, *18*, 135–156.

White, P. C., Mune, T., Rogerson, F. M., Kayes, K. M., & Agarwal, A. K. (1997a). 11 beta-Hydroxysteroid dehydrogenase and its role in the syndrome of apparent mineralocorticoid excess. *Pediatric Research*, *41*, 25–29.

White, P. C., Mune, T., Rogerson, F. M., Kayes, K. M., & Agarwal, A. K. (1997b). Molecular analysis of 11 beta-hydroxysteroid dehydrogenase and its role in the syndrome of apparent mineralocorticoid excess. *Steroids*, *62*, 83–88.

Whorwood, C. B., Mason, J. I., Ricketts, M. L., Howie, A. J., & Stewart, P. M. (1995). Detection of human 11 beta-hydroxysteroid dehydrogenase isoforms using reverse-transcriptase-polymerase chain reaction and localization of the type 2 isoform to renal collecting ducts. *Molecular and Cellular Endocrinology*, *110*, R7–R12.

Wyrwoll, C. S., Seckl, J. R., & Holmes, M. C. (2009). Altered placental function of 11beta-hydroxysteroid dehydrogenase 2 knockout mice. *Endocrinology*, *150*, 1287–1293.

Xiao-feng, Z., Nai-qiang, Q., Jing, Z., Zi, L., & Yang, Z. (2009). Di (n-butyl) phthalate inhibits testosterone synthesis through a glucocorticoid-mediated pathway in rats. *International Journal of Toxicology*, *28*, 448–456.

Yabaluri, N., & Bashyam, M. D. (2010). Hormonal regulation of gluconeogenic gene transcription in the liver. *Journal of Biosciences*, *35*, 473–484.

Yamaguchi, H., Akitaya, T., Yu, T., Kidachi, Y., Kamiie, K., Noshita, T., et al. (2011). Homology modeling and structural analysis of 11beta-hydroxysteroid dehydrogenase type 2. *European Journal of Medicinal Chemistry*, *46*, 1325–1330.

Yamaguchi, H., Akitaya, T., Yu, T., Kidachi, Y., Kamiie, K., Noshita, T., et al. (2012). Molecular docking and structural analysis of cofactor-protein interaction between NAD(+) and 11beta-hydroxysteroid dehydrogenase type 2. *Journal of Molecular Modelling*, *18*, 1037–1048.

Ye, L., Su, Z. J., & Ge, R. S. (2011). Inhibitors of testosterone biosynthetic and metabolic activation enzymes. *Molecules*, *16*, 9983–10001.

Ye, L., Zhao, B., Cai, X. H., Chu, Y., Li, C., & Ge, R. S. (2012). The inhibitory effects of perfluoroalkyl substances on human and rat 11beta-hydroxysteroid dehydrogenase 1. *Chemico-Biological Interactions*, *195*, 114–118.

Yu, Z. H., & Chan, H. C. (1998). Gossypol as a male antifertility agent—Why studies should have been continued. *International Journal of Andrology*, *21*, 2–7.

Yuan, K., Zhao, B., Li, X. W., Hu, G. X., Su, Y., Chu, Y., et al. (2012). Effects of phthalates on 3beta-hydroxysteroid dehydrogenase and 17beta-hydroxysteroid dehydrogenase 3 activities in human and rat testes. *Chemico-Biological Interactions*, *195*, 180–188.

Zhang, Y., Lin, L., Cao, Y., Chen, B., Zheng, L., & Ge, R. S. (2009). Phthalate levels and low birth weight: A nested case–control study of Chinese newborns. *The Journal of Pediatrics*, *155*, 500–504.

Zhang, J., Zuo, Z., He, C., Cai, J., Wang, Y., Chen, Y., et al. (2009). Effect of tributyltin on testicular development in Sebastiscus marmoratus and the mechanism involved. *Environmental toxicology and chemistry*, *28*(7), 1528–1535.

Zhao, B., Chu, Y., Hardy, D. O., Li, X. K., & Ge, R. S. (2010). Inhibition of 3beta- and 17beta-hydroxysteroid dehydrogenase activities in rat Leydig cells by perfluorooctane acid. *Journal of Steroid Biochemistry and Molecular Biology*, *118*, 13–17.

Zhao, B., Chu, Y., Huang, Y., Hardy, D. O., Lin, S., & Ge, R. S. (2010). Structure-dependent inhibition of human and rat 11beta-hydroxysteroid dehydrogenase 2 activities by phthalates. *Chemico-Biological Interactions*, *183*, 79–84.

Zhao, B., Hu, G. X., Chu, Y., Jin, X., Gong, S., Akingbemi, B. T., et al. (2010). Inhibition of human and rat 3beta-hydroxysteroid dehydrogenase and 17beta-hydroxysteroid

dehydrogenase 3 activities by perfluoroalkylated substances. *Chemico-Biological Interactions, 188*, 38–43.
Zhao, B., Lian, Q. Q., Chu, Y., Hardy, D. O., Li, X. K., & Ge, R. S. (2011). The inhibition of human and rat 11beta-hydroxysteroid dehydrogenase 2 by perfluoroalkylated substances. *Journal of Steroid Biochemistry and Molecular Biology, 125*, 143–147.
Zheng, L., Dong, G. H., Jin, Y. H., & He, Q. C. (2009). Immunotoxic changes associated with a 7-day oral exposure to perfluorooctanesulfonate (PFOS) in adult male C57BL/6 mice. *Archives of Toxicology, 83*, 679–689.
Zhou, H. Y., Hu, G. X., Lian, Q. Q., Morris, D., & Ge, R. S. (2012). The metabolism of steroids, toxins and drugs by 11beta-hydroxysteroid dehydrogenase 1. *Toxicology, 292*, 1–12.

CHAPTER FOURTEEN

Cadmium Effects on the Thyroid Gland

Snezana A. Jancic[*,1], **Bojan Z. Stosic**[†]
[*]Department of Pathology, Institute for Pathology, Faculty of Medical Sciences, University of Kragujevac, Kragujevac, Serbia
[†]PhD student (Serbian Armed Forces), Faculty of Medical Sciences, University of Kragujevac, Kragujevac, Serbia
[1]Corresponding author: e-mail address: sjancic@medf.kg.ac.rs

Contents

1. Introduction 392
2. Cadmium 393
   2.1 Exposure sources 393
   2.2 Toxicokinetics 394
   2.3 Toxicodynamics 395
3. Structural and Functional Organization of the Thyroid Gland 397
   3.1 Follicular apparatus 397
   3.2 Neuroendocrine apparatus 400
4. Cadmium and the Thyroid Gland 401
   4.1 Cadmium effects on thyroid follicles 402
   4.2 Cadmium effects on parafollicular C cells 405
   4.3 Cadmium and thyroid hormone peripheral metabolism 407
5. Molecular Mechanism of Cadmium Influence 409
   5.1 Influence of cadmium on cell genome 410
   5.2 Cadmium and apoptosis 411
   5.3 Cadmium and mitochondrial dysfunction 413
   5.4 Cadmium and lipid peroxidation 416
6. Conclusions and Future Directions 417
References 417

Abstract

Cadmium has been listed as one of the 126 priority pollutants and a category I carcinogen. Carcinogenic effects of cadmium on the lungs, testicles, and prostate are widely recognized, but there has been insufficient research on the effect of cadmium on the thyroid gland. Cadmium has the affinity to accumulate not only in the liver, kidneys, and pancreas but also in the thyroid gland. It has been established that cadmium blood concentration correlates positively with its accumulation in the thyroid gland. Women of fertile age have higher cadmium blood and urine concentrations than men. In spite of its redox inertia, cadmium brings about oxidative stress and damage to

Vitamins and Hormones, Volume 94
ISSN 0083-6729
http://dx.doi.org/10.1016/B978-0-12-800095-3.00014-6

the tissue by indirect mechanisms. Mitochondria are considered to be the main intracellular targets for cadmium. Colloid cystic goiter, adenomatoid follicular hyperplasia with low-grade dysplasia and thyroglobulin hypo- and asecretion, and parafollicular cell diffuse and nodular hyperplasia and hypertrophy are often found in chronic cadmium toxicity.

1. INTRODUCTION

The earliest clinical observation of the toxic effect of cadmium (Cd) comes from Sovet (1858) who described acute gastrointestinal and delayed respiratory symptomatology among persons who use cadmium carbonate polishing powder (Nordberg, 2009). Due to its pronounced toxicity and prevalence in nature, the American Environmental Protection Agency has classified it as one of the 126 priority polluters. The most frequent sources of cadmium exposure are considered to be tobacco, contaminated water and food, and professional exposure (Hogervorst et al., 2007; Nordberg, Nogawa, Nordberg, & Friedmann, 2007; Satarug et al., 2003; Waalkes, 2003). Its toxicity originates from the reaction with sulfhydryl groups, by which it changes the activity of many enzymes. Although cadmium is not a redox-active metal, it indirectly leads to oxidative stress and damage of organic tissue structure (Ognjanovic et al., 2008; Zhou, Zhang, Liu, & Cai, 2009). This metal has a long biological half-life of 15–30 years primarily due to its weak excretion and excessive accumulation in the blood, kidneys, liver, and other organs (Castelli et al., 2005). Autopsy research has shown that the biggest individual concentrations of cadmium in the thyroid (and liver) have been found in people aged 40–60. Thereby, it has been established that cadmium concentration in the kidney was 10 times than that of the thyroid gland (Tiran, Karpf, & Tiran, 1995).

Cadmium exposure is joined with increased incidence of various neoplastic and nonneoplastic diseases of the kidneys, liver, lungs, bones, brain, peripheral blood, and other organs (Andujar, Bensefa-Colas, & Descatha, 2010; Huff, Lunn, Waalkes, Tomatis, & Infante, 2007; Liu, Qu, & Kadiiska, 2009; Zhou, Lei, & Wang, 2012). Studies that research the disruptions of the thyroid gland caused by cadmium are very rare, and often even contradictory, and vary depending on experimental model and applied dosage (El Heni, Messaoudi, & Ben Chaouacha-Chekir, 2012; Pilat-Marcinkiewicz, Sawicki, Brzoska, & Jakoniuk, 2002).

In this chapter, we will establish the existing level of knowledge about cadmium's influence on the thyroid gland, the metabolism of thyroid hormones, and the probable mechanisms of action in accordance with new knowledge.

2. CADMIUM

Cadmium (Cd) was discovered by German chemist F. Strohmeyer in 1817. Cadmium is a white and soft metal, similar to silver. In nature, it can usually be found together with zinc and is usually obtained as a by-product of zinc production. Both cadmium sulfide and cadmium oxide are soluble (Nordberg, 2009).

2.1. Exposure sources

Cadmium is classified as a heavy metal, and it can be found in nature as cyanide, nitrite, halogenide, and chloride salts. A large part of cadmium that is found in the environment is the result of professional exposure during ore processing and the melting of metal. Cadmium compounds are used as protection from corrosion in the production of batteries and accumulators. Pure cadmium, or in alloys, is used as pigment in dye, glass, ceramics, and enamel manufacture. It is used in manufacturing plastic masses and in the pesticide industry (as neutron absorber in reactors) (Ognjanovic et al., 2008; Satarug et al., 2003; Waalkes, 2003).

Cadmium is a toxic metal that accumulates in the atmosphere during a gradual erosion process and soil and rock abrasion caused by forest fires and volcanic eruptions (Marcano, Carruyo, Montiel, Morales, & de Soto, 2009). A significant concentration of cadmium in soil and water is the cause of its concentrations in animal meat, fish, fruits, and vegetables, so contaminated food is the primary source of exposure for the population (Hogervorst et al., 2007; Selinus, 2005). Tobacco also has Cd, 0.3–0.5 μg per cigarette, so it is also an important factor for population contamination (Nordberg et al., 2007; Tsutsumi et al., 2009).

The main source of cadmium pollution in professionals is inhalation, but an additional way is via the digestive system and skin. When cadmium enters the circulation, it transports to certain depots. The most important are the kidneys, liver, and muscles. Cadmium is eliminated via digestive tract and urine, but due to small degree of excretion from the body and excessive accumulation in blood and depots, it has a biological half-life of up to 30 years (Castelli et al., 2005).

Cadmium is present in almost every food, but concentration varies significantly, depending on food type and external contamination. A high concentration is present in entrails, crabs, and mollusks such as oysters. Herbal foods contain a higher Cd concentration than meat, eggs, milk and dairy products, and fish muscles (Järup and Åkesson, 2009). It is estimated that more than 80% of Cd food intake comes from cereals, vegetables, and tomatoes (Olsson et al., 2002). In the United States, the average daily food intake of Cd is 18.9 μg. In most other countries, the average daily intake varies from 0.1 to 0.4 μg/kg body weight (IARC, 2012). Cd intake is bigger in certain populations with specific food habits, for instance, vegetarians, and due to increased consumption of oysters. Cd in drinking water contributes less than a few percent to the total Cd intake (Olsson et al., 2002).

Women have a higher level of Cd than men, which manifests as a higher concentration of Cd in the blood, urine, and kidney cortex (Vahter, Akesson, Liden, Ceccatelli, & Berglund, 2007). The main reason is an increased intestinal absorption of Cd from food in low iron depots, which is frequent in women during fertility and pregnancy. The duodenal metal transporter, which is responsible for the intake of iron in a cell's mucus and is hyperexpressed in iron deficiency, has a high cadmium affinity (Vahter et al., 2007).

A second important source of Cd exposure is tobacco. Fifty percent of cadmium is being absorbed into the system from the lungs (Satarug et al., 2003). It is estimated that a person who smokes is exposed to 1.7 μg of cadmium from which about 10% is inhaled while smoking (IARC, 2012).

2.2. Toxicokinetics

After absorption, Cd circulates in erythrocytes or it is transported linked to albumin into the liver where it is taken by hepatocytes. It can induce and link to metallothioneins (MT) in the liver, which are cysteine-rich proteins that can concentrate Cd up to 3000 times (Klaassen, Liu, & Choudhuri, 1999; Nordberg, 2004). Due to numerous cysteines with thiol groups (–SH), MT have a high affinity for various reactions with metals. MT expression is induced by a metal-responsive transcriptional factor 1 (MTF-1) as a response to various stresses via linking with metal-responsive element located in promoting regions of target genes (Bi, Palmiter, Wood, & Ma, 2004) that contain two cysteines and two histidines (Giedroc, Chen, & Apuy, 2001), and in this way, it represents a potential target for cadmium intoxication. Both events, the reduction of MT expression and glutathione level, increase cellular damage due to cadmium exposure. The existence of cadmium-binding protein

(MT) has been known for quite some time, not only in the kidneys, liver, and pancreas but also in the thyroid gland in people (Sato & Takizawa, 1982). At the same time, these organs displayed an affinity to accumulate high levels of cadmium.

Cadmium is not biodegradable and redox is inert when compared to other metals (Fe and Cu). Little is known about Cd's biotransformation except its conjugation with sulfhydryl groups such as MT and glutathione (Klaassen et al., 1999; Nordberg, 2004). Molecules that are different from MT, such as albumin, cysteine, glutathione, and proteins rich with sulfhydryl groups, can also form compounds with Cd (Wimmer, Wang, Georgiev, & Schaffner, 2005).

Thanks to the capability of binding Cd, MT is Cd's efficient intracellular detoxifier. The protective role of MT with cadmium toxicity is confirmed not only with acute Cd poisoning but also with chronic Cd toxicity and Cd carcinogenesis (Klaassen, Liu, & Diwan, 2009). It is well known that MTs modulate three fundamental processes: releasing gas mediators such as hydroxyl radical or NO (nitrogen oxide), apoptosis, and the binding and exchange of heavy metals such as Zn, Cd, and copper (Thirumoorthy et al., 2011).

The presence of MT in all mammal cell types indicates that these MT play an important role in intracellular functions, but it is thought that their role is not vital for survival and reproduction (Vašak & Hasler, 2000). In mammals' cells, MT is located in certain compartments, for instance, cytoplasm, lysosomes, mitochondria, and the nucleus, which indicates a compartmentalized function in health and disease. Many studies have indicated the leading role of cytoplasmic MT in the homeostasis of Zn and Cu (Nordberg & Nordberg, 2009; Petering, Krezoski, & Tabatabai, 2009; Tapia et al., 2004; Vašak & Hasler, 2000) and in the protection of or decrease in oxidative stress induced with toxic metals and other states (Klaassen et al., 2009; Liu et al., 2009; Petering et al., 2009).

2.3. Toxicodynamics

The MT–Cd complex is gradually excreted from the liver and circulates in the kidneys where it can accumulate. Until recently, it was considered that around 50% of the total body deposit of Cd is located in the liver, kidneys, and muscles (Waalkes, 2003). However, research of tissue concentrations in thyroids of Japanese with "itai-itai" has shown that tissue concentration of Cd in thyroids in males is located in another place, behind Cd concentrations in the liver, and in females in a tertiary place, behind the liver and pancreas. At the same time, it has been observed that Cd concentration in the thyroid gland is three times greater in people who live in areas polluted with Cd than people from nonpolluted areas (Uetani et al., 2006). One epidemiological study of the dosage-addictive connection of Cd intake had shown that the total lifetime intake of Cd that brings unwanted effects is 2000 mg (Klaassen, 2001), which will result in submicromolar Cd concentrations in target organs. Two decades ago, it was shown that the physiological level of Cd is in the nanomolar range (Staessen et al., 1991).

Cadmium is considered a nonspecific toxicant that reacts with a wide spectrum of cell components and can easily enter the cell through L-type voltage calcium channels and receptor-modulated Ca channels (Martelli, Rousselet, Dycke, Bouron, & Moulis, 2006). Cadmium is accumulated due to binding with cytoplasmic and nuclear materials (Beyersmann and Hechtenberg, 1997), as well as slow excretion. The biological half-life of cadmium is very long, between 5 and 30 years (Castelli et al., 2005). It accumulates in various organs over time and causes a wide spectrum of negative effects on human health (Järup and Åkesson, 2009), so it is ranked as eighth on the list of 20 primary dangerous substances (ATSDR, 1999).

In chronic cadmium exposure, besides local irritation effects, there are also system effects on the lungs, kidneys, liver, testicles, bones, brain, and peripheral blood (Andujar et al., 2010; Jin et al., 2003; Kocak and Akcil, 2006). It was also established that it has a neurotoxic effect, because it can influence the integrity or permeability of the blood–brain barrier and also CNS (Govel, Chaudhary, Waseem, & Parvez, 2012).

Evidence indicates that cadmium exposure is related to lung, prostate, pancreatic, kidney, breast, and urinary carcinoma in humans (Huff et al., 2007; IARC, 1993; Liu et al., 2009; Schwartz and Reis, 2000; Waalkes, 2003). Cadmium is classified as a category I human carcinogen by the International Agency for Research on Cancer and the National Toxicology Program of the United States (IARC, 1993; NTP, 2011).

Since the mechanism responsible for cellular accumulation of metals is still unclear, a hypothesis was formulated that cadmium uptake includes competition with essential elements such as Ca or Zn for specific transport systems (Gagnon, Hontela, & Fumarie, 2007), and once accumulated, Cd is capable of influencing transcription activity pattern (Sirchia, Longo, & Luparello, 2008) and cellular signalization stimulating various stages of mitogen cascade such as proto-oncogene expression, DNA synthesis, and cell proliferation with various cell systems in mammals, acting like carcinogen (Liu, Yu, & Shaikh, 2008).

Cadmium increases the production of reactive oxygen radicals (ROR) (IARC, 2012) and changes the expression of various genes that halt the cellular cycle (Zhou et al., 2004) and then gene mutation, chromosome damage, cell transformation, and the DNA mechanism repair disruption (NTP, 2011).

3. STRUCTURAL AND FUNCTIONAL ORGANIZATION OF THE THYROID GLAND

The thyroid gland is situated on the frontal part of the neck, in front of the trachea. It is composed of two lateral lobes that are linked by an isthmus. The lobe length is about 5–6 cm, its width is 2–2.5 cm, and its thickness is about 2 cm. The average weight of an adult thyroid gland is 15–25 g. The gland's weight varies depending on human age, constitution, hormonal status, etc. In women, the gland's weight is heaviest during the menstrual cycle (Carcangiu, 2007).

The thyroid gland is enveloped by a thin fibrous capsule, with a narrow septum that divides the thyroid into lobes. The gland is richly vascularized and it is supplied with blood by the upper and lower thyroid artery. Vein drainage is supplied via upper, lower, and middle thyroid veins. Lymph drainage is also well developed and there is pronounced communication between the right and left lobes, via the isthmus. Nerves are formed on capsule, and they come from sympathetic trunks and vagus nerves (Carcangiu, 2007; Murray, 1998).

The embryonic origin of the thyroid gland's cells is diverse. Thyroid follicular cells originate from endoderm and C-parafollicular cells from the neural crest. Thyroid hormone secretion by follicular cells is mostly regulated by the thyroid-stimulated hormone (TSH) from the pituitary gland, which is under control of the thyrotrophic-releasing hormone from the hypothalamus. Parafollicular C cells belong to a diffuse neuroendocrine system (DNES). They secrete calcitonin, a hormone responsible for hypocalcemia and hypophosphatemia. Besides calcitonin, C cells produce other regulatory peptides (Huang, Sun, Moonga, & Zaidi, 2006).

3.1. Follicular apparatus

The thyroid gland's parenchim is composed of thyroid folliculi of a spherical shape, whose size is 150–500 μm. It is estimated that adult gland contains about 3 million folliculi. Folliculi are surrounded with one layer of specialized epithelial cells—follicular cells (thyrocytes). The follicular lumen contains gelatinous, transparent periodic acid–Schiff (PAS)—positive substance—colloid.

Immunohistochemical reactivity to thyroglobulin, triiodothyronine, and thyroxine was observed in the colloid. Parafollicular or C cells are situated among follicular cells (Carcangiu, 2007). Besides follicular and parafollicular cells, the thyroid also contains other cells, parafollicular localizations. They have granular, acidophil cytoplasm and are called oncocytes, oxyphil cells, or Askanazy cells. Surrounding the folliculi, there is a granular fragmentary connective tissue of interstice with rich network of capillaries of fenestrated type, nerve tissues, and lymph vessels (Krause, 2005).

Thyrocytes are the biggest part of the thyroid gland's mass. The shape of thyrocytes can vary from high cubic to flat. Their shape depends on gland stimulation; they become highly cubical during active stimulation, and folliculi have a small amount of colloid, and they become flat with folliculi full of colloid and low-grade hormones, if the gland is inactive. In the inner, luminal thyrocyte surface, there are many offshoots that enter the colloid and increase contact surface between the cells and colloid. The apical part of the cell contains the Golgi apparatus and apical vesicles that contain thyroglobulin that is released with exocytosis into folliculi as a colloid. Folliculi are filled with thyroglobulin, which is synthesized by the thyroid's follicular cells. At the same time, they represent a reservoir of secreted hormones, absorbed by thyrocytes and concurrently to be transferred into the blood. Thyrocytes synthesize and secrete triiodothyronine (T_3) and thyroxine (T_4). Thyrocytes show immunohistochemical reactivity to cytokeratin's small weight molecules, epithelium membrane antigen, and vimentin. They also contain estrogen and progesterone receptors and thyroid transcript factor-1 (Liu, Luthringer, & Easen, 2002; Pilat-Marcinkiewicz et al., 2002).

Physiological activity of thyroid gland is intimately related with iodine metabolism in an organism, which it uses for the synthesis of T_3 and T_4. The synthesis and secretion of T_3 and T_4 can be divided into several stages. First commences the uptake of amino acids, monosaccharides, and iodine from blood and thyroglobulin synthesis. In granular endoplasmic reticulum (grER), amino acids are used for the synthesis of polypeptide chain, which, through glycolysis in the Golgi apparatus, turns into the final product—thyroglobulin, placed in apical vesicles. Iodine, which takes thyrocyte from the blood, in an inactive state becomes oxidized by the thyroperoxidase enzyme. Iodide transfers from inactive to active state—iodine. In the next stage, exocytosis of apical vesicles releases thyroglobulin into the lumen of the thyroid folliculi and is deposited as a colloid (Cormack, 1998). In the presence of enzyme iodase, iodation of thyroglobulin into monoiodotyrosine and diiodotyrosine takes place. Connecting monoiodotyrosine and diiodotyrosine creates triiodothyronine (T_3), and binding two diiodothyronine molecules creates one molecule of tetraiodothyronine (T_4) (Cormack, 1998).

Formed hormones stay in colloid until thyrocytes receive the signal for hormone secretion. When they receive the signal, they become stimulated and import colloid particles by endocytosis and form colloid vacuoles. Connecting colloid vacuoles with primary lysosomes creates phagolysosomes where thyroglobulin is hydrolyzed into globulin. T_3 and T_4 diffuse through the cytosol and thyrocyte membrane to pericapillary areas and then through diffusion reach the bloodstream through capillary walls. Most of the thyroid's normal secretion belongs to thyroxin that converts by deiodination into T_3 when it arrives at the target organ. T_3 is considered a biologically active thyroid hormone, and most circulating T_3 is created through extrathyroid deiodination of T_4, which mostly occurs in the liver. However, T_4 is synthesized only in the thyroid's follicular cells (Nussey & Whitehead, 2001).

Reactions necessary to form T_3 and T_4 are influenced and controlled by the pituitary TSH that stimulates follicular cells in the thyroid gland (Kelly, 2000). Pituitary secretion of TSH is controlled by negative feedback modulated by circulating levels of free T_4 and T_3 as well as conversion of T_4 and T_3 in pituitary thyrotropin cells. TSH secretion is also under TRH's influence (Kelly, 2000).

The effect of thyroid hormones primarily depends on intracellular concentration of 3,5,3′-triodothyronin (T_3) and bonding T_3 to its nuclear receptor (TR) (Harvey & Williams, 2002). The intracellular level of T_3 is regulated by the level of circulating thyroxines (T_4) and T_3 by the conversion of T_4 mostly with deiodination of D2 into T_3, as well as the degradation of T_4 with deiodination of D3 into the reverse T_3 (rT_3) (Fauci et al., 2008). There are three iodothyronine deiodinases, D1, D2, D3, that catalyze external ring-shaped and/or inner-ring deiodination in mammals (Bianco, Salvatore, Gereben, Berry, & Larsen, 2002; Fauci et al., 2008).

T_3 homeostasis is mostly maintained by its production in various extrathyroid tissues through 5′ deiodination catalyzed with D1 and D2. Intracellular T_3 homeostasis in the pituitary gland and brain is maintained only because of D2-modulated T_4 deiodination (Bianco et al., 2002). Activity of D2 deiodination is also regulated by thyroid hormones so that hypothyroidism induces its activity and results in increased conversion of T_4 and T_3 primarily in the brain and pituitary gland (Fauci et al., 2008). This indicates that D_2 plays an important role in the regulation of intracellular T_3

level, especially in the brain and pituitary gland. D3 catalyzes inner-ring deiodination and in that way inactivates T4 and T3 (Bianco et al., 2002).

Serum thyroid hormones also regulate D1 activity from the liver, which is increased in hyperthyroidism, but decreased in hypothyroidism, and as we previously said, the opposite is happening in the case of D2 activity in the brain (Bianco et al., 2002, Fauci et al., 2008). However, it is well known that the conversion of T_4 and T_3 with D2 induces degradation of the D2 enzyme molecule via activation of the ubiquitin–protease system and serves as an important posttranslational feedback mechanism for maintaining T_3 homeostasis (Curcio-Morelli et al., 2003); therefore, D2 activity is increased in hyperthyroidism (Bianco et al., 2002; Fauci et al., 2008).

Thyroid hormones' serum levels, including T_3, T_4, and TSH, are often used as reliable indicators of thyroid function in people and experimental animals. Changes in serum concentration of these hormones reflect changes in their glandular synthesis and/or secretion as well as disruptions in their extrathyroid peripheral metabolism. Thyroid hormones are metabolized in peripheral tissues (deiodination, conjugation, deamination, and decarboxylation). Changes in their metabolism can significantly influence thyroid hormone function on the cellular level (Cormack, 1998; Kelly, 2000).

Iodothyronines (T_3 and T_4) synthesized in follicular cells improve oxidation processes in cells, which increases metabolism of proteins, carbohydrates, fats, and some vitamins. This effect is reflected in the differentiation and increase of tissue and development and maturation of bone, nerve, muscle, and endocrine systems and partly hematopoietic tissues (Vanderpump & Tunbridge, 2008).

3.2. Neuroendocrine apparatus

Parafollicular C cells are situated between the base membrane and thyrocytes, but they do not touch the colloid. They are usually round or polygonal, with a centrally placed round nucleus and bright cytoplasm. The most typical structure of C cells is secretory granules with great electronic mass, 60–550 nm in size. The granules are situated in the base part of the cytoplasm and isolated from the surrounding hyaloplasm by the trilaminar membrane. Two main groups of granules are identified (DeLellis and Wolfe, 1981): type 1, 280 nm in diameter, and type 2, which are smaller, with a diameter of 130 nm. The contents of secretory granules are most frequently the hormones calcitonin and somatostatin, the calcitonin gene-related peptide, chromogranin, neuron-specific enolase (NSE), and synaptophysin and can contain other hormones from the DNES spectrum. Some of them are local stimuli of the thyroid function (serotonin, gastrin-releasing peptide (GRP), and helodermin), while others are inhibitors (somatostatin, TRH, and calcitonin gene-related peptide (cGRP)) (Huang et al., 2006).

Both types of C cells are argyrophilic and immunoreactive on regulatory peptides situated in secretion granules. They are also immunoreactive to carcinoembryonic antigens (Carcangiu, 2007).

The main product of parafollicular C cells is calcitonin. It is composed of 32 amino acids, and its receptor belongs to the family of G protein-bonding receptors. The signal for calcitonin secretion is an increased level of Ca^{2+} in the blood. It decreases the level of calcium in the blood by inhibiting osteoclast activity in bone resorption and increases integration of Ca^{2+} into bone tissue. This effect is quick, direct, and short and is quickly overpowered by the mechanism of the parathyroid hormone. Gastrin and cholecystokinin, which belong to the same hormonal group due to similarities of terminal part, also increase calcitonin secretion (Marzia et al., 2006).

The physiological effects of calcitonin imply a direct influence on osteoclasts, as hypocalcemic agent or potent bone resorption inhibitor. These effects probably reflect the influence on numerous specific surface osteoclast receptors that initiate intracellular signalization using cyclical AMP and calcium commissioned second messenger patterns (Huang et al., 2006).

Although the role of calcitonin in calcium homeostasis and remodeling bones remains unresolved, studies that use calcitonin-null mice show that it could be included in the protection of the skeletal system during a "calcium stress" period, such as growth, pregnancy, or lactation (Woodrow et al., 2006). Also, it is considered that calcitonin prolongs the survival of osteoclast by inhibiting apoptosis (Kuo et al., 2012).

4. CADMIUM AND THE THYROID GLAND

Due to its complex histological structure and functions, the thyroid gland is often the target of many endocrine toxins, including cadmium (Bekheet, 2011; Rinal, Meenu, Viral, Tushar, & Pravin, 2012). Research on autopsies has shown that significantly higher concentrations of cadmium in the human thyroid gland are present after only 20 years of age (Tiran et al., 1995). Investigating the accumulation of cadmium in the thyroid gland in nonsmokers who have not been occupationally exposed and who live in areas with average industrial development has shown that the biggest individual concentration of cadmium in the thyroid (and liver) in the inquiry was in a group aged 40–60 years. Also, it has been established that cadmium concentration in the kidneys was 10 times higher than that of the thyroid gland (Tiran et al., 1995). Rare reports from literature indicate that, in spite of the small retention of Cd in the thyroid, there are proofs of structural and functional damages of the follicular and neuroendocrine apparatus of the thyroid gland (Jancic et al., 2011; Pilat-Marcinkiewicz, Brzóska, Sawicki, & Moniuszko-Jakoniuk, 2003; Pilat-Marcinkiewicz et al., 2002). It had been shown that Cd concentration in blood is in positive correlation with its accumulation in the thyroid gland (Pilat-Marcinkiewicz et al., 2003).

4.1. Cadmium effects on thyroid follicles

Chronic exposure to cadmium causes many histological and metabolic changes in the thyroid gland. Histopathologic changes in the thyroid are dose-dependent and are manifested by flattening follicular cells, by their desquamation inside the folliculi, by increasing interstitial fibrous tissue between folliculi, and by mononuclear cellular infiltration in the stroma around the folliculi (Pilat-Marcinkiewicz et al., 2003). Statistically significant lower follicular epithelium in cadmium toxicosis was also established in fish (Jadhao, Paul, & Rao, 1994).

Our yet-unpublished results of histopathologic and immunohistochemical research of the thyroid glands of albino Wistar rats, which were provided with 15 mg/kg Cd dissolved (as $CdCl_2$) in drinking water for 3 months, are somewhat different from previous research. After sacrificing the animals, we investigated their thyroid glands and found a spectrum of preneoplastic changes on thyroid folliculi. The most frequent find is a diffuse, rarely nodular colloid goiter. Follicular hyperplasia contains cystic folliculi filled with colloid and coated with one-layered atrophic low-cubic thyreocytes (Fig. 14.1). A frequent finding is also a microfollicular hyperplasia with multifocally present hyalinosis and acellular fibrosis with reduplication of the capsule's collagenic fibers (Fig. 14.2). A less frequent find is follicular adenomatoid hyperplasia with thyreocytes with hyperchromatic nuclei, conspicuous nucleoli, and increased mitotic activity (Fig. 14.3). We have verified thyroglobulin hypo- and asecretion, in areas of adenomatoid follicular hyperplasia, using immunohistochemical staining with antibodies to thyroglobulin (Fig. 14.4).

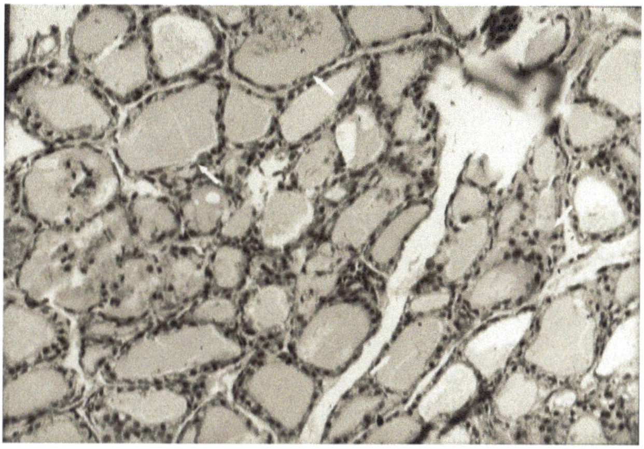

Figure 14.1 Colloid goiter with cystic follicles (arrow) and atrophic thyreocytes (H&E ×200). (See color plate.)

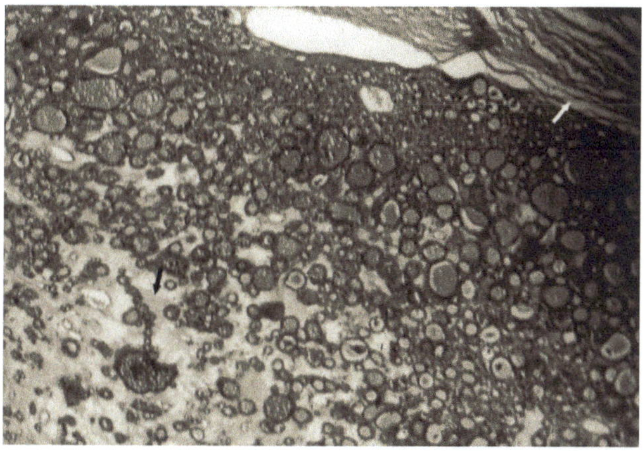

Figure 14.2 Microfollicular hyperplasia with focal hyalinosis (black arrow) and pronounced fibrosis of thyroid gland capsule (white arrow) (H&E ×200). (See color plate.)

Ultrastructural research of a rat's thyroid gland has shown that already after the fifth day of taking Cd, swelling of mitochondria occurs, and the rough surface of the endoplasmic reticulum (ER) decays in thyroid follicular epithelium. Bonding dilation reservoirs of rough grER creates large intracellular vacuoles. Also, the number of thyroglobulin secretory granules in the apical cytoplasm is decreased, which results in a significant decrease of serum levels T_3 and T_4 (Yoshizuka et al., 1991).

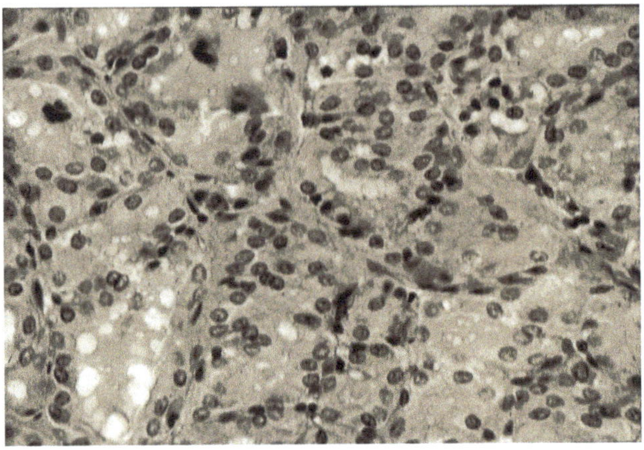

Figure 14.3 Adenomatoid follicular hyperplasia with atypical thyreocytes, nuclei, and conspicuous nucleoli (H&E ×400). (See color plate.)

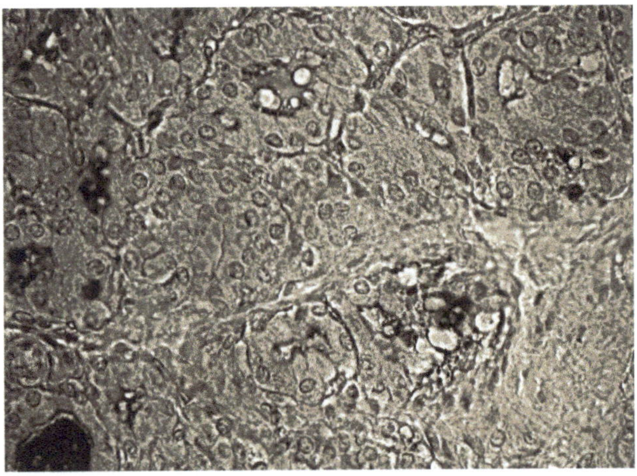

Figure 14.4 Adenomatoid follicular hyperplasia with atypical thyreocytes and thyroglobulin hypo- and asecretion of the rats exposed to cadmium (ABC ×400). (See color plate.)

In-depth information on Cd's influence on the thyroid gland can be found in the study of Hammouda and his associates who have shown that oral intake of Cd during 5 weeks results in its being accumulated in the rat's thyroid along with an increase of relative weight of thyroid gland and significant decrease of the T_4 serum level when compared with the control group. Keeping in mind that T_4 is synthesized only in the thyroid gland's follicular cells, the decrease of its serum level in rats exposed to Cd suggests that Cd influences the synthesis and/or secretion of T_4 follicular cells (Hammouda et al., 2008). The same authors also observed that Cd can disrupt, besides calcium, the metabolism of other essential metals such as Zn, Se, and iodine (Hammouda et al., 2008).

Cadmium thyrotoxicosis creates a significant fall of thyroxin levels (T_4) in serum, which is confirmed in various experiments on rats (Hammouda et al., 2008; Pilat-Marcinkiewicz et al., 2002), sheep (Badiei, Nikghadam, & Mostaghni, 2009), rabbits (Ghosh & Bhattachary, 1992), and fish (Hontela, Daniel, & Ricard, 1996).

When it comes to the level of serum T_3, literature contains many contradictory data. Experiments with rabbits have, at the same time as a significant decrease of thyroxin in serum, registered increased activity of thyroid peroxidases with a subsequent increase level of triiodothyronine (T3). Authors suggested that T_3 toxicosis in this study may be caused by privileged synthesis of T_3 and/or privileged deiodination of T_4 and T_3 (Ghosh & Bhattachary, 1992). The following increase of T_3 plasma levels with a decreased serum level of T_4 was also shown in people that live in areas polluted with cadmium (Nishijo et al., 1994). On the other hand, many studies with a registered decreased plasma level of T_4 did not register any significant change in levels of T_3 (Hontela et al., 1996; Pilat-Marcinkiewicz et al., 2002). The incoherency of the results from these studies indicates that the length of exposure to cadmium, way of entering, dosage, type, and age of experimental animals are important factors that determine endocrine response to this metal.

It was observed that exposure to cadmium decreases the total level of iodine in thyroid and serum and disrupts the metabolism of thyroid hormones. Parallel with this decrease of serum iodine and iodine in the thyroid occurs an increase of the thyroid gland's relative weight (El Heni et al., 2012). As a result of iodine deficiency, there is a decreased production of thyroid hormones, both in people and animals, which leads to morphological and functional changes in the thyroid gland, as well as decreased thyroxin production (ICCIDD, UNICEF, &WHO, 2001).

4.2. Cadmium effects on parafollicular C cells

In experiments with rats, cadmium causes diffuse hyperplasia of C cells with secretion of calcitonin, synaptophysin, chromogranin A, and somatostatin. In these animals, levels of Ca^{2++} in serum were significantly reduced (Pilat-Marcinkiewicz et al., 2002).

Diffuse hyperplasia of C cells in cadmium toxicosis is also described by our authors (Fig. 14.5), but unlike previous research, in the thyroid glands of our experimental animals, we verified nodular hyperplasia of C cells (Fig. 14.6), even C-cell microadenomas besides diffuse hyperplasia, hypertrophy, and C-cell hypergranulation. Testing of secretory activity of C cells, we observed the functional differentiation of these cells. Functional difference is manifested by capability of one type of C cells to secrete more different regulatory peptides (CT, cGRP, ChrA, NSE, and SST) and

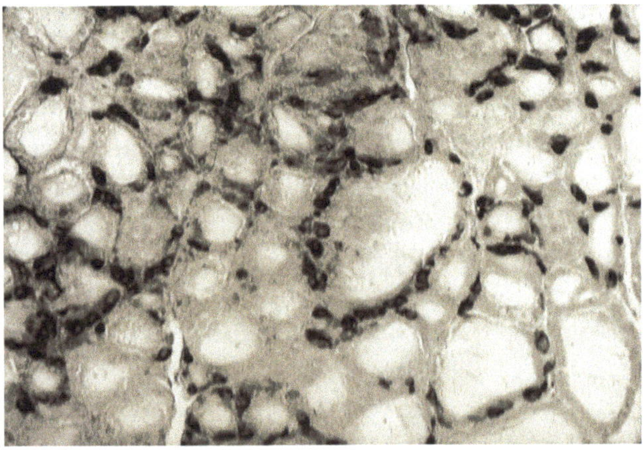

Figure 14.5 Diffuse C-cell hyperplasia in cadmium-exposed rats shows a strong reaction to calcitonin (ABC ×400). (See color plate.)

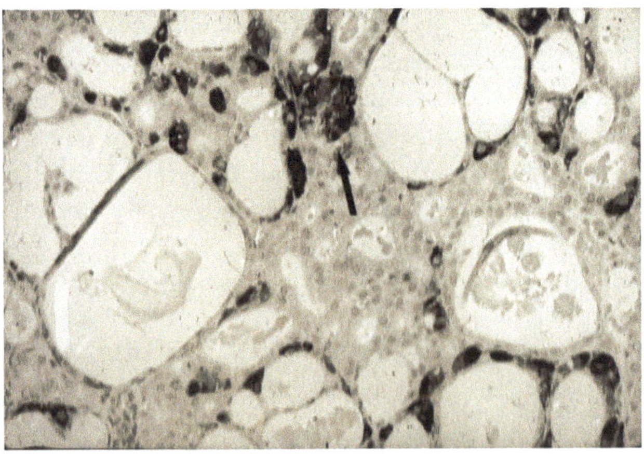

Figure 14.6 Nodular C-cell hyperplasia in cadmium-exposed rats shows a strong reaction to cGRP (ABC ×400). (See color plate.)

other types of C cells, constituents of nodular hyperplasia and microadenomas, that secrete exclusively cGRP (Jancic et al., 2011). Many years ago, DeLellis and associates have reported two ultrastructurally different cell types in C-cellular hyperplasia of thyroid gland. The first cell type was predominantly located in areas of diffuse C-cellular hyperplasia. Cells of this type contain great secretor granules; they have relatively weakly developed grER and Golgi apparatus, which indicates that the secretory cycle of these cells is in a resting phase. This type of C cells is also found in healthy thyroid gland. The second type of C cells contains granules with smaller diameter and characteristically localizes in areas of nodular C-cellular hyperplasia. This cell type is found in cells with cytological proofs of active synthesis of protein and secretion (DeLellis, Nunnemacher, & Wolfe, 1997).

4.3. Cadmium and thyroid hormone peripheral metabolism

Environmental polluters can influence thyroid homeostasis at the receptor or peripheral level, with different mechanisms of action. At the receptor level, atmospheric polluters disrupt thyroid homeostasis by binding onto transport proteins in the cellular uptake mechanism or modifying the metabolism of thyroid hormones (Morreale, Obregon, & Escobar, 2004). The influence of Cd on the peripheral metabolism of thyroid hormones includes an influence on the central nervous system and peripheral extraglandular effect.

There is a thought that alteration in the level of circulating thyroid hormone or TSH level, in relation to exposure to metals such as cadmium, is created due to the influence on various levels of hypothalamic–pituitary–thyroid axis and/or as a result of the disruption of transport of thyroid hormones and peripheral metabolism/deactivation (Boas, Feldt-Rasmussen, Skakkebaek, & Main, 2006; Zoeller, Tan, & Tyl, 2007). Cadmium can cause the disruption of hypothalamic–pituitary–endocrine axis activity by influencing the hypothalamus and also pituitary gland (Pillai, Laxmi Priya, & Gupta, 2002; Pillai, Priya, & Gupta, 2003). It was shown that cadmium accumulates in various regions of brain, which are included in the control of pituitary hormones releasing such as the hypothalamus and the eminentia mediana (Pillai et al., 2003). In experiments with fish, it was observed that exposure to cadmium leads to the significant inactivation of thyrotropin-secreting cells with an accumulation of secretory products (Jadhao et al., 1994).

It is well known that secretion of TSH from the pituitary gland is inversely bound with levels of thyroid hormones that serve as the basis for feedback control of circulating thyroid hormones (Fauci et al., 2008). Cadmium influence creates thyroid dysfunction, which leads to an increase in the thyroid gland's weight, accumulation of Cd on this level, and an increase of serum TSH concentration in rats (Hammouda et al., 2008; Lafuente, Cano, & Esquifino, 2003) and humans (Iijima et al., 2007).

A tendency of increased TSH concentration in serum at a higher level of Cd exposure is probably the answer to the decrease of serum T_4 level. Lack of significant TSH response to the decrease of the serum T4 level may indicate the effects of cadmium on pituitary regulation of production and secretion of thyroid hormones (Pavia, Paier, Noli, Hagmuller, & Zaninovich, 1997).

Thyroid hormones are metabolized in peripheral tissue by various enzymatic reactions like deiodination, conjugation, deamination, and decarboxylation. In this way, changes in these metabolic patterns can significantly influence thyroid hormones and thyroid function at the cellular level (Kelly, 2000). Most of circulating T_3 is created in peripheral extrathyroid tissue by peripheral deiodination of T_4 to T_3, which happens mostly in the liver and is dependent on deiodinase enzyme activity, mostly through type I, which is located in the thyroid, liver, and kidneys (Fauci et al., 2008).

Unlike triiodothyronine (T_3), thyroxin (T_4) is synthesized in the thyroid gland in much greater volume and presents a precursor for the more potent T_3 hormone. Also in relation to type I deiodinase, which has a relatively low affinity for T_4, deiodinase type II has a higher affinity for T_4 and it is primarily located in pituitary gland, CNS, gray fatty tissue, and the thyroid gland (Fauci et al., 2008). In principle, tissue-specific deiodination (D1, D2, and D3) of thyroid hormones greatly determines their fate (Kelly, 2000).

In *in vitro* conditions, it has been observed that Cd inhibits conversion of T_4 to T_3 in several tissues (Paier et al., 1993; Pavia et al., 1997). Paier and associates showed that adding Cd to the homogenate of gray fatty rat tissue significantly blocks *in vitro* conversion of T_4 to T_3. This study used similar concentrations of Cd, which have significantly inhibited deiodination of T_4 in the liver (Paier et al., 1993; Yoshida et al., 1987) and in the pituitary gland (Pavia et al., 1997). An experiment with chickens confirmed that Cd causes a decrease in not only serum T3 but also deiodinase activity (5′D-I), which indicates that Cd disrupts thyroid metabolism primarily on an extrathyroid level in chickens, unlike mammals, where cadmium inhibits the metabolism on both thyroid and extrathyroid levels (Gupta & Kar, 1999).

A probable mechanism of cadmium's effect on 5′-deiodinases can be a strong affinity of Cd for sulfhydryl enzyme groups. It was shown that Cd can inhibit many enzymes by binding to the sulfhydryl groups of the enzyme active sites or via disruptions in forming an enzyme–substrate complex (Vallee & Ullmer, 1972). The activity of 5′deiodinases is highly dependent on the presence of sulfhydryl groups (Chopra, 1978). A positive correlation has been proved between total amount of sulfhydryl groups and activity of 5′-deiodinases in the liver (Brzezińska-Slebodzińska & Pietras, 1997). This understanding is supported by an experiment on rats where a significant decrease of T_4 deiodination occurred after the treatment with Cd, as well as a decrease in the creation of iodine and T_3. Hepatic concentration of nonprotein sulfhydryl groups was also decreased. Serum concentration of T_4 and T_3 decreased significantly, while administration of DTT (dithiothreitol) did not succeed to normalize hormonal levels in serum. These data confirm that Cd probably decreases 5′deiodinase activity via binding with sulfhydryl groups of 5′deiodinases as it does with other enzymes (Brzezińska-Slebodzińska & Pietras, 1997; Paier et al., 1993). It has been suggested that 5′-D activity is an important control point for the regulation of thyroid hormone activity (Visser, 1978) and that change in activity of this enzyme is reflected in the total amount of T4 and T3 hormones present in circulation (Gupta & Kar, 1997).

5. MOLECULAR MECHANISM OF CADMIUM INFLUENCE

Back in the seventies, it was observed that cells exposed to cadmium show significant changes of cellular organelles, which was manifested by disintegrating ribosomes, destroying endoplasmic reticulum (EPRs), and swelling mitochondria (Kawahara, Takashima, Nakamura, & Yamagami, 1975). Subsequent findings established that Cd in cells of mammals and in cell cultures has the following effects:

- Directly inhibits or stimulates activity of various enzymes (Puri & Saha, 2003)
- Disrupts adequate formation of membrane and secretory proteins (Huang, Fang, & Huang, 2011; Kitamura & Hiramatsu, 2010)
- Decreases concentration of intracellular antioxidants (mostly glutathione-GSH) and cleaners of free radicals (vitamins E and C) (Ognjanovic et al., 2008)
- Inhibits activity of antioxidant enzymes (GSH-peroxidases, GSH-reductases, GSH-transferases, catalases, and superoxide dismutase),

directing cytoplasmic redox state to oxidation, with increased reactive oxygen species (ROS) and reactive nitrate compounds (Liu et al., 2009; Petering et al., 2009)

- Liberates essential metals linked with MT (Zn and Cu) and various intracellular membranes and metalloproteins (Zn, Cu, and Fe) (Moulis, 2010; Petering et al., 2009)

Released Cu and Fe promote the development of oxidative stress and creation of free radicals in cells (Bergendi, Benes, Duracková, & Ferencik, 1999; Petering et al., 2009). Released Zn promotes synthesis of new apo-MTs via activation of MTF-1 and antagonism for Cd binding places and reactivity (Andrews, 2000; Powel, 2000). Disruption of homeostasis of transitional metals with cadmium and cellular transport of cadmium via the patterns of these transitional metals (Fe and Zn) contribute to toxic mechanism of cadmium (Moulis, 2010).

5.1. Influence of cadmium on cell genome

All the aforementioned processes lead to induction of both gene groups included in cellular survival, as well as genes included in apoptosis, by cadmium, resulting in balance alteration between cellular survival and death. Balance can be changed by a dose-dependent and time-dependent cadmium effect on the transcription of every Cd-inducible gene (Moulis, 2010; Shin, Park, Lee, Moon, & Lee, 2003).

Cadmium affects the progression of the cell cycle, proliferation, differentiation, DNA replication and repair, and apoptosis patterns (Huff et al., 2007; Oh & Lim, 2006; Waisberg, Joseph, Hale, & Beyersmann, 2003). Cadmium's effect on DNA synthesis and proliferation is dose-dependent (Misra, Gawdi, & Pizzo, 2003).

Due to an affinity to thiol groups and ligands that contain nitrogen (N), Cd can link to a wide spectrum of biological macromolecules (such as proteins and DNA), destroying their structure and disrupting their function. It is thought that Cd at the same time induces DNA damage and inhibits DNA repair mechanisms (Bertin & Averbeck, 2006). It also has a high affinity for sulfhydryl groups, so there is competition with zinc (Zn) in proteins, and it is bound to DNA bases and causes tearing of one DNA chain (McMurray & Tainer, 2003). Cadmium influences the stability of the genome by inducing ROS in cells, but it also inhibits several DNA repair systems, decreases the activity of cellular antioxidants such as glutathione, and alters the apoptosis process (McMurray & Tainer, 2003).

Analysis of gene expression analysis indicates that chronic Cd exposure significantly modifies the expression of 217 regulatory genes (it hyper-expresses 137 genes and decreases expression in 80 genes), apoptosis, oncogenes, and transporters; cellular cycle; stress response and immune response; or metabolism (Dakeshita et al., 2009). Several DNA repair systems that modulate damage on one of the DNA chains are influenced by cadmium toxicity: mismatch repair, nucleotide excision repair, and base excision repair (Bertin & Averbeck, 2006).

A high cytotoxic concentration of Cd is connected to DNA-single-strand break complexes, chromosome aberrations, changes in sister chromatids, and disruptions in binding proteins to DNA in several types of mammal cells (Liu, He, Yan, Qi, & Zhang, 2011).

Cadmium can influence proteins that contain Zn (finger motif) and that are included in maintaining genome stability or DNA repair and damage signalization (Hartwig et al., 2002).

There is overwhelming evidence that Cd is a transcriptional modulator for several cell types, both normal and pathological. For instance, exposure to low Cd concentrations in several cell types changes the level of expression of several gene classes (c-fos, c-jun, c-myc, p53, MT, glutathione, heat shock proteins, tif3.tef-1a, and Nur77) and, in that way, influences intracellular signal patterns leading to an increase in cell proliferation, while higher concentrations are inhibitory and cytotoxic (Hartwig et al., 2002).

Sensitivity to Cd varies from one cell type to another. It is clear that every effect will depend on Cd concentration, duration of exposure, and target tissue/cell (Cannino, Ferruggia, Luparello, & Rinaldi, 2009). Literature takes the prevailing attitude that the main reason for DNA damage is due to Cd's twofold influence, inducing DNA damage and at the same time inhibiting its repair. It is possible that the main reason is cadmium inhibition of DNA repair (Filipic, Fatur, & Vudrag, 2006; Liu et al., 2011).

5.2. Cadmium and apoptosis

On the cellular level, Cd influences proliferation, differentiation, apoptosis, and other cellular activities (Bertin & Averbeck, 2006; Waisberg et al., 2003). Exposure to Cd in relatively high doses causes primarily necrosis and in low doses apoptosis, which indicates that modality of cellular death caused by Cd depends on exposure level (Satoh, Kaji, & Tohyama, 2003). When applied in small or moderate dosage under *in vivo* and *in vitro* conditions, Cd mostly causes apoptosis (Sancho et al., 2006). High doses of cadmium, related to acute exposure, also induce necrosis and apoptosis. Relation between both types of cell death is dose-dependent and also depends on cell type. A proapoptotic cadmium effect is modulated with various signal pathways that activate caspase-dependent or caspase-independent cellular deaths. The latter include loss of mitochondrial membrane potential and translocation into nucleus of apoptosis-induced factor (AIF), as well as endonuclease G (Lemarié et al., 2004; Martelli et al., 2006).

Cellular death induced with Cd occurs via a caspase-dependent pathway joined with the release of cytochrome C or by caspase-independent cellular death joined with ROS and the translocation of AIF (Wang, Shih, Ko, Wei, & Shih, 2008). Significant growth of intracellular calcium was observed in both types of apoptosis. It is known that Cd can also change intracellular calcium concentration (Ca) from outside of the cell, which is a universal and versatile intracellular signal molecule (Martelli et al., 2006). It is also known that the ER is the main depot of Ca in the cell, and earlier, we mentioned that cadmium influences ER as well (Wang et al., 2008).

Since Ca ions play a central role in various biological functions, it is believed that cytotoxicity of Cd is partly connected to the intracellular Ca level. A change in the intracellular Ca level can cause apoptosis. A high concentration of Ca ions can cause disruption of Ca homeostasis in mitochondria, which facilitates the loss of potential of mitochondrial membrane and in the end leads to ROS formation. The exact cellular mechanism by which cadmium includes calcium ions in its toxic effect is not completely understood (Son et al., 2010).

Cadmium induces apoptosis by caspase-dependent or caspase-independent mechanisms depending on cell type (Son et al., 2010). Cadmium induces caspase-dependent apoptosis including two main pathways, extrinsic Fas-FADD caspase-8 initiated by the activation of the death receptor on cell membrane resulting in activation of caspase-8 or caspase-10 (Eichler et al., 2006) and intrinsic that is activated by the signals of cellular stress (such as DNA damage) activating caspase-9. Caspase-8 and caspase-9 are torn and activate effector caspases, caspase-3 and caspase-7, which will kill the cell by tearing many protein substrates (Kondoh et al., 2002).

Apoptosis can also be induced independent of caspases after intoxication or by Cd–calpain complex or translocation of the AIF in the nucleus (Daugas et al., 2000; Shih et al., 2004).

Cadmium initiates a mitochondrial pathway that leads to apoptosis (Belyaeva, Dymkowska, Wieckowski, & Wojtczak, 2006; Su et al., 2008).

Mitochondria cause apoptosis via increased permeability of external mitochondrial membrane, decreased mitochondrial membrane potential, freeing of cytochrome *c*, and the activation of caspases (Susin, Zamzami, & Kroemer, 1998).

It should be stressed that the mechanism of Cd-induced cytotoxicity is not exactly defined and is still under intensive research. Among other things, exposure to cadmium causes necrotic cell death (Ishido, Ohtsubo, Adachi, & Kunimoto, 2002; Sancho et al., 2006). Both apoptosis and necrosis can be induced by increased ROS accumulation (Fleury, Mignotte, & Vayssière, 2002; Hossain, Liu, Nguyen, Shore, & Almazan, 2009) and increased lipid peroxidation, which has been observed several times after Cd exposure (Cuypers et al., 2010; Kotelnikova, Sokolova, & Kotelnikov, 2008; Slyuzova, Stepanova, Temraleeva, Kireev, & Ignatov, 2008).

5.3. Cadmium and mitochondrial dysfunction

Mitochondria are found in almost all eukaryotic cells, and the mitochondrial respiratory chain plays a key role in maintaining energetic homeostasis via oxidative phosphorylation (OXPHOS), which is the most important for ATP generation. These organelles are included in the synthesis of amino acids, nucleotides, lipids, ion homeostasis, cellular proliferation, motility, and programmed death of cells (Ackerman & Tzagoloff, 2005; Cannino et al., 2009).

In 1991, Yoshizuka et al. assumed that Cd accumulated in mitochondria of thyroid follicular epithelial cells can disrupt OXPHOS of the organelles and lead to the loss of energy supply, which likely causes synthesis of inhibition and the release of thyroid hormones (Yoshizuka et al., 1991).

Based on the observation that Cd on mitochondria causes heavy structural and consequential enzyme-functional changes (Tang & Shaikh, 2001), numerous studies emphasize that mitochondrial dysfunction is the earliest event in the cytotoxicity of heavy metals (Belyaeva, Glazunov, & Korotkov, 2004; Liu et al., 2011; Sanni, Williams, Sokolov, & Sokolova, 2008). Divalent heavy-metal cations such as Cd, Hg, and Cu accumulate in mitochondria, which have, it is supposed, a Ca uniporter channel for Ca input (MCU), which activates by change in transmembrane potential, which also transport these cations. Cadmium, besides the capability to be a Ca agonist, has a high affinity for thiol groups. Both of these properties of Cd are responsible for the induction of mitochondrial permeability transition (MPT) pores with this heavy metal (Saris & Carafoli, 2005). MPT pores, voltage-dependent, nonselective high-conductive channels of the internal mitochondrial membrane that enable passage of up to 1500 Da, participate in physiological and pathological processes, including the induction of cellular death of various types (Belyaeva, Korotkov, & Saris, 2011; Lemasters, Theruvath, Zhong, & Nieminen, 2009).

Permeability transition pores of mitochondria are protein complexes that lie on contact side between the inner and outer mitochondrial membrane. Although its exact structure is not clear, it is believed that it contains hexokinase, a voltage-dependent anion channel (VDAC), creatine kinase, adenine nucleotide translocator (ANT), and cyclophilin D. Many inductors and inhibitors of apoptosis influence VDAC or ANT, such as Ca, oxidants, and Bcl-2 family members. It is assumed that Cd influences ANT, which lies on the inner side of mitochondrial membrane and which is probably the trigger for opening pores of transitional permeability (Li et al., 2003; Zazueta, Sanchez, Garcia, & Correa, 2000).

Critical places for binding Cd are thiol groups of proteins. Inactivation of sulfhydryl groups of essential proteins can lead to functional deficit in subcellular organelles, such as the nucleus, mitochondria, and ER (Diep, Denizeau, & Jumarie, 2005).

Cadmium changes activity of many mitochondrial proteins, leading to the inhibition of enzymes of the respiratory chain, collapse of membrane potential, and the swelling of mitochondria, with consequential inhibition of respiration, loss of inner mitochondrial membrane potential, and accumulated Ca. At the same time, mitochondrial swelling occurs together with abnormal acidification due to lactate production, which indicates disruption of oxidative metabolism. Cd increases lipid peroxidation by binding with the inner membrane and disrupts the integrity of the mitochondrial membrane (Cannino et al., 2009).

Production of ROS turned out to be one of the first steps in Cd-induced cytotoxicity that precedes mitochondrial damage. ROS lead the attack on membrane phospholipids and cause a loss of mitochondrial membrane potential, which leads to the increased release of cytochrome C from damaged mitochondria, activation of caspases, and resulting apoptosis (Cuypers et al., 2010; Mao et al., 2005; Szuster-Ciesielska et al., 2000; Zhang et al., 2010).

Through research of mitochondria function in rat liver, two stages that follow Cd intoxication have been defined. In the first stage, after 2.5 min of incubation, occurs scattering of transmembrane electronic potential, changes in membrane permeability, and stimulation of basal respiration, accompanied by a decrease in the level of ATP. The second stage begins 5–10 min after exposure and includes respiratory inhibition, mobilization of iron, and lipid peroxidation of the mitochondrial membrane (Dorta et al., 2003).

Mitochondria contain many potentially damaging proteins. Increased permeability of the mitochondrial membrane is a critical event that results in the release of various molecules crucial for apoptosis. These molecules include enzymes that are called pro-caspases, Cyt-C (a caspase activator), Smac/Diablo (a caspase coactivator), and AIF, which activates nucleases that divide DNA in small fragments. All aerobic cells generate ROS including superoxide, hydrogen peroxide (H_2O_2), and hydroxyl radicals enzymatically and nonenzymatically. The mitochondrial electronic transport chain is the main place for cellular production of ROS. ROS production increases with decreased electronic transport, which happens in pathological conditions. Cd inhibits the electronic transport chain and induces production of ROS, which explicitly explains the correlation between ROS formation and mitochondria dysfunction (Mao et al., 2010).

Most antioxidants and enzymes become inactive when exposed to cadmium due to the direct linking of Cd with active places that contain sulfhydryl groups (−SH) or the ejection of metal cofactors from active places. Mitochondria are sensitive to Cd-induced cellular damage in low micromolar concentrations. Cd can connect tightly to sulfhydryl groups of mitochondrial membrane proteins and in that way induce a change of MPT, as well as disruption of other mitochondrial functions. It means that Cd can lead to various cellular damages by inducing oxidative stress and mitochondrial dysfunction (Liu et al., 2009, 2011). Numerous studies have discovered that besides oxidative stress, cadmium additionally causes stress disruption of the ER *in vitro* and *in vivo*, which also has an important role in the inducing of apoptosis with Cd (Kitamura & Hiramatsu, 2010; Yokouchi et al., 2007, 2008).

Long time ago, it was shown in *in vitro* experiments that cadmium easily connects to mitochondria and that it is capable of inhibiting respiration (75%) and OXPHOS (100%) in concentrations as low as 5×10^{-6} M. Regarding the *in vivo* effect of cadmium on mitochondria, it is known that it depends on synthesis, accessibility, and degradation of Cd MT (Fowler, 1978).

In the literature, there is a consensus that mitochondria are key intracellular targets for Cd due to their capabilities to accumulate Cd and sensitivity of mitochondrial enzymes to damage caused by Cd. Due to the central role of mitochondria and critical cellular processes such as bioenergetics, redox signalization, and cellular death, mitochondrial damage induced by Cd has long-term consequences for cellular function, energetic homeostasis, and organism survival (Cannino et al., 2009; Liu et al., 2011; Sanni et al., 2008).

5.4. Cadmium and lipid peroxidation

Lipid peroxidation is oxidative damage that affects cellular membranes, lipoproteins, and other molecules that contain lipids in conditions with oxidative stress. Cellular membrane lipids represent most often substrates of oxidative attack (Nawrot et al., 2008). Lipid peroxidation is a chain reaction and is created by free radicals influencing unsaturated fatty acids in cell membranes, leading to their damage. Free radicals are initiators and terminators of lipid peroxidation processes. Once activated, reaction continues autocatalytically; it has a progressive course, and its final result is structural and functional changes of substrate (Cuypers et al., 2010; Ognjanovic et al., 2008).

Cadmium-induced oxidative stress causes not only DNA damage (mutations) and protein oxidation but also lipid peroxidation (Bertin & Averbeck, 2006; Cuypers et al., 2010) in many organisms (Bertin & Averbeck, 2006; Cuypers et al., 2010; Thevenod, 2009), which results in damaging various organs (Järup and Åkesson, 2009; Nawrot et al., 2008). Cadmium is bivalent cation and cannot generate free radicals directly, but even in spite of that, the production of ROS after exposure to cadmium has been observed in many studies (Belyaeva et al., 2006; Liu et al., 2009; Pathak & Khandelwal, 2006; Wang, Fang, Leonard, & Rao, 2004; Zhou et al., 2009).

Increasing levels of lipid peroxidation caused by cadmium are connected to increased production of free radicals (Stohs and Bagchi, 1995). The formation of free radicals stimulates lipid peroxidation in biomembranes, and constant fragmentation of fatty acid lateral chains produces aldehydes and hydrocarbonates, which in the end leads to the loss of membrane integrity (Gupta & Kar, 1999). It was observed that chronic intake of lead and cadmium in rats significantly stimulates peroxidative reaction. Metal-induced inhibition of type I iodothyronine 5′-monodediodinase was also observed, with subsequent thyroid dysfunction (Chaurasia, Gupta, Kar, & Maiti, 1996). Several years later, in an experiment with chickens, other authors established that cadmium-induced lipid peroxidation is connected to decreased activity of 5′D-I (deiodinase), which causes a decrease in forming T3 (Gupta & Kar, 1999).

Lipid peroxidation can cause mutual cross-linking and polymerization of membrane components. In this way, the cellular membrane can be modified in its lipid content and thus modify its cellular function. Induction of ROS and lipid oxidation can lead to important changes in membrane function, such as the modification of transmembrane potential (depolarization), release of mitochondrial calcium and division, and activation of caspases-3, DNA fragmentation, and apoptosis (Bertin & Averbeck, 2006).

6. CONCLUSIONS AND FUTURE DIRECTIONS

Chronic Cd exposition disturbs the structure and function of the thyroid gland. Both follicular and parafollicular cells are damaged.

Cadmium causes morphological preneoplastic changes that are manifested as colloid cystic goiter and follicular adenomatoid hyperplasia with low-grade dysplasia. The accompanying functional changes include weaker thyreoglobuline synthesis and T_3 and T_4 hyposecretion.

Cadmium concurrently induces parafollicular C-cell diffuse and nodular hyperplasia and hypertrophy. Chronic Cd exposition produces functional differentiation of the parafollicular cells of the thyroid gland, the first cell type being present in the area of diffuse hyperplasia and secreting various regulatory peptides and the other the constituent of nodular hyperplasia and microadenomas, secreting cGRP exclusively.

The mechanisms of C-cell hyperplasia are complex and call for further research with special emphasis on parathyroid gland morphology and function (unpublished data of the same author). Secondary parathyroidism caused by cadmium kidney damage is probably an important link in C-cell hyperplasia pathogenesis.

REFERENCES

Ackerman, S. H., & Tzagoloff, A. (2005). Function, structure, and biogenesis of mitochondrial ATP synthase. *Progress in Nucleic Acid Research and Molecular Biology*, *80*, 95–133.

Andrews, G. K. (2000). Regulation of metallothionein gene expression by oxidative stress and metal ions. *Biochemical Pharmacology*, *59*, 95–104.

Andujar, P., Bensefa-Colas, L., & Descatha, A. (2010). Acute and chronic cadmium poisoning. *La Revue de Médecine Interne*, *31*, 107–115.

Agency for Toxic Substances and Disease Registry (ATSDR). (1999). Toxicological Profile for Cadmium. Atlanta, GA: U.S. Department of Health and Human Services, *Public Health Service* 1-397. http://www.atsdr.cdc.gov,atsdr,1999.

Badiei, K., Nikghadam, P., & Mostaghni, K. (2009). Effect of cadmium on thyroid function in sheep. *Comparative Clinical Pathology*, *18*, 255–259.

Bekheet, H. M. S. (2011). Comparative effects of repeated administration of cadmium chloride during pregnancy and lactation and selenium protection against cadmium toxicity on some organs in immature rats' offsprings. *Biological Trace Element Research, 144*, 1008–1023.

Belyaeva, E. A., Dymkowska, D., Wieckowski, M. R., & Wojtczak, L. (2006). Reactive oxygen species produced by the mitochondrial respiratory chain are involved in Cd^{2+}-induced injury of rat ascites hepatoma AS-30D cells. *Biochimica et Biophysica Acta, Bioenergetics, 1757*(12), 1568–1574.

Belyaeva, E. A., Glazunov, V. V., & Korotkov, S. M. (2004). Cd^{2+} promoted mitochondrial permeability transition: A comparison with other heavy metals. *Acta Biochimica Polonica, 51*(2), 545–551.

Belyaeva, E. A., Korotkov, S. M., & Saris, N. E. (2011). In vitro modulation of heavy metal-induced rat liver mitochondria dysfunction: A comparison of copper and mercury with cadmium. *Journal of Trace Elements in Medicine and Biology, 25S*, S63–S73.

Bergendi, L., Benes, L., Duracková, Z., & Ferencik, M. (1999). Chemistry, physiology and pathology of free radicals. *Life Sciences, 65*, 1865–1874.

Bertin, G., & Averbeck, D. (2006). Cadmium: Cellular effects, modifications of biomolecules, modulation of DNA repair and genotoxic consequences (a review). *Biochimie, 88*, 1549–1559.

Beyersmann, D., & Hechtenberg, S. (1997). Cadmium, gene regulation, and cellular signalling in mammalian cells. *Toxicology and Applied Pharmacology, 144*, 247–261.

Bi, Y., Palmiter, R. D., Wood, K. M., & Ma, Q. (2004). Induction of metallothionein I by phenolic antioxidants requires metal-activated transcription factor 1 (MTF-1) and zinc. *The Biochemical Journal, 380*, 695–703.

Bianco, A. C., Salvatore, D., Gereben, B., Berry, M. J., & Larsen, P. R. (2002). Biochemistry, cellular and molecular biology, and physiological roles of the iodothyronine selenodeiodinase. *Endocrine Reviews, 23*, 38–89.

Boas, M., Feldt-Rasmussen, U., Skakkebaek, N. E., & Main, K. M. (2006). Environmental chemicals and thyroid function. *European Journal of Endocrinology, 154*, 599–611.

Brzezińska-Slebodzińska, E., & Pietras, B. (1997). The protective role of some antioxidants and scavengers on the free radicals-induced inhibition of the liver iodothyronine 5′-monodeiodinase activity and thiols content. *Journal of Physiology and Pharmacology, 48*(3), 451–459.

Cannino, G., Ferruggia, E., Luparello, C., & Rinaldi, A. M. (2009). Cadmium and mitochondria. *Mitochondrion, 9*, 377–384.

Carcangiu, M. L. (2007). Thyroid. In S. E. Mills (Ed.), *Histology for pathologists* (3rd ed.). (pp. 112–145). Philadelphia: Lippincott Williams & Wilkins.

Castelli, M., Rossi, B., Corsetti, F., Mantovani, A., Spera, G., Lubrano, C., et al. (2005). Levels of cadmium and lead in blood: An application of validated methods in a group of patients with endocrine/metabolic disorders from the Rome area. *Microchemical Journal, 79*, 349–355.

Chaurasia, S. S., Gupta, P., Kar, A., & Maiti, P. K. (1996). Free radical mediated membrane perturbation and inhibition of type-I iodothyronine 5′-monodeiodinase activity by lead and cadmium in rat liver homogenate. *Biochemistry and Molecular Biology International, 39*, 765–770.

Chopra, I. J. (1978). Sulfhydryl groups and the monodeiodination of thyroxine to triiodothyronine. *Science, 199*, 904–906.

Cormack, D. H. (1998). Endocrine and reproductive systems. In *Clinically integrated histology* (pp. 219–275). Philadelphia: Lippincott-Raven.

Curcio-Morelli, C., Zavacki, A. M., Christofollete, M., Gereben, B., de Freitas, B. C. G., Harney, J. W., et al. (2003). Deubiquitination of type 2 iodothyronine deiodinase by von Hippel-Lindau protein-interacting deubiquitinating enzymes regulates thyroid hormone activation. *The Journal of Clinical Investigation, 112*, 189–196.

Cuypers, A., Plusquin, M., Remans, T., Jozefczak, M., Keunen, E., Gielen, H., et al. (2010). Cadmium stress: An oxidative challenge. *Biometals*, *23*, 927–940.

Dakeshita, S., Kawai, T., Uemura, H., Hiyoshi, M., Oguma, E., Horiguchi, H., et al. (2009). Gene expression signatures in peripheral blood cells from Japanese women exposed to environmental cadmium. *Toxicology*, *257*, 25–32.

Daugas, E., Susin, S. A., Zamzami, N., Ferri, K. F., Irinopoulou, T., Larochette, N., et al. (2000). Mitochondrio-nuclear translocation of AIF in apoptosis and necrosis. *The FASEB Journal*, *14*, 729–739.

DeLellis, R. A., Nunnemacher, G., & Wolfe, H. J. (1997). C-cell hyperplasia. An ultrastructural analysis. *Laboratory Investigation*, *36*, 237–248.

DeLellis, R. A., & Wolfe, H. J. (1981). The pathobiology of the human calcitonin (C)-cell: A review. *Pathology Annual*, *61*, 237–248.

Diep, P. T. N., Denizeau, F., & Jumarie, C. (2005). Kinetics of the early subcellular distribution of cadmium in rat hepatocytes. *Biometals*, *18*, 255–267.

Dorta, D. J., Leite, S., DeMarco, K. C., Prado, I. M., Rodrigues, T., Mingatto, F. E., et al. (2003). A proposed sequence of events for cadmium-induced mitochondrial impairment. *Journal of Inorganic Biochemistry*, *97*(3), 251–257.

Eichler, T., Ma, Q., Kelly, C., Mishra, J., Parikh, S., Ransom, R. F., et al. (2006). Single and combination toxic metal exposures induce apoptosis in cultured mutine podocytes exclusively via the extrinsic caspase 8 pathway. *Toxicological Sciences*, *90*, 392–399.

El Heni, J., Messaoudi, I., & Ben Chaouacha-Chekir, R. (2012). Effects of sub-chronic exposure to cadmium on some parameters of calcium and iodine metabolisms in the Shaw's jird Meriones shawi. *Environmental Toxicology and Pharmacology*, *34*, 136–143.

Fauci, A. S., Braunwald, E., Kasper, D. L., Hauser, S. L., Longo, D. L., Jameson, J. L., et al. (2008). *Harrison's principles of internal medicine* (17th ed.). (pp. 2224–2247). Printed in the United States of America: The McGraw-Hill Companies, Inc.

Filipic, M., Fatur, T., & Vudrag, M. (2006). Molecular mechanisms of cadmium induced mutagenicity. *Human and Experimental Toxicology*, *25*, 67–77.

Fleury, C., Mignotte, B., & Vayssière, J. L. (2002). Mitochondrial reactive oxygen species in cell death signalling. *Biochimie*, *84*, 131–141.

Fowler, B. A. (1978). General subcellular effects of lead, mercury, cadmium, and arsenic. *Environmental Health Perspectives*, *22*, 37–41.

Gagnon, E., Hontela, A., & Fumarie, C. (2007). Reciprocal inhibition of Cd and Ca uptake in isolated head kidney cells of rainbow trout (Oncorhynchus mykiss). *Toxicology In Vitro*, *21*, 1077–1086.

Ghosh, N., & Bhattachary, A. S. (1992). Thyrotoxicity of the chlorides of cadmium and mercury in rabbit. *Biomedical and Environmental Sciences*, *5*, 236A–240A.

Giedroc, D. P., Chen, X., & Apuy, J. L. (2001). Metal response element (MRE)-binding transcription factor-1 (MTF-1): Structure, function, and regulation. *Antioxidants & Redox Signaling*, *3*, 577–596.

Govel, N., Chaudhary, S., Waseem, M., & Parvez, S. (2012). Postnuclear supernatant: An in vitro model for assessing cadmium-induced neurotoxicity. *Biological Trace Element Research*, *146*, 402–409.

Gupta, A., & Kar, A. (1997). Role of testosterone in ameliorating the cadmium induced inhibition of thyroid function in adult male mouse. *Bulletin of Environmental Contamination and Toxicology*, *58*, 422–428.

Gupta, P., & Kar, A. (1999). Cadmium induced thyroid dysfunction in chicken: Hepatic type I iodothyronine 5′-monodeiodinase activity and role of lipid peroxidation. *Comparative Biochemistry and Physiology*, *123*, 39–44.

Hammouda, F., Messaoudi, I., El Hani, J., Baati, T., Said, K., & Kerkeni, A. (2008). Reversal of cadmium-induced thyroid dysfunction by selenium, zinc, or their combination in rat. *Biological Trace Element Research*, *126*(1–3), 194–203.

Hartwig, A., Asmuss, M., Blessing, H., Hoffmann, S., Jahnke, G., Khandelwal, S., et al. (2002). Interference by toxic metal ions with zinc-dependent proteins involved in maintaining genomic stability. *Food and Chemical Toxicology, 40*, 1179–1184.

Harvey, C. B., & Williams, G. R. (2002). Mechanism of thyroid hormone action. *Thyroid, 12*, 441–446.

Hogervorst, J., Plusquin, M., Vangronsveld, J., Nawrot, T., Cuypers, A., Van Hecke, E., et al. (2007). House dust as possible route of environmental exposure to cadmium and lead in the adult general population. *Environmental Research, 103*, 30–37.

Hontela, A., Daniel, C., & Ricard, A. C. (1996). Effects of acute and subacute exposures to cadmium on the interrenal and thyroid function in rainbow trout, Oncorhynchus mykiss. *Aquatic Toxicology, 35*, 171–182.

Hossain, S., Liu, H. N., Nguyen, M., Shore, G., & Almazan, G. (2009). Cadmium exposure induces mitochondria-dependent apoptosis in oligodendrocytes. *Neurotoxicology, 30*, 544–554.

Huang, Q. Y., Fang, C. W., & Huang, H. Q. (2011). Alteration of heart tissue protein profiles in acute cadmium-treated scallops Patinopecten yessoensis. *Archives of Environmental Contamination and Toxicology, 60*, 90–98.

Huang, C. L., Sun, L., Moonga, B. S., & Zaidi, M. (2006). Molecular physiology and pharmacology of calcitonin. *Cellular and Molecular Biology (Noisy-le-Grand), 52*(3), 33–43.

Huff, J., Lunn, R. M., Waalkes, M. P., Tomatis, L., & Infante, P. F. (2007). Cadmium-induced cancers in animals and in humans. *International Journal of Occupational Environmental Health, 13*, 202–212.

International Agency for Research on Cancer, (IARC), (1993). Beryllium, cadmium, mercury and exposures in the glass industry. *Monographs on the evaluation of carcinogenic risk to humans.* (pp. 119–237). Lyon, France: IARC, Vol. 58.

International Agency for Research on Cancer, (IARC), (2012). Cadmium and cadmium compounds. *Monographs on the evaluation of carcinogenic risks to humans.* (pp. 121–145). Lyon, France: IARC, Vol. 100C.

ICCIDD, UNICEF, & WHO, (2001). *Assessment of iodine deficiency disorders and monitoring their elimination* (2nd ed.). Geneva: WHO Publication.

Iijima, K., Otake, T., Yoshinaga, J., Ikegami, M., Suzuki, E., Naruse, H., et al. (2007). Cadmium, lead, and selenium in cord blood and thyroid hormone status of newborns. *Biological Trace Element Research, 119*, 10–18.

Ishido, M., Ohtsubo, R., Adachi, T., & Kunimoto, M. (2002). Attenuation of both apoptotic and necrotic actions of cadmium by Bcl-2. *Environmental Health Perspectives, 110*, 37–42.

Jadhao, A. G., Paul, P. L., & Rao, P. D. (1994). Effect of cadmium chloride on the pituitary, thyroid and gonads in the catfish, Clarias batrachus (Linn.). *Functional and Developmental Morphology, 4*(1), 39–44.

Jancic, S., Bojanic, V., Rancic, G., Joksimovic, I., Jancic, N., Zindovic, M., et al. (2011). Calcitonin gene-related peptide (CGRP)—Microadenomas of the thyroid gland induced by cadmium toxicity. Experimental study. *Journal of BUON, 16*(2), 331–336.

Järup, L., & Åkesson, A. (2009). Current status of cadmium as an environmental health problem. *Toxicology and Applied Pharmacology, 238*, 201–208.

Jin, Y. H., Clark, A. B., Slebos, R. J., Al-Refai, H., Taylor, J. A., Kunkel, T. A., et al. (2003). Cadmium as a mutagen that acts by inhibiting mismatch repair. *Nature Genetics, 34*, 326–329.

Kawahara, H., Takashima, Y., Nakamura, M., & Yamagami, A. (1975). Electron microscopic study of the cytotoxicity of cadmium and mercury in vitro. *Journal of Dental Research, 54*(1), 125–130.

Kelly, G. S. (2000). Peripheral metabolism of thyroid hormones: A review. *Alternative Medicine Review, 5*(4), 306–333.

Kitamura, M., & Hiramatsu, N. (2010). The oxidative stress-endoplasmic reticulum stress axis in cadmium toxicity. *BioMetals, 23*, 941–950.

Klaassen, C. D. (2001). *Casarett and Doull's toxicology*. (pp. 822–826). New York: McGraw-Hill Medical Publishing Division.
Klaassen, C. D., Liu, J., & Choudhuri, S. (1999). Metallothionein: An intracellular protein to protect against cadmium toxicity. *Annual Review of Pharmacology and Toxicology*, *39*, 267–294.
Klaassen, C. D., Liu, J., & Diwan, B. A. (2009). Metallothionein protection of cadmium toxicity. *Toxicology and Applied Pharmacology*, *238*, 215–220.
Kocak, M., & Akcil, E. (2006). The effects of chronic cadmium toxicity on the hemostatic system. *Pathophysiology of Haemostasis and Thrombosis*, *35*, 411–416.
Kondoh, M., Araragi, S., Sato, K., Higashimoto, M., Takiguchi, M., & Sato, M. (2002). Cadmium induces apoptosis partly via caspase-9 activation in HL-60 cells. *Toxicology*, *170*, 111–117.
Kotelnikova, S. V., Sokolova, N. G., & Kotelnikov, A. V. (2008). Lipid peroxidation in various organs and tissues of albino rats with cadmium intoxication in winter and summer. *Bulletin of Experimental Biology and Medicine*, *146*(3), 291–292.
Krause, J. W. (2005). Endocrine glands. In J. W. Krause (Ed.), *Essential human histology for medical students* (pp. 258–271). Boca Raton, FL: Universal Publishers.
Kuo, Y. J., Tsuang, F. Y., Sun, J. S., Lin, C. H., Chen, C. H., Li, J. Y., et al. (2012). Calcitonin inhibits SDCP-induced osteoclast apoptosis and increases its efficacy in a rat model of osteoporosis. *PLoS One*, 7(7), e40272.
Lafuente, A., Cano, P., & Esquifino, A. I. (2003). Are cadmium effects on plasma gonadotropins, prolactin, ACTH, GH and TSH levels, dose-dependent? *BioMetals*, *16*, 243–250.
Lemarié, A., Lagadic-Gossmann, D., Morzadec, C., Allain, N., Fardel, O., & Vernhet, L. (2004). Cadmium induces caspase-independent apoptosis in liver Hep3B cells: Role for calcium in signaling oxidative stress-related impairment of mitochondria and relocation of endonuclease G and apoptosis inducing factor. *Free Radical Biology and Medicine*, *36*, 1517–1531.
Lemasters, J. J., Theruvath, T. P., Zhong, Z., & Nieminen, A. L. (2009). Mitochondrial calcium and the permeability transition in cell death. *Biochimica et Biophysica Acta*, *1787*(11), 1395–1401.
Li, M., Xia, T., Jiang, C. S., Li, L. J., Fu, J. L., & Zhou, Z. C. (2003). Cadmium directly induced the opening of membrane permeability pore of mitochondria which possibly involved in cadmium triggered apoptosis. *Toxicology*, *194*, 19–33.
Liu, T., He, W., Yan, C., Qi, Y., & Zhang, Y. (2011). Roles of reactive oxygen species and mitochondria in cadmium-induced injury of liver cells. *Toxicology and Industrial Health*, *27*(3), 249–256.
Liu, S. K., Luthringer, D. J., & Easen, R. N. (2002). Thyroid transcription factor-1: A review. *Applied Immunohistochemistry and Molecular Morphology*, *10*, 97–102.
Liu, J., Qu, W., & Kadiiska, M. B. (2009). Role of oxidative stress in cadmium toxicity and carcinogenesis. *Toxicology and Applied Pharmacology*, *238*, 209–214.
Liu, Z., Yu, X., & Shaikh, Z. A. (2008). Rapid activation of ERK1/2 and AKT in human breast cancer cells by cadmium. *Toxicology and Applied Pharmacology*, *228*, 286–294.
Mao, W. P., Zhang, N. N., Zhou, F. Y., Li, W. X., Liu, H. Y., Feng, J., et al. (2010). Cadmium directly induced mitochondrial dysfunction of human embryonic kidney cells. *Human and Experimental Toxicology*, *30*(8), 920–929.
Mao, W. P., Zhao, J. M., Shi, X. J., Xu, F., Zou, X. S., Jiang, P., et al. (2005). Mitochondrial pathway in cadmium-induced apoptosis in HEK293 cells. *Chinese Journal of Pharmacology and Toxicology*, *19*, 305–307.
Marcano, L. B. C., Carruyo, I. M., Montiel, X. M., Morales, C. B., & de Soto, P. M. (2009). Effect of cadmium on cellular viability in two species of microalgae (Scenedesmus sp. and Dunaliella viridis). *Biological Trace Element Research*, *130*(1), 86–93.
Martelli, A., Rousselet, E., Dycke, C., Bouron, A., & Moulis, J. M. (2006). Cadmium toxicity in animal cells by interference with essential metals. *Biochimie*, *88*, 1807–1814.

Marzia, M., Chiusaroli, R., Neff, L., Kim, N. Y., Chishti, A. H., Baron, R., et al. (2006). Calpain is required for normal osteoclast function and is down-regulated by calcitonin. *The Journal of Biological Chemistry, 281*, 9745–9975.

McMurray, C. T., & Tainer, J. A. (2003). Cancer, cadmium and genome integrity. *Nature Genetics, 34*, 239–241.

Misra, U. K., Gawdi, G., & Pizzo, S. V. (2003). Induction of mitogenic signalling in the 1LN prostate cell line on exposure to submicromolar concentrations of cadmium^{+}. *Cellular Signalling, 15*, 1059–1070.

Morreale, G., Obregon, M. J., & Escobar, F. (2004). Role of thyroid hormone during early brain development. *European Journal of Endocrinology, 151*, 5–37.

Moulis, J. M. (2010). Cellular mechanisms of cadmium toxicity related to the homeostasis of essential metals. *Biometals, 23*, 877–896.

Murray, D. (1998). The thyroid gland. In K. Kovacs & S. L. Asa (Eds.), *Functional endocrine pathology* (2nd ed.). (pp. 295–380). Boston, MA: Blackwell Science.

Nawrot, T. S., Van Hecke, E., Thijs, L., Richart, T., Kuznetsova, T., Jin, Y., et al. (2008). Cadmium related mortality and long-term secular trends in the cadmium body burden of an environmentally exposed population. *Environmental Health Perspectives, 116*(12), 1620–1628.

Nishijo, M., Nakagawa, H., Morikawa, Y., Tabata, M., Senma, M., Miura, K., et al. (1994). A study of thyroid hormone levels of inhabitants of the cadmium-polluted Kakehashi River basin. *Nippon Eiseigaku Zasshi, 49*, 598–605.

Nordberg, G. F. (2004). Cadmium and health in the 21st century-historical remarks and trends for the future. *Biometals, 17*, 485–489.

Nordberg, G. F. (2009). Historical perspectives on cadmium toxicology. *Toxicology and Applied Pharmacology, 238*, 192–200.

Nordberg, G. F., Nogawa, K., Nordberg, M., & Friedmann, J. M. (2007). Cadmium. In G. F. Nordberg, B. A. Fowler, M. Nordberg, & L. Friberg (Eds.), *Handbook on the toxicology of metals* (pp. 445–486). Amsterdam: Elsevier.

Nordberg, M., & Nordberg, G. F. (2009). *Metal Ions in Life Sciences* (5). In A. Sigel, et al. (Eds.), *Metallothioneins: Historical development and overview* (pp. 1–29).

National Toxicology Program (NTP). (2011). 12th Report on carcinogens (pp. 80–82). Research Triangle Park, NC: National Institution of Environmental Health Sciences, U.S. Department of Health and Human Services, Public Health Service.

Nussey, S., & Whitehead, S. (2001). *Endocrinology: An integrated approach.* Chapter 3, The thyroid gland, Oxford: BIOS Scientific Publishers.*http://www.ncbi.nlm.nih.gov/books/NBK28/.*

Ognjanovic, B. I., Markovic, S. D., Pavlovic, S. Z., Zikic, R. V., Stajn, A. S., & Saicic, Z. S. (2008). Effect of chronic cadmium exposure on antioxidant defense system in some tissues of rats: Protective effect of selenium. *Physiological Research, 57*, 403–411.

Oh, S. H., & Lim, S. C. (2006). A rapid and transient ROS generation by cadmium triggers apoptosis via caspase-dependent pathway in HepG2 cells and this is inhibited through N-acetylcysteine mediated catalase upregulation. *Toxicology and Applied Pharmacology, 212*, 212–223.

Olsson, I. M., Bensryd, I., Lundth, T., Ottosson, H., Skerfving, S., & Oskarsson, A. (2002). Cadmium in blood and urine-impact of sex, age, dietary intake, iron status, and former smoking-association of renal effects. *Environmental Health Perspectives, 110*, 1185–1190.

Paier, B., Hagmüller, K., Noli, M. I., Gonzalez, P. M., Stiegler, C., & Zaninovich, A. A. (1993). Changes induced by cadmium administration on thyroxine deiodination and sulfhydryl groups in rat liver. *The Journal of Endocrinology, 138*, 219–224.

Pathak, N., & Khandelwal, S. (2006). Oxidative stress and apoptotic changes in murine splenocytes exposed to cadmium. *Toxicology, 220*(1), 26–36.

Pavia, M. A., Jr., Paier, B., Noli, M. I., Hagmuller, K., & Zaninovich, A. A. (1997). Evidence suggesting that cadmium induces a nonthyroidal illness syndrome in the rat. *Journal of Endocrinology*, *154*, 113–117.

Petering, D. H., Krezoski, S., & Tabatabai, N. M. (2009). Metallothionein toxicology: Metal ion trafficking and cellular protection. *Metal Ions in Life Sciences*, *5*, 353–397.

Pilat-Marcinkiewicz, B., Brzóska, M. M., Sawicki, B., & Moniuszko-Jakoniuk, J. (2003). Structure and function of thyroid follicular cells in female rats chronically exposed to cadmium. *Bulletin of the Veterinary Institute in Pulawy*, *47*, 157–163.

Pilat-Marcinkiewicz, B., Sawicki, B., Brzoska, M. M., & Jakoniuk, J. M. (2002). Effect of chronic administration of cadmium on the rat thyroid: Radioimmunological and immunohistochemical studies. *Folia Histochemica et Cytobiologica*, *40*, 189–190.

Pillai, A., Laxmi Priya, P. N., & Gupta, S. (2002). Effects of combined exposure to lead and cadmium on pituitary membrane of female rats. *Archives of Toxicology*, *76*, 671–675.

Pillai, A., Priya, L., & Gupta, S. (2003). Effects of combined exposure to lead and cadmium on the hypothalamic–pituitary axis function in proestrous rats. *Food and Chemical Toxicology*, *41*, 379–384.

Powel, S. R. (2000). The antioxidant properties of zinc. *The Journal of Nutrition*, *130*, 1447S–1454S.

Puri, V. N., & Saha, S. (2003). Comparison of acute cardiovascular effects of cadmium and captopril in relation to oxidant and angiotensin converting enzyme activity in rats. *Drug and Chemical Toxicology*, *26*(3), 213–218.

Rinal, P. S., Meenu, B. N., Viral, D. T., Tushar, D. R., & Pravin, T. R. (2012). Screening of herbal drugs for heavy metal toxicity with specific reference to arsenic and lead with its therapeutic significance. *International Bulletin of Drug Research*, *1*(2), 10–23.

Sancho, P., Fernández, C., Yuste, V. J., Amrán, D., Ramos, A. M., de Blas, E., et al. (2006). Regulation of apoptosis/necrosis execution in cadmium-treated human promonocytic cells under different forms of oxidative stress. *Apoptosis*, *11*, 673–686.

Sanni, B., Williams, K., Sokolov, E. P., & Sokolova, I. M. (2008). Effects of acclimation temperature and cadmium exposure on mitochondrial aconitase and LON protease from a model marine ectotherm, Crassostrea virginica. *Comparative Biochemistry and Physiology Toxicology & Pharmacology*, *147*, 101–112.

Saris, N. E., & Carafoli, E. (2005). A historical review of cellular calcium handling, with emphasis on mitochondria. *Biochemistry (Mosc)*, *70*, 187–194.

Satarug, S., Baker, J. R., Urbenjapol, S., Haswell-Elkins, M., Reilly, P. E., Williams, D. J., et al. (2003). A global perspective on cadmium pollution and toxicity in non-occupationally exposed population. *Toxicology Letters*, *137*(1–2), 65–83.

Sato, M., & Takizawa, Y. (1982). Cadmium-binding proteins in human organs. *Toxicology Letters*, *11*(3–4), 269–273.

Satoh, M., Kaji, T., & Tohyama, C. (2003). Low dose exposure to cadmium and its health effects. (3) Toxicity in laboratory animals and cultured cells. *Nippon Eiseigaku Zasshi*, *57*, 615–623(in Japanese).

Schwartz, G. G., & Reis, I. M. (2000). Is cadmium a cause of human pancreatic cancer? *Cancer Epidemiology, Biomarkers & Prevention*, *9*, 139–145.

Selinus, O. (2005). *Essentials of medical geology: Impacts of the natural environment on public health.* (p. 187). New York: Academic Press.

Shih, C. M., Ko, W. C., Wu, J. S., Wei, Y. H., Wang, L. F., Chang, E. E., et al. (2004). Mediating of caspase-independent apoptosis by cadmium through the mitochondria-ROS pathway in MRC-5 fibroblasts. *Journal of Cellular Biochemistry*, *91*, 384–397.

Shin, H. J., Park, K. K., Lee, B. H., Moon, C. K., & Lee, M. O. (2003). Identification of genes that are induced after cadmium exposure by suppression subtractive hybridization. *Toxicology*, *191*, 121–131.

Sirchia, R., Longo, A., & Luparello, C. (2008). Cadmium regulation of apoptotic and stress response genes in tumoral and immortalized epithelial cells of the human breast. *Biochimie, 90,* 1578–1590.

Slyuzova, O. V., Stepanova, E. V., Temraleeva, A. D., Kireev, R. A., & Ignatov, V. V. (2008). Effects of prenatal and neonatal cadmium intoxication on the intensity of lipid peroxidation and activity of glutathione system in progeny of albino rats. *Bulletin of Experimental Biology and Medicine, 146*(1), 41–44.

Son, Y. O., Lee, J. C., Hitron, J. A., Pan, J., Zhang, Z., & Shi, X. (2010). Cadmium induces intracellular Ca^{2+} and H_2O_2-dependent apoptosis through JNK- and p53-mediated pathways in skin epidermal cell line. *Toxicological Sciences, 113*(1), 127–137.

Staessen, J., Amery, A., Bernard, A., Bruaux, P., Buchet, J. P., Claeys, F., et al. (1991). Effects of exposure to cadmium on calcium metabolism: A population study. *British Journal of Industrial Medicine, 48,* 710–714.

Stohs, S. J., & Bagchi, D. (1995). Oxidative mechanisms in the toxicity of metal ions. *Free Radical Biology and Medicine, 18,* 321–336.

Su, J. K., Hyun-Ja, J., Noh-Yil, M., Min-chol, K., Jeong-Han, L., Hong-seob, S., et al. (2008). The protective mechanism of antioxidants in cadmium-induced ototoxicity in vitro and in vivo. *Environmental Health Perspectives, 116*(7), 854–862.

Susin, S. A., Zamzami, N., & Kroemer, G. (1998). Mitochondria as regulators of apoptosis: Doubt no more. *Biochimica et Biophysica Acta, 366,* 151–165.

Szuster-Ciesielska, A., Stachura, A., Slotwinska, M., Kaminska, T., Sniezko, R., Paduch, R., et al. (2000). The inhibitory effect of zinc on cadmium-induced cell apoptosis and reactive oxygen species (ROS) production in cell cultures. *Toxicology, 145,* 159–171.

Tang, W., & Shaikh, Z. A. (2001). Renal cortical mitochondrial dysfunction upon cadmium metallothionein administration to Sprague–Dawley rats. *Journal of Toxicology and Environmental Health.* Part A, *63,* 221–235.

Tapia, L., González-Agüero, M., Cisternas, M. F., Suazo, M., Cambiazo, V., Uauy, R., et al. (2004). Metallothionein is crucial for safe intracellular copper storage and cell survival at normal and supra-physiological exposure levels. *The Biochemical Journal, 378*(Pt 2), 617–624.

Thevenod, F. (2009). Cadmium and cellular signaling cascades: To be or not to be? *Toxicology and Applied Pharmacology, 238*(3), 221–239.

Thirumoorthy, N., Shyam Sunder, A., Manisenthil Kumar, K. T., Senthil kumar, M., Ganesh, G. N. K., & Chatterjee, M. A. (2011). Review of metallothionein isoforms and their role in pathophysiology. *World Journal of Surgical Oncology, 9,* 54.

Tiran, B., Karpf, E., & Tiran, A. (1995). Age dependency of selenium and cadmium content in human liver, kidney, and thyroid. *Archives of Environmental Health, 50*(3), 242–246.

Tsutsumi, R., Hiroi, H., Momoeda, M., Hosokawa, Y., Nakazawa, F., Yano, T., et al. (2009). Induction of early decidualization by cadmium, a major contaminant of cigarette smoke. *Fertility and Sterility, 91,* 1614–1617.

Uetani, M., Kobayashi, E., Suwazono, Y., Honda, R., Nishijo, M., Nakagawa, H., et al. (2006). Tissue cadmium (Cd) concentrations of people living in a Cd polluted area, Japan. *BioMetals, 19,* 521–525.

Vahter, M., Akesson, A., Liden, C., Ceccatelli, C., & Berglund, M. (2007). Gender differences in the disposition and toxicity of metals. *Environmental Research, 104,* 85–95.

Vallee, B. L., & Ullmer, D. D. (1972). Biochemical effects of mercury, cadmium and lead. *Annual Review of Biochemistry, 41,* 91–128.

Vanderpump, M., & Tunbridge, M. (2008). *Thyroid disease (the facts).* Oxford: Oxford University Press.

Vašak, M., & Hasler, D. W. (2000). Metallothioneins: New functional and structural insights. *Current Opinion in Chemical Biology, 4,* 177–183.

Visser, T. J. (1978). A tentative review of recent *in vitro* observations of enzymatic deiodination of iodothyronines and its possible physiological implications. *Molecular and Cellular Endocrinology*, *10*, 241–247.

Waalkes, M. P. (2003). Cadmium carcinogenesis. *Mutation Research*, *533*, 107–120.

Waisberg, M., Joseph, P., Hale, B., & Beyersmann, D. (2003). Molecular and cellular mechanisms of cadmium carcinogenesis. *Toxicology*, *192*, 95–117.

Wang, Y., Fang, Y. J., Leonard, Z., & Rao, K. M. (2004). Cadmium inhibits the electron transfer chain and induces reactive oxygen species. *Free Radical Biology & Medicine*, *36*, 1434–1443.

Wang, S. H., Shih, Y. L., Ko, W. C., Wei, Y. H., & Shih, C. M. (2008). Cadmium-induced autophagy and apoptosis are mediated by a calcium signaling pathway. *Cellular and Molecular Life Sciences*, *65*, 3640–3652.

Wimmer, U., Wang, Y., Georgiev, O., & Schaffner, W. (2005). Two major branches of anti-cadmium defense in the mouse: MTF-1/metallothioneins and glutathione. *Nucleic Acids Research*, *33*, 5715–5727.

Woodrow, J. P., Sharpe, C. J., Fudge, N. J., Hoff, A. O., Gagel, R. F., & Kovacs, C. S. (2006). Calcitonin plays a critical role in regulating skeletal mineral metabolism during lactation. *Endocrinology*, *147*(9), 4010–4021.

Yokouchi, M., Hiramatsu, N., Hayakawa, K., Kasai, A., Takano, Y., Yao, J., et al. (2007). Atypical, bidirectional regulation of cadmium-induced apoptosis via distinct signaling of unfolded protein response. *Cell Death and Differentiation*, *14*, 1467–1474.

Yokouchi, M., Hiramatsu, N., Hayakawa, K., Okamura, M., Du, S., Kasai, A., et al. (2008). Involvement of selective reactive oxygen species upstream of proapoptotic branches of unfolded protein response. *The Journal of Biological Chemistry*, *283*, 4252–4260.

Yoshida, K., Sugihira, N., Suzuki, M., Sakurada, T., Saito, S., Yoshinaga, K., et al. (1987). Effect of cadmium on T4 outer ring monodeiodination by rat liver. *Environmental Research*, *42*, 400–405.

Yoshizuka, M., Mori, N., Hamasaki, K., Tanaka, I., Yokoyama, M., Hara, K., et al. (1991). Cadmium toxicity in the thyroid gland of pregnant rats. *Experimental and Molecular Pathology*, *55*, 97–104.

Zazueta, C., Sanchez, C., Garcia, N., & Correa, F. (2000). Possible involvement of the adenine nucleotide translocase in the activation of the permeability transition pore induced by cadmium. *The International Journal of Biochemistry & Cell Biology*, *32*, 1093–1101.

Zhang, C., Yuan, X., Mao, W., Yue, L., Kong, X., Gao, Y., et al. (2010). Inhibition of cadmium-induced apoptosis by glutathione S-transferase P1 via mitogen-activated protein kinases and mitochondrial pathways. *Environmental Toxicology and Pharmacology*, *30*, 202–208.

Zhou, T., Jia, X., Chapin, R. E., Maronpot, R. R., Harris, M. W., Liu, J., et al. (2004). Cadmium at a non-toxic dose alters gene expression in mouse testes. *Toxicology Letters*, *154*, 191–200.

Zhou, Z. H., Lei, Y. X., & Wang, C. X. (2012). Analysis of aberrant methylation in DNA repair genes during malignant transformation of human bronchial epithelial cells induced by cadmium. *Toxicological Sciences*, *125*(2), 412–417.

Zhou, Y. J., Zhang, S. P., Liu, C. W., & Cai, Y. Q. (2009). The protection of selenium on ROS-mediated apoptosis by mitochondria dysfunction in cadmium-induced LLC-PK1 cells. *Toxicology In Vitro*, *23*(2), 288–294.

Zoeller, R. T., Tan, S. W., & Tyl, R. W. (2007). General background on the hypothalamic-pituitary-thyroid (HPT) axis. *Critical Reviews in Toxicology*, *37*, 11–53.

CHAPTER FIFTEEN

A Recombinant PPRE-Driven Luciferase Bioassay for Identification of Potential PPAR Agonists

Feng-Yuan Tsai, Yi-Ting Cheng, Tsui-Chun Tsou[1]
Laboratory of Molecular Toxicology, Division of Environmental Health and Occupational Medicine, National Health Research Institutes, Zhunan, Miaoli, Taiwan
[1]Corresponding author: e-mail address: tctsou@nhri.org.tw

Contents

1. Introduction 428
2. Materials 428
   2.1 Cells and culture medium 428
   2.2 Selection of G-418-resistant cell clones components 429
   2.3 Luciferase assay components 430
3. Methods 431
   3.1 Protocol for establishment of recombinant Huh7-PPRE-Luc cells for PPRE-driven luciferase assay 431
   3.2 Treatments of Huh7-PPRE-Luc cells with chemicals for PPRE-driven luciferase assay 433
   3.3 PPRE-driven luciferase assay 433
4. Notes 433
Acknowledgment 434
References 434

Abstract

A recombinant Huh7-PPRE-Luc cell line, carrying a peroxisome proliferator response element (PPRE)-driven luciferase gene, is an efficient tool for evaluation of potential peroxisome proliferator-activated receptor (PPAR) agonists. The cells exhibited a good dose–response induction in PPRE-driven luciferase activity by three subtypes of PPAR agonists as well as by a retinoid X receptor agonist, 9-*cis*-retinoic acid. Here, the bioassay is fitted into a 96-well plate format for high-throughput screening purpose.

Vitamins and Hormones, Volume 94
ISSN 0083-6729
http://dx.doi.org/10.1016/B978-0-12-800095-3.00015-8

1. INTRODUCTION

Peroxisome proliferator-activated receptor (PPAR), a member of the nuclear hormone receptor family, includes three subtypes (PPARα, PPARβ/δ, and PPARγ) that are encoded by three different genes. PPAR functions as transcription factors regulating the expression of genes (Michalik et al., 2006). When activated by agonists, PPAR bind as heterodimers with a retinoid X receptor and bind to the peroxisome proliferator response element (PPRE) in the promoter region of those downstream target genes. The physiological responses of PPAR relate to lipid/glucose metabolism and energy homeostasis. PPAR also plays critical roles in regulating cellular differentiation and development, as well as in tumorigenesis (Belfiore, Genua, & Malaguarnera, 2009) of higher organisms (Berger & Moller, 2002; Feige, Gelman, Michalik, Desvergne, & Wahli, 2006). Therefore, identification of potential PPAR agonists would be very important to determine their roles in those PPAR-related physiological or pathological consequences.

PPRE-driven reporter genes can be used to assay for the activation of PPAR by PPAR agonists. Luciferase gene is chosen as the reporter because when expressed in culture cells, it is easily analyzed with most of commercially available kits by using a microplate luminometer. Most important, establishment of a recombinant Huh7-PPRE-Luc cell line (Wang et al., 2010), carrying a stable PPRE-driven luciferase gene, does not require the routine transient transfection procedure and thus makes the analysis more convenient and reliable. For high-throughput screening purpose, we have fitted the bioassay into a white 96-well plate format using Huh7-PPRE-Luc cells. The whole procedure, from cell culture, chemical treatments, cell lysis, and finally to luciferase assay, can be carried out in one single plate.

2. MATERIALS

2.1. Cells and culture medium

1. HuH-7 cells (Japanese Collection of Research Bioresources Cell Bank/ Health Science Research Resources Bank, Osaka, Japan).
2. Dulbecco's modified Eagle medium (D-MEM) (high glucose, with L-glutamine) (Invitrogen): Measure out 850 mL sterile dH_2O. Add

powdered media to room-temperature sterile dH_2O with gentle stirring. Rinse out inside of package to remove all traces of powder and add to media. Add 3.7 g of $NaCO_3$ to media. Add dH_2O to 900 mL. Stir for 1 h until dissolved. Adjust pH of media to 7.3 using 1 N NaOH or 1 N HCl (add slowly with stirring). Sterilize immediately by using a 0.22 μm vacuum filter top (Millipore). Store media at 4 °C in the dark for up to 12 months.

3. Complete D-MEM: D-MEM containing 10% fetal bovine serum (FBS) and antibiotics (100 units penicillin and 100 μg streptomycin/mL) (Invitrogen).

2.2. Selection of G-418-resistant cell clones components

1. PPRE ×3-tk-Luc plasmid is a reporter construct containing three copies of PPRE upstream of a thymidine kinase promoter fused to a luciferase gene (Kliewer, Umesono, Noonan, Heyman, & Evans, 1992). The plasmid was kindly provided by Dr Ronald M. Evans (Howard Hughes Medical Institute, Salk Institute for Biological Studies, La Jolla, CA, United States) (Fig. 15.1A).
2. pSUPER-EGFP-neo (Oligoengine), carrying enhanced green fluorescence protein (EGFP) and neo genes, is a selection plasmid (Fig. 15.1B).
3. Lipofectamine™ 2000 Transfection Reagent (Invitrogen).

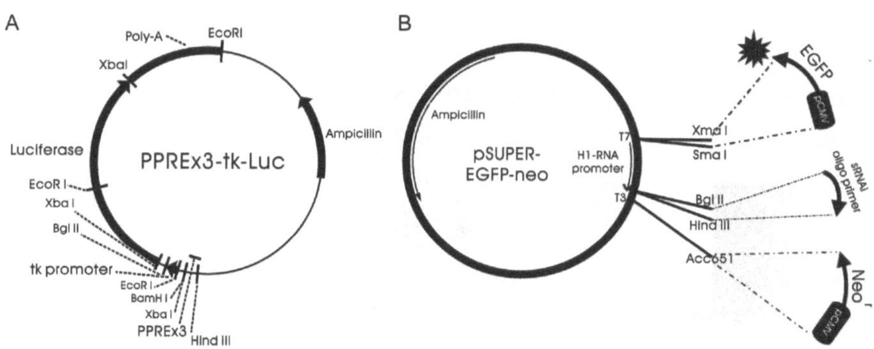

Figure 15.1 Two plasmid constructs for establishing the recombinant Huh7-PPRE-Luc cells. (A) PPRE ×3-tk-Luc plasmid is a reporter construct containing three copies of PPRE (PPRE ×3) upstream of a thymidine kinase (tk) promoter fused to a luciferase gene. (B) pSUPER-EGFP-neo, carrying EGFP and neo genes, is a selection plasmid.

4. Preparation of the DNA–Lipofectamine™ 2000 complexes.
   a. Dilute PPRE ×3-tk-Luc plasmid DNA (2.5 μg) and pSUPER-EGFP-neo plasmid DNA (0.5 μg) in 250 μL of D-MEM without serum. Mix gently (see Note 1).
   b. Mix Lipofectamine™ 2000 gently before use and then dilute 5 μL of Lipofectamine™ 2000 in 250 μL of D-MEM without serum. Mix gently (see Note 2).
   c. Combine the diluted DNA with the diluted Lipofectamine™ 2000 (total volume is 500 μL). Mix gently and incubate for 1 h at room temperature to allow the DNA–Lipofectamine™ 2000 complexes to form (see Note 3).
5. High-selection D-MEM: Complete D-MEM containing 800 μg G418/mL (Infinigen Biotech Inc.). Median-selection D-MEM: Complete D-MEM containing 200 μg G418/mL. Low-selection D-MEM: Complete D-MEM containing 50 μg G418/mL.
6. Dulbecco's Phosphate-Buffered Saline (D-PBS) (Invitrogen): Measure out 1000 mL sterile dH_2O. Add D-PBS powder to room-temperature sterile dH_2O with gentle stirring. Rinse out inside of package to remove all traces of powder and add to the buffered solution. Stir for 1 h until dissolved. Sterilize immediately by autoclaving. The final D-PBS contains 2 g/L KCl, 0.2 g/L KH_2PO_4, 8 g/L NaCl, and 1.15 g/L Na_2HPO_4.
7. Cloning cylinder (6 × 8 mm) (BELLCO).
8. Trypsin-EDTA (10 ×) (Invitrogen): Contains 5.0 g/L trypsin, 2.0 g/L EDTA·4Na, and 8.5 g/L NaCl, but no phenol red. Aseptically prepare 1 × Trypsin-EDTA in D-PBS (see Note 4).

2.3. Luciferase assay components

1. Nunc® FluoroNunc™ 96-well white plate (Nalge Nunc).
2. Luciferase Assay System (Promega).
3. 1 × Reporter Lysis Buffer: Add 4 v of water to 1 v of 5 × Reporter Lysis Buffer (Promega). Equilibrate 1 × Reporter Lysis Buffer to room temperature before use.
4. Incubator/shaker (Labnet VorTemp 56 EVC, Labnet International, Inc.).
5. Programmed microplate luminometer (MicroLumatPlus LB96V, EG&G Berthold).

3. METHODS

3.1. Protocol for establishment of recombinant Huh7-PPRE-Luc cells for PPRE-driven luciferase assay

1. HuH-7 cells are routinely maintained in complete D-MEM in a humidified atmosphere containing 5% CO_2 at 37 °C.
2. One day before transfection, plate 6×10^5 HuH-7 cells in complete D-MEM per 60 mm dish so that the cells will be 90–95% at the time of transfection.
3. Before transfection, the HuH-7 cells were washed with 2 mL of D-MEM (without serum and antibiotics) twice. The cells are cotransfected with a reporter vector, PPRE ×3-tk-Luc, and a selection vector, pSUPER-EGFP-neo, using the Lipofectamine™ 2000 Transfection Reagent (Invitrogen) according to the provided protocol with modifications.
4. Add 500 μL of DNA–Lipofectamine™ 2000 complexes (see Section 2.2) to each dish containing cells and then add another 1 mL of D-MEM (without serum and antibiotics) (total volume is 1.5 mL). Mix gently by rocking the dishes back and forth.
5. Incubate the cells at 37 °C in a CO_2 incubator for 6 h, add another 1.5 mL of D-MEM (with 20% FBS and without antibiotics) (total volume is 3 mL), and then incubate the cells at 37 °C in a CO_2 incubator overnight.
6. Maintain the transfected cells in 2 mL of high-selection D-MEM for 6 days (replace with fresh selection medium every 3 days) and then in median-selection D-MEM for another 4 days.
7. Following the 10-day G418 selection, scrape those G418-resistant/EGFP-negative cell colonies and keep those G418-resistant/EGFP-positive cell colonies. Maintain the G418-resistant/EGFP-positive cell colonies in 2 mL of median-selection D-MEM for 4 days.
8. After the G418 selection, examine those well-isolated cell clones with G418-resistant/EGFP-positive phenotype with an inverted microscope.
9. Draw a circle around the selected colonies on the bottom of the dish with a marking pen.
10. Remove and discard the growth medium. Rinse the dish with D-PBS.

11. Using sterile medium forceps, pick up a cloning cylinder (6 × 8 mm). Gently press the flat bottom of the cylinder into the smooth silicone grease and remove with a sudden vertical motion. If done properly, this will give even distribution of grease on the bottom of the cylinder. Set the cylinder over a colony. Gently press the cylinder down evenly with the forceps (see Note 5).
12. Add about 0.1 mL of the 1 × trypsin–EDTA to the cloning cylinder and then incubate the dish at 37 °C for 5 min.
13. Add a few drops of growth medium to the cylinder and gently aspirate the cells with a micropipettor.
14. Transfer each cell colony to a well in a 24-well dish with 1 mL of complete D-MEM and then incubate the cells in a humidified atmosphere containing 5% CO_2 at 37 °C overnight (see Note 6).
15. Maintain the cells in 1 mL of low-selection D-MEM and replace with fresh medium every 3 days till the cells grow to confluence (in about 1 week).

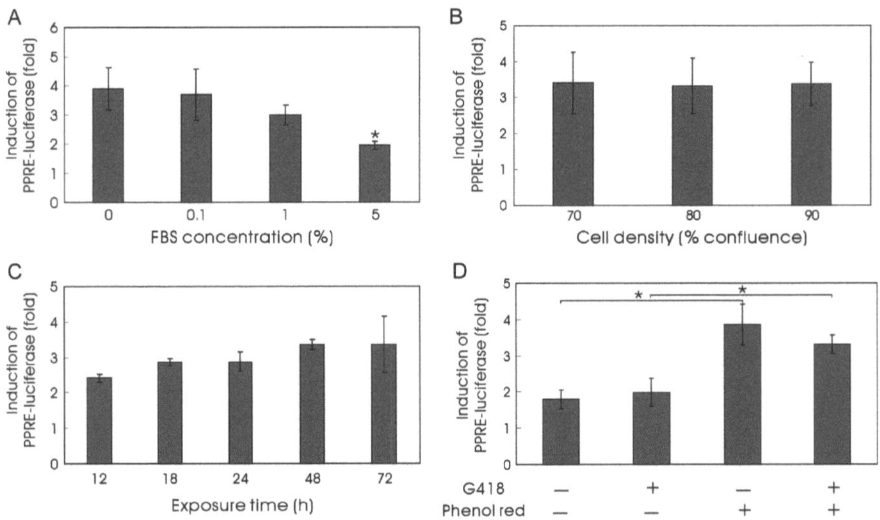

Figure 15.2 Dose–response induction in PPRE-driven luciferase activity by PPAR agonists. Huh7-PPRE-Luc cells were left untreated or treated with (A) WY-14643 (a PPARα agonist), (B) L-165,041 (a PPARβ/δ agonist), (C) Fmoc-Leu (a PPARγ agonist), and (D) troglitazone (a PPARγ agonist) for 24 h. Relative PPRE-driven luciferase activity is expressed as induction of PPRE-driven luciferase activity (fold) as compared with those of untreated controls. All data are presented as means ± SD ($n = 3$). $^{*}p < 0.05$, $^{**}p < 0.01$, and $^{***}p < 0.001$ versus the untreated controls. *Reproduced from Wang et al. (2010) with permission from Springer.*

16. Amplify the cells in low-selection D-MEM and test the cells with the PPRE-driven luciferase activation by different PPAR agonists. As previously described, a Huh7-PPRE-Luc cell clone was established for its sharp dose–response in luciferase induction by PPAR agonists (Fig. 15.2; Wang et al., 2010).

3.2. Treatments of Huh7-PPRE-Luc cells with chemicals for PPRE-driven luciferase assay

1. Routinely maintain Huh7-PPRE-Luc cells in low-selection D-MEM.
2. One day before analysis, plate Huh7-PPRE-Luc cells at a density of 1×10^4 of cells per well on a Nunc® FluoroNunc™ 96-well plate (white) with complete D-MEM medium.
3. For PPRE-driven luciferase assay, replace the culture medium with 90 μL of D-MEM (without FBS), add 10 μL of treated chemicals (10 ×) per well, and then incubate the cells for 24 h (see Note 7).

3.3. PPRE-driven luciferase assay

1. Analyze PPRE-driven luciferase activity using a Luciferase Assay System (Promega) (see Note 8).
2. After treatments, carefully remove as much the growth medium as possible from cells to be assayed (see Note 9), directly add 50 μL of 1 × Reporter Lysis Buffer per well, and then shake the plate in an incubator/shaker (Labnet VorTemp 56 EVC, Labnet International, Inc.) at 900 rpm and 37 °C for 10 min.
3. Program the luminometer for the delay time (2 s) and measurement time (10 s).
4. Place the plate, containing 50 μL of cell lysate per well, into the luminometer with injector. The injector adds 100 μL of Luciferase Assay Reagent per well and then the well is read immediately. The plate is advanced to the next well for a repeat of the inject-then-read process.
5. Measure the light produced for a period of 10 s (see Note 10). Luciferase activity was expressed as relative light units/well.

4. NOTES

1. To eliminate the possibility of spontaneous G418-resistant cell clone, selection of the cell clones was based on two criteria, that is, G418-resistant and EGFP-positive, contributed by pSUPER-EGFP-neo. To increase the probability that the selected G418-resistant/EGFP-positive cell clones

also carried the PPRE ×3-tk-Luc plasmid DNA, we performed transfection using the DNA mixture of 2.5 μg of PPRE ×3-tk-Luc and 0.5 μg of pSUPER-EGFP-neo (PPRE ×3-tk-Luc/pSUPER-EGFP-neo = 5).

2. Combine the diluted Lipofectamine™ 2000 with the diluted DNA within 5 min. Longer incubation times may decrease activity.
3. DNA–Lipofectamine™ 2000 complexes are stable for 6 h at room temperature.
4. Both Ca^{2+} and Mg^{2+} inhibit trypsin activity. Make sure to prepare 1 × Trypsin-EDTA in balanced salt solution without Ca^{2+} and Mg^{2+}.
5. Uneven pressure will cause the grease seal to leak. Be very careful not to slide the cylinder across the colony. This will smear the silicone grease over the cells and prevent the trypsin from contacting them.
6. Smaller colonies or diluting the cells too much will often result in slow or no growth.
7. The chemical-induced cytotoxicity may result in decreases in luciferase activity. For those chemicals dissolved in DMSO, dilute the stock chemicals to 10× of final concentrations with D-MEM (without FBS). Final DMSO concentration in culture medium has to be ≤1%, otherwise results in cytotoxicity.
8. The Luciferase Assay Reagent and samples should be at ambient temperature prior to performing a luciferase assay.
9. Residual growth medium left in the well may decrease the luciferase activity.
10. The light intensity of the reaction is nearly constant for about 1 min and then decays slowly, with a half-life of approximately 10 min. The typical delay time is 2 s, and the typical read time is 10 s. The assay time may be shortened significantly to decrease the total read time if sufficient light is produced.

ACKNOWLEDGMENT

This work was supported by grants from National Health Research Institutes in Taiwan.

REFERENCES

Belfiore, A., Genua, M., & Malaguarnera, R. (2009). PPAR-γ agonists and their effects on IGF-I receptor signaling: Implications for cancer. *PPAR Research*, *2009*. Article ID 830501, 18 pages. http://dx.doi.org/10.1155/2009/830501.

Berger, J., & Moller, D. E. (2002). The mechanisms of action of PPARs. *Annual Review of Medicine*, *53*, 409–435.

Feige, J. N., Gelman, L., Michalik, L., Desvergne, B., & Wahli, W. (2006). From molecular action to physiological outputs: Peroxisome proliferator-activated receptors are nuclear

receptors at the crossroads of key cellular functions. *Progress in Lipid Research, 45*, 120–159.
Kliewer, S. A., Umesono, K., Noonan, D. J., Heyman, R. A., & Evans, R. M. (1992). Convergence of 9-cis retinoic acid and peroxisome proliferator signalling pathways through heterodimer formation of their receptors. *Nature, 358*, 771–774.
Michalik, L., Auwerx, J., Berger, J. P., Chatterjee, V. K., Glass, C. K., Gonzalez, F. J., et al. (2006). International Union of Pharmacology. LXI. Peroxisome proliferator-activated receptors. *Pharmacological Reviews, 58*, 726–741.
Wang, Y. F., Chao, H. R., Wu, C. H., Tseng, C. H., Kuo, Y.-T., & Tsou, T.-C. (2010). A recombinant peroxisome proliferator response element-driven luciferase assay for evaluation of potential environmental obesogens. *Biotechnology Letters, 32*, 1789–1796.

INDEX

Note: Page numbers followed by "*f*" indicate figures and "*t*" indicate tables.

A

Acetochlor, 37
AD. *See* Alzheimer's disease (AD)
Adenine nucleotide translocator (ANT), 287–288
ADHD. *See* Attention-deficit hyperactivity disorder (ADHD)
Adipogenesis, epigenetic perturbations
  adipocyte differentiation, 305
  basal metabolic rate and energy partitioning, 308
  central metabolic regulation, 308
  chemokine and hematopoietic factors, 304–305
  excess fetal glucocorticoid exposure, 306
  fetal programming, 307–308
  gestational growth retardation, 306–307
  glucocorticoid signaling, 307
  human metabolic syndrome diseases, 303
  lineage-tracing studies, 303–304
  maternal stress, 306–307
  mesolimbic reward pathways, 307–308
  metabolic programming, 305–306
  murine embryonic stem cells, 304–305
  neurotoxic organotins, 307
  organotin exposure, 303
  osteogenic differentiation capacity, 304–305
  proinflammatory environment, 303–304
  weight-cycling problems, 303–304
Adulthood, EDCs
  reproductive parameters, 50–51
  sexually dimorphic brain morphology, 51–52
Agricultural pesticides
  acetochlor, 37
  animal and human studies, 37
  DDT and DDE, 34–35
  description, 27–28
  endosulfans, 36
  methoxychlor, 35–36
  proportion, environmental pollutants, 27–28
  puberty (*see* Puberty)
  vinclozolin, 37
Alkylphenols, 11β-HSD2, 369
ALS. *See* Amyotrophic lateral sclerosis (ALS)
Alzheimer's disease (AD), 47
Amyotrophic lateral sclerosis (ALS), 47
Androgenic effects, 64
Androgen receptor (AR)
  AR-deficient mice (AR-KO), 239
  bisphenols
    antiandrogenic activity, 239–240
    estrogenic activity, 240
  complete or partial androgen insensitivity syndromes, 239
  male-*versus*-female hormonal milieu, 239
Antiandrogenic activity, 64
Apoptosis
  biological functions, 412
  caspase-dependent pathway, 412
  Cd-induced cytotoxicity, 413
  cell type, 412
  cellular level, 411–412
  in vivo and *in vitro* conditions, 411–412
  mitochondrial pathway, 412–413
  necrosis, 411–412
  protein substrates, 412
Assisted reproductive technology (ART), 254
Attention-deficit hyperactivity disorder (ADHD), 43, 57

B

Benzbromarone, 20α-HSD (AKR1C1), 377
Benzophenone, 17β-HSD3, 375
B3 integrin (ITGB3), 256–257

Bisphenol A (BPA), 254–255
body and environment, 2–3
drinking water, 15
3β-HSD2, 356
11β-HSD2, 367
17β-HSD3, 374
male reproductive function, 7
maternal/cord blood, 4–5
and prostate: case study
in adulthood, 143–144
developmental exposure, 144
fetal exposures, 143
positive controls, NTP panel, 144
U-shaped dose–response curves, 2–3
Bisphenol-A (BPA), 231
BPA. *See* Bisphenol A (BPA)
BPA exposure, neonatal
animal models, health risks, 260–261
DES exposure, 259–260
early postnatal exposure
ovariectomized (OVX) adult rats model, 264–266, 265*f*
progesterone pathway, 264–266
SMRT expression, 267*f*, 268–269
uterine vascularization, 266–268
VEGF expression, 266–268, 267*f*
EDs (*see also* Endocrine disruptors (EDs))
and developmental programming hypothesis, 259–269
and female fertility, 269
endocrine signaling, preimplantation uterus
ERa and PR, 262–263
higher dose (BPA20), 262–263
lower dose (BPA.05), 262–263
S294 phosphorylation, 262–263
female reproductive disorders, 259
Hoxa10 and *Hoxa11* genes, 260–261
implantation-associated genes
EMX-2 and *ITGB3*, 263, 264*f*
Hoxa10, 263, 264*f*
rat model, 260
reproductive performance, effects
embryo resorptions, 261–262
ovulation rate and CL "activation", 261–262
uterine implantation of embryo
gene expression, 256–257
ovarian steroids and nuclear receptors, 257–258
stromal and endothelial proliferation, 258–259
Brain development
description, 9
disruption, sex steroid, 12–14
thyroid function disruption, 11–12

C

Cadmium (Cd)
exposure sources
classification, 393
erosion process, 393
fertility and pregnancy, 394
food type and external contamination., 393–394
oysters, 393–394
production, batteries and accumulators, 393
source, 393
tobacco, 394
molecular mechanism
and apoptosis, 411–413
cell genome, 410–411
and lipid peroxidation, 416–417
and mitochondrial dysfunction, 413–416
oxidative stress, 392
parafollicular C cells, effects
C-cellular hyperplasia, 406–407
hyperplasia, 405
nodular C-cell hyperplasia, 406–407, 406*f*
testing, secretory activity, 406–407
toxicosis, 406–407, 406*f*
thyroid follicles, effects
adenomatoid follicular hyperplasia, 402, 404*f*
bonding dilation reservoirs, 403
chronic exposure, 402
colloid goiter, 402, 403*f*
histopathologic research, 402
immunohistochemical research, 402
immunohistochemical staining, 402
iodine deficiency, 405
length, exposure, 405
metabolism, thyroid hormones, 405

microfollicular hyperplasia, 402, 403*f*
mononuclear cellular infiltration, 402
thyrotoxicosis, 405
and thyroid hormone peripheral metabolism, 407–409
toxic effect, 392
toxicodynamics, 395–397
toxicokinetics, 394–395
CAMP response element-binding protein (CREB), 299–300
Catalan Health Interview Survey (CHIS), 34–35, 173–174
CCAAT/enhancer-binding protein (C/EBP), 298–299
Cell genome
biological macromolecules, 410
cellular survival and death, 410
cytotoxic concentration, 411
DNA damage, 410
DNA synthesis and proliferation, 410
gene expression analysis, 411
genome stability, 411
induction, gene groups, 410
sensitivity, 411
thiol group, 410
transcriptional modulator, 411
types, 411
Cellular organotin toxicity
bioactive intermediate metabolites, 285–286
bond hybridization, 288
cell's antioxidative defense system, 287
chemical and physical properties, 285–286
chemical reactivity, 287
immuno-and neurotoxic effects, 287
induction, apoptosis, 287–288
lipid peroxidation, 286
modes, organotin covalent bonding, 288–290, 289*f*
molecular level, 285–286
molecule antioxidants, 286
protein thiols, 286
radical initiation, 287
RLS, 286
tetra-substituted organotins, 285–286
tricarboxylic acid cycle, 288–290
triorganotins, 287–288
vicinal thiols, 288–290
Chemical toxicants
chromium, 115–117
cyclophosphamide, 114–115
menadione, 117–118
methoxychlor, 110–112
PAHs, 112–113
phthalates, 109–110
Chromium (Cr)
follicular atresia, 116
industrial and natural sources, 115–116
lipid peroxidation, 116
mitochondrial pathway, 116–117
primary rat granulosa cells, 116–117
Cognitive function
animals, 12
thyroid hormone insufficiency, 11
Constitutive androstane receptor, 66–67
Contaminants, EDCs
environmental sources
fish, 44–45
flame retardants, 45
food chain, 44–45
PCBs, 43, 44–45
pesticides and herbicides, 45
steroid levels and ERs, 43
negative effects, 45
Coumestrol, 20α-HSD (AKR1C1), 377
Cryptorchidism, humans, 336
Cyclophosphamide
anticancer activity, alkylating agents, 114–115
caspase activation, 114–115
oxidative DNA damage, 115
treatment, cancer and autoimmune diseases, 114

D

4,4-Dichlorodiphenyldichloroethylene (DDE), 34–35
Dichlorodiphenyltrichloroethane (DDT), 27–28, 34–35
Diethylstilbestrol, 48–49
Diethylstilbestrol (DES), 131–132
Differentially methylated domains (DMD), 214
Dioxins, 31
Dithiocarbamates, 11β-HSD2, 369
DNA methyl transferases (DNMTs), 214–215

E

Early normal puberty, 29
EDCs. *See* Endocrine-disrupting chemicals (EDCs)
EDS. *See* Ethane-dimethanesulfonate (EDS)
EDs. *See* Endocrine disruptors (EDs)
E_2 metabolism
  AhR, 62–63
  altered rates of estradiol metabolism, 63
  P450 cytochromes (P450/CYP), 62–63
  steroid hormones, 62–63, 62*f*
  in vitro and *in vivo* tests, 63
  whole-animal model approach, 63–64
Empty spiracles homolog 2 (EMX-2), 256–257
Endocrine-active compounds (EACs), 29
Endocrine disrupters
  and antiandrogenic effects
    classical antiandrogens, 336–338
    cryptorchidism, 338–339
    fetal Leydig cell maturation, 336–338
    human fetal xenografts, 338–339
    phthalate-induced inhibition, 338–339
    phthalates, 336–338
    pubertal development, 336–338, 338*f*
    rodent models, 338–339
  cryptorchidism, humans, 336
  and estrogenic compounds, 339–340
Endocrine disrupters (EDs)
  analytical chemical methods
    acid digestion of mixture, 35–36
    detection and quantification, 35–36
    gas chromatography analyses, 35–36
    POPs in serum, 35–36
    total serum lipids (TLs), 35–36
  biomonitoring studies, 187
  chemicals and concentrations, analysis, 32–33
  chemicals at high concentrations, 33–34
  cutoff point
    high concentrations, definitions, 33
    number of POPs at high concentrations, 33
  distribution of concentrations, 186
  human contamination and EDCs (*see* Endocrine disrupting chemicals (EDCs))
  organochlorine pesticides, 186
  POPs, human exposure (*see* Persistent organic pollutants (POPs))
  population distribution, analysis, 32–33
  study population
    CHIS, 34–35, 173–174
    Goldthorpe's scheme, 173–174
    social groups, classification, 173–174
    sociodemographic variables, 173–174
Endocrine disrupting chemicals (EDCs)
  human contamination
    compounds, limited, 28
    DDT, 27–28
    high-dose exposure, 29
    hormone-disrupting chemicals or EACs, 29
    man-made chemicals, 31
    POPs, 27–28
    screening and testing initiatives, 29–30
Endocrine-disrupting chemicals (EDCs)
  and ADHD, 43
  adulthood (*see* Adulthood, EDCs)
  adverse consequences
    behavior, biochemistry/physiology, 46*f*, 47
    cancer, 46
    heart disease, 46–47
    negative effects, steroid sensitive tissues, 45, 46*f*
    neurodegenerative diseases, 47
  androgenic/antiandrogenic effects, 64
  animal studies, 84–85
  autism, 43
  behavioral process, 83–84
  bio-monitoring studies, 130
  bisphenol A (BPA), 130–131
  BPA, 2–3
  brain areas, 67–68
  and brain development, 9–14
  contaminants (*see* Contaminants, EDCs)
  definition, 130
  description, 2
  developmental effects, epigenetics, 16–17
  E_2 metabolism, 62–64
  and energy balance, 14–16
  ERα and ERβ, 66
  estrogenicity of compounds
    additivity, 60
    concentrations, 60

mixtures, 59–60
and fetal growth, 4–5
hormones' effects, 48
in utero, 68
intracellular steroid receptors, 65–67
logistical factors, 81–82
low-dose hypothesis, 130–131
low-dose mixtures, 2–3
male and female, 2
male and female rodents, 68
mechanisms
activational effects, adults, 80
Aroclor 1242, 58
Aroclor 1260, 59
endogenous estradiol, 58
ERs, 57–58
hypothalamus/hippocampus, 59
lead, 59
offspring, organizational and activational effects, 81
PCB 52, 59
PCB 77, 59
PCBs, 58
rate-limiting factors, 58–59
reproductive responses, 57–58
second-generation studies, females, 80–81
neurodevelopmental process, 47–48
non-ER mechanisms, 84
nonreproductive behaviors, 43–44
offspring, 43–44
and PCBs, 83
and puberty, 8–9
reproductive development (*see* Reproductive development)
reproductive dysfunction, 43
and sexual differentiation, 5–8
sexually dimorphic nonreproductive behaviors (*see* Sexually dimorphic nonreproductive behaviors)
steroid hormones, 43–44
tissues, 84–85
uterotropic activity, 60–61
whole-animal estrogenic measurement, 61–62
Endocrine disruptors (EDs)
antiestrogenic and androgenic effects, 31–32, 33
brain, 30
breast development, 33
classification, pesticides, 31–32, 32*t*
and developmental programming hypothesis (*see* BPA exposure, neonatal)
environmental factors, 30
estrogenic effects, 31–32, 33
and female fertility, 269
hormone-like characteristics, 31
hormones/substances with hormone-disrupting capability, 30
and male infertility
CpG-specific effects, methoxychlor, 221–223
environmental factors, 216
methoxychlor, 219–221
pesticides and fungicides, 216
vinclozolin, 217–219
menarcheal age in girls, 30
pesticides, 30–31, 31*t*
steroids from adrenal glands, 30
time period, 32–33
Endosulfans, 36
Energy balance
BPA effects, 16
DES and BPA, 14–15
fetal growth, 14
glucose tolerance, 15
hormone cortisone, 15–16
pharmaceutical estrogen, 14
Environmental pollutants
Environmental pollutants and HSD. *See* Hydroxysteroid dehydrogenases (HSD)
Epigenetics
CpG islands, 213
definition, 212
degree of dysregulation, 213
ERα and ERβ, 66
Estrogen receptors (ER)
bisphenols
BPA activity, 233
TBBPA and TCBPA, estrogenic activity, 233
BP-bound ERs
binding modes, 233–236, 235*f*

Estrogen receptors (ER) (*Continued*)
"BPA-like" or "BPC-like" positioning, 233–236
van der Waals interactions, 233–236
ERα and ERβ, 232
Estrogen-related receptor γ (ERRγ)
bisphenols, 237
BPs
BPA binding, receptor structure, 237–238
LBP rearrangements, 237–238, 238*f*
phenol-hydroxyl groups, BPA and BPZ, 237–238
exogenous overexpression, 236–237
tissue-restricted manner, 236
Ethane-dimethanesulfonate (EDS), 336–338

F

Fetal growth
birth weight, 4–5
PBDEs, 5
placental barrier, 4
serial urinary measurements, 4–5
Follicular apparatus
effect, thyroid hormones, 399
extrathyroid peripheral metabolism., 400
formed hormones, 399
immunohistochemical reactivity, 397–398
iodothyronines (T3 and T4), 400
phagolysosomes, 399
physiological activity, 398–399
pituitary secretion, TSH, 399
T_3 homeostasis, 399–400
thyrocytes, 398
thyroid hormones serum levels, 400

G

Genistein, 3β-HSD2, 357
Gossypol
3β-HSD2, 357
11β-HSD2, 367
17β-HSD3, 374
Granular endoplasmic reticulum (grER), 398–399
GrER. *See* Granular endoplasmic reticulum (grER)

H

Hexachlorobenzene (HCB), 31
Hexachlorocyclohexanes (HCHs), 31
H19/IGF2 imprinting control region 1 (ICR1), 215–216
High concentrations, definitions, 33
High-throughput screening, 428
HPA. *See* Hypothalamic-pituitary-adrenal (HPA)
HPG. *See* Hypothalamic–pituitary–gonadal (HPG)
HPTE, estrogenicity of methoxychlor
in vitro screening assays
antiandrogenic effects, 198
ER-α, 195–196
ER-β, 196–197
HPTE, 198
MCF-7 cells, 197–198, 197*f*
receptor binding assays, 196*f*
in vivo screening assays
serum concentrations, 198–199
uterotrophic assay in rats/mice, 198
3β-HSD2
enzyme reaction, 353
gene, 353–354
inhibition, environmental pollutants
BPA, 356
genistein, 357
gossypol, 357
methoxychlor, 356
organotins, 356–357
perfluoroalkyl substance, 355
phthalates, 357–358
protein structure, 354
tissue localization and function, 355
11β-HSD1
enzyme reaction, 358–360, 359*f*
gene, 360
inhibition, environmental pollutants
BPA, 362–363
gossypol, 363
licorice components, 363–364
methoxychlor, 363
organotins, 363
perfluoroalkyl substance, 362
protein structure, 360–361
tissue localization and function
human and rat livers, 362

Leydig cells, testis, 362
modulation, phosphatidylcholin, 361–362
primary oxidase, 362
surfactant protein synthesis, 361–362
11β-HSD2
enzyme reaction, 359*f*, 364
gene, 364
inhibition, environmental pollutants
alkylphenols, 369
BPA, 367
dithiocarbamates, 369
gossypol, 367
licorice components, 368
methoxychlor, 367
organotins, 367
perfluoroalkyl substance, 366–367
phthalates, 368–369
protein structure, 364–365
tissue localization and function
aldosterone, 365
atherogenesis, 366
gene transcription, 365
Leydig cells, 366
mineralocorticoid receptor, 365
placenta, 365–366
pregnancy and fetal maturation, 365–366
17β-HSD1
enzyme reaction, 370–371, 370*f*
gene, 371
inhibition, environmental pollutants
benzophenones, 372
cattle feed and medical treatment, 371–372
chrysoeriol, 372
diethylstilbestrol, 371–372
flavonoids, 372
scutellarein, 372
protein structure, 371
tissue localization and function, 371
17β-HSD3
enzyme reaction, 370*f*, 372
gene, 373
inhibition, environmental pollutants
benzophenone, 375
BPA, 374
gossypol, 374
methoxychlor, 374
organotins, 374
perfluoroalkyl substance, 373–374
phthalates, 374
protein structure, 373
tissue localization and function, 373
20α-HSD (AKR1C1)
enzyme reaction, 375, 375*f*
gene, 376
inhibition, environmental pollutants
benzbromarone, 377
coumestrol, 377
licorice component glycyrrhetinic acid, 377
phenolphthalein, 376–377
quercitrin, 377
protein structure, 376
tissue localization and function, 376
3β-HSD/isomerase
3β-HSD2, 353–358
isoforms, 352–353
tissue localization, 352–353
Huh7-PPRE-Luc cells, recombinant
with chemicals, 433
protocol, 431–433
Hunger Winter Family Study, 215
Hydroxyphenyltrichloroethane (HPTE). *See* HPTE, estrogenicity of methoxychlor
11β-Hydroxysteroid dehydrogenases (11β-HSD), 295
Hydroxysteroid dehydrogenases (HSD)
biosynthesis and metabolism, 350
classification, 350, 350*t*
endocrine disruptors, 350–352
3β-HSD, 352–358
11β-HSD, 358–369
17β-HSD, 370–375
20α-HSD, 375–377
inhibitors, enzymes, 350–352, 351*t*
steroid hormones, 377
steroidogenic enzymes, 350
types, 350
Hypothalamic-pituitary-adrenal (HPA), 57
Hypothalamic–pituitary–gonadal (HPG), 29–30

I

Imposex, 281–282
Imprinting
  clusters, 214
  defects and male infertility
    DNA methylation, 215–216
    ICR1, 215–216
    PEG1/MEST locus, 215–216
  definition, 213
  DMD, 214
  DNMTs, 214–215
  environmental changes
    in vitro-cultured embryos, 215
    Hunger Winter Family Study, 215
    imprinted gene IGF2, 215
    imprinting reprogramming, 215
  genes in human/mouse, estimation, 213
  germ cell differentiation and maturation, 214
  methoxychlor, effects, 219–221
INSL3. *See* Insulin-like factor 3 (INSL3)
Insulin-like factor 3 (INSL3)
  autocrine and paracrine functions, 334–335
  and bone formation, 336
  cryptorchidism, 328
  and endocrine disrupters, 336–340
  expression and receptor RXFP2, 328–329
  fetal, neonatal, and adult Leydig cells, 329–330
  fetal testosterone production, 328
  germ cell survival, 328
  human fetal testis, 341
  human studies, 334
  Insl3-induced germ cell survival, 334–335
  meiotic germ cells, 334–335
  meiotic progression, 335
  regulation, adult Leydig cells, 330–331
  species differences, testicular descent, 332–334
  testicular descent and hormonal control
    androgen-dependent fashion, 332
    hormonal regulation, 332, 333*f*
    inguinoscrotal phase, 332
    transabdominal phase, 331–332
    transinguinal and inguinoscrotal phases, 332
  testicular functions, 334–335
  testosterone secretion, 335
Intracellular cognate estrogen receptors, 67, 67*f*
Intracellular steroid receptors
  estrogenic compounds, 66
  and membrane, 66–67
  protein proliferation and tissue restructuring, 65–66, 65*f*
  steroid hormones, 65–66
  tissue-specific responses, 66
  transporter protein, 65–66
Ionizing radiation
  antineoplastic drugs, 118
  fetal ovary, 119–120
  GSH synthesis, 119
  melatonin, 119
  temporary amenorrhea, 118

L

LC. *See* Locus coeruleus (LC)
Licorice components
  glycyrrhetinic acid, 20α-HSD (AKR1C1), 377
  11β-HSD2, 368
Lipid peroxidation
  biomembranes, 416
  Cd-induced oxidative stress, 416
  cellular membrane lipids, 416
  depolarization, 417
  oxidative damage, 416
  peroxidative reaction, 416
  thyroid dysfunction, 416
Locus coeruleus (LC), 7–8
Logistical factors, EDCs
  controlling, cohort and maternal behavior effects, 81–82
  random assignment to dependent measurement sets, 82
Long-term potentiation (LTP), 53–54
Low-dose effects, hormones and EDs
  biological changes
    adaptive changes, 148
    adverse effects, 148–149
    end points, 149
    mammary gland carcinogen, 149–150
    sexually dimorphic behaviors, 149
  BPA and prostate (*see* Bisphenol A (BPA))

DES daughters, 131–132
EDC BPA, 133
environmentally exposed individuals, 132–133
high-dose exposures, 131–132
hormones act
activational and organizational effects, 135
EDC exposures, 133
estrogen exposure, 135–136
ppt and ppb range, 133–134
the spare receptor hypothesis, 135
steroid hormones, phases, 134
TSH, 134–135
hormones, principles
conception through aging, 136
interactions with receptors, 137
life stage-dependent, 137–138
low doses, 137
nonlinear and nonmonotonic, effects, 138
laboratory animals and human populations, evidences
BPA, 145–146
DDT, 145
environmental exposures, PCBs, 145–146
industrial chemicals, 145–146
TCDD, 145
nonmonotonic dose responses
EDC exposures, 151–152
NMDRCs, 151
nonmonotonicity, concept, 152
NTP (*see* National Toxicology Program (NTP))
occupational exposures, high dose, 132–133
ppt and ppb range, 132
real world EDC exposures
chemical safety screening, 150
xenoestrogen mixtures, 150–151
traditional toxicology studies
end points, apical, 147
guideline study, 146–147
LOAEL, 146–147
low dose cutoff, definition, 147
'safe' doses, 146–147
toxicology testing, 147–148
Lowest-observable-adverse-effect level (LOAEL), 146–147
LTP. *See* Long-term potentiation (LTP)
Luciferase assay components, 43, 430

M

Male infertility. *See* Endocrine disruptors (EDs)
Menadione, 117–118
MEP. *See* Monoethyl phthalate (MEP)
Metal-responsive transcriptional factor 1 (MTF-1), 394–395
Methoxychlor
effects on domestic/wild animals, 195
endogenous hormone levels
female hormone levels, 204
fertile and infertile females, 204
FSH and LH levels, 203–204
hormonal imbalance, 203–204
estrogenicity and HPTE (*see also* HPTE, estrogenicity of methoxychlor)
in vitro screening assays, 195–198
in vivo screening assays, 195, 198–199
female reproductive organs
estrous cycle lengths, 201–202
hypothalamus–pituitary–gonad feedback system, 199–200
oral or intraperitoneal treatment, 200
ovaries, histopathologic features, 200–201
uterus, 201
vaginal opening, accelerating, 201
fertility and fetal development
chronic/transgenerational exposures, 205
dietary exposure, 205–206
perinatal and juvenile oral gavage study, 205
subcutaneous injection, 206
uterine decidualization, 206
3β-HSD2, 356
11β-HSD2, 367
17β-HSD3, 374
lipid peroxidation, 111–112
male reproductive organs
dietary exposure, 202
perinatal and juvenile oral exposures, 202

Methoxychlor (*Continued*)
suppressed sperm production, 203
testis and spermatogenesis, 203
organochlorine insecticide, 110–111
reproductive and developmental toxicities, 199–206
structures, 194*f*
toxicological features, 195
transitional and primary follicles, 111–112
treatment regimens, 110–111
Methoxychlor (MXC)
CpG-specific effects
CpG sensitivity, 221–223
deleterious effects, mechanisms, 221–223
resistance to reprogramming, 221–223
imprinting and fertility, effects
gestational period, 221
imprinting reestablishment, 221
imprinting unbalance, 221
methylation defects, DMDs, 220
oxidative stress, testes, 220
perinatal exposure, 220
pregnancy, 220
reproductive effects, 221, 222*t*
sperm concentration, 220–221
Mitochondrial dysfunction
antioxidants and enzymes, 415
cellular processes, 415–416
electronic transport chain, 415
enzyme-functional changes, 413–414
in vitro experiments, 415
function, rat liver, 414–415
permeability transition pores, 414
physiological and pathological processes, 413–414
production, ROS, 414
respiratory chain, 413
stress disruption, 415
thyroid follicular epithelial cells, 413
Mitochondrial permeability transition (MPT), 413–414
Monoethyl phthalate (MEP)
breast milk, 6–7
LH/free testosterone ratio, 6–7
MPT. *See* Mitochondrial permeability transition (MPT)
MTF-1. *See* Metal-responsive transcriptional factor 1 (MTF-1)

N

National Toxicology Program (NTP)
NTP panel report, updates, 142–143
Panel's assessment
analysis of anti-androgens, 141
BPA, 141
DES, 140–141, 142
estradiol, 140–141
genistein, 140–141
methoxychlor, 140–141
nonylphenol, 140–141
panel's findings: 2000–2002
intrauterine position, 139
low-dose effects, definition, 138–139
strain and species differences, 139–140
Neuroendocrine apparatus
calcium homeostasis, 401
gastrin and cholecystokinin, 401
parafollicular C cells, 400–401
physiological effects, calcitonin, 401
remodeling bones, 401
secretory granules, 400–401
types, C cells, 401
NMDA receptors, 67, 67*f*
Nonmonotonic dose response curves (NMDRCs), 151
No-observed-adverse-effect level (NOAEL), 133
Nuclear hormone receptors
androgen receptor (AR), 295–296
cell-based transcriptional assay, 291–292
classical steroid receptor signaling pathways, 295–296
competitive displacement-binding, 291–292
covalent lipid interactions, 294–295
direct ligand binding, 291–292
endogenous endocrine hormones, 296
in vitro enzyme-linked coactivator recruitment assay, 291
glucocorticoid signaling, 295
mass spectrometric experiments, 294–295
NR gene networks, 291

NR signaling pathways, 295–296
organotin-dependent activation, 293–294
retinoic acid receptors, 291–292
steroid-binding cavity, 295
synthetic rexinoid ligands, 293
transcriptional responses, 291
Nuclear hormone receptors (NHRs), 230–231

O

Obesogen tributyltin
adipocyte lipid accumulation, 311
animal toxicity studies, 310
bioactive lipid intermediaries, 308–310
biological effects of organotins, 281
cellular organotin toxicity, 285–291
chemical environment, 278
chemical pollutants, 280
cigarette carbon monoxide, 279
differential tissue-specific sensitivity, 310
EDCs, 278
energy homeostasis and metabolic integrity, 310
environmental exposure
bioaccumulation, 282–283
common organotin derivatives, 281, 282*f*
degradation, 282–283
dietary and nonpoint source exposure, 285
health risk assessments, 284
household plastic products, 283–284
human dietary exposure, 283
human liver biopsies, 284–285
human organotin exposure, 285
immune system function, 282–283
Imposex, 281–282
organotin additives, 283–284
sex hormone-dependent endocrine signaling, 282–283
triorganotins, 281–282, 283
epigenetic perturbations, adipogenesis, 303–308
fat accumulation and obesity, 278
food conversion efficiency, 310–311
food production and distribution, 277–278
human metabolic physiology, 277–278
low-dose organotin exposure, 310–311
maternal smoking, 279
metabolic sensors, 310–311
nicotine, 279
nuclear hormone receptors, 291–296
protein modification, 308–310
psychiatric disorders., 279–280
TBT and disrupted adipose biology, 297–303
TBT exposure, 308–310, 309*f*
therapeutic treatment, 279–280
Organized reproductive parameters
adulthood, EDCs, 50–51
androgens/estrogens, 68, 68*f*
biomarker of effects, 75
effects in adults
androgens/estrogens, 72–73, 72*f*
fertility and fecundity, 73–75
manifestation, sexual responsiveness, 73, 74*t*
immature rats
anogenital distance, 69, 69*t*
perinatal androgen surge, 69
peripubertal and maturation measures
accessory structures, 70
E_2 and androgen levels, 70–72, 71*t*
E_2 receptors, 72
estrous cycle/sperm motility, 70
puberty, 70
Organochlorine pesticides, 33–34, 186
Organotins
3β-HSD2, 356–357
11β-HSD2, 367
17β-HSD3, 374
Orphan receptors, 66–67
Ovarian follicles
atresia, 100–102, 101*f*
fluid-filled vesicles, 100
gonadotropin hormone, 102–103
granulosa cell proliferation, 100
and granulosa cells, exogenous H_2O_2, 109
and ovulation, 100–102
stimulation, rodents, 102–103
theca cells, 100
Oxidative stress
biological systems, 103–104
cellular redox balance, 104
enzyme systems, 103–104

Oxidative stress (*Continued*)
normal hormonal support, 108
redox-sensitive cysteine residues, proteins, 104
ROS generation and detoxification, 103–104, 103*f*
steroidogenic tissues, 103–104
xenobiotics, 103–104

P

PAHs. *See* Polycyclic aromatic hydrocarbons (PAHs)
Parkinson's disease, 47
PCBs. *See* Polychlorinated biphenyls (PCBs)
Perfluoroalkyl substance
3β-HSD2, 355
11β-HSD2, 366–367
17β-HSD3, 373–374
Peroxisome proliferator-activated receptor (PPAR)
agonists, 432*f*
cellular differentiation and development, 428
types, 428
Peroxisome proliferator-activated receptor gamma (PPARγ), 286
Peroxisome proliferator response element (PPRE). *See* PPRE-driven luciferase bioassay
Peroxysome proliferator-activated receptor γ (PPARγ)
bisphenols
organotins, 240–241
TBBPA and TCBPA, 240–241
halogenated bisphenols action
structures, TBBPA and TCBPA, 241–243, 242*f*
weak binding affinity, rosiglitazone, 241–243
LBD, 240
Persistent organic pollutants (POPs)
disease–disease associations, 31
elimination or reduction, 31–32
health and well-being, adverse effects, 31
low doses, 31
results
BMI and sex, 178, 180*f*
cutoff percentage, 182*f*, 183
high concentration, primary definition, 182, 182*f*
high/low concentrations, 177–179
number of compounds, analysis, 179–182, 181*f*
number of POPs, detection, 175, 176*f*
PCBs concentrations, 175–176
upper quartile, 175–176, 177*f*, 178, 179*f*
US Fourth National Report, 183, 184*t*, 185*t*
toxic substances, 31
Pesticides. *See* Agricultural pesticides
Phenolphthalein, 20α-HSD (AKR1C1), 376–377
Phthalates
apoptotic and cell cycle regulatory gene expression, 110
di(2-ethylhexyl) phthalate (DEHP), 109–110
estradiol synthesis, 110
3β-HSD2, 357–358
11β-HSD2, 368–369
17β-HSD3, 374
metabolism, estradiol, 109–110
oxidative stress-dependent mechanism, 110
plasticizers, 109–110
Polybrominated diphenyl ethers (PBDEs)
birth weight, 5
flame-retardant chemicals, 5
semivolatile, 12
Polychlorinated biphenyls (PCBs)
Aroclor 1242, 58
Aroclor 1260, 59
cognitive functions, 11–12
congeners and concentrations, 60
and DDT, 46
and dioxin exposure, 54
environmental contaminants, 43, 44
estrogenic/antiestrogenic actions, 58
exposure and cognitive development, 52
industrial compounds, 44–45
intoxication, 49
and lead, 53–54
paradoxical effects, 11–12
PCB 52, 59
PCB 77, 59

and PCDFs, 54
and sperm profile, 51
TCDD activate AhR, 63
thyroid hormone concentration, 11–12
thyroxin replacement, 11–12
Polycyclic aromatic hydrocarbons (PAHs)
BaP fetal ovary toxicity, 113
DMBA-induced oxidative stress, 112–113
fetal ovary, 113
granulosa cell apoptosis, 113
PP. *See* Precocious puberty (PP)
PPAR. *See* Peroxisome proliferator-activated receptor (PPAR)
PPRE-driven luciferase bioassay
cells and culture medium, 428–429
genes, activation of PPAR, 43
G-418-resistant cell clones, components, 429–430, 429*f*
Huh7-PPRE-Luc cells, 43
with chemicals, treatments, 433
protocol for recombinant, 431–433
luciferase assay components, 43, 430
PPAR agonists, 432*f*
Precocious puberty (PP)
characterization, 29
development of secondary sexual characteristics, 29
diagnosis, 29
early puberty, 29
girls within age range, 29
gonadotropin-dependent/gonadotropin-independent, 29–30
and HPG, 29–30
significant problem in girls, 29
Pregnane X receptor (PXR)
activation, 244
bisphenols, 244
Protein kinase C (PKC)-signaling pathway, 53–54
Puberty
animal and human studies, 37
breast development and menarche, 8–9, 10*t*
characterization, 28
description, 8–9
ED effects, 30–33
hypothalamic–pituitary–gonadal axis, 28
hypothalamic–pituitary maturation, 8–9
organochlorine pesticides, 33–34
PP, 29–30
premature, 29
prenatal/early postnatal exposure, EDCs, 8–9, 9*t*

Q

Quercitrin, 20α-HSD (AKR1C1), 377

R

Rapid progressive thelarche variant, 29
Reactive lipid species (RLS), 286
Reactive oxygen species (ROS), 47
chemical toxicants, 109–118
follicular development (*see* Ovarian follicles)
granulosa cells, 109
ionizing radiation, 118–120
ovarian antioxidants, hormonal regulation
antral follicle development and ovulation, 105–106
blastogenesis, 107–108
enzymatic and nonenzymatic, 104–105
γ-glutamyl transpeptidase-1 (Ggt1), 107
levels, vitamin A, 107–108
nonenzymatic antioxidants, 107–108
postimplantation embryonic mortality, 105–106
preimplantation embryonic mortality, 106–107
retinoic acid, 107–108
serum progesterone levels, 105–106
vitamin E, 107–108
and oxidative stress, 103–104
Reproductive development
and behavior
description, 48, 49*f*
diethylstilbestrol, 48–49
measurement, 79
reproductive dysfunction, 49–50
organized reproductive parameters (*see* Organized reproductive parameters)
Reproductive dysfunction
animal models, 49–50
intoxication with PCBs, 49

Reproductive dysfunction (*Continued*)
lactational exposure, 49–50
oil disease, 49
quails, 50
TCDD exposure to rat pups, 49–50
ROS. *See* Reactive oxygen species (ROS)

S

Sex differentiation
BPA and diethylhexyl phthalate, 7
hormonal environment, 5–6
LC and TH neurons, 7–8
masculinization programming window, 5–6
milk MEP levels, 6–7
phthalates, 6–7
testicular testosterone, 7
testosterone, 7–8
Sexually dimorphic brain morphology, 51–52
Sexually dimorphic nonreproductive behaviors
cognitive dysfunction
chronic exposure, 53
LTP, 53–54
pesticide exposure, 53
PKC-signaling pathway, 53–54
prenatal PCB exposure and cognitive development, 52
description, 75
emotional reactivity, 55–56, 78, 78*t*
measurement, 79
rough-and-tumble play, 55, 77, 77*t*
sex dimorphisms, 52
spatial memory, 54–55
spatial performance, 76–77, 76*t*
steroid hormones, 52
stress, 56–57
SIGCs. *See* Spontaneously immortalized granulosa cells (SIGCs)
the Spare receptor hypothesis, 135
Spatial memory, 54–55
Spontaneously immortalized granulosa cells (SIGCs), 116–117
Steroidogenic acute regulatory (StAR) protein expression, 109
Steroid receptor coactivator-3 (SRC-3), 258
Stress
behavioral/emotional disorders, 57
E2's effects, HPA, 57
female rats, 56–57

T

TBT and disrupted adipose biology
adipocyte-specific pattern of gene expression, 298–299
adipogenic lineage dynamics, 302–303
adipogenic stimulation, 297–298
adipose mass and weight gain, 300
adipose tissue architecture, 301–302
adipose tissue biology, 298
chronic exposure, 301–302
ectopic adipocyte formation, 302
genome-wide analyses, 298–299
glucose tolerance, 297–298
liver steatosis, 300–301
mammalian systems, 302
metabolic syndrome diseases, 297–298
molecular mechanism and phenotypes, 302
molecular mechanisms, 298
MSC lineages, 297–298, 297*f*
murine 3T3-L1 preadipocyte cell line model, 299
obesogenic phenotype, 300–301
organotins enhanced food conversion efficiency, 302
preadipocytes, 298–299
transient epigenomic transition, 298–299
triorganotins, 302–303
types, 297–298
visceral fat, obesity, 297–298
TCDD. *See* 2,3,7,8-Tetrachlorodibenzo-*p*-dioxin (TCDD)
Testicular descent
and hormonal control
androgen-dependent fashion, 332
hormonal regulation, 332, 333*f*
inguinoscrotal phase, 332
transabdominal phase, 331–332
transinguinal and inguinoscrotal phases, 332
species differences, 332–334
Tetrabromobisphenol-A (TBBPA), 231–232

Tetrachlorobisphenol-A (TCBPA), 231–232
2,3,7,8-Tetrachlorodibenzo-*p*-dioxin (TCDD), 46–47
TH. *See* Tyrosine hydroxylase (TH)
The organotin tributyltin (TBT), 280
Thyroid gland
  cadmium (*see* Cadmium (Cd))
  molecular mechanism, cadmium influence, 409–417
  structural and functional organization
    follicular apparatus, 397–400
    neuroendocrine apparatus, 400–401
Thyroid hormone peripheral metabolism
  accumulation, secretory products, 407
  Cd influence, 408
  in vitro conditions, 408
  5′deiodinase activity, 409
  eminentia mediana, 407
  environmental polluters, 407
  enzymatic reactions, 408
  peripheral extraglandular effect, 407
  thyroxin (T_4), 408
  TSH concentration, serum, 408
Thyroid receptors
  bisphenols, 243
  halogenated BPAs, 243
Thyroid-stimulating hormone (TSH), 134–135
Thyrotropin-releasing hormone (TRH), 308
Total serum lipids (TLs), 35–36
Toxicodynamics, Cd
  biological half-life, 396
  carcinogen, 396
  cellular accumulation, metals, 396
  local irritation effects, 396
  spectrum, cell components, 396
  tissue concentrations, 395–396
  transcription activity, 396
Toxicokinetics, Cd
  biotransformation, 395
  health and disease, 395
  mammal cell types, 395
  MTF-1, 394–395
  protective role, MT, 395
Tributyltin oxide (TBTO), 281–282
Tyrosine hydroxylase (TH)
  paradoxical effects, 11–12
  rostral periventricular preoptic area, 7–8

U

Uterine implantation of embryo
  embryonic lethality, 255
  gene expression
    Hoxa10, 256
    ITGB3 and *EMX-2*, 256–257
    VEGF, 257
  molecular signaling pathways, 255
  ovarian steroids and nuclear receptors
    ERα or ERβ, 258
    estradiol and progesterone, 257
    PR-A and PR-B, 258
    preimplantation period, 258
  stromal and endothelial proliferation, 258–259

V

Vascular endothelial growth factor (VEGF), 257
Vinclozolin (VCZ)
  imprinting and fertility, effects
    epigenetic reprogramming, DNMTs, 218
    erasure and reprogramming mechanisms, 217
    F1 or F2/F3 generations, 218–219
    imprinted-like gene/DNA sequences, 217, 218
    methylation defects, DMDs, 218
    methylation pattern, Peg3, 218–219
    offspring, 217
    pregnancy, 217
    rodent reproductive system, 219
    sperm imprinting errors, 218

W

Whole-animal model approach, 63–64

X

Xenobiotics, 103–104

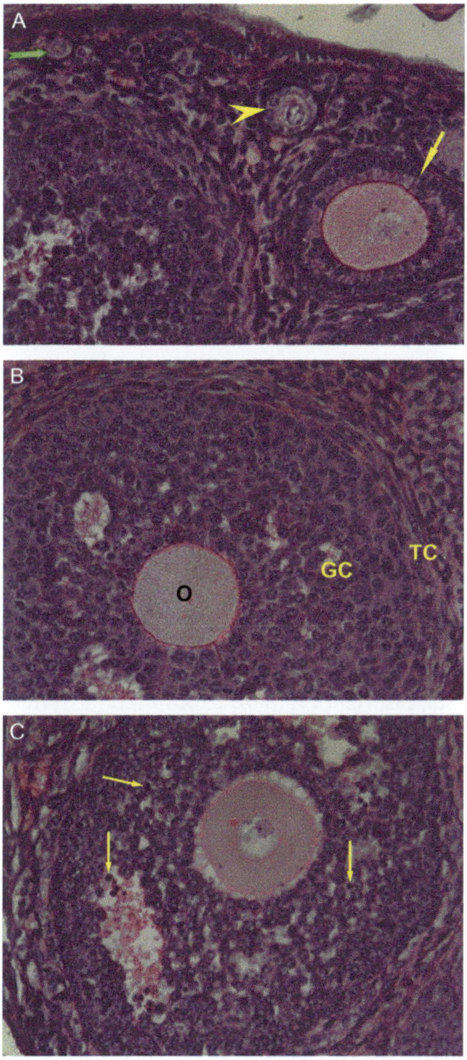

Ulrike Luderer, Figure 4.1 Ovarian follicular development. (A) Ovarian follicles progress from the least mature primordial stage (green arrow in A) through primary (yellow arrowhead in A), secondary (yellow arrow in A), antral (B and C), and preovulatory stages. (B) Portion of a healthy small antral follicle with multiple fluid-filled vesicles that have not yet coalesced. Mitotic figures can be seen in the granulosa cell layer. O, oocyte; G, granulosa cells; T, theca cells. (C) Portion of an atretic antral follicle, characterized by pyknotic granulosa cells (arrows) and loss of intercellular connections between oocyte and granulosa cells and among granulosa cells. Images are hematoxylin and periodic acid Schiff-stained sections from mouse ovary. Original magnification 400 ×.

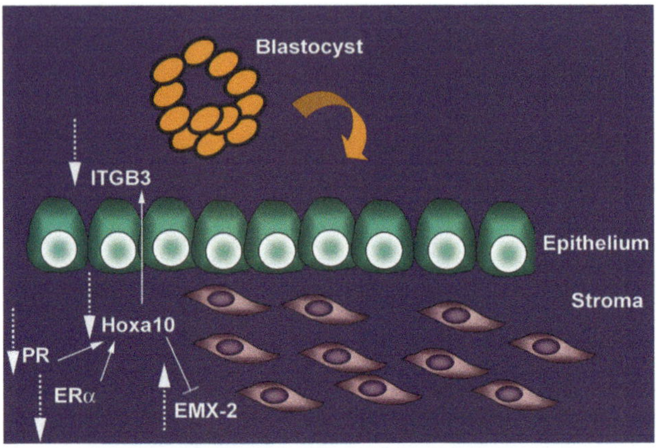

Jorgelina Varayoud *et al.*, Figure 10.1 Schematic representation showing long-lasting effects of early postnatal bisphenol A (BPA) exposure on essential molecular events of the implantation process. In control conditions, the sex steroids estradiol and progesterone and their cognate receptors PR and ERα upregulate *Hoxa10* in the subepithelial uterine stroma, which in turn represses *EMX-2* expression. In addition, *Hoxa10* acting downstream of sex steroids upregulates *ITGB3* expression by endometrial epithelial cells, suggesting terminal differentiation in this cell type in preparation for embryo implantation. Dashed arrows indicate the neonatal BPA effects on implantation-associated gene expression evaluated in the rat uterine tissue on gestation day 5. Alterations in the endocrine-regulated *Hoxa10* gene pathways (steroid receptors–*Hoxa10–ITGB3/EMX-2*) could explain, at least in part, the BPA effects on the implantation process. ----▶ indicates induction and ⊣ indicates repression. PR (progesterone receptor), ERα (estrogen receptor alpha), *ITGB3* (*Beta 3 integrin*), and *EMX-2* (*empty spiracles homolog 2*).

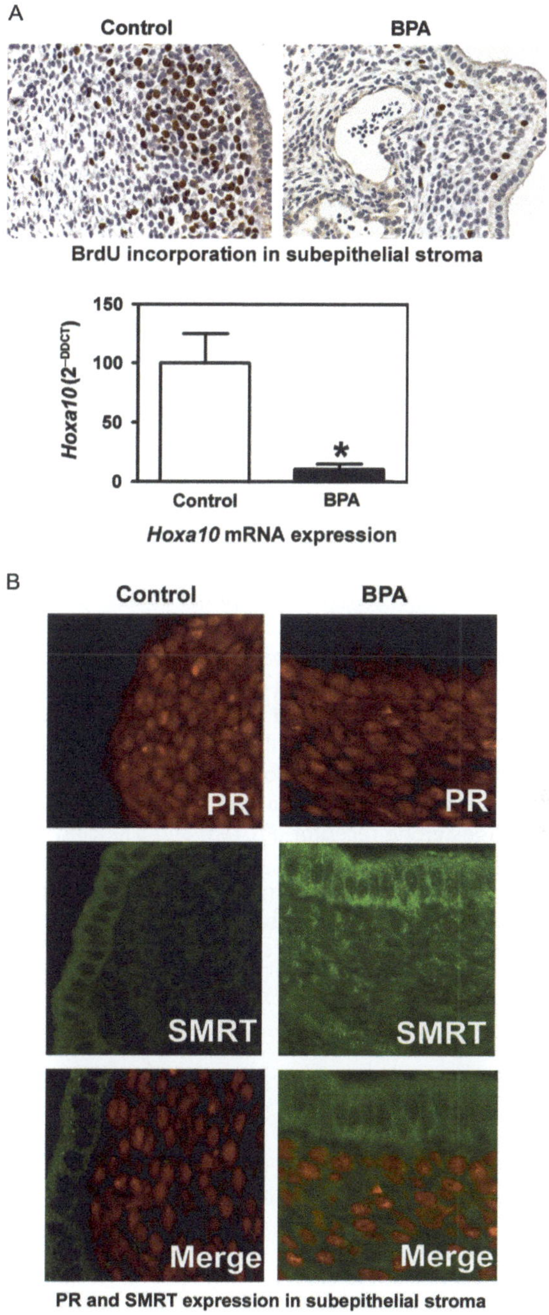
A
Control
BPA
BrdU incorporation in subepithelial stroma
150
100
50
0
Hoxa10 (2^-DDCT)
*
Control
BPA
Hoxa10 mRNA expression
B
Control
BPA
PR
PR
SMRT
SMRT
Merge
Merge
PR and SMRT expression in subepithelial stroma

Jorgelina Varayoud *et al.*, Figure 10.2 Long-term effects of postnatal exposure to BPA in the uterus of adult ovariectomized rats in response to steroid hormone replacement. (A) Subepithelial stromal proliferation detected by bromodeoxyuridine (BrdU) incorporation. Relative *Hoxa10* mRNA expression was measured via real-time quantitative PCR and fold expression from control values was calculated by the equation $2^{-\Delta\Delta CT}$. Control group was assigned to a reference level of 100 and values are given as mean $\pm$ SEM. Ribosomal protein L19 was used as internal control. *Asterisk* indicates $p < 0.05$. ($n = 8$/group). Note that BrdU incorporation and *Hoxa10* mRNA expression decrease in uterine tissue of rats postnatally exposed to BPA. Magnification: $\times 400$. (B) Dual immunofluorescence staining for progesterone receptor (PR, red) and silencing mediator for retinoic acid and thyroid hormone receptor (SMRT, green). An increase in SMRT expression is observed in the subepithelial stroma of postnatally exposed BPA rats. The merge images show that SMRT colocalizes with PR in the subepithelial stroma. Magnification: $\times 1000$. *For methodological details, see Varayoud et al. (2008).*

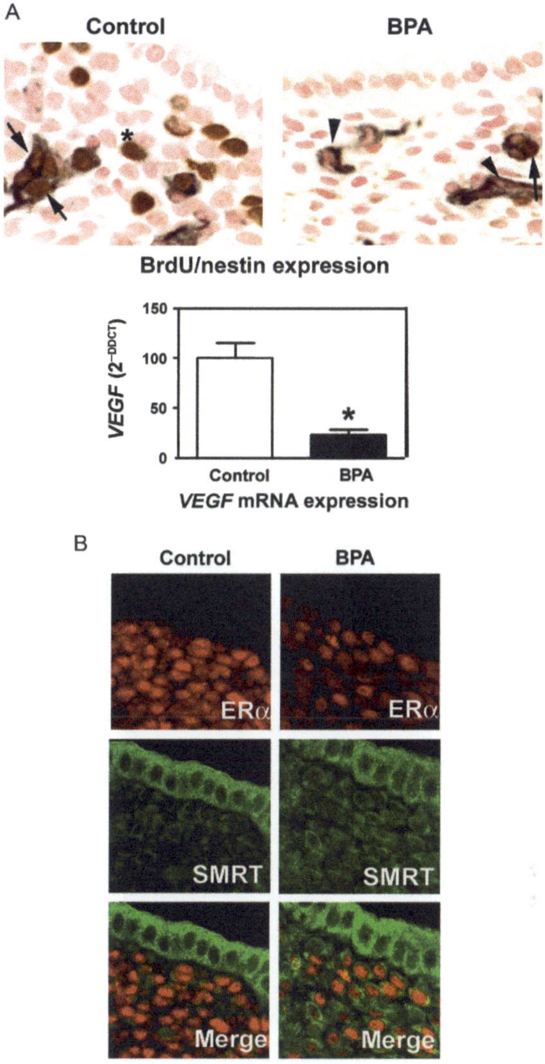

Jorgelina Varayoud *et al.*, Figure 10.3 Effect of neonatal exposure to BPA on steroid regulation of vascular endothelial growth factor expression (*VEGF*) and endothelial cell proliferation. (A) Representative photomicrographs of uterine sections double-immunostained for BrdU (brown nuclei) and nestin (black cytoplasms) to evaluate endothelial proliferation. Arrows indicate double-positive cells (proliferating endothelial cells), and arrowheads indicate nonproliferating endothelial cells (positive for nestin in the cytoplasms with pink nuclei counterstained with nuclear fast red). Asterisk in the control photomicrograph indicates BrdU-positive fibroblastic stromal cell. Magnification: ×1000. Relative *VEGF* mRNA levels were measured by real-time quantitative PCR and fold expression from control values was calculated by the equation $2^{--\Delta\Delta CT}$. Control group was assigned to a reference level of 100 and values are given as mean ± SEM. Ribosomal protein L19 was used as internal control. *Asterisk* indicates $p < 0.05$. ($n = 8$/group). BrdU endothelial incorporation and *Vegf* mRNA expression decreased

(*Continued*)

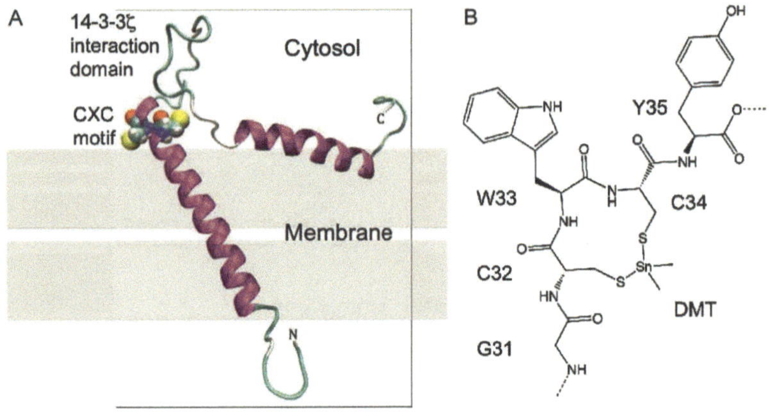

Felix Grün, Figure 11.3 Stannin membrane topology and dimethyltin binding. (A) Solution NMR structure of stannin (Snn) indicates a transmembrane helix, CXC motif, 14-3-3 interaction domain, and helical cytoplasmic tail (Buck, Mascioni, Cramer, & Veglia, 2004; Buck-Koehntop, Mascioni, Buffy, & Veglia, 2005). (B) Dimethyltin (DMT) binding to vicinal cysteine residues (C32 and C34) induces a β-turn disrupting the adjacent 14-3-3ζ interaction domain.

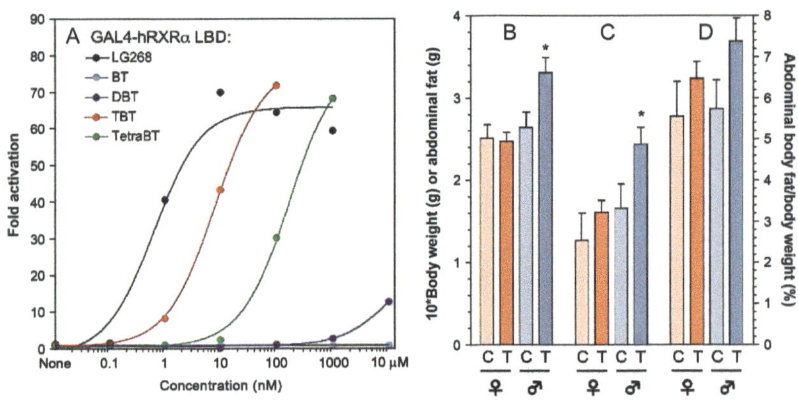

Felix Grün, Figure 11.4 TBT activates RXRs and increases adiposity in mice. (A) Gal-RXR activation reporter assay with butyltins or the rexinoid LG268 control. TBT is a full agonist with $EC_{50} = 5$ nM. Data are redrawn from Grun et al., 2006 with permission. Copyright 2006, The Endocrine Society. (B–D) C58BL6 pregnant dams treated by oral gavage with 0.5 mg TBT/kg bw or vehicle control at E16.5, offspring maintained on normal chow diet and analyzed at 1 year for body weight (B), abdominal fat (C), and adiposity (ratio of abdominal fat/body weight, %). C, vehicle control; T, tributyltin. Data are plotted as means ± SEM, $n = 5$. One-tailed t-test with Welch's correction, $^{*}p$-value <0.05.

Figure 10.3—Cont'd in rats neonatally exposed to BPA. (B) Dual immunofluorescence staining for estrogen receptor alpha (ERα, red) and silencing mediator for retinoic acid and thyroid hormone receptor (SMRT, green). An increase in SMRT expression is observed in the subepithelial stroma of BPA neonatally exposed rats. The merge images show that SMRT colocalizes with ERα in the subepithelial stroma. Magnification: ×1000. *For methodological details, see Bosquiazzo et al. (2010).*

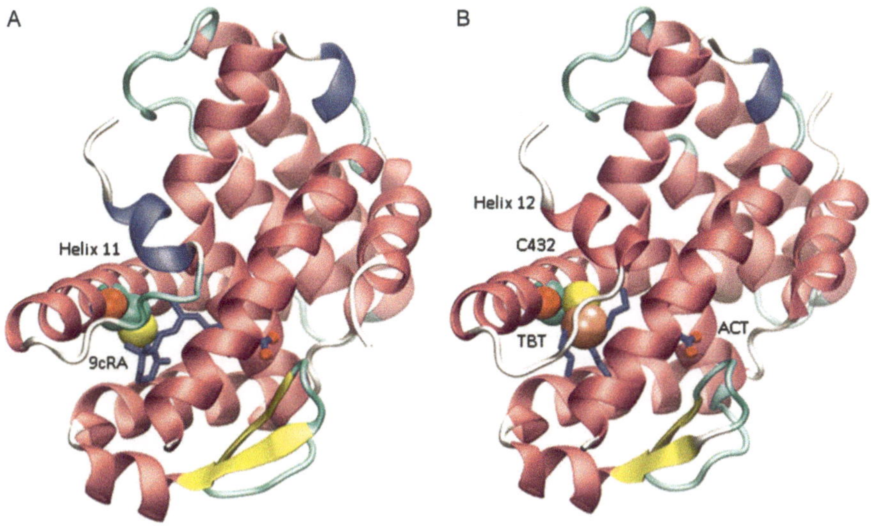

Felix Grün, Figure 11.5 TBT is an agonist ligand of RXRs. (A) 3D crystal structure of RXRα ligand binding domain (LBD) bound to its agonist ligand 9-*cis* RA (blue). (B) 3D crystal structure of TBT bound to RXRα LBD via a thio–Sn bond with C432 in helix 11; an acetate molecule (ACT) is cocrystallized in the TBT–RXR structure. Helix 12 is positioned for coactivator peptide binding. TPHT binds and activates RXRα in a similar manner (le Maire et al., 2010, 2009). Color key: α-helix, purple; β-sheet, yellow; 9-*cis* RA ligand, blue stick; C432 residue, space filled with sulfur atom, yellow; 9-*cis* RA carboxylate group or acetate molecule, blue/red stick; TBT ligand, butyl carbon bonds, blue stick; Sn atom, space filled pink. Models derived from PDB: 1FBY and 3E94.

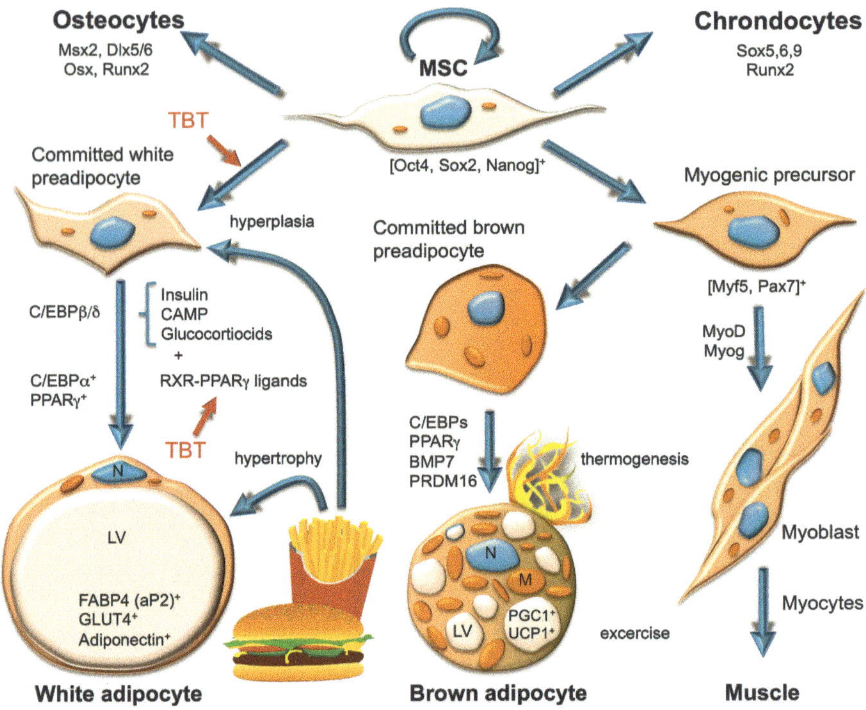

Felix Grün, Figure 11.6 MSC lineages: Adipose mesenchymal stem cells (MSCs) give rise to osteocytes, chondrocytes, myocytes, and adipocyte lineages. Adipogenic signals act on committed white preadipocytes to induce a switch to C/EBPα and PPARy transcriptional regulation that causes terminal differentiation into mature white adipocytes. WAT secretes a variety of adipokine hormones and responds to metabolic cues to regulate the flow of lipid nutrients for storage or mobilization. Brown adipocytes are derived from a myogenic lineage precursor ($Myf5^{+}Pax7^{+}$), are rich in mitochondria (M) and multilocular lipid vesicles (LV), and express genes that control thermogenic responses. The obesogen tributyltin (TBT) promotes adipocyte differentiation by acting as a dual agonist ligand of RXR and PPARγ. In addition, TBT can skew cell fate decisions in favor of the adipogenic lineage at the expense of osteo-chondrogenesis.

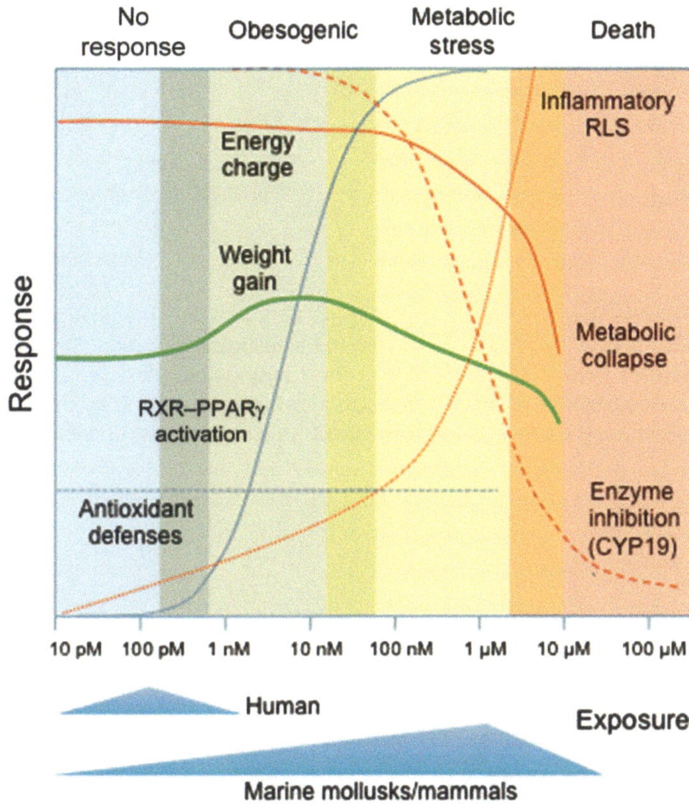

Felix Grün, Figure 11.7 Conceptual overview of responses to TBT exposure. Low-dose obesogenic effects mediated by high-affinity targets, for example, RXR–PPARγ transcriptional regulation of adipogenic GRNs; $EC_{50} = 5$ nM (solid blue). Disruption of mitochondrial integrity (cell energy charge, solid red) and production of inflammatory reactive lipid species (RLS) by organotin-mediated peroxidation (dotted red) contribute to metabolic and chronic inflammatory signals. Beyond the threshold of cellular antioxidant capacity (dotted blue), TBT and RLS accumulation is cytotoxic, contributes to metabolic collapse, and triggers apoptosis and eventually death. Above micromolar levels, TBT directly inhibits biosynthetic enzymes of steroidogenesis and metabolism, for example, CYP19 and 11β-HSD2 (hashed red), but sensitivity to transcriptional misregulation may shift endocrine-disruptive responses 100-fold lower. Combinations of these factors likely contribute to the obesogenic response (increased adiposity and weight gain) at low environmental exposures that produces a nonmonotonic dose–response curve (inverted U-shape, solid green). Bioaccumulation by marine organisms can result in significant organotin exposures that disrupt endocrine systems (imposex) and are immunotoxic/cytotoxic and biocidal. Average human exposure is typically subnanomolar, although serum and tissues levels in the range of 10–100 nM are reported for some individuals.

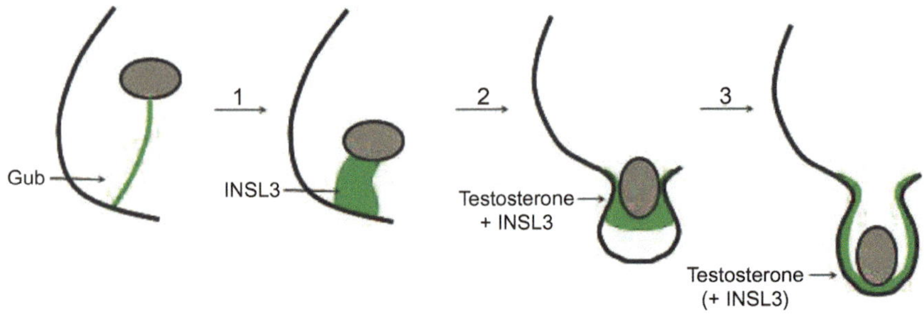

Katrine Bay and Ravinder Anand-Ivell, Figure 12.1 Hormonal regulation of testicular descent. INSL3 is essential for the initial abdominal testis translocation (1) via outgrowth of gubernaculum (gub). Important steps in the transinguinal passage (2) involve both INSL3 and testosterone. The final, inguinoscrotal testis descent (3) is mediated primarily by androgens, though INSL3 may also be involved. *Modified from Bay and Andersson (2011).*

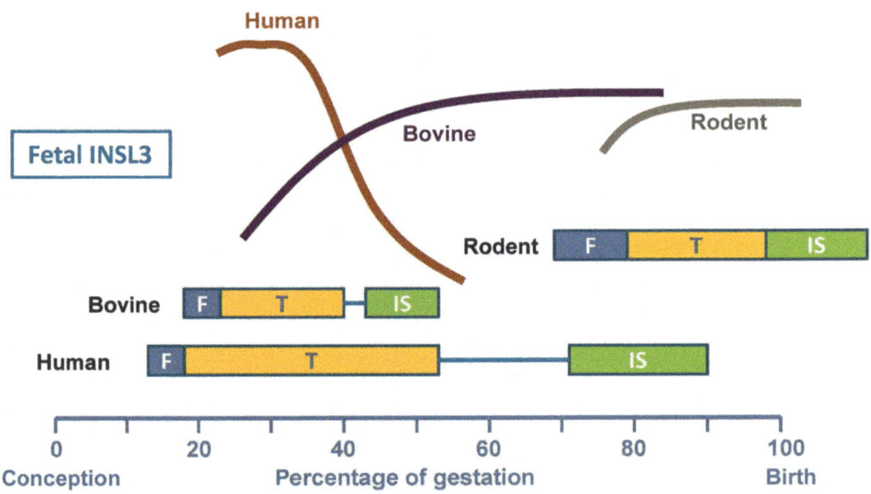

Katrine Bay and Ravinder Anand-Ivell, Figure 12.2 Scheme to indicate the relative timing of testis formation (F), the transabdominal (TA), and inguinoscrotal (IS) phases of testicular descent in humans, cows, and rodents (Amann & Veeramachaneni, 2007; Hughes & Acerini, 2008). Full-term gestation is indicated as 100%. Above this scheme are indicated the approximate levels of fetal INSL3 in male embryos based on amniotic fluid samples (Anand-Ivell et al., 2008; Bay et al., 2008) or fetal and/or maternal blood concentrations (R. Anand-Ivell and R. Ivell, unpublished data).

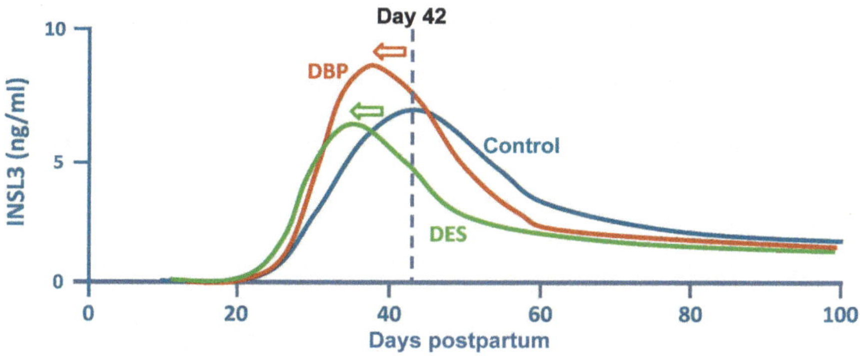

Katrine Bay and Ravinder Anand-Ivell, Figure 12.3 Effect on subsequent pubertal development of brief maternal exposure to dibutyl phthalate (DBP) or diethylstilbestrol (DES) in late pregnancy and the commencement of lactation in developing male rats. Early exposure of adult-type Leydig stem cells to these endocrine disruptors leads to a shift in the dynamics of later Leydig cell differentiation during puberty, as assessed by circulating INSL3 concentrations. Whereas in control rats there is a peak in INSL3 concentration on day 42, concomitant with the first appearance of sperm in the epididymis, DES and DBP advance this time, without, however, influencing later mature levels of INSL3 (Ivell et al., 2013). Very similar results were obtained also using the EDS model of adult-type Leydig cell regeneration (Heng et al., 2012).

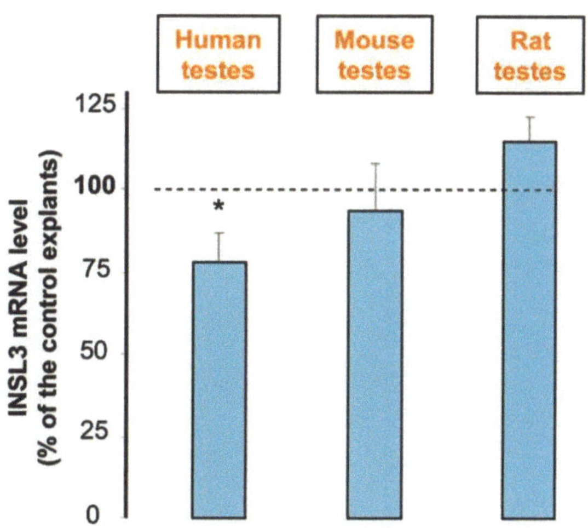

Katrine Bay and Ravinder Anand-Ivell, Figure 12.4 Effect of 10^{-8} M bisphenol A on *INSL3* mRNA levels in human, mouse, and rat fetal testes explants. Values are the mean $\pm$ SEM of *INSL3* mRNA levels normalized to β-actin one and expressed as percentage of control values from seven (human), five (mouse), and six (rat) independent experiments. $^{*}p < 0.05$ in the statistical comparison between BPA-treated and control testes (Wilcoxon's nonparametric paired test). *The figure is originally from N'tumba-Byn et al. (2012). For details of the experimental setup, please see this chapter.*

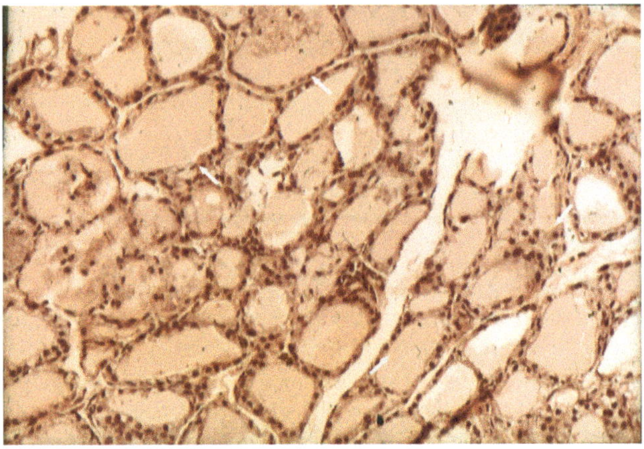

Snezana A. Jancic and Bojan Z. Stosic, Figure 14.1 Colloid goiter with cystic follicles (arrow) and atrophic thyreocytes (H&E ×200).

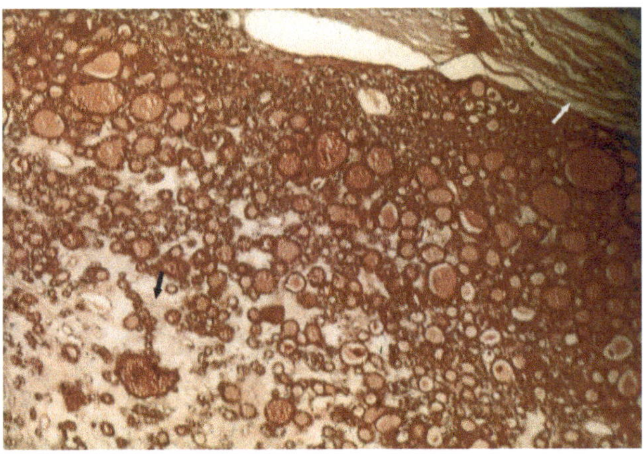

Snezana A. Jancic and Bojan Z. Stosic, Figure 14.2 Microfollicular hyperplasia with focal hyalinosis (black arrow) and pronounced fibrosis of thyroid gland capsule (white arrow) (H&E ×200).

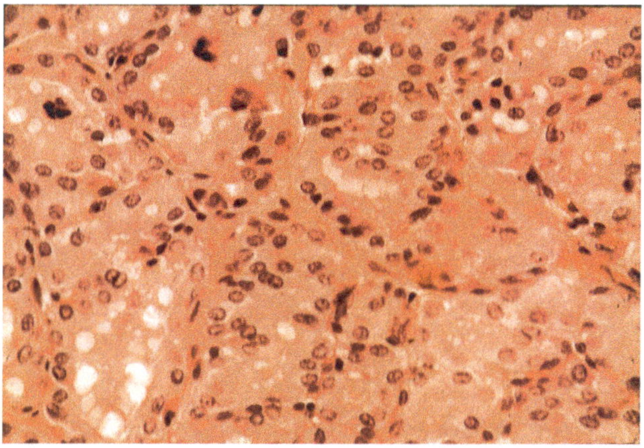

Snezana A. Jancic and Bojan Z. Stosic, Figure 14.3 Adenomatoid follicular hyperplasia with atypical thyreocytes, nuclei, and conspicuous nucleoli (H&E ×400).

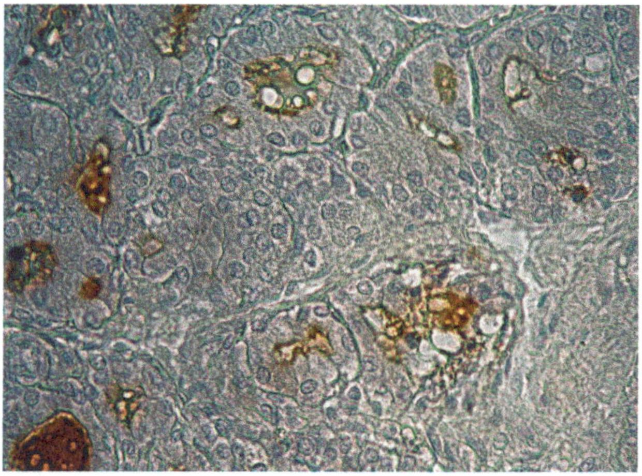

Snezana A. Jancic and Bojan Z. Stosic, Figure 14.4 Adenomatoid follicular hyperplasia with atypical thyreocytes and thyroglobulin hypo- and asecretion of the rats exposed to cadmium (ABC ×400).

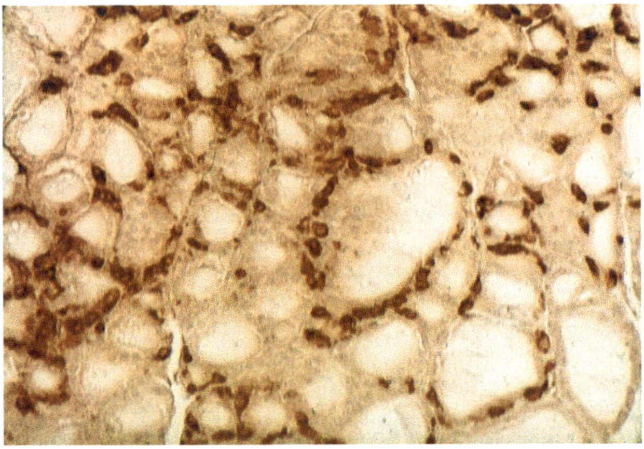

Snezana A. Jancic and Bojan Z. Stosic, Figure 14.5 Diffuse C-cell hyperplasia in cadmium-exposed rats shows a strong reaction to calcitonin (ABC ×400).

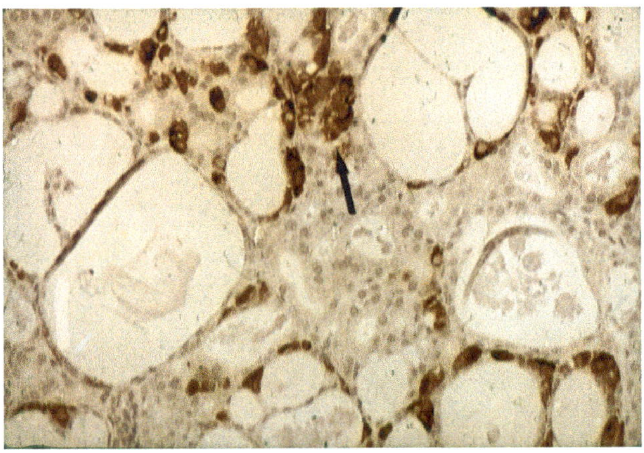

Snezana A. Jancic and Bojan Z. Stosic, Figure 14.6 Nodular C-cell hyperplasia in cadmium-exposed rats shows a strong reaction to cGRP (ABC ×400).

FSC
www.fsc.org
MIX
Papier | Fördert gute Waldnutzung
FSC® C083411

Kolibri 360 GmbH
Ferdinand-Jühlke-Straße 7
99095 Erfurt, Deutschland
produktsicherheit@kolibri360.de